Current Technological Advancements in Ophthalmology Research

Current Technological Advancements in Ophthalmology Research

Edited by Philip Watts

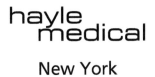

hayle
medical

New York

Hayle Medical,
750 Third Avenue, 9th Floor,
New York, NY 10017, USA

Visit us on the World Wide Web at:
www.haylemedical.com

ISBN: 978-1-64647-513-1

Cataloging-in-Publication Data

Current technological advancements in ophthalmology research / edited by Philip Watts.
    p. cm.
Includes bibliographical references and index.
ISBN 978-1-64647-513-1
1. Ophthalmology. 2. Eye--Diseases. 3. Eye--Diseases--Treatment. I. Watts, Philip.
RE46 .C55 2023
617.7--dc23

Table of Contents

Preface

The specialty within the field of medicine which focuses on the diagnosis and treatment of eye diseases is known as ophthalmology. It comprises both medical and surgical components. Some of its major subspecialties are anterior segment surgery, neuro-ophthalmology and ocular oncology. New technological advancements within this field have various beneficial impacts such as improving outcomes and providing new treatment options. One of the prominent technological advancements applied within this field is artificial intelligence. Its application in studying various eye diseases can help in expanding and extending the usage of digital ophthalmology. It will be helpful in the enhancement of productivity, accessibility, and availability of various resources and will enhance the effectiveness of eye care services. One of the significant applications of artificial intelligence includes computer vision and image recognition. This book unravels the recent studies on technological advancements in ophthalmology research. It will serve as a reference to a broad spectrum of readers.

This book is a comprehensive compilation of works of different researchers from varied parts of the world. It includes valuable experiences of the researchers with the sole objective of providing the readers (learners) with a proper knowledge of the concerned field. This book will be beneficial in evoking inspiration and enhancing the knowledge of the interested readers.

In the end, I would like to extend my heartiest thanks to the authors who worked with great determination on their chapters. I also appreciate the publisher's support in the course of the book. I would also like to deeply acknowledge my family who stood by me as a source of inspiration during the project.

Editor

1

Deep Learning-Based Estimation of Axial Length and Subfoveal Choroidal Thickness from Color Fundus Photographs

Li Dong[1†], Xin Yue Hu[2†], Yan Ni Yan[1], Qi Zhang[3], Nan Zhou[1], Lei Shao[1], Ya Xing Wang[3], Jie Xu[3], Yin Jun Lan[1], Yang Li[1], Jian Hao Xiong[2], Cong Xin Liu[2], Zong Yuan Ge[4,5], Jost. B. Jonas[6] and Wen Bin Wei[1]*

[1] Beijing Key Laboratory of Intraocular Tumor Diagnosis and Treatment, Beijing Ophthalmology and Visual Sciences Key Laboratory, Medical Artificial Intelligence Research and Verification Key Laboratory of the Ministry of Industry and Information Technology, Beijing Tongren Eye Center, Beijing Tongren Hospital, Capital Medical University, Beijing, China, [2] Beijing Eaglevision Technology Co., Ltd., Beijing, China, [3] Beijing Ophthalmology and Visual Science Key Laboratory, Beijing Tongren Eye Center, Beijing Tongren Hospital, Beijing Institute of Ophthalmology, Capital Medical University, Beijing, China, [4] eResearch centre, Monash University, Melbourne, VIC, Australia, [5] ECSE, Faculty of Engineering, Monash University, Melbourne, VIC, Australia, [6] Department of Ophthalmology, Medical Faculty Mannheim, Heidelberg University, Mannheim, Germany

*Correspondence:
Wen Bin Wei
weiwenbintr@163.com

[†] These authors have contributed equally to this work and share the first authorship

This study aimed to develop an automated computer-based algorithm to estimate axial length and subfoveal choroidal thickness (SFCT) based on color fundus photographs. In the population-based Beijing Eye Study 2011, we took fundus photographs and measured SFCT by optical coherence tomography (OCT) and axial length by optical low-coherence reflectometry. Using 6394 color fundus images taken from 3468 participants, we trained and evaluated a deep-learning-based algorithm for estimation of axial length and SFCT. The algorithm had a mean absolute error (MAE) for estimating axial length and SFCT of 0.56 mm [95% confidence interval (CI): 0.53,0.61] and 49.20 μm (95% CI: 45.83,52.54), respectively. Estimated values and measured data showed coefficients of determination of $r^2 = 0.59$ (95% CI: 0.50,0.65) for axial length and $r^2 = 0.62$ (95% CI: 0.57,0.67) for SFCT. Bland–Altman plots revealed a mean difference in axial length and SFCT of −0.16 mm (95% CI: −1.60,1.27 mm) and of −4.40 μm (95% CI, −131.8,122.9 μm), respectively. For the estimation of axial length, heat map analysis showed that signals predominantly from overall of the macular region, the foveal region, and the extrafoveal region were used in the eyes with an axial length of < 22 mm, 22–26 mm, and > 26 mm, respectively. For the estimation of SFCT, the convolutional neural network (CNN) used mostly the central part of the macular region, the fovea or perifovea, independently of the SFCT. Our study shows that deep-learning-based algorithms may be helpful in estimating axial length and SFCT based on conventional color fundus images. They may be a further step in the semiautomatic assessment of the eye.

Keywords: deep learning, convolution neural network, axial length, subfoveal choroidal thickness, fundus photography, fundus image

INTRODUCTION

Axial length and subfoveal choroidal thickness (SFCT) belong to the most important biometric parameters of the eye and are directly or indirectly associated with axial ametropias and maculopathies such as myopic macular degeneration and pachychoroid-associated macular diseases, to name only a few (Fujiwara et al., 2009; Spaide, 2009; Saka et al., 2010; Cheung et al., 2013; Shao et al., 2014; Ohno-Matsui et al., 2015; Tideman et al., 2016; Yan et al., 2018a,b; Lim et al., 2020; Peng et al., 2020). Although both parameters can relatively easily and non-invasively be determined with relative high precision, their measurements necessitate costly ophthalmological devices and equipment, which are not readily available and the use of which are personal dependent and time consuming. Incentives have, therefore, started to assess axial length and SFCT by other means than the conventional measurement devices. Since fundus photographs can be taken with easily available devices including smartphones (Bastawrous et al., 2016; Toy et al., 2016; Muiesan et al., 2017; Mamtora et al., 2018), we conducted this study to assess whether readily taken photographs of the ocular fundus could serve for an estimation of both biometric parameters with the application of deep-learning-based algorithms. In previous studies, artificial intelligence has already been shown to be helpful in the assessment of medical images and diagnosis of diseases (Ting et al., 2017; Biousse et al., 2020; Milea et al., 2020). Deep learning, known as a subset of artificial intelligence, allows computational systems to learn representations directly from a large number of images without designing explicit hand-crafted features (LeCun et al., 2015). The applications of deep-learning techniques trained on color fundus images have produced systems with competitive or close-to-expert performance for an automatic detection of ophthalmic diseases, including diabetic retinopathy (Cao et al., 2020; Gargeya and Leng, 2017; Ting et al., 2017), age-related macular degeneration (Burlina et al., 2017; Grassmann et al., 2018; González-Gonzalo et al., 2020), retinopathy of prematurity (Wang et al., 2018; Mao et al., 2020), glaucoma (Hemelings et al., 2020), and other disorders (Shah et al., 2020); assessment of ocular and systemic risk factors such as age, gender, body mass index, and blood pressure; estimation of the refractive error (Poplin et al., 2018; Varadarajan et al., 2018; Chun et al., 2020).

MATERIALS AND METHODS

The Beijing Eye Study 2011 was a population-based, cross-sectional study conducted in Northern China (Wei et al., 2013; Yan et al., 2015). The Medical Ethics Committee of the Beijing Tongren Hospital approved the study protocol, and all participants gave an informed consent. The study was carried out in five communities in the urban area of Haidian district and three communities in the village area of Daxing District. The only eligibility criterion for inclusion in the study was an age group of ≥ 50 years. In total, 3468 individuals (1963 female, 56.6%) participated in the eye examination. Optical low-coherence reflectometry (Lensstar 900 Optical Biometer, Haag-Streit, 3098

Koeniz, Switzerland) was used for biometry of the right eyes for the measurement of axial length. After medical mydriasis, photographs of the macula and optic disk were taken using a 45° fundus camera (Type CR6-45NM, Canon Inc, Lake Success, NY, United States). The SFCT was measured using spectral-domain optical coherence tomography (SD-OCT) (Spectralis, wavelength of 870 nm; Heidelberg Engineering Co, Heidelberg, Germany) applying the enhanced depth imaging (EDI) modality. Seven OCT sections, each comprising 100 averaged scans, were obtained in a rectangle measuring 5° × 30°, centered onto the fovea. The horizontal section running through the center of the fovea was selected for further analysis. SFCT was defined as the vertical distance between the hyperreflective line of the Bruch's membrane to the hyperreflective line of the inner surface of the sclera. The measurements were performed using the Heidelberg Eye Explorer software (v. 5.3.3.0; Heidelberg Engineering Co, Heidelberg, Germany) (**Figure 1**). Only the right eye of each study participant was assessed. The interobserver agreement between two ophthalmologists in measuring the SFCT had been assessed in a previous study and had shown correlation coefficient of $r^2 = 0.98$ (Shao et al., 2013).

We split the dataset into a development dataset and a validation dataset. The division was performed randomly with a ratio of 9:1 for the development/validation dataset. The development dataset consisted of a training set and a tuning set with the proportion of 8:1 (**Table 1**).

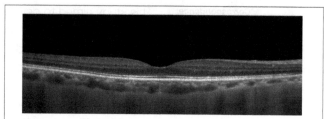

FIGURE 1 | Optical coherence tomographic image (enhanced depth imaging mode) showing the retina and the choroid. Red line: subfoveal choroidal thickness.

TABLE 1 | Baseline characteristics (mean ± standard deviation) of participants in the development group and validation group.

	Development set	Validation set	P value
Axial length (mm)	23.24 ± 1.15	23.29 ± 1.17	0.49
Number of participants	2,811	313	–
Number of images	5,688	616	–
< 22 mm	506 (8.9%)	55 (8.9%)	–
≥ 22 mm and < 26 mm	5004 (88.0)	546 (88.6%)	–
≥26 mm	178 (3.1%)	15 (2.4%)	–
SFCT (μm)	258.13 ± 106.46	247.65 ± 105.55	0.16
Number of participants	2,672	300	–
Number of images	5,436	592	–
< 150 μm	887 (16.3%)	119 (20.1%)	–
≥ 150 μm and < 350 μm	3498 (64.3%)	364 (61.5%)	–
≥350 μm	1051 (19.3%)	109 (18.4%)	–

SFCT, subfoveal choroidal thickness.

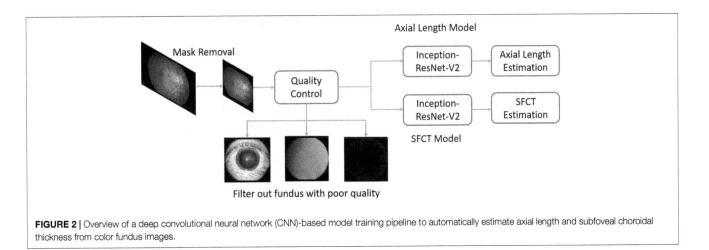

FIGURE 2 | Overview of a deep convolutional neural network (CNN)-based model training pipeline to automatically estimate axial length and subfoveal choroidal thickness from color fundus images.

For the development of the algorithm, we used a convolutional neural network (CNN), a specialized deep-learning model (Krizhevsky et al., 2012), to analyze the digitized fundus images. The models employed the same configurations and CNN architecture as Inception-Resnet-v2 (Szegedy et al., 2016). Based on this architecture, a modified 164-layer CNN was employed to estimate axial length and SFCT. We initialized the parameters of the neural network with the ImageNet classification pretrained model.

Before the analysis, we preprocessed the images to improve the CNN-based analysis. We removed the dark background by detecting a circular mask of the photographs, and the images were resized to the size of 500×500 pixels. A quality control module was implemented after the mask removal to assess the image quality and to filter out unqualified images (**Figure 2**). The standard for excluding poor quality images followed the procedures used in previous investigations (Zago et al., 2018) and utilized parameters such as the readable region ratio, illumination, blurriness, and image contents. The pixel values of the selected images applied to a linear mapping with a pixel value ranging from (0, 255) to (0, 1). In the training stage, a batch of images, called the training batch, was generated and fed back to the network. The Huber loss was calculated based on this batch (Huber, 2004). The corresponding gradients of the loss were back-propagated to update the network parameters. We set the batch size (also known as mini-batch size) as 14. The stochastic gradient descent was used for the mini-batch optimization with the learning rate of 0.0001.

To implement and deploy the network, an open-source software library (Keras, V2.2.2[1]) was used for training and evaluation. The model was trained on a dual-GPU of NVIDIA Titan-X with CUDA version 9.0 and cuDNN 7.0. The Inception-ResNet-V2 network architecture used in this work was publicly available in the Keras-Application package.

Since axial length and SFCT are continuous values, the metrics used for the assessment of the model performance were the mean absolute error and the coefficient of determination (r^2). We calculated the mean absolute error and r^2 with their 95%

confidence intervals (CIs) with an evaluation of 2000 times. Bland–Altman plotting was used to visualize the agreement between the estimated values and the measured values.

To illustrate the fundus region predominantly used by the CNN to generate and apply the algorithm, we implanted another convolutional visualization layer into our network architecture (Zhou et al., 2016). The layer takes image features learned by the preceding layers and gives each feature a weight indicating its importance. It is shown in heat maps.

RESULTS

Out of the 3468 participants of the Beijing Eye Study, fundus images of 3124 (90.1%) individuals were eventually included into the present study, after the images of 344 (9.9%) individuals had been excluded due to the exclusion criteria detailed above. Among the included photographs, 3239 images were centered on the macula, and 3065 images were centered on the optic nerve head. For the estimation of axial length, the development group used 5688 retinal fundus images from 2811 participants, and the validation group consisted of 616 images from 313 participants. Since some participants had not undergone OCT imaging, the development group for the estimation of SFCT used 5436 fundus images of the macula from 2672 participants and validated the model using 592 images from 300 participants (**Table 1**). The mean axial length was 23.24 mm (median, 23.12 mm; range, 18.96–30.88 mm), and the mean SFCT was 257 μm (median, 252 μm; range, 12–854 μm). An axial length between 22 mm and 26 mm was measured for 5550 (88.0%) images, and a SFCT between 150 μm and 350 μm was determined for 3862 (64.1%) images. The development group and the validation group did not differ significantly in axial length ($P = 0.488$) and SFCT ($P = 0.163$).

The mean absolute error (MAE) of the algorithm for the estimation of axial length and SFCT was 0.56 mm (95% CI, 0.53–0.61) and 49.20 μm (95% CI, 45.83–52.54), respectively, with coefficients of determination values of r^2 of 0.59 (95% CI, 0.50–0.65) for axial length and r^2 of 0.62 (95% CI, 0.57–0.67) for SFCT (**Table 2**). The estimated values and the measured values showed

---

[1]https://github.com/fchollet/keras

TABLE 2 | Algorithm performance in the validation set.

Parameters	Performance (95% CI)
Axial length (_n_ = 616)	
MAE (95% CI), mm	0.56 (0.53, 0.61)
r^2 (95% CI)	0.59 (0.50, 0.65)
SFCT (_n_ = 592)	
MAE (95% CI), μm	49.20 (45.83, 52.54)
r^2 (95% CI)	0.62 (0.57, 0.67)

MAE, mean absolute error; CI, confidence interval; SFCT, subfoveal choroidal thickness.

a relatively linear relationship for both parameters (**Figure 3**). In Bland–Altman plots, the mean difference of axial length was −0.16 mm (95% CI, −1.60–1.27 mm), with 3.7% (23/616) measurement points located outside the 95% limits of agreement (**Figure 4**). The mean difference of SFCT was −4.40 μm (95% CI, −131.8–122.9 μm), and 4.9% (29/592) of the measurement points were located outside the 95% limits of agreement in the Bland–Altman plots. Subgroup analysis showed the MAE of the algorithm for the estimation of axial length ranged from 22 to 26 mm was 0.50 mm (95% CI, 0.47–0.53), and the MAE for the estimation of SFCT was 42.47 μm (95% CI, 38.80–46.32).

For the estimation of axial length, the heat map analysis showed that signals from overall of the macular region were used by the CNN in the eyes with an axial length of < 22 mm, while in the eyes with an axial length ranging between 22 mm and < 26 mm, the CNN used signals mostly from the foveal region, and in the eyes with an axial length of > 26 mm, the CNN used signals from the extrafoveal region within the macular (**Figures 5A–F**). For the estimation of SFCT, the CNN used mostly the central part of the macular region, the fovea or perifovea, independently of the SFCT (**Figures 5G–L**).

DISCUSSION

In our population-based study, the CNN-based algorithm had a mean absolute error for estimating axial length and SFCT of 0.56 mm and 49.20 μm, respectively, and the Bland–Altman plots revealed a mean difference in axial length and SFCT of −0.16 mm and −4.40 μm, respectively.

These results of our study with respect to the estimation of axial length cannot directly be compared with the results of other investigations, since axial length has not been included in a study on deep learning yet. Komuku et al. (2020) used an adaptive binarization method to analyze choroidal vessels on color fundus photographs and a deep-learning-based method to estimate the SFCT based on the binarization-generated choroidal vessel images. The correlations between choroidal vasculature appearance index and choroidal thickness were −0.60 for normal eyes (_P_ < 0.01) and −0.46 for eyes with central serous chorioretinopathy (CSC) (_P_ < 0.01), respectively. For the deep-learning system, the correlation coefficients between the value estimated from the color images and the true choroidal thickness were 0.68 for normal eyes (_P_ < 0.01) and 0.48 for the eyes with CSC (_P_ < 0.01), respectively. These values are comparable with the value of $r^2 = 0.62$ found in our study with a larger study population and a population-based recruitment.

The difference between the estimated values and measured values of the axial length measurements was lower than that between axial length measurements by optical low-coherence reflectometry and sonographic axial length determinations [mean difference, −0.72 mm (95% CI, −0.75, −0.69 mm)] (Gursoy et al., 2011). In that context, it has to be taken into account that it is not the mean difference but the scattering of the difference between two methods that markedly influence the clinical reliability and validity of a technique. The algorithm in our study overestimated axial length for the eyes with a

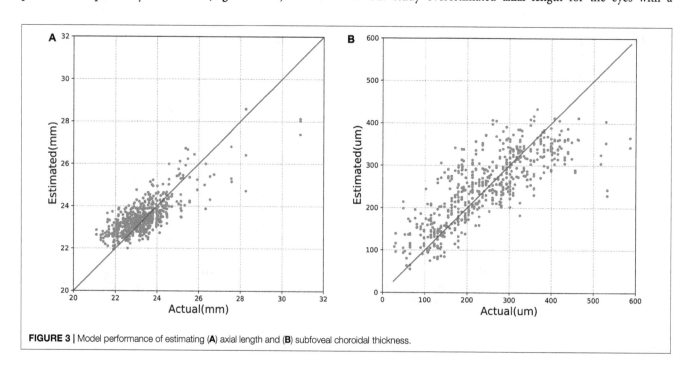

FIGURE 3 | Model performance of estimating (**A**) axial length and (**B**) subfoveal choroidal thickness.

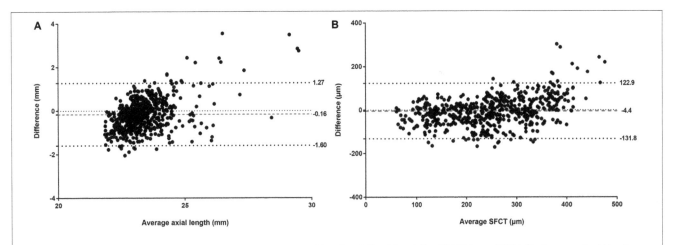

FIGURE 4 | Bland–Altman plots comparing the (**A**) actual and estimated axial length and (**B**) subfoveal choroidal thickness (SFCT). X-axis: mean of axial length or SFCT. Y-axis: measured values minus the estimated values. The mean differences and the 95% confidence limits of the difference are shown by the three dotted lines.

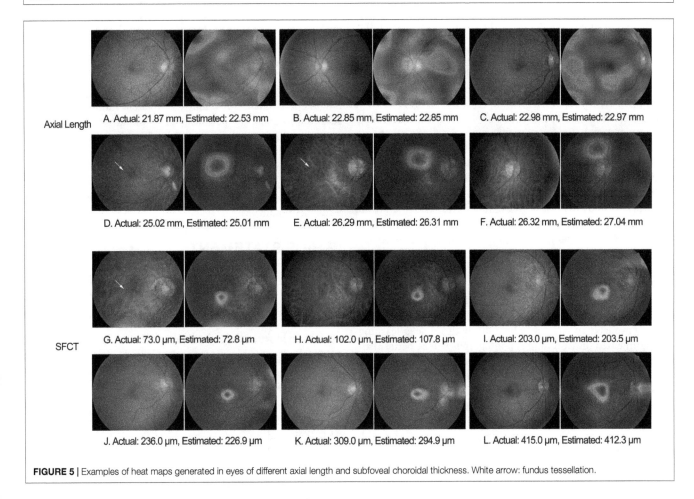

FIGURE 5 | Examples of heat maps generated in eyes of different axial length and subfoveal choroidal thickness. White arrow: fundus tessellation.

small axial length, and the model underestimated the SFCT in the eyes with a thick SFCT. The findings may be related to an underrepresentation of eyes with a small axial length and eyes with a thick SFCT in the study population. Most eyes included into the study had an axial length ranging between 22 and 26 mm and a SFCT ranging between 150 μm and 350 μm. The advantage of our study population being recruited in a population-based level was combined with the disadvantage of a relative lack of eyes in the extreme range of measurements of axial length and SFCT. Future studies may include preferably such eyes to further improve the algorithm.

The observations made in our study agree with the findings made in other investigations and with clinical experience that axially elongated eyes differ in the appearance of their posterior fundus from the eyes with a short axial length. In a parallel manner, it holds true for the SFCT, since it is strongly correlated with axial length (Fujiwara et al., 2009; Wei et al., 2013). A main feature of an axially elongated eye is an increased degree of fundus tessellation, which is also strongly correlated with a decreasing thickness of the SFCT (Yan et al., 2015). Other features of an increasing axial elongation in non-highly myopic eyes include a shift of the Bruch's membrane (BM) opening, usually into the temporal direction, leading to an overhanging of BM into the intrapapillary compartment at the nasal optic disk and, correspondingly, an absence of BM at the temporal disk border in the form of a parapapillary gamma zone; an ovalization of the ophthalmoscopically detectable optic disk shape and a decrease in the ophthalmoscopical horizontal disk diameter due to the temporal BM shift; and an increase in the disk–fovea distance due to the development of parapapillary gamma zone and, correspondingly, a decrease in the angle kappa between the two temporal vascular arcades (Jonas et al., 2015, 2017, 2019; Guo et al., 2018). In view of this long list of axial elongation-associated morphological changes in the posterior fundus, it might have been expected that besides ophthalmologists, also deep-learning-based algorithms can estimate axial length. Interestingly, the heat map analysis revealed that signals predominantly from overall of the macular region, the foveal region, and the extrafoveal region were used in eyes with an axial length of < 22 mm, 22–26 mm, and > 26 mm, respectively. For the estimation of SFCT, the CNN used mostly the central part of the macular region, the fovea or perifovea, independently of the SFCT. It agrees with the finding of a previous study that the degree of fundus tessellation assessed in the macular region or in parapapillary region can be used to estimate SFCT and that a high degree of fundus tessellation is a surrogate for a leptochoroid (Yan et al., 2015).

The practical importance of an algorithm estimating the axial length may be in a combination of portable and cheap fundus cameras with such an algorithm (Bastawrous et al., 2016; Toy et al., 2016; Muiesan et al., 2017; Mamtora et al., 2018). Based on the data available so far, it may be unlikely that a deep-learning algorithm based only on fundus photographs will be better than biometry for the measurement of axial length. The same may hold true for the assessment of SFCT.

When the results of our study are discussed, its limitations should be taken into account. First, the study population included only subjects aged $\geq$ 50 years, so the results of our study cannot directly be transferred to younger individuals. Second, by the same token, the study population consisted only of Chinese so that future studies may address study population of different ethnicity. Third, the use of both optic-disk-centered fundus images and macula-centered fundus photographs, for the training and validation of the algorithm, might have led to some scattering in estimations. However, it should be noticed that the fovea was visible also on the optic nerve head images, and vice versa, the optic disk was visible on the macula-centered photographs. It indicates that the fovea, as the most important part for the estimation of the SFCT and axial length, was assessable in both types of photographs. In addition, the optic nerve head shows characteristic of axial-length-related particularities, so that the inclusion of its full image in the optic-disk-centered images might only have supported finding a best fitting algorithm. It also holds true for the estimation of the SFCT since the SFCT is strongly correlated with axial length (Liu et al., 2018). Adding the optic nerve head photographs to the study, furthermore, increased the sample size for the training of the model. Fourth, the attention maps did not rule out that other features in the images were also used, and we did not perform a quantitative validation of the heat maps. Fifth, although the study population as a real-world group also included eyes with disorders of the macula and optic nerve, we did not analyze whether the inclusion of eye with disorders influenced the performance of the algorithm. Sixth, we did not include a second data set of a completely different study population so that the validation of the algorithm can still be further refined. Further research may include data sets from populations of different age ranges and ethnicities and may use different fundus cameras. In addition, to boost the performance of the model, one may use more data for the development of the algorithm and improve the training schemes, such as using data augmentation.

In conclusion, deep-learning-based algorithms may be helpful for estimating axial length and SFCT based on conventional color fundus images. They may be a further step in the semiautomatic assessment of the eye.

ETHICS STATEMENT

The studies involving human participants were reviewed and approved by the Ethics Committee of Beijing Tongren Hospital. The patients/participants provided their written informed consent to participate in this study. Written informed consent was obtained from the individual(s) for the publication of any potentially identifiable images or data included in this article.

AUTHOR CONTRIBUTIONS

LD, YNY, QZ, NZ, YXW, and WBW: design of the study. XYH, JHX, CXL, and ZYG: development of the algorithm. YNY, QZ, YXW, JX, LS, YJL, and YL: gathering the data. LD, XYH, YNY, QZ, NZ, YXW, JX, and JBJ: performing the data analysis. LD, XYH, and JHX: drafting the first version of the manuscript. All authors: revision and approval of the manuscript.

REFERENCES

Bastawrous, A., Giardini, M. E., Bolster, N. M., Peto, T., Shah, N., Livingstone, I. A., et al. (2016). Clinical validation of a smartphone-based adapter for optic disc imaging in Kenya. *JAMA Ophthalmol.* 134, 151–158. doi: 10.1001/jamaophthalmol.2015.4625

Biousse, V., Newman, N. J., Najjar, R. P., Vasseneix, C., Xu, X., Ting, D. S., et al. (2020). Optic disc classification by deep learning versus expert neuro-ophthalmologists. *Ann. Neurol.* 88, 785–795. doi: 10.1002/ana.25839

Burlina, P. M., Joshi, N., Pekala, M., Pacheco, K. D., Freund, D. E., and Bressler, N. M. (2017). Automated grading of age-related macular degeneration from color fundus images using deep convolutional neural networks. *JAMA Ophthalmol.* 135, 1170–1176. doi: 10.1001/jamaophthalmol.2017.3782

Cao, J., You, K., Jin, K., Lou, L., Wang, Y., Chen, M., et al. (2020). Prediction of response to anti-vascular endothelial growth factor treatment in diabetic macular oedema using an optical coherence tomography-based machine learning method. *Acta Ophthalmol.* 99, e19–e27. doi: 10.1111/aos.14514

Cheung, C. M., Loh, B. K., Li, X., Mathur, R., Wong, E., Lee, S. Y., et al. (2013). Choroidal thickness and risk characteristics of eyes with myopic choroidal neovascularization. *Acta Ophthalmol.* 91, e580–e581. doi: 10.1111/aos.12117

Chun, J., Kim, Y., Shin, K. Y., Han, S. H., Oh, S. Y., Chung, T. Y., et al. (2020). Deep learning-based prediction of refractive error using photorefraction images captured by a smartphone: model development and validation study. *JMIR Med. Inform.* 8:e16225. doi: 10.2196/16225

Fujiwara, T., Imamura, Y., Margolis, R., Slakter, J. S., and Spaide, R. F. (2009). Enhanced depth imaging optical coherence tomography of the choroid in highly myopic eyes. *Am. J. Ophthalmol.* 148, 445–450. doi: 10.1016/j.ajo.2009.04.029

Gargeya, R., and Leng, T. (2017). Automated identification of diabetic retinopathy using deep learning. *Ophthalmology* 124, 962–969. doi: 10.1016/j.ophtha.2017.02.008

González-Gonzalo, C., Sánchez-Gutiérrez, V., Hernández-Martínez, P., Contreras, I., Lechanteur, Y. T., Domanian, A., et al. (2020). Evaluation of a deep learning system for the joint automated detection of diabetic retinopathy and age-related macular degeneration. *Acta Ophthalmol.* 98, 368–377. doi: 10.1111/aos.14306

Grassmann, F., Mengelkamp, J., Brandl, C., Harsch, S., Zimmermann, M. E., Linkohr, B., et al. (2018). A deep learning algorithm for prediction of age-related eye disease study severity scale for age-related macular degeneration from color fundus photography. *Ophthalmology* 125, 1410–1420. doi: 10.1016/j.ophtha.2018.02.037

Guo, Y., Liu, L. J., Tang, P., Feng, Y., Wu, M., Lv, Y. Y., et al. (2018). Optic disc-fovea distance and myopia progression in school children: the Beijing Children Eye Study. *Acta Ophthalmol.* 96, e606–e613. doi: 10.1111/aos.13728

Gursoy, H., Sahin, A., Basmak, H., Ozer, A., Yildirim, N., and Colak, E. (2011). Lenstar versus ultrasound for ocular biometry in a pediatric population. *Optom. Vis. Sci.* 88, 912–919. doi: 10.1097/OPX.0b013e31821cc4d6

Hemelings, R., Elen, B., Barbosa-Breda, J., Lemmens, S., Meire, M., Pourjavan, S., et al. (2020). Accurate prediction of glaucoma from colour fundus images with a convolutional neural network that relies on active and transfer learning. *Acta Ophthalmol.* 98, e94–e100. doi: 10.1111/aos.14193

Huber, P. J. (2004). *Robust Statistics*, Vol. 523. Hoboken, NJ: John Wiley & Sons.

Jonas, J. B., Ohno-Matsui, K., Jiang, W. J., and Panda-Jonas, S. (2017). Bruch membrane and the mechanism of myopization. A new theory. *Retina* 37, 1428–1440. doi: 10.1097/IAE.0000000000001464

Jonas, J. B., Ohno-Matsui, K., and Panda-Jonas, S. (2019). Myopia: anatomic changes and consequences for its etiology. *Asia Pac. J. Ophthalmol.* 8, 355–359. doi: 10.1097/01.APO.0000578944.25956.8b

Jonas, J. B. A., Wang, Y. X., Yang, H., Li, J. J., Xu, L., Panda-Jonas, S., et al. (2015). Optic disc-fovea distance, axial length and parapapillary zones. The Beijing Eye Study. *PLoS One* 10:e0138701. doi: 10.1371/journal.pone.0138701

Komuku, Y., Ide, A., Fukuyama, H., Masumoto, H., Tabuchi, H., Okadome, T., et al. (2020). Choroidal thickness estimation from colour fundus photographs by adaptive binarisation and deep learning, according to central serous chorioretinopathy status. *Sci. Rep.* 10:5640. doi: 10.1038/s41598-020-62347-7

Krizhevsky, A., Sutskever, I., and Hinton, G. E. (2012). Imagenet classification with deep convolutional neural networks. *Adv. Neural Inf. Process. Syst.* 25, 1097–1105. doi: 10.1259/bjr.20180028

LeCun, Y., Bengio, Y., and Hinton, G. (2015). Deep learning. *Nature* 521, 436–444.

Lim, H. B., Kim, K., Won, Y. K., Lee, W. H., Lee, M. W., and Kim, J. Y. (2020). A comparison of choroidal thicknesses between pachychoroid and normochoroid eyes acquired from wide-field swept-source OCT. *Acta Ophthalmol.* 99, e117–e123. doi: 10.1111/aos.14522

Liu, B., Wang, Y., Li, T., Lin, Y., Ma, W., Chen, X., et al. (2018). Correlation of subfoveal choroidal thickness with axial length, refractive error, and age in adult highly myopic eyes. *BMC Ophthalmol.* 18:127. doi: 10.1186/s12886-018-0791-5

Mamtora, S., Sandinha, M. T., Ajith, A., Song, A., and Steel, D. H. W. (2018). Smart phone ophthalmoscopy: a potential replacement for the direct ophthalmoscope. *Eye* 32, 1766–1771. doi: 10.1038/s41433-018-0177-1

Mao, J., Luo, Y., Liu, L., Lao, J., Shao, Y., Zhang, M., et al. (2020). Automated diagnosis and quantitative analysis of plus disease in retinopathy of prematurity based on deep convolutional neural networks. *Acta Ophthalmol.* 98, e339–e345. doi: 10.1111/aos.14264

Milea, D., Najjar, R. P., Zhubo, J., Ting, D., Vasseneix, C., Xu, X., et al. (2020). Artificial intelligence to detect papilledema from ocular fundus photographs. *N. Engl. J. Med.* 382, 1687–1695. doi: 10.1056/NEJMoa1917130

Muiesan, M. L., Salvetti, M., Paini, A., Riviera, M., Pintossi, C., Bertacchini, F., et al. (2017). Ocular fundus photography with a smartphone device in acute hypertension. *J. Hypertens.* 35, 1660–1665. doi: 10.1097/HJH.0000000000001354

Ohno-Matsui, K., Kawasaki, R., Jonas, J. B., Cheung, C. M., Saw, S. M., Verhoeven, V. J., et al. (2015). International classification and grading system for myopic maculopathy. *Am. J. Ophthalmol.* 159, 877–883. doi: 10.1016/j.ajo.2015.01.022

Peng, C., Li, L., Yang, M., Teng, D., Wang, J., Lai, M., et al. (2020). Different alteration patterns of sub-macular choroidal thicknesses in aquaporin-4 immunoglobulin G antibodies sero-positive neuromyelitis optica spectrum diseases and isolated optic neuritis. *Acta Ophthalmol.* 98, 808–815. doi: 10.1111/aos.14325

Poplin, R., Varadarajan, A. V., Blumer, K., Liu, Y., McConnell, M. V., Corrado, G. S., et al. (2018). Prediction of cardiovascular risk factors from retinal fundus photographs via deep learning. *Nat. Biomed. Eng.* 2, 158–164. doi: 10.1038/s41551-018-0195-0

Saka, N., Ohno-Matsui, K., Shimada, N., Sueyoshi, S., Nagaoka, N., Hayashi, W., et al. (2010).). Long-term changes in axial length in adult eyes with pathologic myopia. *Am. J. Ophthalmol.* 150, 562.e1–568.e1. doi: 10.1016/j.ajo.2010.05.009

Shah, M., Roomans Ledo, A., and Rittscher, J. (2020). Automated classification of normal and Stargardt disease optical coherence tomography images using deep learning. *Acta Ophthalmol.* 98, e715–e721. doi: 10.1111/aos.14353

Shao, L., Xu, L., Chen, C. X., Yang, L. H., Du, K. F., Wang, S., et al. (2013). Reproducibility of subfoveal choroidal thickness measurements with enhanced depth imaging by spectral-domain optical coherence tomography. *Invest. Ophthalmol. Vis. Sci.* 54, 230–233. doi: 10.1167/iovs.12-10351

Shao, L., Xu, L., Wei, W. B., Chen, C. X., Du, K. F., Li, X. P., et al. (2014). Visual acuity and subfoveal choroidal thickness: the Beijing Eye Study. *Am. J. Ophthalmol.* 158, 702.e1–709.e1. doi: 10.1016/j.ajo.2014.05.023

Spaide, R. F. (2009). Age-related choroidal atrophy. *Am. J. Ophthalmol.* 147, 801–810.

Szegedy, C., Vanhoucke, V., Ioffe, S., Shlens, J., and Wojna, Z. (2016). "Rethinking the inception architecture for computer vision," in *Proceedings of the IEEE Conference on Computer Vision and Pattern Recognition*, (New York, NY: IEEE), 2818–2826.

Tideman, J. W., Snabel, M. C., Tedja, M. S., van Rijn, G. A., Wong, K. T., Kuijpers, R. W., et al. (2016). Association of axial length with risk of uncorrectable visual impairment for Europeans with myopia. *JAMA Ophthalmol.* 134, 1355–1363. doi: 10.1001/jamaophthalmol.2016.4009

Ting, D. S. W., Cheung, C. Y., Lim, G., Tan, G. S. W., Quang, N. D., Gan, A., et al. (2017). Development and validation of a deep learning system for diabetic retinopathy and related eye diseases using retinal images from multiethnic populations with diabetes. *JAMA* 318, 2211–2223. doi: 10.1001/jama.2017.18152

Toy, B. C., Myung, D. J., He, L., Pan, C. K., Chang, R. T., Polkinhorne, A., et al. (2016). Smartphone-based dilated fundus photography and near visual acuity testing as inexpensive screening tools to detect referral warranted diabetic eye disease. *Retina* 36, 1000–1008. doi: 10.1097/IAE.0000000000000955

Varadarajan, A. V., Poplin, R., Blumer, K., Angermueller, C., Ledsam, J., Chopra, R., et al. (2018). Deep learning for predicting refractive error from retinal fundus images. *Invest. Ophthalmol. Vis. Sci.* 59, 2861–2868. doi: 10.1167/iovs.18-23887

Wang, J., Ju, R., Chen, Y., Zhang, L., Hu, J., Wu, Y., et al. (2018). Automated retinopathy of prematurity screening using deep neural networks. *EBioMedicine* 35, 361–368. doi: 10.1016/j.ebiom.2018.08.033

Wei, W. B., Xu, L., Jonas, J. B., Shao, L., Du, K. F., Wang, S., et al. (2013). Subfoveal choroidal thickness: the Beijing Eye Study. *Ophthalmology* 120, 175–180.

Yan, Y. N., Wang, Y. X., Xu, L., Xu, J., Wei, W. B., and Jonas, J. B. (2015). Fundus tessellation: prevalence and associated factors: the Beijing Eye Study 2011. *Ophthalmology* 122, 1873–1880. doi: 10.1016/j.ophtha.2015.05.031

Yan, Y. N., Wang, Y. X., Yang, Y., Xu, L., Xu, J., Wang, Q., et al. (2018a). Long-term progression and risk factors of fundus tessellation in the Beijing Eye Study. *Sci. Rep.* 8:10625. doi: 10.1038/s41598-018-29009-1

Yan, Y. N., Wang, Y. X., Yang, Y., Xu, L., Xu, J., Wang, Q., et al. (2018b). Ten-year progression of myopic maculopathy: the Beijing Eye Study 2001-2011. *Ophthalmology* 125, 1253–1263. doi: 10.1016/j.ophtha.2018.01.035

Zago, G. T., Andreão, R. V., Dorizzi, B., and Teatini Salles, E. O. (2018). Retinal image quality assessment using deep learning. *Comput. Biol. Med.* 103, 64–70. doi: 10.1016/j.compbiomed.2018.10.004

Zhou, B., Khosla, A., Lapedriza, A., Oliva, A., and Torralba, A. (2016). "Learning deep features for discriminative localization," in *Proceedings of the IEEE Conference on Computer Vision and Pattern Recognition*, (New York, NY: IEEE), 2921–2929.

2

Detection of Fuchs' Uveitis Syndrome from Slit-Lamp Images using Deep Convolutional Neural Networks in a Chinese Population

Wanyun Zhang[1†], Zhijun Chen[1†], Han Zhang[2], Guannan Su[1], Rui Chang[1], Lin Chen[1], Ying Zhu[1], Qingfeng Cao[1], Chunjiang Zhou[1], Yao Wang[1] and Peizeng Yang[1]*

[1] *The First Affiliated Hospital of Chongqing Medical University, Chongqing Key Laboratory of Ophthalmology and Chongqing Eye Institute, Chongqing Branch of National Clinical Research Center for Ocular Diseases, Chongqing, China,* [2] *School of Computer Science and Technology, Harbin Institute of Technology, Harbin, China*

Correspondence:
Peizeng Yang
peizengycmu@126.com

[†] *These authors have contributed equally to this work*

Fuchs' uveitis syndrome (FUS) is one of the most under- or misdiagnosed uveitis entities. Many undiagnosed FUS patients are unnecessarily overtreated with anti-inflammatory drugs, which may lead to serious complications. To offer assistance for ophthalmologists in the screening and diagnosis of FUS, we developed seven deep convolutional neural networks (DCNNs) to detect FUS using slit-lamp images. We also proposed a new optimized model with a mixed "attention" module to improve test accuracy. In the same independent set, we compared the performance between these DCNNs and ophthalmologists in detecting FUS. Seven different network models, including Xception, Resnet50, SE-Resnet50, ResNext50, SE-ResNext50, ST-ResNext50, and SET-ResNext50, were used to predict FUS automatically with the area under the receiver operating characteristic curves (AUCs) that ranged from 0.951 to 0.977. Our proposed SET-ResNext50 model (accuracy = 0.930; Precision = 0.918; Recall = 0.923; F1 measure = 0.920) with an AUC of 0.977 consistently outperformed the other networks and outperformed general ophthalmologists by a large margin. Heat-map visualizations of the SET-ResNext50 were provided to identify the target areas in the slit-lamp images. In conclusion, we confirmed that a trained classification method based on DCNNs achieved high effectiveness in distinguishing FUS from other forms of anterior uveitis. The performance of the DCNNs was better than that of general ophthalmologists and could be of value in the diagnosis of FUS.

Keywords: Fuchs' uveitis syndrome, diffuse iris depigmentation, slit-lamp images, deep convolutional neural model, deep learning

INTRODUCTION

Fuchs' uveitis syndrome (FUS) is a chronic, mostly unilateral, non-granulomatous anterior uveitis, accounting for 1–20% of all cases of uveitis at referral centers, and is the second most common form of non-infectious uveitis (Yang et al., 2006; Kazokoglu et al., 2008; Abano et al., 2017). It is reported to be one of the most under- or misdiagnosed uveitis entities, with its diagnosis often delayed for years (Norrsell and Sjödell, 2008; Tappeiner et al., 2015; Sun and Ji, 2020). Patients with FUS generally present with an asymptomatic mild inflammation of the anterior segment of the eye (Sun and Ji, 2020). The syndrome is featured by characteristic keratic precipitates (KPs), depigmentation in the iris with or without heterochromia, and absence of posterior synechiae (Tandon et al., 2012). Heterochromia is a striking feature of FUS in white people (Bonfioli et al., 2005). However, iris depigmentation may be absent or subtle, especially in patients from Asian or African populations, who have a higher melanin density in their iris (Tabbut et al., 1988; Arellanes-García et al., 2002; Yang et al., 2006; Tugal-Tutkun et al., 2009). In a previous study on Chinese FUS patients, we described the presence of varying degrees of diffuse iris depigmentation without posterior synechiae rather than heterochromia (Yang et al., 2006). Degrees of diffuse iris depigmentation may be considered as the most sensitive and reliable signs of FUS in Chinese as well as in other highly pigmented populations (Mohamed and Zamir, 2005; Yang et al., 2006). The subtle iris depigmentation is however often neglected, leading to a misdiagnosis (Tappeiner et al., 2015). Many undiagnosed FUS patients are unnecessarily treated chronically or intermittently with topical or systemic corticosteroids or even other immunosuppressive agents, which may lead to cataract formation and severe glaucoma (Menezo and Lightman, 2005; Accorinti et al., 2016; Touhami et al., 2019). Until now, the diagnosis is highly dependent on the skills of the uveitis specialist with broad experience in the detection of subtle iris pigmentation abnormalities in a patient with mild anterior uveitis.

Deep learning (DL), one of the most promising artificial intelligence technologies, has been demonstrated to learn from and make predictions on data sets (He et al., 2019). Deep convolutional neural network (DCNN), a subtype of DL, has proven to be a useful method in image-centric specialties, especially in ophthalmology (Hogarty et al., 2019). The capability of DCNN to learn a complicated representation of the data makes it useful for solving the classification problem to facilitate accurate diagnosis of various diseases (Kapoor et al., 2019; Ting et al., 2019). To offer assistance for ophthalmologists in the screening and diagnosis of FUS, we decided to develop DCNNs to classify slit-lamp images automatically and in this report we show its feasibility in the detection of FUS.

MATERIALS AND METHODS

Data Sets

We designed a retrospective study based on the slit-lamp images of 478 Fuchs patients and 474 non-FUS controls from the uveitis center of the First Affiliated Hospital of Chongqing Medical University during January 2015 to October 2020. The diagnosis of FUS was made according to the criteria by La Hey et al. (1991) in combination with the description for Chinese FUS patients in a previous report from our group (Yang et al., 2006). Non-FUS patients with other uveitis entities (**Table 1**), who presented with signs and symptoms of anterior uveitis and had images comparable with those in FUS patients, served as controls. All enrolled patients were diagnosed by more than two

TABLE 1 | Uveitis entities in the Non-Fuchs' uveitis syndrome group.

Entity	Total	Number (%)	
		The training and validation set	The test set
Idiopathic chronic anterior uveitis	124	100 (26.2)	24 (26.1)
Posner–Schlossman syndrome	83	66 (17.3)	17 (18.5)
Presumed viral anterior uveitis	74	60 (15.7)	14 (15.2)
Acute anterior uveitis	66	53 (13.9)	13 (14.1)
Sarcoidosis	62	51 (13.3)	11 (12.0)
Vogt–Koyanagi–Harada disease	35	28 (7.3)	7 (7.6)
Behcet's disease	30	24 (6.3)	6 (6.5)
Total	474	382	92

specialists from referring hospitals and then verified by uveitis specialists from our center. The slit-lamp images of each patient were collected using a digital slit-lamp microscope (Photo-Slit Lamp BX 900; Haag-Streit, Koeniz, Switzerland). These images were taken with a 30° angle using direct illumination and focused on the iris with varying degrees of magnification (10, 16, or 25). To highlight the diffusion and uniformity of the iris depigmentation, only images that covered about half of the iris appearance were included.

A total of 2,000 standard slit-lamp images were collected anonymously and removing all personal data except types of disease. These images were used as the basis for training DCNNs consisting of 872 slit-lamp images of affected eyes showing the diffuse and uniform iris depigmentation without posterior synechiae from FUS patients (FUS group) and 1,128 images of control eyes from non-FUS patients (non-FUS group). Then, the 20% aggregate images were set as an independent test set to evaluate the effectiveness and generalization ability of DCNNs. The remaining 80% images were randomly and respectively assigned to the training set and the validation set in an 8:2 ratio. The training set was used to train DCNNs, whereas the validation set was utilized to optimize learnable weights and parameters of DCNNs. The images collected from the same patient (left and right eyes or from multiple sessions) could ensure to be not separated between the test set and the other two sets. The study was approved by the Ethical Committee of First Affiliated Hospital of Chongqing Medical University (No. 2019356) and was conducted in accordance with the Declaration of Helsinki for research involving human subjects.

Development of the DL Algorithm

The slit-lamp images were initially preprocessed to derive data for developing the DCNNs. Each image was resized to 224×224 pixels to be compatible with the original dimensions of the experiment networks. Then, the pixel values were scaled to range from 0 to 1. To increase the diversity of the data set and reduce the risk of overfitting, we applied several augmentations to each image, involving random cropped, random rotation, random brightness change, and random flips. Data augmentation is an essential approach to automatically generate new annotated training samples and improve the generalization of DL models (Tran et al., 2017). We obtained samples with shearing with ranges of $[-15\%, +15\%]$ of the image width, with rotation $[0°, 360°]$, with brightness change with ranges of $[-10\%, +10\%]$, and with or without flipping, thereby generating 10 images per photograph.

Resnet, as a residual deep neural network, was widely used because it is easy to optimize and can gain accuracy from significantly increased depths (He et al., 2016). There are various depths of Resnet structures (Resnet50, Resnet101, and Resnet152), and in this study we used Resnet50 as the experimental models. ResNext, as a new network derived on the basis of Resnet, was included since it can improve accuracy while maintaining Resnet's high-portability benefits (Xie et al., 2017). Moreover, we introduced a new "attention" unit: the Squeeze-and-Excitation (SE) module. This module allows the network to selectively emphasize informative features and suppresses less useful ones (Hu et al., 2017). After uniting data with the SE module, four different networks (Resnet50, SE-Resnet50, ResNext50, and SE-ResNext50) were included. For comparison, we also selected the Xception network, containing a new convolutional structure named depth-wise separable convolutions that used less parameters and were defined or modified easily (Chollet, 2017). These five classical DCNNs were pre-trained to running the detection of FUS.

To improve test accuracy, we constructed a new optimized model, using ResNext50 as the backend. Considering the ResNext50 lack of ability to be spatially invariant to the input data, we introduced a "Spatial Transformer (ST)" module, which is another "attention" unit to provide explicit spatial transformation capabilities. This module performs the ability to learn invariance to translation, scale, rotation, and more generic warping, resulting in state-of-the-art performance (Jaderberg et al., 2015). Applying a mixed "attention" module (SE and ST module), our new model (SET-ResNext50) could not only learn the informative features but also focus on the informative location. We also conducted ablation experiments (ST-ResNext50: ResNext50 with ST module) to verify the effectiveness of our proposed mixed "attention" module. Moreover, we manually tuned various combinations of the hyper-parameters to ensure that the trained models met our experimental requirements. The architecture of SET-ResNext50 is shown in **Figure 1**.

We developed DCNNs to classify the slit-lamp images into two categories: FUS and Non-FUS. To optimize the models and achieve a better training effect, each model was pre-trained in a classification dataset Imagenet (Deng et al., 2009) to initialize its parameters. Then, we used a 2080 Ti GPU and mini-batches of 96 inputs. The cross entropy was used as a loss function to update all the parameters of the network. The Adam optimizer was used as an optimization function with a learning rate of 10^{-4}. The last layer of DCNNs was modified to output a two-dimension vector. We applied fivefold cross-validation for each DCNN to test the statistical significance of the developed models. The heat maps highlighted lesions and showed the location on which the decision of the algorithm was based (Zhou et al., 2016).

Evaluation of the DL Algorithm

The performance of our experimental models was evaluated in an independent test data set. Images obtained from the same patient could ensure to be not split across the test set and the other two sets. The fivefold cross-validation binary classification results of each model were used to calculate the mean and standard deviation for testing the statistical significance of the developed models. We used receiver operating characteristic (ROC) curves, with calculations of an area under the receiver operating characteristic curves (AUCs), as an index of the performance of our automated models (Carter et al., 2016). AUCs were computed for each finding with 95% confidence intervals computed by the exact Clopper–Pearson method using the Python scikit-learn package version 0.18.2. Precision, accuracy, and recall were used to evaluate the FUS classification performance of our developed models. To make a trade-off between precision and accuracy, F1 measures were added to assess the effectiveness. SPSS version 24.0 (IBM) was used to compare quantitative variables by Student's t-test.

Comparison of the Networks With Human Ophthalmologists

We compared the performance between seven DCNNs and the clinical diagnosis of ophthalmologists. We chose six ophthalmologists in two different levels (attending ophthalmologists with at least 5 years of clinical training in uveitis from our center: Dr. Zi Ye, Shenglan Yi, and Handan Tan; resident ophthalmologists with 1–3 years of clinical training in ophthalmology from other eye institutes: Dr. Jun Zhang, Yunyun Zhu, and Liang Chen). None of them has participated in the current research. The slit-lamp images were subjected to each ophthalmologist alone and were requested to assign one of three labels to each image, i.e., FUS, uncertain, non-FUS. They were strongly advised not to choose the uncertain label because it is considered as a wrong answer for final evaluation.

RESULTS

Baseline Characteristics

A total of 2,000 slit-lamp images from 478 FUS patients and 474 non-FUS controls were collected and assessed during the study period. The non-FUS group included various forms of anterior uveitis and panuveitis with a presentation of anterior uveitis. The types and proportion of non-FUS cases are listed in **Table 1**. The 2,000 images were assigned to the training set, the validation set, and the test set. The training and validation set (1,600 images) included 698 images from 380 FUS patients and 902 images from 382 non-FUS patients, and the test set (400 images) consisted of 174 images from 98 FUS patients and 226 images from 92 non-FUS patients.

Performance of the DL Algorithm

After applying fivefold cross-validation, we calculated the mean value and standard deviation to evaluate the performance of our developed models. Performance results are reported in

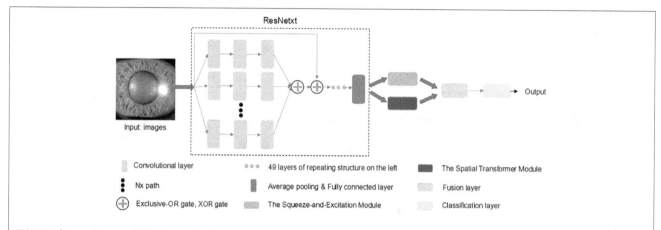

FIGURE 1 | The architecture of SET-ResNext50. We used ResNext50 as backend uniting a mixed "attention" module (the Squeeze-and-Excitation module and the Spatial Transform module). This network was pre-trained in a classification dataset Imagenet to initialize its parameters. Then, we modified the last layer to output a two-dimension vector and updated all the parameters by using the cross entropy.

Table 2. In aggregate, the performance of all trained models showed promising outcomes when considering the selected metrics including accuracy, precision, F1 measure, and recall. In the test set of 400 images, seven DCNNs achieved the accuracy of 0.883–0.930, while F1 measures were 0.866–0.920. We found that the performance of ResNext50 was better than that of SE-ResNext50 or ST-ResNext50, demonstrating that the combination of SE or ST modules with the model would not improve the effectiveness of our networks. However, after uniting with the mixed "attention" module, our SET-ResNext50 model consistently outperformed other network models with its performance (accuracy = 0.930; Precision = 0.918; Recall = 0.923; F1 = 0.920). There were significant differences in accuracy between SET-ResNext50 and the other models except ResNext50 ($p < 0.05$). The F1 measure of SET-ResNext50 was higher than that of ResNext50 ($p = 0.043$), which showed that SET-ResNext50 is more superior than other models.

The ROCs and AUCs are reported in **Figure 2**. AUCs were 0.951–0.977 of DCNNs, which also demonstrate good performance of the developed models. SET-ResNext50 with its AUC of 0.977 showed that this model could be the optimal choice to facilitate the diagnosis of FUS among seven networks. The other metrics in **Table 2** also echoed these observations.

Figures 3, 4 present the examples of heat maps of SET-ResNext50 model for each finding, accompanied by the corresponding original image. The heat maps showed the most apparently affected region in slit-lamp images. This region was the most important indicator to distinguish FUS from non-FUS. In **Figure 3**, the affected area of FUS accounted for nearly half of the total iris appearance and was mostly located in the pupillary collar. In contrast, the affected area of non-FUS images (**Figure 4**) was unevenly distributed, including in the pupil or around the periphery of the iris. The affected areas of our SET-ResNext50 model correspond to those identified by the clinicians for diagnosis. In summary, SET-ResNext50 showed the best level of performance in our study and emphasized the most important clues of the image that pointed to the classification results.

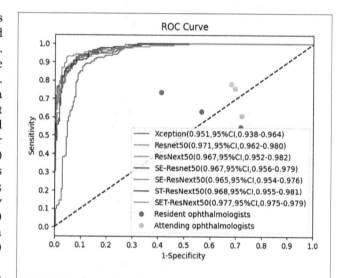

FIGURE 2 | Receiver operating characteristic curves of the performance for diagnosis of Fuchs uveitis syndrome in the test set. SET-ResNext50 achieved an AUC of 0.977 (95%CI, 0.975–0.979), which outperformed other developed networks and outperformed all the ophthalmologists by a large margin.

Comparison With Ophthalmologists

Three resident ophthalmologists and three attending ophthalmologists were included to detect FUS. The average accuracy is 0.709 for attending ophthalmologists from our uveitis center, which is higher than that (0.597) for resident ophthalmologists from other eye institutes. There is significant difference in accuracy between these two groups ($p = 0.024$). Moreover, there was a huge performance gap between ophthalmologists and DCNNs (**Table 2**). The average accuracy of ophthalmologists is significantly lower than that of DCNNs ($p < 0.01$). As shown in **Table 2**, comparing the accuracy of ophthalmologists (0.597 and 0.709), the SET-ResNext50 model with the accuracy of 0.930 shows that the latter is superior for detecting FUS.

TABLE 2 | Performance of the deep convolutional neural networks with fivefold cross-validation and the compared methods in the test set.

		Accuracy (SD)	Precision (SD)	Recall (SD)	F1-measure (SD)	*P*-value*
The classical DCNNs	Xception	0.883 (0.007)	0.861 (0.039)	0.875 (0.047)	0.866 (0.008)	<0.01
	Resnet50	0.903 (0.016)	0.879 (0.047)	0.905 (0.044)	0.890 (0.016)	0.044
	SE-Resnet50	0.893 (0.025)	0.855 (0.040)	0.909 (0.052)	0.880 (0.028)	0.007
	ResNext50	0.904 (0.015)	0.889 (0.019)	0.890 (0.048)	0.889 (0.020)	0.052
	SE-ResNext50	0.893 (0.024)	0.897 (0.038)	0.852 (0.045)	0.873 (0.029)	<0.01
Ablation experiments	ST-ResNext50	0.896 (0.013)	0.885 (0.036)	0.879 (0.068)	0.880 (0.021)	0.014
Our proposed model	SET-ResNext50	0.930 (0.005)	0.918 (0.028)	0.923 (0.027)	0.920 (0.004)	–
Ophthalmologists	Resident	0.597 (0.045)	0.539 (0.054)	0.638 (0.095)	0.578 (0.009)	<0.01
	Attending	0.709 (0.032)	0.648 (0.018)	0.722 (0.100)	0.681 (0.056)	<0.01

Comparison of accuracy with the SET-ResNext50.
SD, standard deviation; SE, Squeeze-and-Excitation; ST, Spatial Transformer.

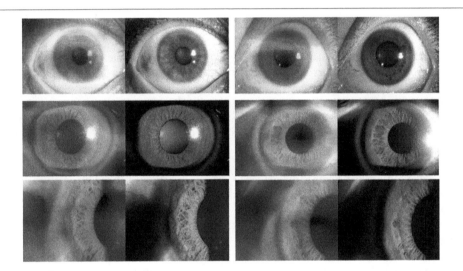

FIGURE 3 | The heat maps of the SET-ResNext50 model in slit-lamp image with Fuchs uveitis syndrome demonstrating representative findings, shown in the original slit-lamp image (right) and corresponding heat map for target areas (left).

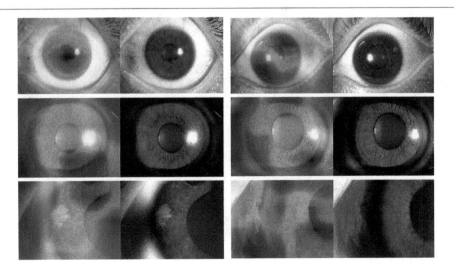

FIGURE 4 | The heat maps of the SET-ResNext50 model in slit-lamp image with non-Fuchs uveitis syndrome demonstrating representative findings, shown in the original slit-lamp image (right) and corresponding heat map for target areas (left).

DISCUSSION

In this study, we developed DCNNs to prove a well-trained DL method for distinguishing FUS from various anterior uveitis and even identify the diagnostic clues that many clinical ophthalmologists neglect. Our study includes three meaningful conclusions. Firstly, to our knowledge, this is the first initiative to assist ophthalmologists in making a correct diagnosis of FUS using slit-lamp images. Secondly, we trained seven DCNNs and developed a new optimized model (SET-ResNext50). SET-ResNext50 achieved both high accuracy and precision, consistently outperforming other models and the general ophthalmologists. Thirdly, our study provided heat maps that highlighted and showed the location of lesions in slit-lamp images. Applying the DCNNs to assist the detection of hidden lesions can facilitate the clinical diagnosis and treatment process.

Recently, DCNNs have been rapidly popularized in clinical practice to make predictions of diseases automatically. Schlegl et al. (2018) achieved excellent accuracy for the detection and quantification of macular fluid in OCT images by using DL in retinal image analysis. Several studies have suggested that applying a DCNN-based automated assessment of age-related macular degeneration from fundus images can produce results that are similar to human performance levels (Burlina et al., 2017; Grassmann et al., 2018; Russakoff et al., 2019). Intensive efforts to develop automated methods highlight the attraction of these tools for advanced management of clinical disease, especially for diseases like FUS. The slit-lamp microscope is the most widely used auxiliary instrument in clinical practice (Jiang et al., 2018). In busy clinics, taking a mass of slit-lamp images into consideration is inherently impractical and error-prone for ophthalmologists. Therefore, automated DCNNs could be used to screen slit-lamp image data sets, direct the ophthalmologists' attention to the lesion, and in the near future perform diagnosis independently. Our presented DCNNs with high accuracy for the detection of FUS highlighted the location of lesions and may become widely applicable.

Building and optimizing a new DCNN may require a substantial amount of hyper-parameter tuning time. Therefore, many studies have used classical networks such as Resnet as the backend (Wu et al., 2017). In this study, as the basis of ResNext50, we proposed a mixed "attention" module combining informative attention and spatial attention in our optimized model architecture. We found that SET-ResNext50 with a mixed "attention" module outperformed the models combining with one of the SE and ST modules, indicating that there is mutual promotion between the SE module and ST module. The innovative method of using this mixed module may be useful in other areas of ophthalmology. With too few images or too many training steps, the DL classifier may show overfitting, resulting in the poor generalization of results (Treder et al., 2018). In this study, we used data augmentation to generate new annotated training samples and set an independent test set to evaluate the generalization ability of DCNNs. We found that the performance of our DCNNs was consistently good in

the test set, indicating that the models had the generalization ability without overfitting. We compared the effectiveness of DCNNs against ophthalmologists with different experience levels. The performance of attending ophthalmologists was better than that of the resident ophthalmologists, indicating that the misdiagnosis of FUS may be due to a lack of accumulation of clinical experience. As expected, the DCNNs achieving the highest sensitivity while keeping high specificity outperformed the resident and attending ophthalmologists by a large margin. Moreover, our model produced the heat map visualizations to identify the existence of the target areas in images and then generated the output of the classification. In the heat maps, the most apparently affected regions of FUS images were mainly located in the depigmentation of the pupil collar and accounted for nearly half of the overall iris appearance (**Figure 3**), which generally proved the characteristic of diffuse and uniform iris depigmentation in the vicinity of the pupil in FUS patients. Other uveitis entities like the Posner–Schlossman syndrome may show heterogeneous and uneven iris depigmentation. Iris depigmentation can also be detected in patients with herpetic uveitis, but it usually displays a local appearance. Those signs correspond to the irregular affected areas on the heat maps of non-FUS (**Figure 4**). Some affected areas in non-FUS cases (like idiopathic chronic anterior uveitis) that were located in the pupil may arise from the presentation of posterior synechiae without iris depigmentation. However, the heat maps produced by DCNNs are challenging and difficult to interpret (Ramanishka et al., 2017). In image-based diagnostic specialties, interpreting the heat map may facilitate a better understanding of the diagnosis.

We realize that our study has several limitations. First, our data of slit-lamp images only included Chinese patients with highly pigmented iris and our findings therefore need to be validated in other ethnic populations. Unfortunately, there is no other public dataset of the FUS patients from different populations to validate our models. Such a dataset would be a significant value for further research and expected to evaluate the performance of other DCNNs in the future. Second, the available data set is relatively small for training or validation. Unlike in other common eye diseases such as age-related macular degeneration or diabetic retinopathy, there are a relatively smaller number of cases with FUS. Third, the program we developed could only distinguish FUS from non-FUS according to the iris change. Further research is expected to combine DCNNs with other clinical findings in the diagnosis of complex diseases. Anyhow, we believe that the method presented here is a meaningful step toward the automated analysis of slit-lamp images and may aid in the detection of FUS.

CONCLUSION

In conclusion, we have developed various DCNNs and validated a sensitive automated model (SET-ResNext50) to detect FUS using slit-lamp images. Our presented models achieved both high accuracy and precision, and outperformed general ophthalmologists by a large margin. The SET-ResNext50 model may be the optimal choice to facilitate the diagnosis of FUS. Moreover, the heat map could extract important features from the iris, which proved that DCNNs could be trained to detect specific disease-related changes. The DCNNs are expected to be applied to auxiliary imaging instruments for preliminary screening of diseases, which is of value in future clinical practices.

ETHICS STATEMENT

The studies involving human participants were reviewed and approved by the Ethical Committee of First Affiliated Hospital of Chongqing Medical University (No. 2019356). The patients/participants provided their written informed consent to participate in this study. Written informed consent was obtained from the individual(s) for the publication of any potentially identifiable images or data included in this article.

AUTHOR CONTRIBUTIONS

PY, WZ, and ZC: had full access to all of the data in the study and took responsibility for the integrity of the data and the accuracy of the data analysis. WZ, ZC, and HZ: acquisition, analysis, or interpretation of data. RC, LC, and GS: statistical analysis. YZ, QC, CZ, and YW: methodology supervision. WZ and ZC: writing—review and editing. PY: funding acquisition. All authors contributed to the article and approved the submitted version.

ACKNOWLEDGMENTS

We thank Dr. Zi Ye, Handan Tan, Shenglan Yi, Jun Zhang, Yunyun Zhu, and Liang Chen for their helpful and valuable discussions.

REFERENCES

Abano, J. M., Galvante, P. R., Siopongco, P., Dans, K., and Lopez, J. (2017). Review of epidemiology of uveitis in Asia: pattern of uveitis in a tertiary hospital in the Philippines. *Ocul. Immunol. Inflamm.* 25(suppl. 1), S75–S80. doi: 10.1080/09273948

Accorinti, M., Spinucci, G., Pirraglia, M. P., Bruschi, S., Pesci, F. R., and Iannetti, L. (2016). Fuchs' Heterochromic Iridocyclitis in an Italian tertiary referral centre: epidemiology, clinical features, and prognosis. *J. Ophthalmol.* 2016:1458624. doi: 10.1155/2016/1458624

Arellanes-García, L., del Carmen Preciado-Delgadillo, M., and Recillas-Gispert, C. (2002). Fuchs' heterochromic iridocyclitis: clinical manifestations in dark-eyed Mexican patients. *Ocul. Immunol. Inflamm.* 10, 125–131. doi: 10.1076/ocii.10.2.125.13976

Bonfioli, A. A., Curi, A. L., and Orefice, F. (2005). Fuchs' heterochromic cyclitis. *Semin. Ophthalmol.* 20, 143–146. doi: 10.1080/08820530500231995

Burlina, P. M., Joshi, N., Pekala, M., Pacheco, K. D., Freund, D. E., and Bressler, N. M. (2017). Automated grading of age-related macular degeneration from color fundus images using deep convolutional neural networks. *JAMA Ophthalmol.* 135, 1170–1176. doi: 10.1001/jamaophthalmol.2017.3782

Carter, J. V., Pan, J., Rai, S. N., and Galandiuk, S. (2016). ROC-ing along: evaluation and interpretation of receiver operating characteristic curves. *Surgery* 159, 1638–1645. doi: 10.1016/j.surg.2015.12.029

Chollet, F. (2017). "Xception: deep learning with depthwise separable convolutions," in *Proceedings of the 2017 IEEE Conference on Computer Vision and Pattern Recognition (CVPR)*, (Honolulu, HI: IEEE), 1800–1807. doi: 10.1109/CVPR.2017.195

Deng, J., Dong, W., Socher, R., Li, L. J., Li, K., and Fei-Fei, L. (2009). "Imagenet: a large-scale hierarchical image database," in *Proceedings of IEEE Computer Vision & Pattern Recognition*, Miami, FL, 248–255. doi: 10.1109/CVPR.2009.5206848

Grassmann, F., Mengelkamp, J., Brandl, C., Harsch, S., Zimmermann, M. E., Linkohr, B., et al. (2018). A deep learning algorithm for prediction of age-related eye disease study severity scale for age-related macular degeneration from color fundus photography. *Ophthalmology* 125, 1410–1420. doi: 10.1016/j.ophtha.2018.02.037

He, J., Baxter, S. L., Xu, J., Xu, J., Zhou, X., and Zhang, K. (2019). The practical implementation of artificial intelligence technologies in medicine. *Nat. Med.* 25, 30–36. doi: 10.1038/s41591-018-0307-0

He, K., Zhang, X., Ren, S., and Sun, J. (2016). "Deep residual learning for image recognition," in *Proceedings of the IEEE Conference on Computer Vision & Pattern Recognition*, (Las Vegas, NV: IEEE Computer Society). doi: 10.1109/CVPR.2016.90

Hogarty, D. T., Mackey, D. A., and Hewitt, A. W. (2019). Current state and future prospects of artificial intelligence in ophthalmology: a review. *Clin. Exp. Ophthalmol.* 47, 128–139. doi: 10.1111/ceo.13381

Hu, J., Shen, L., Sun, G., and Albanie, S. (2017). "Squeeze-and-excitation networks," in *Proceedings of the IEEE Transactions on Pattern Analysis and Machine Intelligence*, Salt Lake City, 7132–7141. doi: 10.1109/TPAMI.2019.2913372

Jaderberg, M., Simonyan, K., Zisserman, A., and Kavukcuoglu, K. (2015). "Spatial transformer networks," in *Proceedings of the Advances in neural information processing systems*, London, 2017–2025.

Jiang, J., Liu, X., Liu, L., Wang, S., Long, E., Yang, H., et al. (2018). Predicting the progression of ophthalmic disease based on slit-lamp images using a deep temporal sequence network. *PLoS One* 13:e0201142. doi: 10.1371/journal.pone.0201142

Kapoor, R., Walters, S. P., and Al-Aswad, L. A. (2019). The current state of artificial intelligence in ophthalmology. *Surv. Ophthalmol.* 64, 233–240. doi: 10.1016/j.survophthal.2018.09.002

Kazokoglu, H., Onal, S., Tugal-Tutkun, I., Mirza, E., Akova, Y., Ozyazgan, Y., et al. (2008). Demographic and clinical features of uveitis in tertiary centers in Turkey. *Ophthalmic Epidemiol.* 15, 285–293. doi: 10.1080/09286580802262821

La Hey, E., Baarsma, G. S., De Vries, J., and Kijlstra, A. (1991). Clinical analysis of Fuchs' heterochromic cyclitis. *Doc. Ophthalmol.* 78, 225–235. doi: 10.1007/BF00165685

Menezo, V., and Lightman, S. (2005). The development of complications in patients with chronic anterior uveitis. *Am. J. Ophthalmol.* 139, 988–992. doi: 10.1016/j.ajo.2005.01.029

Mohamed, Q., and Zamir, E. (2005). Update on Fuchs' uveitis syndrome. *Curr. Opin. Ophthalmol.* 16, 356–363. doi: 10.1097/01.icu.0000187056.29563.8d

Norrsell, K., and Sjödell, L. (2008). Fuchs' heterochromic uveitis: a longitudinal clinical study. *Acta Ophthalmol.* 86, 58–64. doi: 10.1111/j.1600-0420.2007.00990.x

Ramanishka, V., Das, A., Zhang, J., and Saenko, K. (2017). "Top-down visual saliency guided by captions," in *Proceedings of the 2017 IEEE Conference on Computer Vision and Pattern Recognition (CVPR)*, Honolulu, HI, 3135–3144. doi: 10.1109/CVPR.2017.334

Russakoff, D. B., Lamin, A., Oakley, J. D., Dubis, A. M., and Sivaprasad, S. (2019). Deep learning for prediction of AMD progression: a pilot study. *Invest. Ophthalmol. Vis. Sci.* 60, 712–722. doi: 10.1167/iovs.18-25325

Schlegl, T., Waldstein, S. M., Bogunovic, H., Endstraßer, F., Sadeghipour, A., Philip, A. M., et al. (2018). Fully automated detection and quantification of macular fluid in OCT using deep learning. *Ophthalmology* 125, 549–558. doi: 10.1016/j. ophtha.2017.10.031

Sun, Y., and Ji, Y. (2020). A literature review on Fuchs uveitis syndrome: an update. *Surv. Ophthalmol.* 65, 133–143. doi: 10.1016/j.survophthal

Tabbut, B. R., Tessler, H. H., and Williams, D. (1988). Fuchs' heterochromic iridocyclitis in blacks. *Arch. Ophthalmol.* 106, 1688–1690. doi: 10.1001/ archopht.1988.01060140860027

Tandon, M., Malhotra, P. P., Gupta, V., Gupta, A., and Sharma, A. (2012). Spectrum of Fuchs uveitic syndrome in a North Indian population. *Ocul. Immunol. Inflamm.* 20, 429–433. doi: 10.3109/09273948.2012.723113

Tappeiner, C., Dreesbach, J., Roesel, M., Heinz, C., and Heiligenhaus, A. (2015). Clinical manifestation of Fuchs uveitis syndrome in childhood. *Graefes Arch. Clin. Exp. Ophthalmol.* 253, 1169–1174. doi: 10.1007/s00417-015-2960-z

Ting, D. S. W., Peng, L., Varadarajan, A. V., Keane, P. A., Burlina, P. M., Chiang, M. F., et al. (2019). Deep learning in ophthalmology: the technical and clinical considerations. *Prog. Retin Eye Res.* 72:100759. doi: 10.1016/j.preteyeres.2019. 04.003

Touhami, S., Vanier, A., Rosati, A., Bojanova, M., Benromdhane, B., Lehoang, P., et al. (2019). Predictive factors of intraocular pressure level evolution over time and glaucoma severity in Fuchs' heterochromic iridocyclitis. *Invest. Ophthalmol. Vis. Sci.* 60, 2399–2405. doi: 10.1167/iovs.18-24597

Tran, T., Pham, T., Carneiro, G., Palmer, L., and Reid, I. (2017). "A Bayesian data augmentation approach for learning deep models," in *Proceedings of the Advances in Neural Information Processing Systems*, Long Beach, CA, 2794–2803.

Treder, M., Lauermann, J. L., and Eter, N. (2018). Automated detection of exudative age-related macular degeneration in spectral domain optical coherence tomography using deep learning. *Graefes Arch. Clin. Exp. Ophthalmol.* 256, 259–265. doi: 10.1007/s00417-017-3850-3

Tugal-Tutkun, I., Güney-Tefekli, E., Kamaci-Duman, F., and Corum, I. (2009). A cross-sectional and longitudinal study of Fuchs uveitis syndrome in Turkish patients. *Am. J. Ophthalmol.* 148, 510–515.e1. doi: 10.1016/j.ajo.2009. 04.007

Wu, S., Zhong, S., and Liu, Y. (2017). Deep residual learning for image steganalysis. *Multimedia Tools Appl.* 77, 10437–10453. doi: 10.1007/s11042-017-4440-4

Xie, S., Girshick, R., Dollar, P., Tu, Z., and He, K. (2017). "Aggregated residual transformations for deep neural networks," in *Proceedings of the 2017 IEEE Conference on Computer Vision and Pattern Recognition (CVPR)*, (Honolulu, HI: IEEE), 5987–5995. doi: 10.1109/cvpr.2017.634

Yang, P., Fang, W., Jin, H., Li, B., Chen, X., and Kijlstra, A. (2006). Clinical features of Chinese patients with Fuchs' syndrome. *Ophthalmology* 113, 473–480. doi: 10.1016/j.ophtha

Zhou, B., Khosla, A., Lapedriza, À, Oliva, A., and Torralba, A. (2016). "Learning deep features for discriminative localization," in *Proceedings of the 2016 IEEE Conference on Computer Vision and Pattern Recognition (CVPR)*, (Las Vegas, NV), 2921–2929. doi: 10.1109/CVPR.20 16.319

3

Changes in the Gut Microbiome Contribute to the Development of Behcet's Disease *via* Adjuvant Effects

Qingfeng Wang[1], Shenglan Yi[1], Guannan Su[1], Ziyu Du[1], Su Pan[1], Xinyue Huang[1], Qingfeng Cao[1], Gangxiang Yuan[1], Aize Kijlstra[2] and Peizeng Yang[1]*

[1] The First Affiliated Hospital of Chongqing Medical University, Chongqing Key Laboratory of Ophthalmology, Chongqing Eye Institute, Chongqing Branch of National Clinical Research Center for Ocular Diseases, Chongqing, China, [2] University Eye Clinic Maastricht, Maastricht, Netherlands

*Correspondence:
Peizeng Yang
peizengycmu@126.com

Behcet's disease (BD) is associated with considerable gut microbiome changes. However, it still remains unknown how the composition of the gut microbiome exactly affects the development of this disease. In this study, transplantation of stool samples from patients with active ocular BD to mice *via* oral gavage was performed. This resulted in decreases of three short chain fatty acids (SCFAs) including butyric acid, propionic acid and valeric acid in the feces of the BD-recipient group. Intestinal barrier integrity of mice receiving BD feces was damaged as shown by a decreased expression of tight junction proteins and was associated with the release of Lipopolysaccharides (LPS) in the circulation. The mice also showed a higher frequency of splenic neutrophils as well as an enrichment of genes associated with innate immune responses in the neutrophils and CD4 + T cells as identified by single cell RNA sequencing. Analysis of neutrophils and T cells functions in these mice showed an enhanced mesenteric lymph node and splenic Th1 and Th17 cell differentiation in association with activation of neutrophils. Transplantation of BD feces to mice and subsequent induction of experimental uveitis (EAU) or encephalomyelitis (EAE) led to an exacerbation of disease in both models, suggesting a microbial adjuvant effect. These findings suggest that the gut microbiome may regulate an autoimmune response *via* adjuvant effects including increased gut permeability and enhancement of innate immunity.

Keywords: gut microbiome, autoimmune disease, Behcet's disease, fecal transplantation, T cells, neutrophils

INTRODUCTION

Behcet's disease (BD) is a chronic, multisystemic inflammatory disorder (Zeidan et al., 2016), characterized by recurrent oral and genital ulcers, skin lesions, as well as a sight-threatening intraocular inflammation called panuveitis (Takeuchi et al., 2015). BD is thought to share both autoimmune and autoinflammatory disease features caused by an aberrant population of Th1 and Th17 cells in combination with hyper-activated neutrophils (Yamashita, 1997; Nanke et al., 2008). The exact etiology of the disease is however not yet clear.

Changes in the gut microbiome composition are thought to contribute to the development of various immune and infectious diseases (Bevins and Salzman, 2011; de Oliveira et al., 2017; Russler-Germain et al., 2017; Domingue et al., 2020). Dysbiosis of the gut microbiota has been found in rheumatoid arthritis (RA) and type 1 diabetes (T1D) using metagenomic sequence (MGS) and 16S rDNA gene sequence analysis (Zhang et al., 2015; Vatanen et al., 2018). Studies dealing with the pathogenesis of autoimmunity have suggested that the composition of the gut microbiota plays a crucial role in the development of auto-reactive lymphocytes and the recruitment of neutrophils (Littman and Rudensky, 2010). Some opportunistic intestinal pathogens have been shown to produce the effector pathogen-associated molecular pattern (PAMP) and microbe-associated molecular pattern (MAMP) molecules which can trigger an inflammatory response *via* host cell receptors such as toll like receptors (TLRs) (Fraiture and Brunner, 2014). An impaired gut barrier function caused by metabolites released from the gut microbiota may facilitate this response (Wang et al., 2012; Furusawa et al., 2013).

We recently started investigating the role of the gut microbiome in the development of ocular BD (Consolandi et al., 2015; Ye et al., 2018). Recent studies provided strong evidence that the gut microbiome contains triggers and/or amplification signals for autoreactive T cells that can drive spontaneous uveitis in mice (Horai et al., 2015). These findings may also have implications for the contribution of the gut microbiome to the etiology of human uveitis. However, the mechanisms underlying the contribution of the gut microbiome to the development of clinical uveitis is still unclear. In the present study, we provide evidence that the BD gut microbiome may contribute to the development of intraocular inflammation *via* a complex mechanism including altered gut permeability and immunological adjuvant effects.

MATERIALS AND METHODS

Study Participants

For fecal transplantation, five active BD patients along with 5 sex- and age-matched healthy controls were recruited for this study. The active patients included for the study showed active ocular inflammation and had stopped taking immunosuppressive medicines except topical corticosteroids and cycloplegics for at least 1 month, prior to sampling when they visited our clinic. Healthy controls with diabetes, cardiovascular diseases, systemic disease and other inflammatory diseases were excluded. Additionally, the subjects enrolled for sample collection had not received antibiotics or probiotics for at least 1 month (BD patients are generally not treated with antibiotics). Stool samples from five untreated active BD patients and five healthy controls (the metadata of samples for fecal transplantation are shown in **Supplementary Table 1**) were used to colonize mice. Diagnosis of BD was based on the diagnostic criteria of the international study group for BD (Criteria for diagnosis of Behcet's disease, 1990). Active BD was defined according to the presence of active intraocular inflammation. The study was approved by the Ethics Committee of Chongqing Medical University. Signed informed consent was obtained from all participants at the beginning of the study. All procedures were performed in accordance with the Declaration of Helsinki.

Fecal Microbiome Transplantation in Mice

A fecal sample from each donor was resuspended in sterile PBS to a final concentration of 200 mg/ml and then equal volumes of five donor suspensions were pooled. The suspensions were divided in 1 ml portions per centrifuge tube and stored at −80°C until use. The same batch of fecal samples from BD patients and controls was used for the entire study. Each mouse was orally administered with 200 μl of the pooled fecal suspension once a day for 1 week as described in our previous study after being treated with an antibiotic cocktail containing ampicillin (1 mg/ml), neomycin (1 mg/ml), metronidazole (1 mg/ml), and vancomycin (0.5 mg/ml) (all purchased from Sigma-Aldrich) for 3 weeks (Ye et al., 2018).

Autoimmune Animal Models: Induction, Clinical and Histological Assessment

B10.RIII mice and C57BL/6 mice were purchased from Jackson Laboratory (Bar Harbor, ME, United States) and maintained under specific pathogen free (SPF) conditions. EAU induction was induced in B10.RIII mice using 25 μg of interphotoreceptor retinoid binding protein $(IRBP)_{161-180}$, which is half the dose of peptide for experimental uveitis (EAU) induction as used in earlier studies, in complete Freund's adjuvant (CFA) (Sigma-Aldrich, St. Louis, MO, United States) supplemented with 1.0 mg/ml *Mycobacterium tuberculosis* strain (MTB) (Jiang et al., 2008). For experimental encephalomyelitis (EAE) induction, female C57BL/6 mice were immunized with 100 μg of myelin Oligodendrocyte Glycoprotein (MOG) 35–55 (half dose of peptide for EAE induction before) emulsified in CFA. 200 ng of pertussis toxin (List Biological, Campbell, CA, United States) was injected intraperitoneally (i.p.) 0 and 48 h later (Constantinescu et al., 2011). Low doses of peptides were used to obtain a milder form of the disease so as to enable experiments showing a worsening effect of our experimental conditions on both the EAU as well as the EAE model. To obtain clinical and histological scores of the EAU model, animals were scored at day 14 as described previously (Cortes et al., 2008). The clinical score and body weight of EAE mice was measured starting at 16 days after immunization (Badawi et al., 2012). The animal study was approved by the Ethics Committee of the First Affiliated Hospital of Chongqing Medical University.

Isolation of Lymphocytes and Cytokine Secretion Assays

Lymphocytes from mouse spleen were filtered with cell strainers and purified by mouse Ficoll–Hypaque density gradient centrifugation. The cells were cultured in culture medium consisting of RPMI medium 1640, 100 U/ml penicillin/streptomycin and 10% fetal bovine serum (Invitrogen, CA, United States). For cytokine secretion assays, cells

$(5 \times 10^5/500\ \mu l)$ were seeded into each well of a 48-well plate. The supernatants of lymphocytes after stimulation with peptides were collected after 3 days. The production of IFN-γ and IL-17 in the supernatants was quantified using Duoset ELISA development kits (R&D Systems, MN, United States) according to the manufacturer's instructions. For statistical analysis, concentrations below the detection limit were converted to a value of 50% of the lowest point of the calibration curve (de Jager et al., 2005).

Assessment of Intestinal Barrier Function and LPS in Serum

The colon and serum samples were collected from mice at day 7 after fecal transplantation. Three tight junction proteins were detected by real-time PCR as described above and Western Blotting (WB) analysis. Protein was extracted from colon tissues by radio immunoprecipitation assay (RIPA) lysis buffer (Beyotime, Shanghai, China) including 1% protease inhibitor (Beyotime). WB analysis was performed as described previously (Yang et al., 2014). Bands were analyzed using Image J software, version 1.43. Analysis was normalized against β-actin. Specific primary antibodies used included: Claudin-1 (1/1,000, ImmunoWay, United States), Claudin-4 (1/1,000, ImmunoWay, United States), Occludin (1/1,000, ImmunoWay, United States) and β-actin (1/10,000, ABclonal, United States). The level of Lipopolysaccharide (LPS) in serum was quantified using an Instant ELISA Kit for LPS in accordance with the manufacturer instructions (USCN, Wuhan, China).

Neutrophil Isolation and Neutrophil Extracellular Traps Detection

Neutrophils were isolated from mouse spleen, filtered with cell strainers and purified by Ficoll–Hypaque density gradient centrifugation. After centrifugation, red blood cell (RBC) lysis was performed to obtain pure neutrophils (Coquery et al., 2012). For mesenteric lymph node, we isolated total cells from tissues and filtered by cell strainers. For eye tissue, we dissected the retina from eye balls after removing the cornea, sclera and choroid, and then we isolated total cells from retina by filtering through cell strainers. 1×10^6 cells from these tissues were seeded into each well of a 48-well plate and stimulated with 100 nM phorbol 12-myristate 13-acetate (PMA) for 4 h at 37°C. After stimulation with PMA, slides with neutrophils were washed by PBS and fixed with 4% paraformaldehyde in PBS. Blocking was performed with 10% normal goat serum. Neutrophil extracellular traps (NETs) were detected with rabbit anti-NE (Abcam, Cambridge, MA, United States) and rabbit anti-MPO (Abcam, Cambridge, MA, United States) in 10% normal goat serum. Slides were incubated with goat anti-rabbit IgG secondary antibody (Alexa Fluor 555, ImmunoWay, Plano, TX, United States) and (FITC, ImmunoWay, Plano, TX, United States) in PBS. Images were obtained with a confocal microscope (Nikon, Japan). The supernatants of neutrophil cultures after stimulation were collected for NETs secretion assays. The levels of NE and MPO were quantified in the supernatants of neutrophils using Duoset ELISA development

kits (R&D Systems, MN, United States) in accordance with the manufacturer instructions. For co-culture experiments, 1×10^6 lymphocytes were seeded into each well of a 48-well plate and co-cultured with 500 μl neutrophil culture supernatants and 1 μl cell activation cocktail with Brefeldin A for 6 h before flow cytometry.

Single Cell RNA Sequencing of Splenic Cells

Splenic cells were isolated from mice at day 7 after fecal transplantation. Before loading onto chromium microfluidic chips, red blood cells (RBCs) were removed from the splenic cells by RBC lysis. Sequencing was performed with Illumina (HiSeq 2000) according to the manufacturer's instructions (Illumina). In the quality control of the raw reads, low-quality reads (the average quality per base drops below 10), trailing low quality or N bases (below quality 3), adapters and drop reads below 26 bases long were removed from raw reads by fastq. Then the raw reads were demultiplexed and mapped to the reference genome by 10X Genomics Cell Ranger pipeline[1] using default parameters. The SingleR[2] and Seurat[3] packages were performed to cluster and annotate cell populations and types. After annotating these cells populations, functional enrichment analysis of differential genes in the different cell types was performed by Gene Ontology (GO) and Kyoto Encyclopedia of Genes and Genomes (KEGG) analysis (Ashburner et al., 2000; Kanehisa and Goto, 2000).

Flow Cytometry, Reagents and Antibodies

For flow cytometry, cells were isolated from tissues as described before and seeded into each well of a 48-well plate and treated with 1 μl cell activation cocktail with Brefeldin A (Biolegend, San Diego, CA, United States) for 6 h at 37°C. Then cells were washed, fixed and permeabilized using fixation buffer (Biolegend, San Diego, CA, United States) and permeabilization buffer (Biolegend, San Diego, CA, United States) according to the manufacturer's instructions. The cells were stained with fluorescent antibodies including anti-mouse CD4-APC, anti-mouse IFN-γ-PE-Cy7 and anti-mouse IL-17-PE (all antibodies were purchased from Biolegend, San Diego, CA, United States) for 20 min.

Real-Time PCR

Total RNA was isolated by TRIzol reagent (Invitrogen, Carlsbad, CA, United States) from PBMCs and colon tissue. The PrimeScript RT kit (Takara Biotechnology, Dalian, China) was used to reverse the extracted RNA into complementary DNA. The ABI Prism 7500 system on the SYBR Premix (BIO-RAD, CA, United States) was used to detect and analyze the expression. The relative expression of target genes was quantified by using the $2^{-\Delta\Delta Ct}$ method with β-actin as the internal reference. The sequences of target genes and β-actin PCR primer pairs are shown in **Supplementary Table 2**.

---

[1]https://support.10xgenomics.com/single-cellgeneexpression/software/pipelines/latest/what-is-cell-ranger

[2]https://github.com/dviraran/SingleR

[3]https://satijalab.org/seurat/

16S rDNA Gene Sequence Analysis

DNA was extracted from the mice fecal pellets using the QIAamp Fast DNA Stool Mini Kit (Qiagen, Hilden, Germany) according to the manufacturer's instructions and was subjected to amplification of polymerase chain reaction (PCR) using primers directed at hypervariable region 3–4 (V3–V4) of the 16S rRNA gene (341F and 806R). The PCR products were quantified using Qubit (Invitrogen, Carlsbad, CA, United States). The resulting raw reads matched to sequences spanning the entire V3–V4 amplicon using PANDAseq. The annotation of bacteria was performed by RDP Classifier (version 2.2). The differential abundance of bacteria between groups was analyzed by Wilcoxon test. *P*-value was corrected by False Discovery Rate (FDR). LEfSe analysis was used to explain the features of microbiome composition between the BD and healthy control group. According to the normalized OTU abundance table, PCoA was applied to visualize similarities or dissimilarities of the microbiota of samples in the BD-recipient mice and healthy controls-recipient mice groups and displayed by QIIME2 and ggplot2 package. In brief, a distance matrix of unweighted Unifrac in the samples was transformed to a new set of orthogonal axes. The maximum variation factor was demonstrated by first principal coordinate and the second maximum one by the second principal coordinate. Shannon index was applied to the difference of microbial diversity between the BD-recipient mice with and healthy controls-recipient mice groups. GC-MS analysis was performed using an Agilent 7890B gas chromatograph system coupled with a Agilent 5977B mass spectrometer. This analysis was performed at the Shanghai Biotree Biomedical Technology Co., Ltd., (Shanghai, China).

Statistical Analyses

The results were analyzed by GraphPad Prism V 7.0. The statistical significance between two independent groups was analyzed with the Mann–Whitney U test. The data are shown as mean $\pm$ SEM. A p-value less than 0.05 was considered as statistically significant.

RESULTS

Fecal Transplantation of Stool Samples Obtained From Active BD Patients to Mice

To study the role of the gut microbiome in the development of ocular Behcet's disease, we used a previously established method of transplanting pooled stool samples obtained from five active ocular BD patients and healthy individuals to B10.RIII mice (Ye et al., 2018). Gut microbiome composition in the recipient mice was tested by the ACE index, Shannon index and principle coordination analysis (PCoA) (**Supplementary Figure 1** and **Figures 1A,B**). The PCoA showed that there was a segregation of gut microbiome composition between these two groups. However, we found that there was no statistical significance in ACE index and Shannon index between these groups. After false discovery rate (FDR) correction

(FDR < 0.2), gut microbiome composition was different when comparing BD-recipient mice with healthy controls-recipient mice as shown by analysis of the relative abundances of 11 genera and 14 species (**Supplementary Tables 3, 4**). Up to eight genera and 10 species were enriched in the BD-recipient mice. More importantly, we observed an enrichment in opportunistic pathogen *Parabacteroides* species, sulfate-reducing bacteria (SRB) *Bilophila* species and *Desulfovibrionaceae* species in the BD-treated group. Moreover, there was a reduction in butyrate-producing bacteria (BPB) *Clostridium* species in this group. LDA Effect Size (LEfSe) was used to determine the microbiome most likely to explain differences between these two groups. The results showed 14 genera including *Bilophila* were positively associated with BD-recipient mice, whereas four genera were negatively associated with BD-recipient mice (**Figure 1C**). Because the human fecal samples used for transplanation in the present study were randomly selected from the samples used in our previous MGS study (Ye et al., 2018), we compared the data of 16S rDNA gene sequence analysis in the present study with those of our previous MGS study. The present results were in line with the data of MGS analysis on Behcet and healthy individuals that *Bilophila* and *Parabacteroides* were enriched in BD patients, whereas the level of *Clostridium* was decreased. Because an aberrant abundance of SRB and BPB was found in the BD-recipient mice, we also investigated the changes of short chain fatty acids (SCFAs) in the stool samples after fecal transplantation by gas chromatography-mass spectrometer analysis (GC-MS). Three kinds of SCFAs including butyric acid, propionic acid and valeric acid concentrations were decreased in the BD-recipient mice (**Figure 1D**). These data showed that the gut microbiome composition in the BD-recipient mice may contribute to a concomitant SCFA change.

Dysfunction of the Intestinal Barrier in Mice Following Transplantation of BD Feces

To investigate the effect of BD feces transplantation on intestinal barrier function in mice, we performed the following experiment. Colon tissue was separated from mice after BD feces transplantation and analyzed for mRNA and protein expression. We found that the expression of three tight junction proteins (Epple et al., 2009), Claudin1 (CLDN1), Claudin4 (CLDN4) and Occludin (OCLN) in the colon tissue from the BD-recipient group was significantly decreased as compared to the healthy control-recipient group (**Figures 2A–G**). We subsequently investigated whether the altered gut microbial composition in the mice following BD feces transplantation could lead to the release of lipopolysaccharides (LPS) into the blood circulation of these animals. Serum was collected from the two groups after gut microbiome transplantation and the results showed that the level of LPS in the serum of the BD-recipient group was significantly increased as compared to that of the healthy control-recipient group (**Figure 2H**).

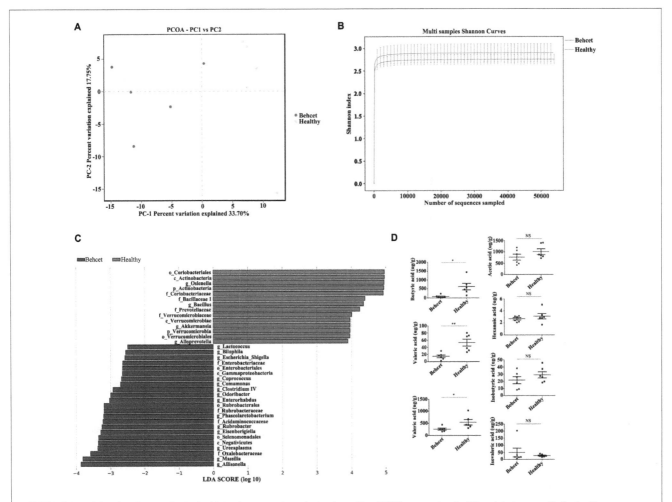

FIGURE 1 | The relative abundances of gut microbiota at genus and species levels and fecal SCFAs comparing the BD-recipient group with the healthy controls-recipient group. **(A)** PCoA analysis of BD-recipient and healthy controls-recipient mice. *n* = 5 for each group; **(B)** Shannon index analysis comparing the BD-recipient and healthy controls-recipient group. *n* = 5 for each group; **(C)** Histogram of the LDA scores computed for taxa differentially abundant between BD-recipient mice and healthy controls-recipient mice. **(D)** The concentrations of SCFAs in the feces comparing BD-recipient mice and healthy controls-recipient mice. ******P < 0.01, *P < 0.05, NS, not significant. *n* = 6 for each group.

The Effect of Transplantation of BD Feces on Th1 and Th17 Cell Differentiation in Mice

Since BD feces transplantation affected intestinal permeability, we further investigated whether the gut microbiome from BD patients could influence Th1 and Th17 cell differentiation in mice. BD feces was transplanted to mice and on day 7, the animals were sacrificed and mesenteric lymph node, splenic lymphocytes as well as retinal tissue were separated. The IFN-γ and IL-17 mRNA expression was significantly increased in the mesenteric lymph node and spleen of the BD-recipient group as compared with the healthy control-recipient group, whereas IL-10 mRNA expression was decreased in the mesenteric lymph node and spleen (**Figures 3A,B**). In addition, the mRNA expression of MCP-1 was found to be increased following BD feces transplantation in the splenic lymphocytes (**Figure 3B**). The transplantation did not lead to ocular inflammation in these non-immunized mice, as shown by real-time PCR analysis of

retinal tissue (**Figure 3C**). The percentages of Th1 cells and Th17 cells in the mesenteric lymph node and splenic lymphocytes of BD-recipient group were higher than that in the healthy control-recipient group (**Figures 3D,E**). These data indicate that transplantation of the gut microbiome from BD patients to mice induces Th1 and Th17 cell differentiation in the mesenteric lymph node and spleen cells.

Single Cell RNA Sequencing of Spleen From Mice Following Transplantation of BD Feces

To investigate the mechanisms underlying the contributions of the gut microbiome from BD patients to the induction of Th1 and Th17 cell differentiation, we performed single cell RNA sequencing of splenic cells from mice after transplantation of BD feces. Twenty six cell clusters were characterized as 10 cell types including B cells, macrophages, T cells, DC, monocytes, neutrophils, NK cells, stem cells, NKT cells and

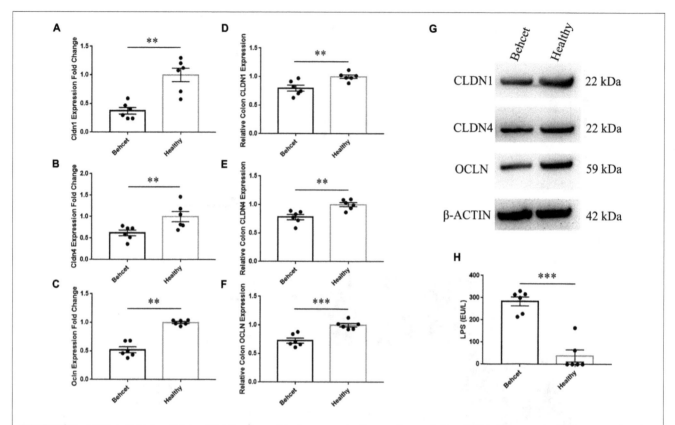

FIGURE 2 | The mRNA and protein expression of tight junction proteins in mouse colon tissue and concentration of LPS in the serum after BD feces transplantation. **(A–C)** Comparison of CLDN1, CLDN4 and OCLN mRNA expression in the colon tissue between BD-recipient and healthy controls-recipient mice. Expression was normalized to β-actin and calculated relative to the healthy control group that was taken as 1.0. **P < 0.01. Data was analyzed by the Mann–Whitney *U* test. *n* = 6 for each group; **(D–G)** Comparison of CLDN1, CLDN4 and OCLN protein expression in the colon tissue between BD-recipient and healthy controls-recipient mice, **P < 0.01. **(H)** The concentration of LPS in the serum of BD-recipient and healthy controls-recipient mice. ***P < 0.001. Data was analyzed by the Mann–Whitney *U* test. *n* = 6 for each group.

basophils after annotation (**Figure 4A**). The ratio of neutrophils (cluster 12) was increased in BD-recipient mice as compared to healthy control-recipient mice (**Figure 4B**). After comparing the mRNA expression levels of neutrophils between these two groups, the expression of 1,321 genes was increased in the BD-recipient mice, whereas 177 genes were decreased (**Figure 4C**). More importantly, the mRNA expression of Mpo and Elane, the components of NETs, were increased in the BD-recipient mice. In addition, the mRNA expression of S100a8 and S100a9, two antimicrobial proteins, were also significantly increased in the BD-recipient mice (**Supplementary Table 5**). Functional enrichment analysis of these differential mRNAs *via* KEGG showed bacterial invasion of epithelial cells and leukocyte transendothelial migration was significantly up-regulated in the neutrophils from BD-recipient mice (**Figure 4D** and **Supplementary Table 6**). Based on GO enrichment analysis, these differential mRNAs were enriched in the ATP metabolic process, oxidative phosphorylation and several terms associated with neutrophils function, such as neutrophil chemotaxis and neutrophil mediated immunity (**Supplementary Figure 2** and **Supplementary Table 7**).

We also compared the mRNA expression of CD4 + T cells from T cell populations between BD-recipient and healthy control-recipient mice. The expression of 1,378 genes was increased in the BD-recipient mice, whereas 276 genes were decreased (**Figure 4E**). Among them, IL-17 mRNA expression was significantly increased in the CD4 + T cells from BD-recipient animals (**Supplementary Table 8**), which was consistent with the results mentioned before. Through KEGG analysis, these differential mRNAs were found enriched in antigen processing and presentation and in Systemic Lupus Erythematosus (SLE, **Figure 4F** and **Supplementary Table 9**). GO enrichment analysis was also performed on these differentially expressed mRNAs. The results showed that the mRNAs were enriched in the innate immune response, positive regulation of immune response, T cell activation, lymphocyte differentiation and response to bacteria (**Supplementary Figure 3** and **Supplementary Table 10**).

Neutrophil Activation Following Fecal Transplantation and the Role of Activated Neutrophils on Th1 and Th17 Differentiation

Neutrophils are found to be hyper-activated in patients with BD (Nelson et al., 2018). Numerous factors from the gut microbiome are found to induce neutrophil activation,

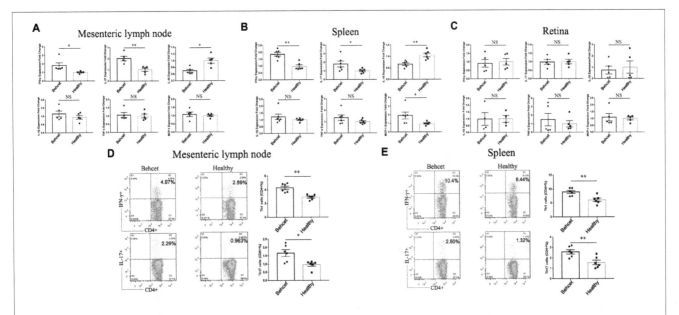

FIGURE 3 | The mRNA expression of IFN-γ, IL-17, IL-10, MCP-1, IL-1β and TNF-α as well as Th1 and Th17 cells in the mesenteric lymph node, splenic lymphocytes and retina after transplantation of BD feces to mice. **(A–C)** Comparison of IFN-γ, IL-17, IL-10, MCP-1, IL-1β and TNF-α mRNA expression in the mesenteric lymph node, splenic lymphocytes and retina between BD-recipient and healthy controls-recipient mice, relative to the healthy control group (taken as 1.0). ******P < 0.01, *****P < 0.05, NS, not significant, data was analyzed by the Mann–Whitney U test. n = 5–6 for each group; **(D,E)** the percentages of CD4 + IFN-γ + Th1 cells and CD4 + IL-17 + Th17 cells in the mesenteric lymph node and splenic lymphocytes in the BD-recipient and healthy controls-recipient group. ******P < 0.01, *****P < 0.05. Data was analyzed by the Mann–Whitney U test. n = 6 for each group.

including LPS (Alexis et al., 2001). Based on the above findings, we hypothesized that the activation of neutrophils in BD patients could be associated with the composition of their gut microbiome. To investigate whether neutrophils can be activated after fecal transplantation, we isolated the total cells from mesenteric lymph nodes and neutrophils from spleens of mice and detected the level of NETs secreted by activated neutrophils after fecal transplantation. After immunostaining neutrophils, we found that NE and MPO were more prominently expressed by neutrophils from the BD-recipient group (**Figure 5A**). The levels of the NETs components, NE and MPO were significantly increased in the cells from mesenteric lymph nodes and neutrophils from spleens from the BD-recipient group as compared to the healthy control-recipient group (**Figures 5B,C**). We also co-cultured lymphocytes the mesenteric lymph nodes of normal B10.RIII mice with neutrophil supernatants of the BD-recipient or healthy control-recipient group, respectively. The percentages of Th1 cells and Th17 cells in the BD-recipient neutrophils co-culture group were higher than in the healthy control-recipient neutrophil co-culture group (**Figure 5D**). These results indicate that the gut microbiome in BD patients might induce Th1 and Th17 cell differentiation *via* activated neutrophils.

The Effect of Fecal Transplantation With BD Patients Gut Microbiome on the Severity of EAU and EAE Models

In our previous study, we demonstrated that feces from active BD patients could exacerbate the development and

severity of uveitis in EAU mice (Ye et al., 2018). In this study, we repeated the experiment concerning the effect of BD patients' gut microbiome on EAU and expanded these earlier studies by also analyzing the cytokine response and lymphocyte differentiation. B10.RIII mice were immunized with 25 μg IRBP161–180 combined with CFA for EAU induction after fecal transplantation (**Figure 6A**). At 14 days after immunization, BD-recipient mice showed a more severe clinical and histological uveitis than the healthy control-recipient group (**Figure 6B**). In line with these observations, we found that the IFN-γ and IL-17 mRNA expression was also significantly increased in the mesenteric lymph node, splenic lymphocytes and retinas of the BD-recipient group as compared with the healthy control-recipient group (**Supplementary Figures 2A,B,D**). IL-10 mRNA expression was decreased in the splenic lymphocytes of the BD-recipient group but not in the mesenteric lymph nodes and retina (**Supplementary Figures 2A,B,D**). The mRNA expression of MCP-1, IL-1β and TNF-α was also increased in the BD-recipient group (**Supplementary Figures 2A,B,D**). The protein levels of IFN-γ and IL-17 in the splenic lymphocytes of the BD-recipient group were also higher than that in the healthy control-recipient group (**Supplementary Figure 2C**). We then investigated the activation of neutrophils, Th1 and Th17 cells differentiation in the mesenteric lymph node, spleen and eye between these two groups. In line with the results mentioned before, NE and MPO were significantly increased in the neutrophils from the mesenteric lymph node, splenic lymphocytes and eyes of the BD-recipient group as compared to the healthy control-recipient group (**Figures 6C–E**). The increased Th1 and Th17

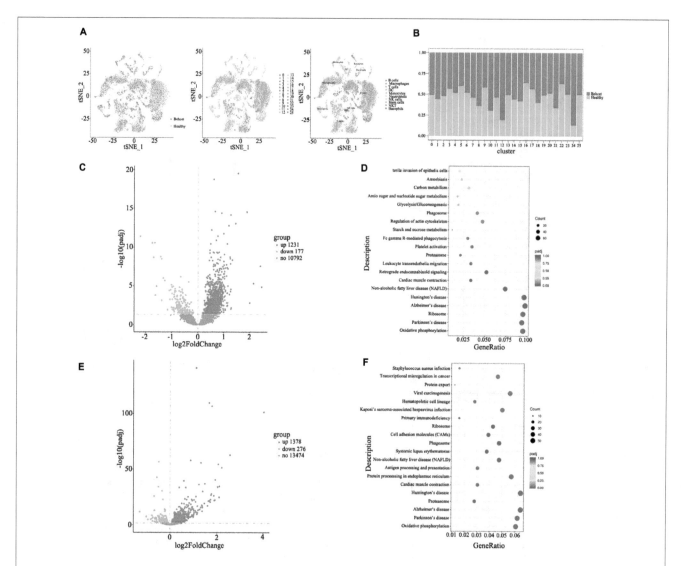

FIGURE 4 | Single cell RNA sequencing of splenic cells from mice after feces transplantation. **(A)** Characterization of cell types in the splenic cells in the tSNE plot; **(B)** The relative ratios of different cell types in the splenic cells between BD-recipient mice and healthy control-recipient mice; **(C)** The volcano plot of differential genes in the neutrophils between BD-recipient and healthy controls-recipient mice; **(D)** KEGG analysis of differential genes in the neutrophils between BD-recipient and healthy controls-recipient mice. Top twenty pathways with the most significant differences are listed; **(E)** The volcano plot of differential genes in the CD4 + T cells between BD-recipient and healthy controls-recipient group; **(F)** KEGG analysis of differential genes in the CD4 + T cells between BD-recipient and healthy controls-recipient mice. Top twenty pathways with the most significant differences are listed.

cell percentages were also found in the mesenteric lymph node, spleen and eyes of the BD-recipient group (**Figures 6F,G** and **Supplementary Figure 2E**).

To investigate whether the effect of BD patient gut microbiome composition was a general effect or whether it was specific for EAU, we also tested fecal transplantation in mice undergoing EAE (**Figure 6A**). We therefore immunized C57/BL6 mice with 100 µg Myelin Oligodendrocyte Glycoprotein (MOG) 35–55 combined with CFA after BD feces transplantation to determine its effect on the severity of EAE. The results showed that the BD-recipient mice also showed a more severe clinical manifestation that began at day 19 following immunization (**Figure 6H**). The expression of pro-inflammatory cytokines, including IFN-γ, IL-17 and MCP-1 was increased

in the lymphocytes from the BD-recipient group, whereas the expression of IL-10 was decreased (**Supplementary Figures 3A–F**). A similar result was also observed in the BD-recipient group concerning the protein expression of IFN-γ and IL-17 (**Supplementary Figures 3G,H**). These results demonstrated that BD patients' feces not only exacerbated the severity of EAU but also of EAE, suggesting an immunological adjuvant effect.

DISCUSSION

In this report, we provide evidence showing that the gut microbiome may affect the development of BD *via* a complex

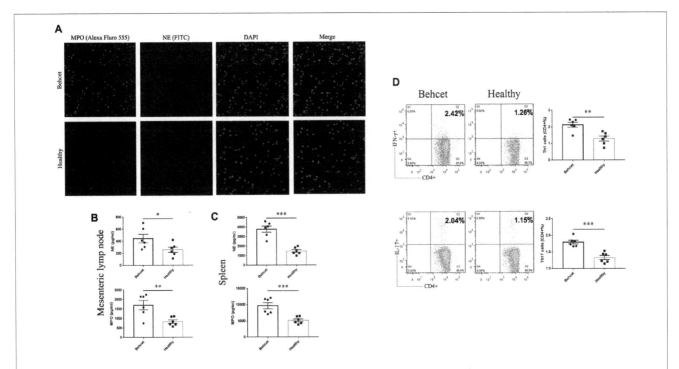

FIGURE 5 | NETs secretion as well as Th1 and Th17 cell differentiation after co-culture with neutrophils. **(A)** Fluorescent images of NETs (MPO and NE) in the BD-recipient group and healthy controls-recipient group. **(B,C)** The protein levels of NE and MPO in the supernatants of mesenteric lymph nodes and splenic neutrophils from the BD-recipient and healthy controls-recipient group. ***P < 0.001, **P < 0.01, *P < 0.05. Data was analyzed by the Mann–Whitney U test. $n = 6$ for each group. **(D)** the percentages of CD4 + IFN-γ + Th1 cells and CD4 + IL-17 + Th17 cells after co-culture with neutrophil supernatants from the BD-recipient and healthy controls-recipient group. ***P < 0.001, *P < 0.01, NS, not significant. Data was analyzed by the Mann–Whitney U test. $n = 5$–6 for each group.

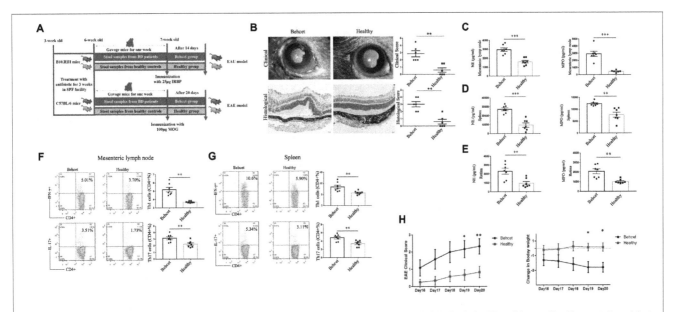

FIGURE 6 | Clinical and histological scores of EAU mice as well as clinical score and weight changes of EAE mice in the BD-recipient and healthy controls-recipient group. **(A)** The experimental scheme of mice experiment; **(B)** Clinical and histological scores of the EAU model in the BD-recipient and healthy controls-recipient group. **P < 0.01. Data was analyzed by the Mann–Whitney U test. $n = 6$ for each group; **(C–E)** The protein levels of NE and MPO in the supernatants of mesenteric lymph nodes, splenic neutrophils and retina from the BD-recipient and healthy controls-recipient group. ***P < 0.001, **P < 0.01. Data was analyzed by the Mann–Whitney U test. $n = 6$–7 for each group. **(F,G)** The percentages of CD4 + IFN-γ + Th1 cells and CD4 + IL-17 + Th17 cells in the mesenteric lymph node and splenic lymphocytes from the BD-recipient and healthy controls-recipient group. **P < 0.01, *P < 0.05. Data was analyzed by the Mann–Whitney U test. $n = 6$–7 for each group. **(H)** Clinical score and weight changes of EAE mice in the BD-recipient and healthy controls-recipient group. **P < 0.01, *P < 0.05. Data was analyzed by the Mann–Whitney U test. $n = 6$ for each group.

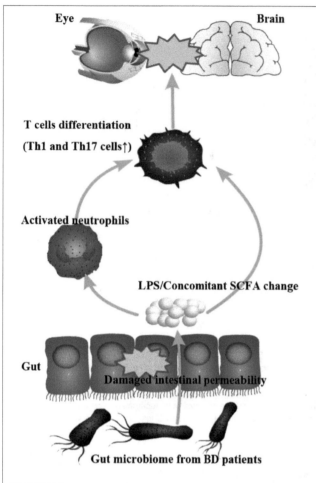

FIGURE 7 | Schematic model demonstrating how the gut microbiome may contribute to the autoimmune response *via* complex mechanisms involving a damaged intestinal barrier leading to the transfer of immuno-stimulatory factors resulting in a state of immune hyper-reactivity.

mechanism that includes an enhanced gut permeability and stimulation of innate immunity (**Figure 7**).

Transplantation of clinical fecal samples to mice provides evidence for a role of the gut microbiome in the pathogenesis of various diseases which are found to be associated with a dysbiosis of gut microbiota (De Palma et al., 2017). The differential abundance of bacteria between the BD-recipient group and healthy control-recipient group were not exactly in line with the data of MGS analysis showed in our previous study, which might be due to differences between humans and mice in their indigenous microbial community, the limited sample size and batch effects of microbiome sequencing (De Palma et al., 2017; Ye et al., 2018). It might also be due to the fact that we used SPF mice in this study, although we did treat mice with antibiotics for 3 weeks before fecal transplantation. Using germ-free mice, in future experiments, may solve the issue. On the other hand, we did find that the *Parabacteroides* species, *Bilophila* species and *Desulfovibrionaceae* species were

enriched and *Clostridium* species were reduced in the BD-treated group which was in line with our earlier results on the gut microbiome in ocular BD (Ye et al., 2018). *Parabacteroides* species are generally considered as opportunistic pathogens in infectious diseases and are associated with changes in the inflammatory response, T cell differentiation and altered abundance of short-chain fatty acid producers (Claesson et al., 2012; Bindels et al., 2016). *Bilophila* species and *Desulfovibrionaceae* species are two kinds of SRB which inhibit butyrate β-oxidation and degrade butyrate (Dostal Webster et al., 2019). A lower level of BPB such as the *Clostridium* species in the BD-treated group might lead to a reduction of butyrate in the host. Butyrate is a beneficial metabolite that maintains host immune homeostasis and protects the integrity of the intestinal epithelial barrier (Furusawa et al., 2013; Geirnaert et al., 2017; Goncalves et al., 2018). Furthermore, SRB produce cytotoxic molecules such as hydrogen sulfide (H_2S) as well as immune stimulating factors like LPS (Muyzer and Stams, 2008). These factors can exacerbate intestinal epithelial barrier damage and produce innate immune triggering signals finally leading to an aberrant Th1 and Th17 cell differentiation (Muyzer and Stams, 2008; Leal Rojas et al., 2017; Stevens et al., 2018). Recently, propionic acid and valeric acid (decreased in the BD-treated group) were also reported as SCFAs that can regulate the function of Th1 and Th17 cells (Bottcher et al., 2000; Duscha et al., 2020). We hypothesize that the concomitant SCFA change caused by the gut microbiome from patients may contribute to the development of autoimmune uveitis.

Using the fecal transplantation model, we showed that it could affect intestinal permeability leading to the leakage of bacterial factors such as LPS into the systemic circulation. Although intestinal manifestations are common (3–60%) in BD patients from Eastern Asia (Ananthakrishnan, 2015), it should be noted that none of the ocular BD patients that donated their stool samples for our study had obvious intestinal problems. Intestinal barrier dysfunction has been observed in several immune-mediated diseases such as ankylosing spondylitis (AS), whereas these patients did not have obvious intestinal problems or intestinal inflammation (Vaile et al., 1999). Intestinal barrier function in ocular BD patients has not yet been investigated and is indeed an interesting area for further research. LPS is one of the most potent gram-negative derived factors that can stimulate Th1 and Th17 cell differentiation and is able to exacerbate experimental autoimmune disease models such as EAU and EAE (Fang et al., 2010; Klaska et al., 2017; Mardiguian et al., 2017). These findings are also consistent with previous studies in which LPS/TLR4 pathways are involved in the aberrant immune response observed in BD and our result showing a higher abundance of SRB (such as *Bilophila* species) in the BD-recipient mice (Liang et al., 2013). Whether other microbe-associated molecular patterns induced by the gut microbiome may also contribute to Th1 and Th17 differentiation needs to be addressed in future experiments. It should be noted that the specificity of the Th1 and Th17 cells in the BD-recipient mice was not investigated and it would be interesting to study whether feces transplantation affected the population of autoreactive cells. However, the increase of Th1 and Th17 cells in the BD-recipient mice might lead to an augmented secretion of pro-inflammatory cytokines including IFN-γ, TNF- α, IL-6 and IL-17 that may contribute to the development of disease (Tang et al., 2009; Pattarini et al., 2017).

Previous studies have implied a role for infections in the pathogenesis of BD, including streptococcus species (Lellouche et al., 2003; Oh et al., 2008). In the study presented here, we provide additional evidence that gut microbiota from BD patients can induce innate immune responses and that this response might play a role in the stimulation of pathogenic T cell populations. An alternative mechanism is also possible where IL-17 triggers neutrophil production and release from the bone marrow (Chuammitri et al., 2019). IL-17 has been shown to recruit neutrophils at the site of T cell activation by inducing the production of chemokines and other cytokines, such as TNF-α (Isailovic et al., 2015). Further studies are needed to show how Th17 cells and neutrophils interact and how this is affected by gut microbiota. The results of single cell sequencing on splenic cells from mice after fecal transplantation also provided evidence that the gut microbiome from BD patients has effects on both neutrophil activation as well as on T cell differentiation. We found that the differential mRNAs in neutrophils were enriched in the oxidative phosphorylation, neutrophil chemotaxis and neutrophil mediated immunity, which all play critical roles in the activation of neutrophils (Li et al., 2019). When analyzing CD4 + T cells, we found that the IL-17 mRNA level was increased in CD4 + T cells from BD-recipient mice. Differentially expressed mRNAs in CD4 + T cells were found enriched in antigen processing and presentation. It is well established that antigen processing and presentation induces activation and differentiation of naïve T cells into Th1 and Th17 cells (Mascanfroni et al., 2013). These results indicate that the gut microbiome in BD-recipient mice might contribute to both neutrophil activation and regulation of T cell differentiation. It should also be mentioned that other cell clusters, such as cluster 24 in B cells, appear to be distinct between BD and healthy-recipient mice. It would be interesting to study the contributions of these cell clusters to disease in future studies. To investigate whether the gut microbiome regulates the function of neutrophils or CD4 + T cells directly, single cell sequencing analysis on intestinal tissue or MLN from mice and human blood is also needed to address this issue in future longitudinal studies.

To our knowledge, this is the first report that directly links a dysbiotic gut microbiome to the activation of neutrophils in BD. There is evidence in the literature that the link between neutrophil activation and the induction of Th1 and Th17 cell differentiation may be mediated by dendritic cells (Warnatsch et al., 2015; Papadaki et al., 2016). Taken together these findings support our hypothesis that a combination of gut metabolites and immune-stimulatory factors behave as an adjuvant leading to a hyperactive immune system.

We realize that our study suffers from several limitations concerning the protocol of fecal transplantation. First of all, we didn't perform a comparison between recipient mice and original donors in the present manuscript due to sample size limitations in the original donors used for transplantation. To further validate our study, further longitudinal studies with a larger sample size are needed to address this issue. Secondly, fecal transplantation was done with pooled patient or healthy control fecal samples in the present study. Gut microbiome diversity could be very different between individuals. Thus, the pooled samples may not be a faithful representation of a real-world individual gut microbiome composition. Fecal transplantation using individual samples may be a favorable method in future experiments. In addition, the donors included in this study had stopped taking immunosuppressive and antibiotic treatment for at least 1 month. However, several studies have suggested that past treatment, such as with antibiotics, may have contributed to the observed changes in the gut microbiome composition of host (Palleja et al., 2018). Using samples from the first-episode BD patients without treatment may solve this issue in future studies. Thirdly, the immunization in the mice may also affect the gut microbiome (Janowitz et al., 2019). To evaluate whether immunization has an influence on the transplanted microbiome, analysis of microbiome composition should be performed before and after immunization.

In conclusion, we show that the gut microbiome may contribute to the development of BD *via* complex mechanisms involving a damaged intestinal barrier leading to the transfer of immuno-stimulatory factors resulting in a state of immune hyper-reactivity. The observations shown in this paper are focused on the eye but similar mechanisms may be operative in other autoimmune diseases and manipulation of the gut microbiome may be a feasible approach to treat these disorders.

ETHICS STATEMENT

The animal study was reviewed and approved by the animal study was approved by the Ethics Committee of The First Affiliated Hospital of Chongqing Medical University.

AUTHOR CONTRIBUTIONS

QW and PY conceived and directed the study. QW, SY, GS, ZD, SP, and XH analyzed the data. PY made the clinical diagnoses. QC collected the samples. QW and XH extracted the fecal DNA and performed the 16S rRNA gene amplicon sequencing, *in vitro* experiment, and animal experiment. GY evaluated histology slides. QW drafted the manuscript. PY and AK reviewed the data interpretation and helped revise the final versions of the manuscript. All authors read and approved the final manuscript.

SUPPLEMENTARY MATERIAL

Supplementary Figure 1 | ACE index analysis results comparing the BD-recipient and healthy controls-recipient group.

Supplementary Figure 2 | The mRNA expression of IFN-γ, IL-17, IL-10, MCP-1, IL-1β and TNF-α from mesenteric lymph node, splenic neutrophils and retina, the protein levels of IFN-γ and IL-17 from splenic lymphocytes as well as Th1 and Th17 cells differentiation from the retina in the EAU models from BD-recipient and healthy controls-recipient mice. **(A,B)** Comparison of IFN-γ, IL-17, IL-10, MCP-1, IL-1β and TNF-α mRNA expression from mesenteric lymph nodes, splenic neutrophils and retina in the EAU models in BD-recipient and healthy controls-recipient mice, ***$P < 0.001$, **$P < 0.01$, *$P < 0.05$, NS, not significant. Data was analyzed by the Mann–Whitney U test. $n = 6$ for each group; **(C)** IRBP161-180-induced production of IFN-γ and IL-17 at the protein level in the BD-recipient and healthy controls-recipient group. ***$P < 0.001$, Data was analyzed by the Mann–Whitney U test. $n = 6$ for each group. **(D)** Comparison of IFN-γ, IL-17, IL-10, MCP-1, IL-1β and TNF-α mRNA expression from the retina of EAU mice between the BD-recipient and healthy controls-recipient group, **$P < 0.01$, *$P < 0.05$, NS, not significant. **(E)** The percentages of CD4 + IFN-γ + Th1 cells and CD4 + IL-17 + Th17 cells in the retina from the BD-recipient and healthy controls-recipient group.*$P < 0.05$. About 2,000–4,000 CD4 + T cells from the eye were collected from the retina for each sample. Retinas of 2 mice from each group were pooled as one sample. Data was analyzed by the Mann–Whitney U test. $n = 4$ for each group (eight mice).

Supplementary Figure 3 | Go analysis of differential genes in the neutrophils between BD-recipient and healthy controls-recipient mice. Top ten terms with the most significant differences are listed. MF, molecular function; BP, biological process; CC, cellular component.

Supplementary Figure 4 | Go analysis of differential genes in the CD4 + T cells between BD-recipient and healthy controls-recipient mice. Top ten terms with the most significant differences are listed. MF, molecular function; BP, biological process; CC, cellular component.

Supplementary Figure 5 | The mRNA expression of IFN-γ, IL-17, IL-10, MCP-1, IL-1β and TNF-α as well as the protein levels of IFN-γ and IL-17 from splenic lymphocytes in the EAE mice of the BD-recipient and healthy controls-recipient group. **(A–F)** Comparison of IFN-γ, IL-17, IL-10, MCP-1, IL-1β and TNF-α mRNA expression in the EAE mice of the BD-recipient and healthy controls-recipient group, **$P < 0.01$, *$P < 0.05$, NS, no significant. Data was analyzed by the Mann–Whitney U test. $n = 6$ for each group; **(G,H)** IRBP161-180-induced production of IFN-γ and IL-17 at the protein level in the BD-recipient and healthy controls-recipient group. *$P < 0.05$, Data was analyzed by the Mann–Whitney U test. $n = 6$ for each group.

REFERENCES

Alexis, N., Eldridge, M., Reed, W., Bromberg, P., and Peden, D. B. (2001). CD14-dependent airway neutrophil response to inhaled LPS: role of atopy. *J. Allergy Clin. Immunol.* 107, 31–35. doi: 10.1067/mai.2001.111594

Ananthakrishnan, A. N. (2015). Epidemiology and risk factors for IBD. *Nat. Rev. Gastroenterol. Hepatol.* 12, 205–217. doi: 10.1038/nrgastro.2015.34

Ashburner, M., Ball, C. A., Blake, J. A., Botstein, D., Butler, H., Cherry, J. M., et al. (2000). Gene ontology: tool for the unification of biology. the gene ontology consortium. *Nat. Genet.* 25, 25–29.

Badawi, A. H., Kiptoo, P., Wang, W. T., Choi, I. Y., Lee, P., Vines, C. M., et al. (2012). Suppression of EAE and prevention of blood-brain barrier breakdown after vaccination with novel bifunctional peptide inhibitor. *Neuropharmacology* 62, 1874–1881. doi: 10.1016/j.neuropharm.2011.12.013

Bevins, C. L., and Salzman, N. H. (2011). Paneth cells, antimicrobial peptides and maintenance of intestinal homeostasis. *Nat. Rev. Microbiol.* 9, 356–368. doi: 10.1038/nrmicro2546

Bindels, L. B., Neyrinck, A. M., Claus, S. P., Le Roy, C. I., Grangette, C., Pot, B., et al. (2016). Synbiotic approach restores intestinal homeostasis and prolongs survival in leukaemic mice with cachexia. *ISME J.* 10, 1456–1470. doi: 10.1038/ismej.2015.209

Bottcher, M. F., Nordin, E. K., Sandin, A., Midtvedt, T., and Bjorksten, B. (2000). Microflora-associated characteristics in faeces from allergic and nonallergic infants. *Clin. Exp. Allergy* 30, 1590–1596.

Chuammitri, P., Wongsawan, K., Pringproa, K., and Thanawongnuwech, R. (2019). Interleukin 17 (IL-17) manipulates mouse bone marrow-derived neutrophils in response to acute lung inflammation. *Comp. Immunol. Microbiol. Infect. Dis.* 67:101356. doi: 10.1016/j.cimid.2019.101356

Claesson, M. J., Jeffery, I. B., Conde, S., Power, S. E., O'Connor, E. M., Cusack, S., et al. (2012). Gut microbiota composition correlates with diet and health in the elderly. *Nature* 488, 178–184.

Consolandi, C., Turroni, S., Emmi, G., Severgnini, M., Fiori, J., Peano, C., et al. (2015). Behcet's syndrome patients exhibit specific microbiome signature. *Autoimmun. Rev.* 14, 269–276. doi: 10.1016/j.autrev.2014.11.009

Constantinescu, C. S., Farooqi, N., O'Brien, K., and Gran, B. (2011). Experimental autoimmune encephalomyelitis (EAE) as a model for multiple sclerosis (MS). *Br. J. Pharmacol.* 164, 1079–1106. doi: 10.1111/j.1476-5381.2011.01302.x

Coquery, C. M., Loo, W., Buszko, M., Lannigan, J., and Erickson, L. D. (2012). Optimized protocol for the isolation of spleen-resident murine neutrophils. *Cytometry A* 81, 806–814. doi: 10.1002/cyto.a.22096

Cortes, L. M., Mattapallil, M. J., Silver, P. B., Donoso, L. A., Liou, G. I., Zhu, W., et al. (2008). Repertoire analysis and new pathogenic epitopes of IRBP in C57BL/6 (H-2b) and B10.RIII (H-2r) mice. *Invest. Ophthalmol. Vis. Sci.* 49, 1946–1956.

Criteria for diagnosis of Behcet's disease (1990). Criteria for diagnosis of Behcet's disease, international study group for Behcet's disease. *Lancet* 335, 1078–1080.

de Jager, W., Prakken, B. J., Bijlsma, J. W., Kuis, W., and Rijkers, G. T. (2005). Improved multiplex immunoassay performance in human plasma and synovial fluid following removal of interfering heterophilic antibodies. *J. Immunol. Methods* 300, 124–135. doi: 10.1016/j.jim.2005.03.009

de Oliveira, G. L. V., Leite, A. Z., Higuchi, B. S., Gonzaga, M. I., and Mariano, V. S. (2017). Intestinal dysbiosis and probiotic applications in autoimmune diseases. *Immunology* 152, 1–12. doi: 10.1111/imm.12765

De Palma, G., Lynch, M. D., Lu, J., Dang, V. T., Deng, Y., Jury, J., et al. (2017). Transplantation of fecal microbiota from patients with irritable bowel syndrome alters gut function and behavior in recipient mice. *Sci. Transl. Med.* 9:eaaf6397.

Domingue, J. C., Drewes, J. L., Merlo, C. A., Housseau, F., and Sears, C. L. (2020). Host responses to mucosal biofilms in the lung and gut. *Mucosal Immunol.* 13, 413–422. doi: 10.1038/s41385-020-0270-1

Dostal Webster, A., Staley, C., Hamilton, M. J., Huang, M., Fryxell, K., Erickson, R., et al. (2019). Influence of short-term changes in dietary sulfur on the relative abundances of intestinal sulfate-reducing bacteria. *Gut Microbes* 10, 447–457. doi: 10.1080/19490976.2018.1559682

Duscha, A., Gisevius, B., Hirschberg, S., Yissachar, N., Stangl, G. I., Eilers, E., et al. (2020). Propionic acid shapes the multiple sclerosis disease course by an immunomodulatory mechanism. *Cell* 180, 1067–1080.e16.

Epple, H. J., Schneider, T., Troeger, H., Kunkel, D., Allers, K., Moos, V., et al. (2009). Impairment of the intestinal barrier is evident in untreated but absent in suppressively treated HIV-infected patients. *Gut* 58, 220–227. doi: 10.1136/gut.2008.150425

Fang, J., Fang, D., Silver, P. B., Wen, F., Li, B., Ren, X., et al. (2010). The role of TLR2, TRL3, TRL4, and TRL9 signaling in the pathogenesis of autoimmune disease in a retinal autoimmunity model. *Invest. Ophthalmol. Vis. Sci.* 51, 3092–3099. doi: 10.1167/iovs.09-4754

Fraiture, M., and Brunner, F. (2014). Killing two birds with one stone: trans-kingdom suppression of PAMP/MAMP-induced immunity by T3E from enteropathogenic bacteria. *Front. Microbiol.* 5:320. doi: 10.3389/fmicb.2014.00320

Furusawa, Y., Obata, Y., Fukuda, S., Endo, T. A., Nakato, G., Takahashi, D., et al. (2013). Commensal microbe-derived butyrate induces the differentiation of colonic regulatory T cells. *Nature* 504, 446–450. doi: 10.1038/nature12721

Geirnaert, A., Calatayud, M., Grootaert, C., Laukens, D., Devriese, S., Smagghe, G., et al. (2017). Butyrate-producing bacteria supplemented in vitro to Crohn's disease patient microbiota increased butyrate production and enhanced intestinal epithelial barrier integrity. *Sci. Rep.* 7: 11450.

Goncalves, P., Araujo, J. R., and Di Santo, J. P. (2018). a cross-talk between microbiota-derived short-chain fatty acids and the host mucosal immune system regulates intestinal homeostasis and inflammatory bowel disease. *Inflamm. Bowel Dis.* 24, 558–572. doi: 10.1093/ibd/izx029

Horai, R., Zarate-Blades, C. R., Dillenburg-Pilla, P., Chen, J., Kielczewski, J. L., Silver, P. B., et al. (2015). Microbiota-dependent activation of an autoreactive T cell receptor provokes autoimmunity in an immunologically privileged site. *Immunity* 43, 343–353. doi: 10.1016/j.immuni.2015.07.014

Isailovic, N., Daigo, K., Mantovani, A., and Selmi, C. (2015). Interleukin-17 and innate immunity in infections and chronic inflammation. *J. Autoimmun.* 60, 1–11. doi: 10.1016/j.jaut.2015.04.006

Janowitz, C., Nakamura, Y. K., Metea, C., Gligor, A., Yu, W., Karstens, L., et al. (2019). Disruption of intestinal homeostasis and intestinal microbiota during experimental autoimmune uveitis. *Invest. Ophthalmol. Vis. Sci.* 60, 420–429. doi: 10.1167/iovs.18-24813

Jiang, G., Ke, Y., Sun, D., Han, G., Kaplan, H. J., and Shao, H. (2008). Reactivation of uveitogenic T cells by retinal astrocytes derived from experimental autoimmune uveitis-prone B10RIII mice. *Invest. Ophthalmol. Vis. Sci.* 49, 282–289. doi: 10.1167/iovs.07-0371

Kanehisa, M., and Goto, S. (2000). KEGG: kyoto encyclopedia of genes and genomes. *Nucleic Acids Res.* 28, 27–30.

Klaska, I. P., Muckersie, E., Martin-Granados, C., Christofi, M., and Forrester, J. V. (2017). Lipopolysaccharide-primed heterotolerant dendritic cells suppress experimental autoimmune uveoretinitis by multiple mechanisms. *Immunology* 150, 364–377. doi: 10.1111/imm.12691

Leal Rojas, I. M., Mok, W. H., Pearson, F. E., Minoda, Y., Kenna, T. J., Barnard, R. T., et al. (2017). Human blood CD1c(+) dendritic cells promote Th1 and Th17 effector function in memory CD4(+) T cells. *Front. Immunol.* 8:971. doi: 10.3389/fimmu.2017.00971

Lellouche, N., Belmatoug, N., Bourgoin, P., Logeart, D., Acar, C., Cohen-Solal, A., et al. (2003). Recurrent valvular replacement due to exacerbation of Behcet's disease by Streptococcus agalactiae infection. *Eur. J. Intern. Med.* 14, 120–122. doi: 10.1016/s0953-6205(03)00019-0

Li, Y., Jia, A., Wang, Y. X., Dong, L., Wang, Y. F., He, Y., et al. (2019). Immune effects of glycolysis or oxidative phosphorylation metabolic pathway in protecting against bacterial infection. *J. Cell. Physiol.* 234, 20298–20309. doi: 10.1002/jcp.28630

Liang, L., Tan, X., Zhou, Q., Zhu, Y., Tian, Y., Yu, H., et al. (2013). IL-1beta triggered by peptidoglycan and lipopolysaccharide through TLR2/4 and ROS-NLRP3 inflammasome-dependent pathways is involved in ocular Behcet's disease. *Invest. Ophthalmol. Vis. Sci.* 54, 402–414. doi: 10.1167/iovs.12-11047

Littman, D. R., and Rudensky, A. Y. (2010). Th17 and regulatory T cells in mediating and restraining inflammation. *Cell* 140, 845–858. doi: 10.1016/j.cell.2010.02.021

Mardiguian, S., Ladds, E., Turner, R., Shepherd, H., Campbell, S. J., and Anthony, D. C. (2017). The contribution of the acute phase response to the pathogenesis of relapse in chronic-relapsing experimental autoimmune encephalitis models of multiple sclerosis. *J. Neuroinflammation* 14:196.

Mascanfroni, I. D., Yeste, A., Vieira, S. M., Burns, E. J., Patel, B., Sloma, I., et al. (2013). IL-27 acts on DCs to suppress the T cell response and autoimmunity by inducing expression of the immunoregulatory molecule CD39. *Nat. Immunol.* 14, 1054–1063. doi: 10.1038/ni.2695

Muyzer, G., and Stams, A. J. (2008). The ecology and biotechnology of sulphate-reducing bacteria. *Nat. Rev. Microbiol.* 6, 441–454. doi: 10.1038/nrmicro1892

Nanke, Y., Kotake, S., Goto, M., Ujihara, H., Matsubara, M., and Kamatani, N. (2008). Decreased percentages of regulatory T cells in peripheral blood of patients with Behcet's disease before ocular attack: a possible predictive marker of ocular attack. *Mod. Rheumatol.* 18, 354–358. doi: 10.3109/s10165-008-0064-x

Nelson, C. A., Stephen, S., Ashchyan, H. J., James, W. D., Micheletti, R. G., and Rosenbach, M. (2018). Neutrophilic dermatoses: pathogenesis, sweet syndrome, neutrophilic eccrine hidradenitis, and Behcet disease. *J. Am. Acad. Dermatol.* 79, 987–1006.

Oh, S. H., Lee, K. Y., Lee, J. H., and Bang, D. (2008). Clinical manifestations associated with high titer of anti-streptolysin O in Behcet's disease. *Clin. Rheumatol.* 27, 999–1003. doi: 10.1007/s10067-008-0844-x

Palleja, A., Mikkelsen, K. H., Forslund, S. K., Kashani, A., Allin, K. H., Nielsen, T., et al. (2018). Recovery of gut microbiota of healthy adults following antibiotic exposure. *Nat. Microbiol.* 3, 1255–1265. doi: 10.1038/s41564-018-0257-9

Papadaki, G., Kambas, K., Choulaki, C., Vlachou, K., Drakos, E., Bertsias, G., et al. (2016). Neutrophil extracellular traps exacerbate Th1-mediated autoimmune responses in rheumatoid arthritis by promoting DC maturation. *Eur. J. Immunol.* 46, 2542–2554. doi: 10.1002/eji.201646542

Pattarini, L., Trichot, C., Bogiatzi, S., Grandclaudon, M., Meller, S., Keuylian, Z., et al. (2017). TSLP-activated dendritic cells induce human T follicular helper cell differentiation through OX40-ligand. *J. Exp. Med.* 214, 1529–1546. doi: 10.1084/jem.20150402

Russler-Germain, E. V., Rengarajan, S., and Hsieh, C. S. (2017). Antigen-specific regulatory T-cell responses to intestinal microbiota. *Mucosal Immunol.* 10, 1375–1386. doi: 10.1038/mi.2017.65

Stevens, B. R., Goel, R., Seungbum, K., Richards, E. M., Holbert, R. C., Pepine, C. J., et al. (2018). Increased human intestinal barrier permeability plasma biomarkers zonulin and FABP2 correlated with plasma LPS and altered gut microbiome in anxiety or depression. *Gut* 67, 1555–1557.

Takeuchi, M., Kastner, D. L., and Remmers, E. F. (2015). The immunogenetics of Behcet's disease: a comprehensive review. *J. Autoimmun.* 64, 137–148.

Tang, J., Zhou, R., Luger, D., Zhu, W., Silver, P. B., Grajewski, R. S., et al. (2009). Calcitriol suppresses antiretinal autoimmunity through inhibitory effects on the Th17 effector response. *J. Immunol.* 182, 4624–4632. doi: 10.4049/jimmunol.0801543

Vaile, J. H., Meddings, J. B., Yacyshyn, B. R., Russell, A. S., and Maksymowych, W. P. (1999). Bowel permeability and CD45RO expression on circulating CD20+ B cells in patients with ankylosing spondylitis and their relatives. *J. Rheumatol.* 26, 128–135.

Vatanen, T., Franzosa, E. A., Schwager, R., Tripathi, S., Arthur, T. D., Vehik, K., et al. (2018). The human gut microbiome in early-onset type 1 diabetes from the TEDDY study. *Nature* 562, 589–594. doi: 10.1038/s41586-018-0620-2

Wang, H. B., Wang, P. Y., Wang, X., Wan, Y. L., and Liu, Y. C. (2012). Butyrate enhances intestinal epithelial barrier function via up-regulation of tight junction protein Claudin-1 transcription. *Dig. Dis. Sci.* 57, 3126–3135. doi: 10.1007/s10620-012-2259-4

Warnatsch, A., Ioannou, M., Wang, Q., and Papayannopoulos, V. (2015). Inflammation. Neutrophil extracellular traps license macrophages for cytokine production in atherosclerosis. *Science* 349, 316–320. doi: 10.1126/science.aaa8064

Yamashita, N. (1997). Hyperreactivity of neutrophils and abnormal T cell homeostasis: a new insight for pathogenesis of Behcet's disease. *Int. Rev. Immunol.* 14, 11–19. doi: 10.3109/08830189709116841

Yang, H., Zheng, S., Qiu, Y., Yang, Y., Wang, C., Yang, P., et al. (2014). Activation of liver X receptor alleviates ocular inflammation in experimental autoimmune uveitis. *Invest. Ophthalmol. Vis. Sci.* 55, 2795–2804. doi: 10.1167/iovs.13-13323

Ye, Z., Zhang, N., Wu, C., Zhang, X., Wang, Q., Huang, X., et al. (2018). A metagenomic study of the gut microbiome in Behcet's disease. *Microbiome* 6:135.

Zeidan, M. J., Saadoun, D., Garrido, M., Klatzmann, D., Six, A., and Cacoub, P. (2016). Behcet's disease physiopathology: a contemporary review. *Auto Immun. Highlights* 7:4.

Zhang, X., Zhang, D., Jia, H., Feng, Q., Wang, D., Liang, D., et al. (2015). The oral and gut microbiomes are perturbed in rheumatoid arthritis and partly normalized after treatment. *Nat. Med.* 21, 895–905. doi: 10.1038/nm.3914

4

Gut Microbiota Composition and Fecal Metabolic Profiling in Patients with Diabetic Retinopathy

Zixi Zhou[†], Zheng Zheng[†], Xiaojing Xiong, Xu Chen, Jingying Peng, Hao Yao, Jiaxin Pu, Qingwei Chen and Minming Zheng*

The Second Affiliated Hospital of Chongqing Medical University, Chongqing, China

*Correspondence:
Minming Zheng
381393002@qq.com

[†] These authors have contributed equally to this work

Recent evidence suggests there is a link between metabolic diseases and gut microbiota. To investigate the gut microbiota composition and fecal metabolic phenotype in diabetic retinopathy (DR) patients. DNA was extracted from 50 fecal samples (21 individuals with type 2 diabetes mellitus-associated retinopathy (DR), 14 with type 2 diabetes mellitus but without retinopathy (DM) and 15 sex- and age-matched healthy controls) and then sequenced by high-throughput 16S rDNA analysis. Liquid chromatography mass spectrometry (LC-MS)-based metabolomics was simultaneously performed on the samples. A significant difference in the gut microbiota composition was observed between the DR and healthy groups and between the DR and DM groups. At the genus level, *Faecalibacterium*, *Roseburia*, *Lachnospira* and *Romboutsia* were enriched in DR patients compared to healthy individuals, while *Akkermansia* was depleted. Compared to those in the DM patient group, five genera, including *Prevotella*, were enriched, and *Bacillus*, *Veillonella*, and *Pantoea* were depleted in DR patients. Fecal metabolites in DR patients significantly differed from those in the healthy population and DM patients. The levels of carnosine, succinate, nicotinic acid and niacinamide were significantly lower in DR patients than in healthy controls. Compared to those in DM patients, nine metabolites were enriched, and six were depleted in DR patients. KEGG annotation revealed 17 pathways with differentially abundant metabolites between DR patients and healthy controls, and only two pathways with differentially abundant metabolites were identified between DR and DM patients, namely, the arginine-proline and α-linolenic acid metabolic pathways. In a correlation analysis, armillaramide was found to be negatively associated with *Prevotella* and *Subdoligranulum* and positively associated with *Bacillus*. Traumatic acid was negatively correlated with *Bacillus*. Our study identified differential gut microbiota compositions and characteristic fecal metabolic phenotypes in DR patients compared with those in the healthy population and DM patients. Additionally, the gut microbiota composition and fecal metabolic phenotype were relevant. We speculated that the gut microbiota in DR patients may cause alterations in fecal metabolites, which may contribute to disease progression, providing a new direction for understanding DR.

Keywords: diabetic retinopathy, gut microbiota, fecal metabolic phenotype, metabolomics, correlation analysis

INTRODUCTION

Diabetic retinopathy (DR) is one of the most common complications of diabetes mellitus and leads to vision-threatening damage to the retina, eventually leading to blindness. It was estimated that the number of people with DR would increase globally from 126.6 million in 2010 to 191.0 million by 2030. If urgent action was not taken, the number with vision-threatening diabetic retinopathy (VTDR) would increase from 37.3 to 56.3 million (Zheng et al., 2012). DR is a vascular and neurodegenerative disease with complex pathogenesis and progression that is mainly characterized by recurrent episodes of capillary occlusion and progressive local retinal ischemia. Previous studies have revealed that activated CCR5 + CD11b + mononuclear macrophages were involved in early DR (Serra et al., 2012). NLR family pyrin domain containing 3 (NLRP3) inflammasome disorder might cause diabetic retinal damage and destruction via the proinflammatory cytokines IL-1β and IL-18 (Raman and Matsubara, 2020). P2 × 7R, a member of the P2XR family of ATP-gated plasma membrane receptors, has been verified to regulate inflammatory and immune responses. P2 × 7R stimulation or overexpression triggered VEGF secretion and promoted diabetic retinopathy (Raman and Matsubara, 2020). The above mentioned studies suggested that an abnormal immune response and the release of inflammatory factors may play an important role in DR progression. Notably, the human gut microbiota and its effects on the metabolic phenotypes have been shown to play a critical role in the maintenance of immune homeostasis (Scher et al., 2015) and anti-inflammation (Al Bander et al., 2020).

The intestinal microbiota played an important role in the metabolic health of the human host and was implicated in the pathogenesis of many common metabolic diseases, including obesity, type 2 diabetes and non-alcoholic liver disease (Fan and Pedersen, 2021). Studies have shown that people with type 2 diabetes mellitus (T2DM) have malnutrition-associated changes in their gut microbiota (Qin et al., 2012; Karlsson et al., 2013). Previous animal studies have found that intermittent fasting-mediated changes could prevent DR by restructuring the microbiota toward species producing taurochenodeoxycholate (TUDCA) and subsequent retinal protection by TGR5 activation (Beli et al., 2018). Therefore, TGR5, the TUDCA receptor, could be a new therapeutic target for DR, which suggested that gut microbial changes may be associated with DR. Besides, dysbiosis occurs in the gut microbiota of people with T2DM and DR more frequently than in healthy individuals, and the interaction of fungal genera differs between them (Jayasudha et al., 2020).

Metabolomics is based on genomics, transcriptomics and proteomics to identify and quantify low-molecular-weight metabolites in biological samples, thus revealing physiological changes influenced by external stimuli or interventions. An abundance of studies applying metabolomic approaches have been used to identify specific metabolic phenotypes in intraocular fluid (vitreous humor, aqueous humor) and blood samples (Jin et al., 2019; Zhu et al., 2019; Wang H. et al., 2020). However, to our knowledge, few metabolomic studies have investigated fecal metabolic phenotypes in DR. To identify the role of the microbiota and metabolites in DR progression, we analyzed the gut microbiota composition and the fecal metabolic phenotype in the study groups using 16S rDNA sequencing and LC-MS-based metabolomics. Our study explored the composition of the gut microbiota and its associated fecal metabolic phenotype in patients with DR. We hypothesized that the gut microbiota of DR patients may lead to altered fecal metabolites, which may contribute to disease progression.

MATERIALS AND METHODS

Study Participants and Sample Collection

The study included 50 individuals who were enrolled from the Second Affiliated Hospital of Chongqing Medical University (Chongqing, China) from December 2019 to December 2020. 50 individuals were divided into three groups: 21 T2DM DR patients (14 men and 7 women), 14 T2DM DR patients with type 2 DM only, and 15 healthy controls. The three groups were closely matched in terms of age (59.57 ± 9.09, 56.13 ± 8.88, 61.93 ± 6.20). The study received the approval of the Ethics Committee of the Second Affiliated Hospital of Chongqing Medical University (2019(012)) and all participants signed informed consents. All procedures in this study followed the Declaration of Helsinki. All 21 subjects met the following inclusion criteria: (a) patients with DR diagnosed by previous slit-lamp biomicroscopy and fluorescein angiography examinations; and (b) patients without other eye diseases or systemic diseases with ocular complications, such as glaucoma, uveitis, ocular trauma, and age-related macular degeneration. All 14 T2DM patients met the following inclusion criteria: (a) all met the 2018 American Diabetes Association Medical Diagnostic Criteria for Diabetes (American Diabetes Association, 2018); and (b) diabetic retinopathy was ruled out by fundus photography and ocular optical coherence tomograph (OCT) examination. The exclusion criteria for each group were as follows: recent treatment with probiotics, antibiotics, or corticosteroids; gastrointestinal tract surgery (<1 month prior to sample collection); a history of autoimmune diseases including rheumatoid arthritis, psoriatic arthritis, systemic lupus erythematosus and inflammatory bowel disease; type 1 diabetes or unclear etiology of diabetes; and hypertension, obesity, malignant tumors or a history of organ transplantation.

DR and DM patients took metformin with or without insulin injections for glycemic control (duration >3 months). Individuals enrolled in our study had a normal diet and regular bowel movements.

Morning fecal samples were collected after defecation at hospital. Then stool samples were placed into two cryotubes and immediately transported on dry ice within 10 min. All samples were collected by a designated doctor. Fecal samples were stored at −80°C until processing.

Fecal DNA Extraction and 16S Sequencing

According to the manufacturer's recommendation, microbial DNA was extracted from fecal samples using a Power Soil DNA Isolation Kit (MoBio Laboratories). Total genomic DNA from samples was extracted using the CTAB method, and the DNA quality and quantity were assessed by the ratios of 260 nm/280 nm and 260 nm/230 nm. The ratios ranged from 1.7 to 1.9 of 260 nm/280 nm and exceed 2.0 of 260 nm/230 nm were considered good. The 16S rRNA V3-V4 region was amplified using the specific primers 341F (CCTACGGGRSGCAGCAG) and 806R (GGACTACV VGGGTATCTAATC). PCR amplification was conducted in a total volume of 50 μl, which included 0.2 μl Q5 High-Fidelity DNA Polymerase, 10 μl Buffer, 1 μl dNTP, 10 μl High GC Enhancer, 10 μM of each primer and 60 ng genome DNA. Thermal cycling conditions were performed as follows: an initial denaturation at 95°C for 5 min, followed by 15 cycles at 95°C for 1 min, 50°C for 1 min and 72°C for 1 min, with a final extension at 72°C for 7 min. The PCR products from the first step PCR were purified through VAHTSTM DNA Clean Beads. A second round PCR was then performed in a 40 μl reaction which contained 20 μl 2 × Phμsion HF MM, 8 μl ddH2O, 10 μM of each primer and 10 μl PCR products from the first step. Thermal cycling conditions were as follows: an initial denaturation at 98°C for 30 s, followed by 10 cycles at 98°C for 10 s, 65°C for 30 s min and 72°C for 30 s, with a final extension at 72°C for 5 min. Finally, all PCR products were quantified by Quant-iT dsDNA HS Reagent and pooled together. Then, the PCR products were purified with a Qiagen Gel Extraction Kit (Qiagen, Germany). The samples were sequenced on an Illumina NovaSeq platform (Illumina, California, United States), and 250 bp paired-end reads were generated.

Sequencing Data Analysis

After Illumina NovaSeq sequencing, we obtained paired-end reads, which were merged using FLASH (V1.2.7)[1] (Magoč and Salzberg, 2011). Then, quality filtering of raw tags was performed to obtain high-quality tag data (clean tags) under strict filtering conditions according to QIIME (V1.9.1)[2] (Bokulich et al., 2013). The clean tags obtained were further filtered to detect the chimera sequence by UCHIME software. Next, we clustered all the effective tags, and those for which similarity >97% were grouped as operational taxonomic units (OTUs). The Silva database[3] (Quast et al., 2013) was used based on the Mothur algorithm to annotate taxonomic information. We have uploaded the sequencing data to the NCBI for general scientific community access. The microbial alpha and beta diversities in our samples were calculated in QIIME software and displayed in R software. Alpha diversity was applied to analyze the complexity of species diversity through indexes, including the Chao1 index and Shannon index. Rank sum test analysis was applied to analyze significant differences in alpha diversity. Beta diversity

analysis, which was used to evaluate differences in species complexity among the samples, was performed with weighted and unweighted UniFrac distances in QIIME software. Principal coordinates analysis (PCoA) was performed with the stats R package to visualize the distance matrix among all the samples. AMOVA and ADONIS analyses were used to assess significant differences in beta diversity among the three groups.

Linear discriminant analysis (LDA) coupled with effect size (LEfSe) was performed with the LEfSe tool (Hess et al., 2011), and the p value was determined by Metastats analysis with the stats R package to discriminate bacterial taxa with significantly different abundances. Only colonies that showed a P value <0.05 and a log LDA score >2 were included. A P value <0.05 was considered significant.

Liquid Chromatography Mass Spectrometry/Mass Spectrometry Analysis

The ultra-high performance liquid chromatography coupled with mass spectrometry detection (UHPLC-MS) was applied in our research for the composition of metabolites in the gut and was performed by Shanghai Biotree Biomedical Technology Co., Ltd, China. Fifty milligrams of stool from each sample were weighed in an Eppendorf (EP) tube and then mixed with 1,000 μL of extraction solution [acetonitrile:methanol:water = 2:2:1 (V/V/V)] containing an isotope-labeled internal standard mixture. After 30 s of vortexing, all the samples were homogenized at 35 Hz for 4 min and then sonicated for 5 min in an ice-water bath. After that, the samples were centrifuged at 12,000 rpm for 15 min at 4°C. The resulting supernatant was transferred to a fresh glass vial for analysis. We collected the same amount of supernatant from all samples and prepared QC samples. Untargeted fecal metabolomics analysis was performed with an UHPLC system (Vanquish, Thermo Fisher Scientific) with a UPLC BEH Amide column (2.1 mm × 100 mm, 1.7 μm) coupled to a Q Exactive HFX mass spectrometer (Orbitrap MS, Thermo). The mobile phase consisted of 25 mmol/L ammonium acetate and 25 mmol/L ammonia hydroxide in water (pH = 9.75) (A) and acetonitrile (B). The elution gradient was set as follows: 0~0.5 min, 95% B; 0.5~7.0 min, 95%~65% B; 7.0~8.0 min, 65%~40% B; 8.0~9.0 min, 40% B; 9.0~9.1 min, 40%~95% B; and 9.1~12.0 min, 95% B. The column temperature was 30°C. The autosampler temperature was 4°C, and the injection volume was 3 μL. All MS1 and MS2 data were obtained with acquisition software (Xcalibur, Thermo).

Data Analysis

The raw data was transformed to mzXML format using ProteoWizard and processed by XCMS for peak detection, extraction, alignment, and integration (Smith et al., 2006). Then, we applied an in-house MS2 database for metabolite annotation. Individual peaks were filtered to remove noise by filtering the deviation value using the relative standard deviation method. Subsequently, the missing values missing up to the minimum value were simulated in the raw data. Finally, 4233 peaks remained after the data were processed by the internal

---

[1] http://ccb.jhu.edu/software/FLASH/

[2] http://qiime.org/scripts/split_libraries_fastq.html

[3] http://www.arb-silva.de/

standard normalization method. To obtain high-dimensional metabolomic datasets, the final dataset was imported into the SIMCA16.0.2 software package (Sartorius Stedim Data Analytics AB, Umea, Sweden) for principal component analysis (PCA) and orthogonal partial least square discriminant analysis (OPLS-DA) after logarithmic transformation and Pareto scaling. In addition to multivariate statistical methods, Student's t-test was used to identify the altered metabolites in DR patients at univariate level. Metabolites with a variable importance in projection (VIP) value >1 in OPLS-DA analysis and $P < 0.05$ in univariate analysis were considered altered metabolites. In addition, the differential metabolites were mapped into their biochemical pathways through metabolic pathway enrichment and pathway analysis based on MetaboAnalyst 5.0[4], which uses the high-quality Kyoto Encyclopedia of Genes and Genomes metabolic pathways as the backend knowledge base (Liu et al., 2019; Wang T. et al., 2020). All raw data has been uploaded to NCBI (SUB9930154) and MetaboLights website (MTBLS3012).

Statistical Analysis

The levels of fecal metabolites and the relative abundances of genera were calculated using Spearman correlation analysis to obtain the corresponding correlation coefficient (Corr) matrix and correlation P value matrix. We determined the correlation between only those genera and metabolites for which $P < 0.05$. In all statistical tests, $P < 0.05$ was considered significant.

RESULTS

Participant Characteristics

None of the statistics presented in **Table 1** for participants recruited in this study was considered significant including hypertension, body mass index (BMI), diabetes duration, glycosylated hemoglobin (HbA1c), total cholesterol, triglyceride or estimated glomerular filtration rate.

Gut Microbiota Alterations in Patients With Diabetic Retinopathy, Diabetes Mellitus Patients Without Diabetic Retinopathy, and Controls

A total of 2,638,100 effective tags were obtained from the fecal samples of 21 patients with DR, 14 patients with DM and 15 healthy controls, with a mean of 52,762 per sample (ranging from 32,140 to 69,867). The sequences were clustered into OTUs with 97% identity, yielding a total of 2,226 OTUs, and then the OTU sequences were annotated with the Silva 132 database for species annotation. Based on the rarefaction curve (**Figure 1A**) and the species accumulation boxplot (**Figure 1B**), the current sequencing and samples were sufficient to identify taxa. The Shannon indexes observed in all three groups (healthy control, T2DM, and DR) were not significantly different (**Supplementary Figure 1C**). The OTU and Chao1 indexes observed were significantly different between DR patients and DM patients. In

addition, the OTU and Chao1 indexes observed between DM patients and healthy controls were also significantly different according to the Wilcoxon test (**Supplementary Figure 1**), which suggested that the number of microbial communities in DR patients differed from that in DM patients and normal subjects; however, their diversity was not significantly different. In the beta diversity analysis, the gut microbiota could be distinguished among the three groups by PCoA (**Figure 1C**), which was significant according to ADONIS and AMOVA analyses (**Supplementary Table 1**). In comparing the boxplots of beta diversity between the groups, when calculated using weighted UniFrac distance, a difference in the gut microbiota was detected between DR patients and healthy controls ($p = 0$), and further comparison of the gut microbiota between DR patients and DM patients likewise produced statistically significant results ($p = 0.0183$) (**Figure 1D**).

To determine the differentially abundant bacterial groups in DR patients, we compared them with healthy controls and then performed LEfSe. The results showed that 21 bacterial taxa were enriched in the DR patients, while 17 bacterial taxa were enriched in healthy controls (**Figure 2A**). Branching maps at six different levels (from kingdom to genus) were obtained by the LEfSe analysis method. The classes Verrucomicrobiae and Clostridia played important roles in the gut microbiota of DR patients. Additionally, not only the orders Verrucomicrobiales and Oscillospirales but also the families Akkermansiaceae and Oscillospiraceae had a greater effect in DR patients (**Figure 2B**). We also performed lefse analysis between DR and DM and among the three groups (**Supplementary Figure 3**). Comparison of the relative abundance of microbiota constituents was performed with Metastats analysis and log LDA score, which revealed differences in the gut microbiota between DR patients and healthy controls. The results revealed that at the family level, differences in gut microorganisms existed between DR patients and healthy controls in four families: Oscillospiraceae, Lactobacillaceae, Ruminococcaceae and Lachnospiraceae. At the genus level, *Faecalibacterium*, *Roseburia*, *Lachnospira* and *Romboutsia* were depleted in DR patients compared with healthy controls, and only *Akkermansia* was enriched in DR patients (**Supplementary Table 2**).

Notably, the use of glucose-lowering drugs, especially metformin, might affect the gut microbiota and could be a confounding factor in this study (Forslund et al., 2015). Based on this possibility, we included all DR and DM patients who received long-term regular oral metformin treatment. To investigate whether the characteristics of the gut microbiota were related just to DR, not to DM, we further compared the composition of the gut microbiota of DR patients with that of DM patients. We discovered that compared to DM patients, DR patients had elevated *Prevotella*, *Faecalibacterium*, *Subdoligranulum*, *Agathobacteria*, and *Olsenella* and reduced *Bacillus*, *Veillonella*, and *Pantoea* abundances at the genus level (**Supplementary Table 3**). Moreover, we found that *Faecalibacterium* and *Lachnospira* were depleted in DM patients compared with healthy controls at the genus level, and *Klebsiella* and *Enterococcus* were enriched (**Supplementary Table 4**), which was consistent with Zhao's study (Zhao et al., 2020).

---

[4]http://www.metaboanalyst.ca

TABLE 1 | Demographic and clinical characteristics of DR patients, DM patients, and healthy controls.

Characteristic	DR patients	Healthy control	DM patients	Total	F/H//z/χ^2	P value	Power
Patient number (n)	21	15	14	50	–	–	–
Age (years)	59.57 ± 9.09	56.13 ± 8.88	61.93 ± 6.20	59.20 ± 8.46	1.790^F	0.178	0.343
Gender (F/M)	7/14	8/7	6/8	21/29	1.443χ^2	0.486	0.108
BMI (kg/m^2)	22.79 ± 2.43	21.23 ± 2.07	22.20 ± 1.65	22.16 ± 2.19	2.326^F	0.109	0.431
Diastolic BP (mm Hg)	133.95 ± 18.15	120.6 ± 14.64	130.29 ± 15.97	129.00 ± 17.14	2.930^F	0.065	0.542
Systolic BP (mm Hg)	82.24 ± 11.86	75.73 ± 6.03	79.79 ± 8.55	79.6 ± 9.73	2.041^F	0.141	0.376
Glycated hemoglobin (HbA1c%)	6.44 ± 0.92	5.79 ± 1.14	6.55 ± 1.19	6.29 ± 1.10	2.301^F	0.111	0.44
Total cholesterol (mmol/L)	4.4 (3.43, 5.04)	3.8 (3.24, 4.51)	4.36 (3.66, 4.36)	4.33 (3.4, 4.9)	2.929^H	0.231	0.275
Low density lipoprotein (mmol/L)	2.34 ± 0.8	2.48 ± 0.71	2.91 ± 0.62	2.56 ± 0.75	3.069^F	0.055	0.5
High density lipoprotein (mmol/L)	1.21 ± 0.26	1.37 ± 0.35	1.25 ± 0.22	1.27 ± 0.28	1.600^F	0.212	0.301
Triglyceride (mmol/L)	1.29 (0.94, 1.73)	1.24 (0.87, 1.34)	1.43 (0.96, 2.08)	1.27 (0.93, 1.58)	2.484^H	0.289	0.273
Duration of diabetes (years)	13 (5, 19.5)	/	11.5 (2.75, 16.25)	5.5 (0, 15)	−0.76^z	0.447	0.169
Estimated glomerular filtration rate (ml/min)	98.00 ± 14.65	99.97 ± 8.65	95.67 ± 14.18	97.81 ± 12.94	0.435^F	0.65	0.134

The superscript F denotes the F statistic of one-way analysis of variance.
χ^2 Analyzed by χ^2 statistic of chi-square test.
^{H} Analyzed by the statistic of non-parametric Kruskal-Wallis test.
^{Z} Analyzed by the statistic of non-parametric Mann-Whitney test.
The results of multiple comparisons between groups at the 0.05 level are marked using lowercase letters (abc), the same letter indicates the difference between the two groups is not significant (p > 0.05), and different letters indicate that the difference between the two groups is significant (p < 0.05).
Using pwr.f2.test() in the pwr package (Champely, 2018) in R (Chang and Kwon, 2020; R Development Core Team, 2020).

Metabolic Alterations in Patients With Diabetic Retinopathy, Diabetes Mellitus Patients Without Diabetic Retinopathy, and Controls

Many studies on the metabolomics of blood and intraocular fluid from DR patients have been conducted (Chen et al., 2016; Haines et al., 2018; Jin et al., 2019). However, stool samples from DR patients have rarely been studied. Hence, we performed a metabolomic analysis of stool samples to discover metabolomic changes in patients with DR. In the OPLS-DA model, significant differences were found in metabolic phenotypes among DR patients, DM patients and healthy controls, suggesting that DR patients may have a unique metabolic profile (**Figures 3A,B**). The model between DR patients and healthy controls proved to be differential after randomization (n = 200) (**Supplementary Figure 2A**). However, the validity of the model between DR patients and DM patients disappeared after verification (**Supplementary Figure 2B**), which might mean that the metabolite differences between the two were not significant. As DR was one of the common complications of DM, the two diseases were closely related, which could explain the above results. A volcano map was drawn to depict trends in differentially abundant metabolites (**Figure 3C**). Four enriched metabolites in DR patients with $p < 0.05$, VIP > 1 and FC (fold change) <0.5 were considered differentially abundant when compared to healthy controls. In addition, 42 metabolites were depleted in the DR samples. By comparing DM patients with healthy controls, seven enriched metabolites and 35 depleted metabolites were found (**Supplementary Table**).

To further determine the metabolic phenotype of DR, we compared the metabolites between DR patients and DM patients. We found that DR patients had significantly decreased levels of traumatic acid, thromboxane B3, salicyluric acid, pyro-L-glutaminyl-L-glutamine, harman, flazine, butylparaben, betonicin, and β-carboline and increased levels of N-gamma-L-glutamyl-D-alanine, N-acetyl-L-methionine, L-threo-3-phenylserine, D-proline, armillaramide, and (R)-pelletierine in fecal samples (**Table 2**).

To identify the metabolic pathways involved in DR, we conducted KEGG annotation and combined the results of powerful pathway enrichment analysis with topological analysis. Metabolic pathway analysis identified 17 pathways with differentially abundant metabolites in DR patients compared with those in the healthy population. The results of the metabolic pathway analysis are shown in bubble plots, revealing β-alanine metabolism, phenylalanine metabolism and nicotinamide metabolism (**Figure 4A**). In addition, arginine-proline metabolism and α-linolenic acid metabolism pathways showed differentially abundant metabolites between DR and DM patients as detected by KEGG.

Correlation of the Gut Microbiota and Metabolic Phenotype in Diabetic Retinopathy Patients

To investigate whether gut microbiota composition was associated with the fecal metabolic phenotype in patients with DR, Spearman correlation was performed between the DR and DM groups (**Figure 4B**). The results showed that *Prevotella* was negatively correlated with armillaramide ($p = 0.02$, $r = -0.39$). *Subdoligranulum* was positively correlated with thromboxane B3 ($p = 0.01$, $r = 0.42$) but negatively correlated with armillaramide ($p = 0.046$, $r = -0.33$). *Bacillus* was positively correlated with armillaramide ($p = 0.0294$, $r = 0.36$) but negatively correlated with traumatic acid ($p = 0.0248$, $r = -0.37$).

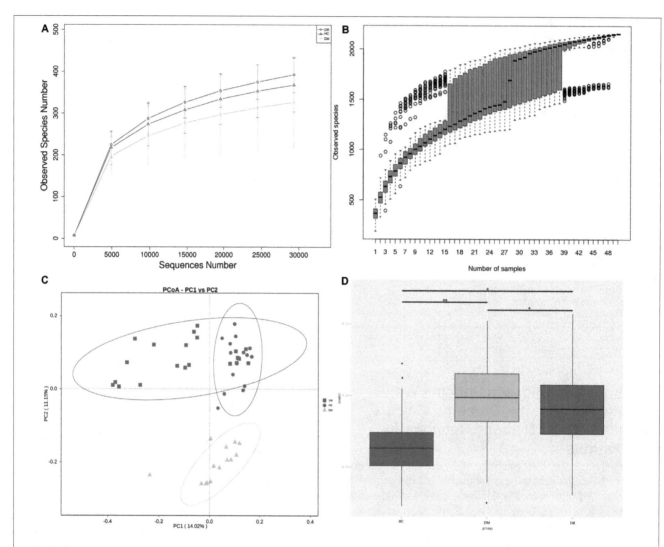

FIGURE 1 | (A) Reflectance curve based on OTU count in healthy control group, DR patients and DM patients. DR, DR patients (orange); HC, healthy people (blue); DM, DM patients (green). **(B)** The horizontal coordinate is the sample size; the vertical coordinate is the number of OTUs after sampling. **(C)** The PCoA ordination of Bray-Curtis distances among DR patients, DM patients and healthy controls from 16S rDNA sequencing data. The first three axes of PCoA showed a clear separation. **(D)** Beta diversity between-group difference box plots are based on weighted unifrac distances for the multi-group non-parametric wilcox test. *$p < 0.05$, **$p < 0.01$.

DISCUSSION

In the present study, we identified a distinctive gut microbiota profile in DR patients. Although the gut microbiota alpha diversity and richness analyses did not show significant differences between DR patients and controls, the structure of the microbiome of DR patients changed significantly according to the beta diversity analysis. This research demonstrated dysbiosis of the gut microbiomes in people with DM and DR compared to those in healthy controls. Compared to healthy controls, *Akkermansiaceae* was enriched significantly at the genus level, while *Faecalibacterium* and *Roseburia* were depleted significantly in DR patients. The intestinal bacterium *Akkermansia muciniphila* (an *Akkermansia* species) can specifically degrade mucin (Derrien et al., 2017). Previous studies have suggested that sugar-fed mice have enriched

A. muciniphila content in the intestine and reduced inner mucus layer thickness, disrupting the intestinal barrier and triggering an inflammatory response (Khan et al., 2020). *A. muciniphila* has been reported to improve glucose tolerance (Greer et al., 2016), prevent fatty liver development and maintain intestinal homeostasis (Kim et al., 2020); however, many studies have confirmed that *A. muciniphila* erodes the intestinal mucus barrier, which could contribute to colitis progression (Desai et al., 2016; Seregin et al., 2017). The significant reduction in the abundances of *Faecalibacterium* spp. and *Roseburia* spp. in the intestines of DR patients is consistent with findings in ulcerative colitis patients (Machiels et al., 2014). Butyrate, which produced by *Faecalibacterium* spp. and *Roseburia* spp., has been shown to block IL-6-induced signal transduction (Yuan et al., 2004). Serving as a vital inflammation pathway, IL-6/STAT3 signaling pathway had been reported to be activated

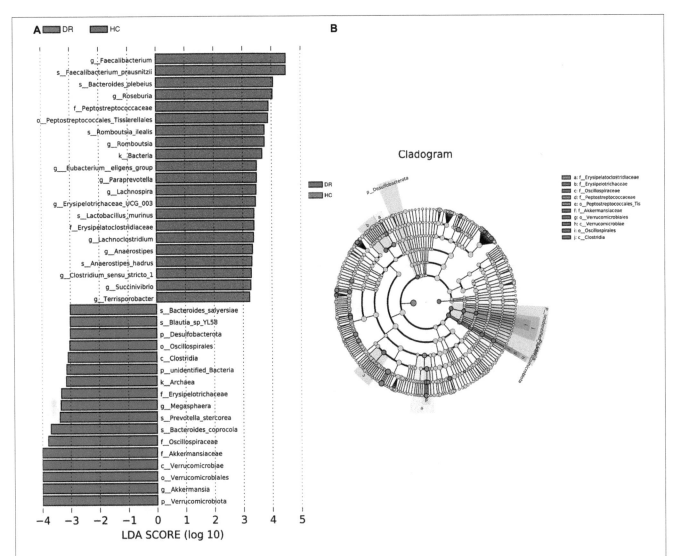

FIGURE 2 | (A) Taxa difference between DR patients and healthy controls. LefSe (LDA > 2logs) was used to detect major differences of bacterial taxa between DR patients and normal individuals. 21 bacterial taxa were enriched in healthy controls (green bars) and 17 were enriched in DR patients (red bars). X-axis shows the log LDA scores. (B) The cladograms of six different taxonomic levels (from kingdom to genus) were constructed. Red circles and shadings show the significantly enriched bacterial taxa were obtained in DR patients. Green circles and shadings show the significantly enriched bacterial taxa obtained in healthy controls.

to trigger inflammatory response of the body in ulcerative colitis (Mitsuyama et al., 1995). Similarly, another research had proved that the activation of the NDRG2/IL-6/STAT3 signaling pathway had credible correlation with the development of DR in rats, and protective effect had been confirmed by inhibiting such an important pathway (Wang Y. et al., 2020). The resemblance may suggest that the reduction in *Faecalibacterium* spp. and *Roseburia* spp. abundances in the intestines of DR patients may cause intestinal pathological changes similar to those found in ulcerative colitis patients.

As DR is one of the important complications of DM, we further compared the gut microbiota of DR and DM patients. Compared with DM patients, DR patients exhibited enrichment of gut microbiota constituents such as *Prevotella* and *Subdoligranulum* at the genus level. The genus *Prevotella* is one of the three representative bacteria of the human gut microbiota and is also one of the core genera of human gut microbes (Arumugam et al., 2011; Costea et al., 2018). Previous studies have confirmed a credible correlation of *Prevotella* with inflammatory diseases. *Prevotella* primarily activates Toll-like receptor 2, which can lead to the production of Th17 inflammatory cytokines (Larsen, 2017). IL-17A was originally derived from Th17 cell lineage which was a subtype of CD4 + T cells (Matsuzaki and Umemura, 2018). Studies have confirmed that IL-17A contributed to the development of DR through the IL-17R-Act1-Fas-activated death domain(FADD)axis, which caused endothelial cell death and capillary degeneration in the retina of diabetic patients (Lindstrom et al., 2019). Consequently, we inferred the occurrence of DR was associated with the interaction between *Prevotella* and IL-17R-Act1-Fas-activated death domain axis, further experimental studies are needed to confirm this hypothesis. *Subdoligranulum* is a strictly

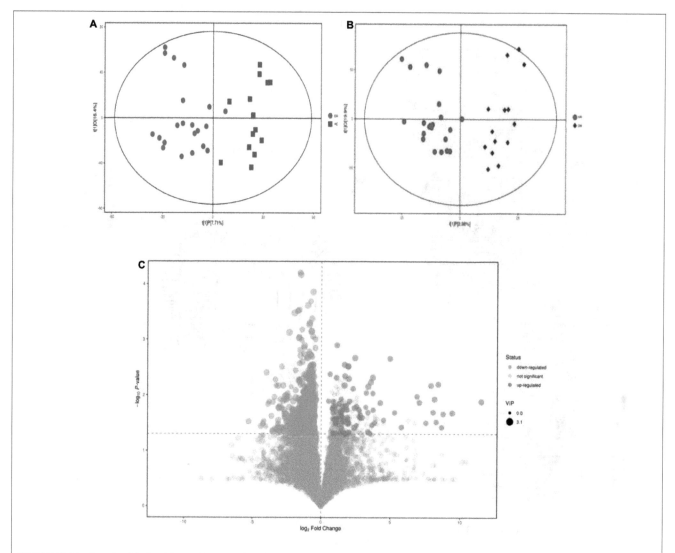

FIGURE 3 | Alteration of metabolites Changes between DR patients and healthy people and between DR patients and DM patients. **(A)** OPLS-DA score samples of fecal samples from DR patients (red circle) and healthy controls (blue square). **(B)** OPLS-DA of fecal samples from DR patients (blue circle) and DM patients (purple square). **(C)** The variation tendencies of fecal metabolites between DR patients and healthy people. The red circles indicate the up-regulated metabolites and blue circles indicate the down-regulated metabolites.

anaerobic, non-spore-forming gram-negative bacterium that has been shown to be associated with poor metabolism and chronic inflammation, which also lead to disturbances in host metabolism (Yu et al., 2020). *Faecalibacterium*, which has previously been confirmed to have anti-inflammatory effects (Xu et al., 2020), was found to be depleted in DR patients in our study. We speculated that the lack of *Faecalibacterium* could aggravate DR development. At present, there is no direct evidence that *Subdoligranulum* and *Faecalibacterium* is related to the pathogenesis of DR. Likewise, we speculated that the dysregulation of *Subdoligranulum* and *Faecalibacterium* could lead to DR through immune mechanism. Further research could consider to verify our hypothesis.

The above results highlight the potential association of the gut microbiota with DR. However, the altered gut microbiota and its effects on the metabolic phenotype in the host under

DR conditions remain unknown and could be a focal point to interpret the possible mechanisms of DR. Therefore, we aimed to assess the impact of the gut microbiota on the fecal metabolic phenotype in DR patients. We found altered fecal metabolite levels in DR patients. Carnosine was depleted in DR patients compared to healthy controls. Carnosine (β-alanyl-l-histidine) is highly abundant in human muscle and brain tissue (Mahootchi et al., 2020) and has strong antioxidant capacity and chelating effects (Boldyrev et al., 2013). Previous studies have also confirmed that various diseases and dysfunctions are associated with alterations in β-alanine and carnosine metabolism, while supplementation with carnosine may be beneficial in multiple sclerosis, diabetic complications and some age-related and neurological diseases (Kirkland and Meyer-Ficca, 2018; Artioli et al., 2019). The levels of succinate, nicotinic acid and niacinamide were decreased

TABLE 2 | Identified differential Fecal metabolites between DR patients and DM patients.

Metabolites	Mean DR	Mean DM	VIP	P-value[a]	FC
Traumatic acid	1.9968E-05	2.59259E-06	1.73	0.025	7.70
Thromboxane B3	1.60099E-05	3.2986E-06	2.06	0.030	4.85
Salicyluric acid	2.52096E-05	9.68573E-06	2.47	0.014	2.60
Pyro-L-glutaminyl-L-glutamine	6.43769E-06	2.58308E-06	1.18	0.032	2.49
N-gamma- L-Glutamyl-D-alanine	2.03928E-05	3.82827E-05	2.64	0.007	0.53
N-Acetyl-L-methionine	1.36203E-05	3.75546E-05	3.47	0.019	0.36
L-Threo-3-Phenylserine	0.000166407	0.000297864	2.97	0.017	0.56
Harman	0.00061641	0.000132657	1.57	0.003	4.65
Flazine	3.60815E-05	1.54617E-05	1.49	0.033	2.33
D-Proline	2.51415E-05	3.99343E-05	2.58	0.010	0.63
Butylparaben	0.000642486	0.000151561	1.47	0.044	4.24
Betonicine	3.06462E-05	1.10492E-05	1.19	0.045	2.77
Beta-Carboline	0.00031619	0.000119	1.67	0.021	2.66
Armillaramide	1.80033E-05	3.58778E-05	1.96	0.003	0.50
(R)-Pelletierine	6.98284E-06	1.10485E-05	2.05	0.048	0.63

VIP, variable importance in the projection; FC, fold change.
[a]P-value was calculated by Student's t-test.

in patients with DR. Succinate is an intermediate of the tricarboxylic acid (TCA) cycle and plays a crucial role in adenosine triphosphate (ATP) generation in mitochondria (Mills and O'Neill, 2014). Some studies have confirmed that abnormal mitochondrial function is closely associated with DR (Dehdashtian et al., 2018), which explains the relationship between DR pathogenesis and energy metabolism. Nicotinic acid (niacin or vitamin B3) is a functional group present in the coenzymes nicotinamide adenine dinucleotide (NAD) and nicotinamide adenine dinucleotide phosphate (NADP),which are important cofactors for most cellular redox reactions (Kirkland and Meyer-Ficca, 2018). NAD + , which serves as a regulator of inflammation by acting through sirtuins, has been suggested to play a crucial role in NLRP3 inflammasome activation (He et al., 2012). A variety of NLRP3 activators can inhibit mitochondrial function and therefore limit NAD + concentrations (Misawa et al., 2013). Dysregulation of the NLRP3 inflammasome could act as a contributing factor to the constellation of tissue insults evident in the diabetic retina (Raman and Matsubara, 2020).

Furthermore, two pathways involved in the differential abundance of metabolites between DR and DM patients were found, namely, arginine-proline metabolism and α-linolenic acid metabolism. D-Proline was significantly lower in DR patients than in DM patients and is involved in the arginine-proline metabolic pathway. Evidence suggested that proline was an important nutrient for the retinal pigment epithelium (RPE),which could promot RPE maturation, regulate glucose metabolism and increase the ability of the RPE to withstand oxidative stress (Yam et al., 2019). Recent evidence suggests that the most important nerve cells (photoreceptors) in the retina and the adjacent retinal pigment epithelium (RPE) play an important role in the development of DR (Tonade and Kern, 2021). Therefore, we hypothesize that a decrease in proline content may lead to RPE impairment and thus to the development of DR. Notably, traumatic acid is enriched during α-linolenic acid metabolism. Traumatic acid, which is regarded as an oxidative derivative of unsaturated fatty acids, has been considered to enhance caspase 7 activity, membrane lipid peroxidation and reactive oxygen species (ROS) levels and to play a crucial role in growth and development (Jabłońska-Trypuć et al., 2019). ROS can be maintained in equilibrium and participate in redox reactions in the body. However, when the balance is disturbed, ROS produce retinal cell damage through interactions with cellular components, which could lead to DR development

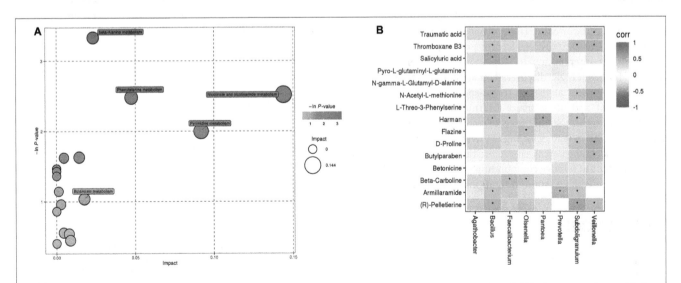

FIGURE 4 | (A) Bubble chart of differential metabolic pathways between DR patients and healthy controls. Each bubble in the bubble chart represents a metabolic pathway. **(B)** The relationship between gut microbiota and fecal metabolites in patients with DR. Red indicates that the flora is positively correlated with metabolites, and purple indicates that the flora is negatively correlated with metabolites. "*" indicates a significant difference between the two groups (p-value < 0.05).

(Calderon et al., 2017). In addition, in the correlation analysis, we found that Bacillus was negatively correlated with traumatic acid. Therefore, we speculate that the decrease in Bacillus abundance leads to an increase in traumatic acid levels, thus leading to DR progression.

We also discovered that armillaramide was negatively correlated with *Prevotella* and *Subdoligranulum* but positively correlated with *Bacillus*. Armillaramide is a lipid-like molecule (Gao et al., 2001) that plays a vital role in maintaining the stability of the membrane structure and is also involved in apoptosis and lipid metabolism pathways (Pruett et al., 2008). However, the exact mechanism of armillaramide in DR is unclear, and we inferred that dysregulation of the intestinal flora could lead to changes in armillaramide content, which contribute to DR occurrence. Further studies are needed to elucidate the specific role of gut dysbiosis and metabolites in the pathogenesis of DR. For instance, we can colonize *Prevotella* and *Subdoligranulum* in the intestine of mice to verify the exact mechanism involved in pathway. We can also conduct targeted analysis on differential metabolites to clarify the relevant role in the pathogenesis.

It is worth noting that, although the permutation test of OPLS-DA model overfit between DR and DM was mentioned above, this was not the only criterion used to determine whether the differences were existed between DR and DM. The student-t test has been widely used in previous studies on metabolomics (Huang et al., 2018; He et al., 2020). When the Student-t test was used to compare metabolites between the DR-DM groups, 15 metabolites were found to be different between the groups. In the future, more evidence should be obtained to validate the accuracy of the differential metabolites by expanding the sample size and performing targeted metabolomics analysis.

To the best of our knowledge, few studies concerning the gut microbiota profile and the analysis of fecal metabolites and their correlation in DR patients have been performed. Plentiful evidence suggests a link between the gut microbiome and hypertension (Li et al., 2017; Yan et al., 2017). A study previously confirmed that gut microbiota-dependent metabolites of trimethylamine n-oxide (tMaO) and its nutrient precursors (choline and l-carnitine) could improve insulin sensitivity during a weight-loss intervention for obese patients (Heianza et al., 2019). Hermes et al. discovered that some gut microbiota patterns were associated with tissue-specific insulin sensitivity in overweight and obese males (Hermes et al., 2020). Hence, we tried to avoid the influence of these confounding factors on the results when selecting individuals. Meanwhile, the demographic and clinical characteristics were simultaneously kept consistent to remove confounding variables such as diabetes duration. Undeniably, some limitations remain in our study.

We used R packages to perform power analysis in **Table 1**. As shown in **Table 1**, the study was statically underpowered, and a larger sample size will be required in future studies. The heterogeneity of genetic factors, environmental factors, dietary habits, antibiotics regimen, age, sex and ethnicity may lead to changes in the gut microbiota, which could influence the results of our study. Confounding factors could be eliminated by stratified analysis. Of the 50 fecal samples we collected, 48 had been free of antibiotics for more than 3 months in our research. In order to expedite the collection of samples, we selected two samples that had not been on antibiotics for 1–3 months, whose selection criteria also refer to certain literature (He et al., 2020). However, in order to eliminate the interference of antibiotics on the research results, samples free of antibiotics for more than 3 months, even 6 months should be selected in future studies. Research on the exact mechanisms of the gut microbiota and metabolites in DR patients is also needed, which may help provide new ideas for potential treatment.

ETHICS STATEMENT

The studies involving human participants were reviewed and approved by The Ethics Committee of the Second Affiliated Hospital of Chongqing Medical University. The patients/participants provided their written informed consent to participate in this study. Written informed consent was obtained from the individual(s) for the publication of any potentially identifiable images or data included in this article.

AUTHOR CONTRIBUTIONS

MZ and ZZo conceived the idea and designed the experiments. ZZo, MZ, and ZZe collected the sample, analyzed the data, and wrote the manuscript. XX, XC, JnP, HY, and JaP interpreted data and revised the manuscript. All authors contributed to the article and approved the submitted version.

ACKNOWLEDGMENTS

The authors thank all participants in this study. The authors also would like to thank the technical support for the BIOTREE company in Shanghai, China.

REFERENCES

Al Bander, Z., Nitert, M. D., Mousa, A., and Naderpoor, N. (2020). The gut microbiota and inflammation: an overview. *Int. J. Environ. Res. Public Health* 17:7618. doi: 10.3390/ijerph17207618

American Diabetes Association (2018). 2 classification and diagnosis of diabetes: standards of medical care in diabetes-2018. *Diabetes Care* 41, S13–S27. doi: 10.2337/dc18-S002

Artioli, G. G., Sale, C., and Jones, R. L. (2019). Carnosine in health and disease. *Eur. J. Sport Sci.* 19, 30–39. doi: 10.1080/17461391.2018.1444096

Arumugam, M., Raes, J., Pelletier, E., Le Paslier, D., Yamada, T., Mende, D. R., et al. (2011). Enterotypes of the human gut microbiome. *Nature* 473, 174–180. doi: 10.1038/nature09944

Beli, E., Yan, Y., Moldovan, L., Vieira, C. P., Gao, R., Duan, Y., et al. (2018). Restructuring of the gut microbiome by intermittent fasting prevents retinopathy and prolongs survival in db/db Mice. *Diabetes* 67, 1867–1879. doi: 10.2337/db18-0158

Bokulich, N. A., Subramanian, S., Faith, J. J., Gevers, D., Gordon, J. I., Knight, R., et al. (2013). Quality-filtering vastly improves diversity estimates from Illumina amplicon sequencing. *Nat. Methods* 10, 57–59. doi: 10.1038/nmeth.2276

Boldyrev, A. A., Aldini, G., and Derave, W. (2013). Physiology and pathophysiology of carnosine. *Physiol. Rev.* 93, 1803–1845. doi: 10.1152/physrev.00039.2012

Calderon, G. D., Juarez, O. H., Hernandez, G. E., Punzo, S. M., and De la Cruz, Z. D. (2017). Oxidative stress and diabetic retinopathy: development and treatment. *Eye (Lond.)* 31, 1122–1130. doi: 10.1038/eye.2017.64

Champely, S. (2018). *Pwr: Basic Functions for Power Analysis [R Package]. Version 1.2-2.* Available online at: http://cran.r-project.org/web/packages/pwr/index. html (accessed April 1, 2018).

Chang, C. B., and Kwon, S. (2020). The contributions of crosslinguistic influence and individual differences to nonnative speech perception. *Languages* 5:49. doi: 10.3390/languages5040049

Chen, L., Cheng, C. Y., Choi, H., Ikram, M. K., Sabanayagam, C., Tan, G. S., et al. (2016). Plasma metabonomic profiling of diabetic retinopathy. *Diabetes* 65, 1099–1108. doi: 10.2337/db15-0661

Costea, P. I., Hildebrand, F., Arumugam, M., Bäckhed, F., Blaser, M. J., Bushman, F. D., et al. (2018). Enterotypes in the landscape of gut microbial community composition. *Nat. Microbiol.* 3, 8–16. doi: 10.1038/s41564-017-0072-8

Dehdashtian, E., Mehrzadi, S., Yousefi, B., Hosseinzadeh, A., Reiter, R. J., Safa, M., et al. (2018). Diabetic retinopathy pathogenesis and the ameliorating effects of melatonin; involvement of autophagy, inflammation and oxidative stress. *Life Sci.* 193, 20–33. doi: 10.1016/j.lfs.2017.12.001

Derrien, M., Belzer, C., and de Vos, W. M. (2017). Akkermansia muciniphila and its role in regulating host functions. *Microb. Pathog.* 106, 171–181. doi: 10.1016/j.micpath.2016.02.005

Desai, M. S., Seekatz, A. M., Koropatkin, N. M., Kamada, N., Hickey, C. A., Wolter, M., et al. (2016). A dietary fiber-deprived gut microbiota degrades the colonic mucus barrier and enhances pathogen susceptibility. *Cell* 167, 1339–1353.e21. doi: 10.1016/j.cell.2016.10.043

Fan, Y., and Pedersen, O. (2021). Gut microbiota in human metabolic health and disease. *Nat. Rev. Microbiol.* 19, 55–71. doi: 10.1038/s41579-020-0433-9

Forslund, K., Hildebrand, F., Nielsen, T., Falony, G., Le Chatelier, E., Sunagawa, S., et al. (2015). Disentangling type 2 diabetes and metformin treatment signatures in the human gut microbiota. *Nature* 528, 262–266. doi: 10.1038/nature15766

Gao, J. M., Yang, X., Wang, C. Y., and Liu, J. K. (2001). Armillaramide, a new sphingolipid from the fungus *Armillaria mellea*. *Fitoterapia* 72, 858–864. doi: 10.1016/S0367-326X(01)00319-7

Greer, R. L., Dong, X., Moraes, A. C., Zielke, R. A., Fernandes, G. R., Peremyslova, E., et al. (2016). Akkermansia muciniphila mediates negative effects of IFNγ on glucose metabolism. *Nat. Commun.* 7:13329. doi: 10.1038/ncomms13329

Haines, N. R., Manoharan, N., Olson, J. L., D'Alessandro, A., and Reisz, J. A. (2018). Metabolomics analysis of human vitreous in diabetic retinopathy and rhegmatogenous retinal detachment. *J. Proteome Res.* 17, 2421–2427. doi: 10.1021/acs.jproteome.8b00169

He, J., Chan, T., Hong, X., Zheng, F., Zhu, C., Yin, L., et al. (2020). Microbiome and metabolome analyses reveal the disruption of lipid metabolism in systemic lupus erythematosus. *Front. Immunol.* 11:1703. doi: 10.3389/fimmu.2020. 01703

He, W., Newman, J. C., Wang, M. Z., Ho, L., and Verdin, E. (2012). Mitochondrial sirtuins: regulators of protein acylation and metabolism. *Trends Endocrinol. Metab.* 23, 467–476. doi: 10.1016/j.tem.2012.07.004

Heianza, Y., Sun, D., Li, X., DiDonato, J. A., Bray, G. A., Sacks, F. M., et al. (2019). Gut microbiota metabolites, amino acid metabolites and improvements in insulin sensitivity and glucose metabolism: the POUNDS lost trial. *Gut* 68, 263–270. doi: 10.1136/gutjnl-2018-316155

Hermes, G. D. A., Reijnders, D., Kootte, R. S., Goossens, G. H., Smidt, H., Nieuwdorp, M., et al. (2020). Individual and cohort-specific gut microbiota patterns associated with tissue-specific insulin sensitivity in overweight and obese males. *Sci. Rep.* 10:7523. doi: 10.1038/s41598-020-64574-4

Hess, M., Sczyrba, A., Egan, R., Kim, T. W., Chokhawala, H., Schroth, G., et al. (2011). Metagenomic discovery of biomass-degrading genes and genomes from cow rumen. *Science* 331, 463–467. doi: 10.1126/science.1200387

Huang, X., Ye, Z., Cao, Q., Su, G., Wang, Q., Deng, J., et al. (2018). Gut microbiota composition and fecal metabolic phenotype in patients with acute anterior uveitis. *Invest. Ophthalmol. Vis. Sci.* 59, 1523–1531. doi: 10.1167/iovs.17-22677

Jabłońska-Trypuć, A., Krętowski, R., Wołejko, E., Wydro, U., and Butarewicz, A. (2019). Traumatic acid toxicity mechanisms in human breast cancer MCF-7 cells. *Regul. Toxicol. Pharmacol.* 106, 137–146. doi: 10.1016/j.yrtph.2019.04.023

Jayasudha, R., Das, T., Kalyana Chakravarthy, S., Sai Prashanthi, G., Bhargava, A., Tyagi, M., et al. (2020). Gut mycobiomes are altered in people with type 2 diabetes mellitus and diabetic retinopathy. *PLoS One* 15:e0243077. doi: 10.1371/journal.pone.0243077

Jin, H., Zhu, B., Liu, X., Jin, J., and Zou, H. (2019). Metabolic characterization of diabetic retinopathy: an (1)H-NMR-based metabolomic approach using human aqueous humor. *J. Pharm. Biomed. Anal.* 174, 414–421. doi: 10.1016/j.jpba.2019.06.013

Karlsson, F. H., Tremaroli, V., Nookaew, I., Bergström, G., Behre, C. J., Fagerberg, B., et al. (2013). Gut metagenome in European women with normal, impaired and diabetic glucose control. *Nature* 498, 99–103. doi: 10.1038/nature12198

Khan, S., Waliullah, S., Godfrey, V., Khan, M. A. W., Ramachandran, R. A., Cantarel, B. L., et al. (2020). Dietary simple sugars alter microbial ecology in the gut and promote colitis in mice. *Sci. Transl. Med.* 12:eaay6218. doi: 10.1126/scitranslmed.aay6218

Kim, S., Lee, Y., Kim, Y., Seo, Y., Lee, H., Ha, J., et al. (2020). Akkermansia muciniphila prevents fatty liver disease, decreases serum triglycerides, and maintains gut homeostasis. *Appl. Environ. Microbiol.* 86:e03004-19. doi: 10.1128/AEM.03004-19

Kirkland, J. B., and Meyer-Ficca, M. L. (2018). Niacin. *Adv. Food Nutr. Res.* 83, 83–149. doi: 10.1016/bs.afnr.2017.11.003

Larsen, J. M. (2017). The immune response to prevotella bacteria in chronic inflammatory disease. *Immunology* 151, 363–374. doi: 10.1111/imm.12760

Li, J., Zhao, F., Wang, Y., Chen, J., Tao, J., Tian, G., et al. (2017). Gut microbiota dysbiosis contributes to the development of hypertension. *Microbiome* 5:14. doi: 10.1186/s40168-016-0222-x

Lindstrom, S. I., Sigurdardottir, S., Zapadka, T. E., Tang, J., Liu, H., Taylor, B. E., et al. (2019). Diabetes induces IL-17A-Act1-FADD-dependent retinal endothelial cell death and capillary degeneration. *J. Diabetes Complications* 33, 668–674. doi: 10.1016/j.jdiacomp.2019.05.016

Liu, W., Wang, Q., and Chang, J. (2019). Global metabolomic profiling of trastuzumab resistant gastric cancer cells reveals major metabolic pathways and metabolic signatures based on UHPLC-Q exactive-MS/MS. *RSC Adv.* 9, 41192–41208. doi: 10.1039/C9RA06607A

Machiels, K., Joossens, M., Sabino, J., De Preter, V., Arijs, I., Eeckhaut, V., et al. (2014). A decrease of the butyrate-producing species *Roseburia hominis* and *Faecalibacterium prausnitzii* defines dysbiosis in patients with ulcerative colitis. *Gut* 63, 1275–1283. doi: 10.1136/gutjnl-2013-304833

Magoč, T., and Salzberg, S. L. (2011). LASH: fast length adjustment of short reads to improve genome assemblies. *Bioinformatics* 27, 2957–2963. doi: 10.1093/bioinformatics/btr507

Mahootchi, E., Cannon Homaei, S., Kleppe, R., Winge, I., Hegvik, T. A., Megias-Perez, R., et al. (2020). GADL1 is a multifunctional decarboxylase with tissue-specific roles in β-alanine and carnosine production. *Sci. Adv.* 6:eabb3713. doi: 10.1126/sciadv.abb3713

Matsuzaki, G., and Umemura, M. (2018). Interleukin-17 family cytokines in protective immunity against infections: role of hematopoietic cell-derived and non-hematopoietic cell-derived interleukin-17s. *Microbiol. Immunol.* 62, 1–13. doi: 10.1111/1348-0421.12560

Mills, E., and O'Neill, L. A. (2014). Succinate: a metabolic signal in inflammation. *Trends Cell Biol.* 24, 313–320. doi: 10.1016/j.tcb.2013.11.008

Misawa, T., Takahama, M., Kozaki, T., Lee, H., Zou, J., Saitoh, T., et al. (2013). Microtubule-driven spatial arrangement of mitochondria promotes activation of the NLRP3 inflammasome. *Nat. Immunol.* 14, 454–460. doi: 10.1038/ni.2550

Mitsuyama, K., Toyonaga, A., Sasaki, E., Ishida, O., Ikeda, H., Tsuruta, O., et al. (1995). Soluble interleukin-6 receptors in inflammatory bowel disease: relation to circulating interleukin-6. *Gut* 36, 45–49. doi: 10.1136/gut.36.1.45

Pruett, S. T., Bushnev, A., Hagedorn, K., Adiga, M., Haynes, C. A., Sullards, M. C., et al. (2008). Biodiversity of sphingoid bases ("sphingosines") and related amino alcohols. *J. Lipid Res.* 49, 1621–1639. doi: 10.1194/jlr.R800012-JLR200

Qin, J., Li, Y., Cai, Z., Li, S., Zhu, J., Zhang, F., et al. (2012). A metagenome-wide association study of gut microbiota in type 2 diabetes. *Nature* 490, 55–60. doi: 10.1038/nature11450

Quast, C., Pruesse, E., Yilmaz, P., Gerken, J., Schweer, T., Yarza, P., et al. (2013). The SILVA ribosomal RNA gene database project: improved data processing and web-based tools. *Nucleic Acids Res.* 41, D590–D596. doi: 10.1093/nar/gks1219

R Development Core Team (2020). *R: A Language and Environment for Statistical Computing. Version 4.0.2.* Available online at: http://www.r-project.org (accessed June 22, 2020).

Raman, K. S., and Matsubara, J. A. (2020). Dysregulation of the NLRP3 inflammasome in diabetic retinopathy and potential therapeutic targets. *Ocul. Immunol. Inflamm.* 7, 1–9. doi: 10.1080/09273948.2020.1811350

Scher, J. U., Ubeda, C., Artacho, A., Attur, M., Isaac, S., Reddy, S. M., et al. (2015). Decreased bacterial diversity characterizes the altered gut microbiota in patients with psoriatic arthritis, resembling dysbiosis in inflammatory bowel disease. *Arthritis Rheumatol.* 67, 128–139. doi: 10.1002/art.38892

Seregin, S. S., Golovchenko, N., Schaf, B., Chen, J., Pudlo, N. A., Mitchell, J., et al. (2017). NLRP6 protects Il10(−/−) mice from colitis by limiting colonization of *Akkermansia muciniphila*. *Cell Rep.* 19:2174.

Serra, A. M., Waddell, J., Manivannan, A., Xu, H., Cotter, M., and Forrester, J. V. (2012). CD11b+ bone marrow-derived monocytes are the major leukocyte subset responsible for retinal capillary leukostasis in experimental diabetes in mouse and express high levels of CCR5 in the circulation. *Am. J. Pathol.* 181, 719–727.

Smith, C. A., Want, E. J., O'Maille, G., Abagyan, R., and Siuzdak, G. (2006). XCMS: processing mass spectrometry data for metabolite profiling using nonlinear peak alignment, matching, and identification. *Anal. Chem.* 78, 779–787.

Tonade, D., and Kern, T. S. (2021). Photoreceptor cells and RPE contribute to the development of diabetic retinopathy. *Prog. Retin. Eye Res.* 83:100919.

Wang, H., Fang, J., Chen, F., Sun, Q., Xu, X., Lin, S. H., et al. (2020). Metabolomic profile of diabetic retinopathy: a GC-TOFMS-based approach using vitreous and aqueous humor. *Acta Diabetol.* 57, 41–51.

Wang, T., Bai, S., Wang, W., Chen, Z., Chen, J., Liang, Z., et al. (2020). Diterpene ginkgolides exert an antidepressant effect through the NT3-TrkA and Ras-MAPK pathways. *Drug Des. Devel. Ther.* 14, 1279–1294.

Wang, Y., Zhai, W. L., and Yang, Y. W. (2020). Association between NDRG2/IL-6/STAT3 signaling pathway and diabetic retinopathy in rats. *Eur. Rev. Med. Pharmacol. Sci.* 24, 3476–3484.

Xu, J., Liang, R., Zhang, W., Tian, K., Li, J., Chen, X., et al. (2020). *Faecalibacterium prausnitzii*-derived microbial anti-inflammatory molecule regulates intestinal integrity in diabetes mellitus mice via modulating tight junction protein expression. *J. Diabetes* 12, 224–236.

Yam, M., Engel, A. L., Wang, Y., Zhu, S., Hauer, A., Zhang, R., et al. (2019). Proline mediates metabolic communication between retinal pigment epithelial cells and the retina. *J. Biol. Chem.* 294, 10278–10289.

Yan, Q., Gu, Y., Li, X., Yang, W., Jia, L., Chen, C., et al. (2017). Alterations of the gut microbiome in hypertension. *Front. Cell. Infect. Microbiol.* 7:381. doi: 10.3389/fcimb.2017.00381

Yu, H. J., Jing, C., Xiao, N., Zang, X. M., Zhang, C. Y., Zhang, X., et al. (2020). Structural difference analysis of adult's intestinal flora basing on the 16S rDNA gene sequencing technology. *Eur. Rev. Med. Pharmacol. Sci.* 24, 12983–12992.

Yuan, H., Liddle, F. J., Mahajan, S., and Frank, D. A. (2004). IL-6-induced survival of colorectal carcinoma cells is inhibited by butyrate through down-regulation of the IL-6 receptor. *Carcinogenesis* 25, 2247–2255.

Zhao, X., Zhang, Y., Guo, R., Yu, W., Zhang, F., Wu, F., et al. (2020). The alteration in composition and function of gut microbiome in patients with Type 2 diabetes. *J. Diabetes Res.* 2020: 8842651.

Zheng, Y., He, M., and Congdon, N. (2012). The worldwide epidemic of diabetic retinopathy. *Indian J. Ophthalmol.* 60, 428–431.

Zhu, X. R., Yang, F. Y., Lu, J., Zhang, H. R., Sun, R., Zhou, J. B., et al. (2019). Plasma metabolomic profiling of proliferative diabetic retinopathy. *Nutr. Metab. (Lond.)* 16:37.

5

High Ambient Temperature Aggravates Experimental Autoimmune Uveitis Symptoms

Su Pan[1†], Handan Tan[1†], Rui Chang[1], Qingfeng Wang[1], Ying Zhu[1], Lin Chen[1], Hongxi Li[1], Guannan Su[1], Chunjiang Zhou[1], Qingfeng Cao[1], Aize Kijlstra[2] and Peizeng Yang[1*]

[1] The First Affiliated Hospital of Chongqing Medical University, Chongqing Key Lab of Ophthalmology, Chongqing Eye Institute, Chongqing Branch of National Clinical Research Center for Ocular Diseases, Chongqing, China, [2] University Eye Clinic Maastricht, Maastricht, Netherlands

Correspondence:
Peizeng Yang
peizengycmu@126.com

[†] *These authors have contributed equally to this work*

Whether ambient temperature influences immune responses leading to uveitis is unknown. We thus tested whether ambient temperature affects the symptoms of experimental autoimmune uveitis (EAU) in mice and investigated possible mechanisms. C57BL/6 mice were kept at a normal (22°C) or high temperature (30°C) housing conditions for 2 weeks and were then immunized with human interphotoreceptor retinoid-binding protein (IRBP651–670) peptide to induce EAU. Histological changes were monitored to evaluate the severity of uveitis. Frequency of Th1 cells and Th17 cells was measured by flow cytometry (FCM). The expression of IFN-γ and IL-17A mRNA was measured by real-time qPCR. The generation of neutrophil extracellular traps (NETs) was quantified by enzyme-linked immunosorbent assay (ELISA). Differential metabolites in the plasma of the mice kept in the aforementioned two ambient temperatures were measured via ultra-high-performance liquid chromatography triple quadrupole mass spectrometry quadrupole time of flight mass spectrometry (UHPLC-QQQ/MS). The differential metabolites identified were used to evaluate their effects on differentiation of Th1 and Th17 cells and generation of NETs in vitro. The results showed that EAU mice kept at high temperature experienced a more severe histopathological manifestation of uveitis than mice kept at a normal temperature. A significantly increased frequency of Th1 and Th17 cells in association with an upregulated expression of IFN-γ and IL-17A mRNA was observed in the splenic lymphocytes and retinas of EAU mice in high temperature. The expression of NETs as evidenced by myeloperoxidase (MPO) and neutrophil elastase (NE), was significantly elevated in serum and supernatants of neutrophils from EAU mice kept at high temperature compared to the normal temperature group. The metabolites in the plasma from EAU mice, fumaric acid and succinic acid, were markedly increased in the high temperature group and could induce the generation of NETs via the NADPH oxidase-dependent pathway, but did not influence the frequency of Th1 and Th17 cells. Our findings suggest that an increased ambient temperature is a risk factor for the development of uveitis. This is associated with the induction of Th1 and Th17 cells as well as the generation of NETs which could be mediated by the NADPH oxidase-dependent pathway.

Keywords: experimental autoimmune uveitis, inflammation, fumaric acid, succinic acid, ambient temperature

INTRODUCTION

Uveitis is an intraocular inflammation which can be caused by infectious and non-infectious mechanisms. Non-infectious uveitis is thought to be caused by an autoimmune or auto-inflammatory response and is often difficult to diagnose and if not appropriately managed may lead to irreversible blindness, causing a heavy burden to patients and their families (Yang et al., 2005). Th1 and Th17 cells and activated neutrophils play an important role in the pathogenesis of uveitis (Balkarli et al., 2016; Safi et al., 2018; Chang et al., 2020).

Both genetic as well as environmental factors can influence the risk of developing an autoimmune disease such as uveitis (Zhou et al., 2014; Tan et al., 2020). Known environmental factors in uveitis include cigarette smoking and vitamin D status (Yuen et al., 2015; Chiu et al., 2020). One of the environmental factors that has not been looked at in detail is the role of climate. Climate change is currently recognized as a serious, worldwide public health concern and some diseases have been shown to be associated with environmental temperature and humidity (Burke et al., 2018; Gao et al., 2019). For example, relatively cool ambient housing temperature could induce suppression of the antitumor immune response and promotes tumor growth and higher temperature may accelerate atherosclerosis (Kokolus et al., 2013; Tian Xiao et al., 2016). To date, only few studies have addressed whether ambient temperature can influence the occurrence of autoimmune disease. We recently reported on the role of climate change in mainland China and showed that a gradual increase in temperature is associated with an increased incidence of uveitis and found that a 1°C increase in monthly temperature was associated with a rise in approximately two uveitis reports per 1,000 individuals (Tan et al., 2020). How temperature affects the development of uveitis is not clear and was therefore the subject of the study presented here, where we used an experimental autoimmune uveitis (EAU) model in mice (Agarwal et al., 2012). We studied the effect of temperature on the autoimmune response to a retinal peptide and focused on the role of T cells and neutrophils as well as the differential expression of metabolites. Our results show that housing mice at a higher temperature is associated with a more severe uveitis. Analysis of the involved mechanisms show that an increase of the ambient temperature is associated with a higher Th1 and Th17 cell response and an increased generation of neutrophils extracellular traps (NETs). Analysis of metabolites suggests important roles for fumaric acid and succinic acid.

MATERIALS AND METHODS

Housing Mice at Different Temperatures

Female, 4-week old C57BL/6J mice were obtained from the Chongqing Medicine University, Department of Laboratory Animal Resources. The mice were housed 6 to a cage in manual climatic boxes (Wanfeng Instrument, Jiangsu, China) maintained at a normal (22°C) or high temperature (30°C) environment. Humidity was controlled at 40 to 50%. Lights were adjusted to 12 h of daylight and 12 h of darkness. Mice were kept under these conditions for 14 days prior to the induction of uveitis (Kokolus et al., 2013).

Experimental Autoimmune Uveoretinitis Model

The mice above were immunized with 350 μg human IRBP peptide (IRBP651–670, LAQGAYRTAVDLESLASQLT) in Complete Freund's adjuvant (CFA) (Mattapallil et al., 2015). The peptide was purchased from Sangon Biotech (Sangon Biotech, Shanghai, China). Simultaneously, the mice were injected intraperitoneally with pertussis toxin (1 μg, Sigma-Aldrich, St. Louis, MO, United States) (Van den Broeck et al., 2006; Agarwal et al., 2012). After immunization, the mice were continuously housed in their previous environments, normal or high temperature environments, respectively. In some experiments, mice were housed under normal temperature conditions and transferred to a high temperature environment after immunization with IRBP, and this group was called the heat stress group. The normal temperature group was regarded as the control group in this study. Experimental Autoimmune Uveoretinitis (EAU) mice were euthanized, and spleens, serum and retina were collected on day 14 following immunization. Earlier experiments showed that this was the peak of inflammation in EAU (Mattapallil et al., 2015; Huang et al., 2018). In total we used 64 mice and actual numbers used in the various experiments are shown in the figure legends.

The protocols were approved by the Animal Care and Use Committee of The First Affiliated Hospital of Chongqing Medical University. Efforts were made to minimize animal discomfort.

Histological Scoring of EAU

Hematoxylin and eosin (H&E) staining. Eyeballs from EAU mice (day 14 after IRBP immunization) were dissected and fixed with paraformaldehyde. Eyes were then washed, dehydrated and embedded in paraffin wax. Serial 6 μm sections were stained with H&E and scored according to Caspi's criteria (Agarwal et al., 2012). H&E images were made using an inverted fluorescence microscope (LEICA, DMIL4000, Germany). The severity of EAU was scored on a scale of 0 (no disease) to 4 (severe disease) by an independent ophthalmologist in a masked fashion.

Isolation of Serum, Neutrophils and CD4$^+$ T Cells

The mice were anesthetized with pentobarbital (10 mg/ml) and blood was collected from the retro-orbital plexus on day 14 after IRBP immunization. Blood was clotted at room temperature for 2 h and centrifuged at 3000 rpm for 10 min. Serum was separated and stored at −80°C and used later for enzyme-linked immunosorbent assay (ELISA).

To isolate splenic neutrophils and CD4$^+$ T cells, anaesthetized mice were euthanized by cervical dislocation and splenic cell suspensions were obtained on day 14 after IRBP immunization. Lymphocyte separation solution (TBD, Tianjin, China) was used to isolate lymphocytes from the middle layer and neutrophils from the lower layer after removing erythrocytes with RBC lysis buffer (Absin, abs9101, Shanghai, China). CD4$^+$ T cells were isolated from splenic lymphocytes with CD4 microbeads (Miltenyi Biotec, Bergisch Gladbach, Germany).

Neutrophil Stimulation

Neutrophils were plated in 24-well plates at a density of 1×10^6 cells/well in 1 ml RPMI 1640 complete medium containing fumaric acid (173 μM), succinic acid (500 μM) or PMA (200 ng/ml). Concentrations were based on previous studies, and cells were incubated at 37°C with 5% CO2 for 4 h (Rubic et al., 2008; Wang et al., 2017; Hoffmann et al., 2018). In other experiments, neutrophils were blocked with diphenyleneiodonium chloride (DPI, 5 μM. Selleck, United States), the inhibitor of NADPH oxidase, for 30 min prior to stimulation with fumaric acid or succinic acid (Dabrowska et al., 2016; Wang L. et al., 2019). The supernatants were collected for ELISA.

CD4$^+$ T cells were plated at a density of 1×10^6 cells/well in 24-well plates in 1 ml RPMI 1640 complete medium containing fumaric acid (173 μM) or dimethyl sulfoxide (DMSO,ST038, BYT, Shanghai, China) as a vehicle control. Cells were stimulated with anti-CD3/CD28 (BioLegend, 100201 and 102101, San Diego, United States) and incubated for 72 h (Huang et al., 2020). CD4$^+$ T cells were collected for flow cytometry (FCM).

ELISA

To quantify NET release, the concentrations of MPO and NE in the serum or neutrophil supernatants were assayed with an ELISA kit (R&D Systems, DY3667 and DY4517, MN, United States) according to the manufacturer's instructions.

Immunofluorescence Detection of NET Formation

The eyeballs from EAU mice were dissected and paraffin-embedded for further experiments. After sections were dewaxed and hydrated, a primary antibody against MPO (Abcam, ab9535, Cambridge, United Kingdom) was used to stain the NETs and DAPI (Absin, abs9235) was used to stain the nuclei overnight at 4°C avoiding light. Sections were then incubated with secondary antibodies (Alexa Fluor 555, ab150078) for 2 h at room temperature. The location of NETs in retinal tissue was detected using immunofluorescence microscopy (NIKON Eclipse ci, Japan).

FCM

For IL-17A and IFN-γ staining, splenic lymphocytes were stimulated with ionomycin, PMA and brefeldin A (Biolegend, 423304) for 6 h, then washed, fixed and permeabilized. Fluorescent anti-mouse CD4-FITC (11-0041-82), anti-mouse IL-17A-PE (12-7177-81) and anti-mouse IFN-γ-PE-cy7 (25-7311-82) were purchased from eBiosciences (California, United States). Cells were stained with antibodies at 4°C for 30 or 60 min. The following markers were used to identify different immune cell subsets: Th1: CD4$^+$IFN-γ$^+$, Th17: CD4$^+$IL-17A$^+$. Stained cells were analyzed with CytExpert cytometry analysis software (Beckman Coulter, United States).

RT-qPCR

RNA was extracted from splenic lymphocytes (1×10^7 cells) or retinal tissue with the TRIzol reagent (Roche, 11667165001, Mannheim, Germany). The PrimeScript RT reagent Kit (MedChemExpress, HY-K0511, United States) was used to generate cDNA. Real-time qPCR was performed with the ABI Prism 7500 system (Applied Biosystems, CA, United States) by using the iTaq Universal SYBR Green Supermix (MedChemExpress, HY-K0522, United States) (Chang et al., 2018). PCR primers employed were as follows: IFN-γ: 5′-CTGCTGATGGGAGGAGATGT-3′(forward) and 5′-TTTGTCATTCGGGTGTAGTCA-3′(reverse); IL-17A: 5′-GGACTCTCCACCGCAATGA-3′(forward) and 5′-TCAGGCTCCCTCTTCAGGAC-3′(reverse) (Meng et al., 2017). PCR primers and mouse GAPDH endogenous reference gene primers were designed and purchased from Sangon Biotech (Sangon, Shanghai, China). Relative mRNA expression was calculated utilizing the $2^{-\Delta\Delta Ct}$ method.

Liquid Chromatography-Mass Spectrometry (LC-MS)

The metabolomics analysis of plasma from mice kept at high or normal temperature was tested by UHPLC-QQQ/MS and was performed by the BIOTREE company (Shanghai, China). Each group had 10 samples. In brief, mice were anesthetized with pentobarbital and blood was collected from the retro-orbital plexus in heparin sodium anticoagulant tubes and centrifuged at 3000 rpm for 10 min. Plasma was separated and stored at −80°C for future LC/MS analysis. The quality control sample, was a pooled preparation, made by mixing an equal aliquot of the supernatants from all samples. The data were analyzed by the SIMCA15.0.2 software package (Sartorius Stedim Data Analytics AB, Umea, Sweden). Metabolite composition was analyzed by calculating the variable importance in the projection (VIP) of the first principal component in orthogonal partial least squares discrimination analysis (OPLS-DA). A metabolite was considered to be differentially expressed when VIP > 1 and $P < 0.05$ (Student t-test).

Statistical Analysis

The results are shown as mean $\pm$ standard deviation (SD). Results that did not assume a Gaussian distribution are shown as median. One-way ANOVA and Kruskal–Wallis tests were used to perform multiple group comparisons. The unpaired t-test and Mann Whitney test were used to analyze two independent groups. Statistical analyses were performed with GraphPad Prism 7.0 software (GraphPad Software, Inc., CA, United States). Significance at each comparison point was indicated as: $^*p < 0.05$, $^{**}p < 0.01$, and $^{***}p < 0.001$.

RESULTS

High Temperature Worsens EAU Manifestation

To investigate whether a higher housing temperature can influence the inflammatory response during EAU, we kept mice at normal (22 degrees Celsius) or high temperature conditions (30 degrees Celsius) for 14 days and then immunized them with the retinal IRBP peptide to induce EAU. Histological scores of EAU were examined by H&E staining. The high temperature EAU mice developed significant inflammation with higher histological scores as compared to animals kept at a normal temperature (**Figure 1**).

In a separate experiment where we tested the effect of short duration of high temperature treatment on EAU, the mice were housed under normal temperature conditions and were then transferred to a high temperature environment after immunization with IRBP (heat stress). There was no statistical difference between the normal temperature group and heat stress group (**Figure 1**). Therefore, the subsequent experiments were done in mice kept at either normal or high temperature housing conditions for at least 14 days before inducing EAU.

High Temperature Is Associated With Increased Frequencies of Th1 and Th17 Cells in EAU Mice

Previous studies have demonstrated that the spleen is an important immune organ and as such hosts a wide range of immunological functions (Lewis et al., 2019). We therefore focused on the effect of housing temperature conditions on the frequencies of lymphocyte subpopulations in the spleen of mice with EAU. The frequencies of Th1 and Th17 cells were significantly higher in the high temperature group when compared to the normal temperature group (**Figures 2A,B**). The expression of IFN-γ and IL-17A mRNA in splenic lymphocytes was also significantly increased in the high temperature group (**Figure 2C**). Analysis of retinal samples also showed that the expression of IFN-γ and IL-17A mRNA was significantly increased in the high temperature group (**Figure 2D**). During

dissection, we found that the spleens of EAU mice kept at high temperatures were clearly smaller and lighter than in the normal temperature group (**Figure 2E**).

High Temperature Increases the Formation of NETs

To investigate changes in neutrophil function following an increased housing temperature we tested MPO and NE as NET markers in serum and neutrophils from EAU animals kept at normal and high temperatures. The results showed that there was a significantly increased generation of NETs both in the serum and neutrophil supernatants from EAU mice kept under high temperature conditions (**Figures 3A–D**). To investigate the expression of NETs in the retinas of EAU mice, we stained the sections with antibodies against MPO. MPO immunoreactivity was more prominently detected in the high temperature group and was distributed in the vitreous, inner plexiform layer (IPL) and inner nuclear layer (INL). In the normal temperature group, a light MPO staining was observed in the vitreous and sites with neovascularization (**Figure 3E**). However, the staining for MPO in retinal tissues was very light and the differences were not easily quantified. Collectively, these results suggest that a high temperature environment can up-regulate the generation of NETs in EAU mice.

High Temperature Is Associated With Higher Levels of Fumaric Acid and Succinic Acid

To determine the change in metabolism associated with the housing temperature conditions we analyzed plasma samples with LC-MS in two groups of 10 EAU mice (normal and high temperature). Using the OPLS-DA model, we found a significant difference in the metabolic phenotype between the two groups, suggesting that a distinct metabolic profile might exist in mice at the two different temperatures investigated (**Supplementary Figure 1**). Among the 141 metabolites detected in plasma, we found 17 differentially expressed metabolites as shown in volcano plots (**Figure 4A**). Each point in the volcanic map represents a metabolite, and the size of the scatter represents the OPLS-DA value. The larger the scatter, the greater the VIP. Higher levels of fumaric acid and succinic acid were found in the high temperature environment (**Figures 4B,C**). Fumaric acid and succinic acid are metabolites originating from the TCA cycle and subsequent experiments were performed to investigate whether these metabolites might affect neutrophil function.

Fumaric Acid or Succinic Acid Promotes the Formation of NETs *in vitro*

Previous research has shown that metabolites of the TCA cycle, especially succinic acid and fumaric acid may play an important role in inflammation (Sudarshan et al., 2009; Mills and O'Neill, 2014). We therefore investigated the effect of fumaric acid or succinic acid on the generation of NETs in vitro. Splenic neutrophils from normal mice were stimulated with PMA following incubation with fumaric acid or succinic acid, but this did not affect the generation of NETs (**Supplementary Figure 2**).

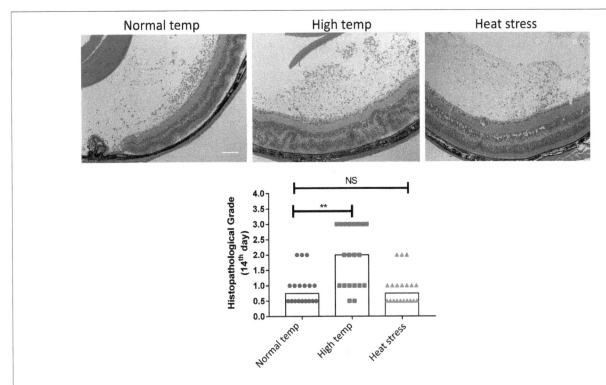

FIGURE 1 | A high temperature environment aggravates ocular inflammation in EAU mice. Left, representative hematoxylin and eosin images of eye sections from EAU mice (day 14 after IRBP immunization) kept at normal temperature, high temperature or a so-called heat stress environment. Scale bar, 10 μm. Quantification of the histopathological score. Representative data from 3 independent experiments ($n_{normal\ temp}$ = 18, $n_{high\ temp}$ = 20, $n_{heat\ stess}$ = 20; median; **p < 0.01; NS, no statistical differences; differences were assessed by the Kruskal–Wallis test).

To exclude the possible influence from PMA and to test the individual effect of fumaric acid or succinic acid on the formation of NETs, we isolated neutrophils and incubated them in medium with fumaric acid or succinic acid alone, to investigate the correlation between NET formation and these two metabolites. During the 4 h of incubation under fumaric acid or succinic acid conditions, a significantly increased NET expression was observed as evidenced by the higher release of MPO and NE (**Figure 5**). These data indicate that fumaric acid and succinic acid can induce NET generation by neutrophils and confirm the correlation found between intermediate metabolites of the TCA cycle and NET production.

Fumaric Acid or Succinic Acid Induces the Formation of NETs via the NADPH Oxidase-Dependent Pathway

Previous research has shown that accumulation of fumaric acid or succinic acid can induce activation of NADPH-oxidase and production of ROS (Sudarshan et al., 2009; Chouchani et al., 2014). To investigate whether a similar mechanism was operative in our system, experiments were performed with DPI, a classic inhibitor of NADPH-oxidase, which was used to block neutrophils before fumaric acid or succinic acid stimulation. NET formation was analyzed by quantifying MPO and NE in neutrophil supernatants after stimulation or inhibition. The results showed that DPI was able to inhibit the effect of fumaric

acid or succinic acid on the generation of NETs (**Figure 6**). Taken together, these data confirmed that NET formation could be regulated by fumaric acid and succinic acid via the NADPH oxidase-dependent pathway.

Fumaric Acid Does Not Activate Th1 and Th17 Cells *in vitro*

Earlier studies have shown that succinic acid does not affect CD4$^+$ T cell activation in vitro, although it can promote the proliferation and activation of CD4$^+$ T cells in vitro following antigen presentation by dendritic cells (Rubic et al., 2008). We confined our experiments to the effect of fumaric acid on CD4$^+$ T cells in vitro, and were not able to show a detectable effect on CD4$^+$ T cell differentiation into Th1 or Th17 cells (**Supplementary Figure 3**).

DISCUSSION

This study shows that an increase in the housing temperature worsens the development of autoimmune uveitis in mice immunized with a retinal peptide (IRBP). This was associated with an increased frequency of Th1 cells and Th17 cells as well as a higher level of neutrophil activation. Plasma metabolomics showed that under our experimental conditions an increased temperature was shown to increase fumaric acid and succinic acid which were intermediate metabolites of the TCA cycle. Further

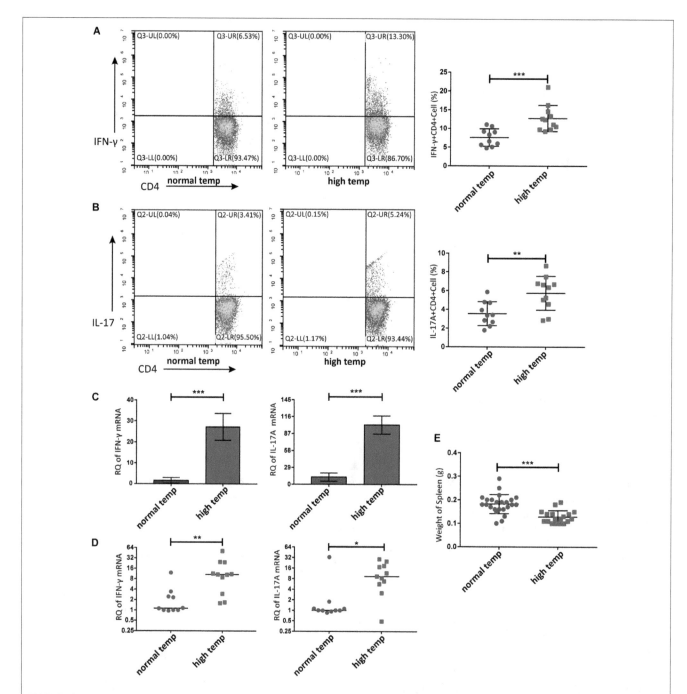

FIGURE 2 | A high temperature environment changes the frequencies of Th1 and Th17 cells in the spleen and retinas of EAU mice (day 14 after IRBP immunization). **(A)** Representative flow cytometry and quantification of IFN-γ+CD4$^+$ T cells in splenic lymphocytes of EAU mice ($n_{normal\ temp}$ = 10, $n_{high\ temp}$ = 11; mean ± SD; ***p < 0.001; Unpaired t-test). **(B)** Representative and quantification of IL-17A+CD4$^+$ T cells in the splenic lymphocytes of EAU mice ($n_{normal\ temp}$ = 10, $n_{high\ temp}$ = 11; mean ± SD; **p < 0.01; Unpaired t-test). **(C)** The expression of IFN-γ, IL-17A mRNA were detected by real-time qPCR in splenic lymphocytes from EAU mice housed under normal or high temperature conditions (n = 5/group; mean ± SD; ***p < 0.001; Unpaired t-test). **(D)** The expression of IFN-γ and IL-17A mRNA was detected by real-time qPCR in the retina from EAU mice ($n_{normal\ temp}$ = 10; $n_{high\ temp}$ = 11; data were not normally distributed; median; **p < 0.01, *p < 0.05; Differences were assessed by Mann Whitney test). **(E)** Weight of spleens were compared between EAU mice under high or normal temperature housing conditions ($n_{normal\ temp}$ = 24, $n_{high\ temp}$ = 18; mean ± SD; ***p < 0.001; Differences were assessed by Unpaired t-test).

experiments showed that these metabolites were able to activate neutrophils as evidenced by an increased generation of NETs.

Uveitis can be caused by infectious or non-infectious mechanisms. Non-infectious uveitis is thought to involve a

dysregulation of the immune response and can be divided into entities with an autoimmune or autoinflammatory etiology (Yang et al., 2005). Risk factors for the development of uveitis include an interplay between genetic and environmental factors

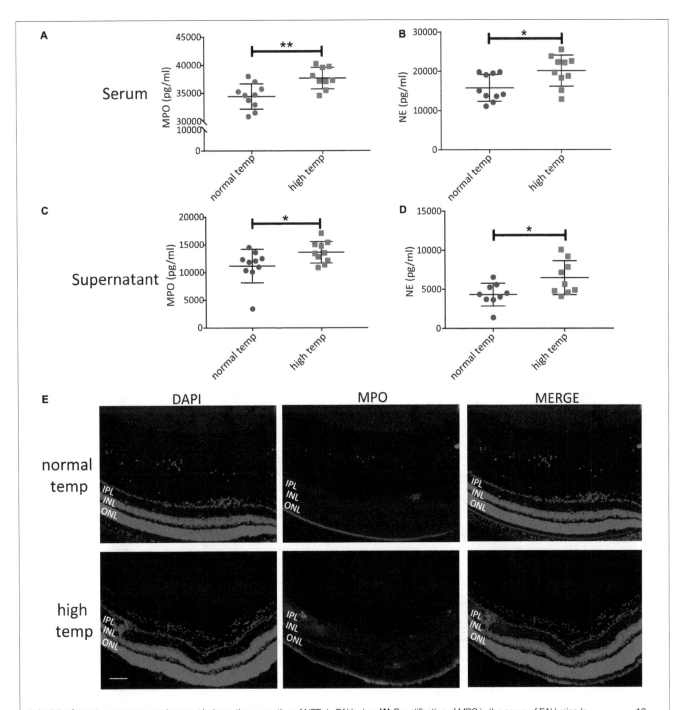

FIGURE 3 | A high temperature environment induces the generation of NETs in EAU mice. **(A)** Quantification of MPO in the serum of EAU mice ($n_{normal\ temp}$ = 10; $n_{high\ temp}$ = 9; mean ± SD; **p < 0.01, *p < 0.05; Differences were assessed by Unpaired t-test). **(B)** Quantification of NE in the serum of EAU mice (n = 10/group; mean ± SD; **p < 0.01, *p < 0.05; Differences were assessed by Unpaired t-test). **(C)** Quantification of MPO in neutrophil supernatants of EAU mice (n = 10/group; mean ± SD; *p < 0.05; Differences were assessed by Unpaired t-test). **(D)** Quantification of NE in neutrophil supernatants of EAU mice (n = 9/group; mean ± SD; *p < 0.05; Differences were assessed by Unpaired t-test). **(E)** Immunofluorescence analysis of MPO to label the location of NETs in the retinas of EAU mice. Scale bar, 106 μm (IPL: inner plexiform layer, INL: inner nuclear layer, ONL: outer nuclear layer).

(Zhou et al., 2014; Yuen et al., 2015; Tan et al., 2020). However, little is known concerning the environmental factors. We recently addressed the role of climate change in mainland China and showed that a high ambient temperature is associated with an increased incidence of uveitis (Tan et al., 2020). In the study presented here, we set out to identify the possible mechanisms that might explain the role of ambient temperature on the development of non-infectious uveitis, whereby we used a well-established animal model of autoimmune uveitis (Agarwal et al., 2012).

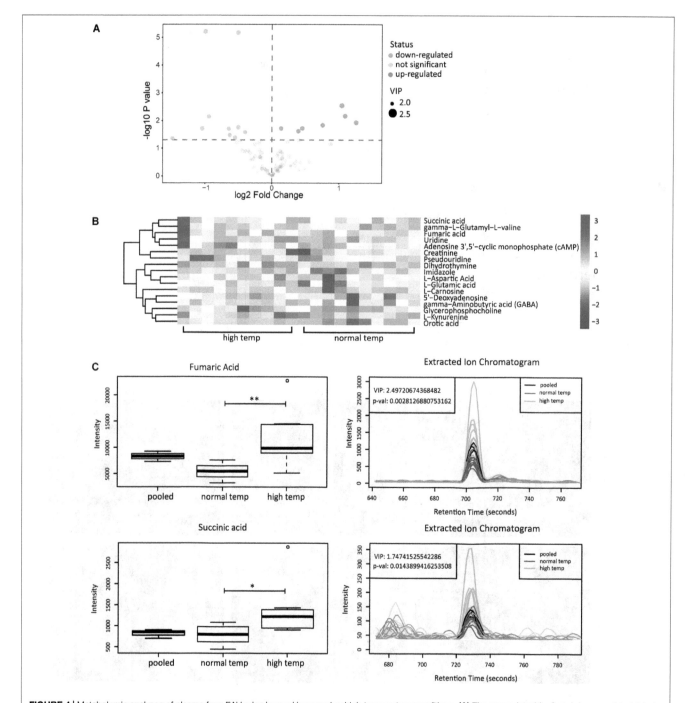

FIGURE 4 | Metabolomic analyses of plasma from EAU mice housed in normal or high temperature conditions. **(A)** The upregulated (red) and downregulated (blue) metabolites between the high and normal temperature group are shown in the volcano plots. **(B)** Heatmap of the 17 significantly differential metabolites. The color is positively correlated with the intensity of change in metabolites, with red indicating up-regulation and blue indicating down-regulation. **(C)** The response of fumaric acid and succinic acid in the sample (left) and extracted ion chromatogram (right) between the high (green) and normal temperature (red) group. The relative quantitative results and extracted ion chromatogram are shown. Pooled represents the quality control sample ($n = 10$/group; **$p < 0.01$, *$p < 0.05$).

Several experimental studies have addressed the role of temperature at which animals are housed on their immune response. These studies showed that a high housing temperature could not only affect the growth of animals, but also affected the immune functions and could aggravate inflammation (Tomiyama et al., 2015; Giles et al., 2016; Koch et al., 2019;

Moriyama and Ichinohe, 2019). Our data are in agreement with observations from these studies. However, in most research, animal models of heat stress are kept at 30°C, 39°C or even higher temperature. In preliminary experiments we found if the ambient temperature was elevated to 39°C or higher it caused an increased mortality rate of the EAU mice during

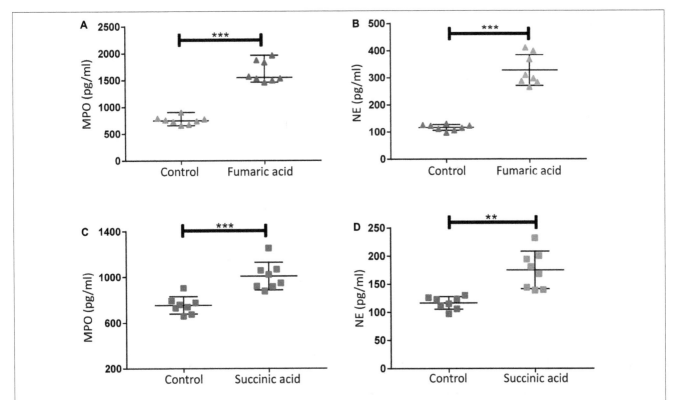

FIGURE 5 | Fumaric acid or succinic acid can promote formation of NETs. **(A,B)** Quantification of MPO and NE in the supernatants of neutrophils from normal mice treated with fumaric acid or DMSO as control ($n = 8$/group; mean ± SD; ***$p < 0.001$; Differences were assessed by Unpaired t-test). **(C,D)** Quantification of MPO and NE in the supernatants of neutrophils from normal mice treated with succinic acid or DMSO as control ($n = 8$/group; mean ± SD; ***$p < 0.001$, **$p < 0.01$; Differences were assessed by Unpaired t-test).

the experiments (Nonaka et al., 2018; Wang J. et al., 2019). We assume that increased mortality in EAU mice exposed to much higher temperatures might be due to heat exhaustion, heatstroke, or hyperthermia. However, we did not record these phenomena objectively and did not evaluate whether these systemic effects had an effect on the ocular inflammation. Instead, a 30°C environment could reduce the death rate of EAU mice induced by anesthesia. This is why we chose a temperature of 30°C, a relatively mild high temperature environment. In our experiments where EAU mice were treated very shortly at a high temperature (30 degrees), the animals also had obvious inflammation of their eyes, but the manifestation was milder, and nearly the same as seen in mice kept in a normal temperature environment. We assume that a short duration of temperature stimulation has no impact on inflammation and only prolonged high temperature conditions had an effect on the ocular autoimmune response.

Our data are in agreement with previous studies which suggested that the frequencies of CD4[+] and CD8[+] T cells could be increased by chronic heat stress (Kokolus et al., 2013; Huo et al., 2019). We also observed that a high ambient temperature could induce higher frequencies of Th1 and Th17 cells, with a concomitant increase of the expression of IFN-γ and IL-17A mRNA -in the spleens and retinas of the EAU.

In addition to helper T cells, macrophages and neutrophils play an important role in autoimmune diseases such as

EAU (Merida et al., 2015; Balkarli et al., 2016). According to previous studies on innate immunity and high ambient temperature, macrophages can be activated by heat stress to present autoantigens to T cells and polarize to the so-called M1 subtype (Slawinska et al., 2016; Koch et al., 2019). Little is known, however, on the mechanisms whereby high environmental temperature influences neutrophil function. NET generation, triggered by activated neutrophils, has recently received an increased attention in several autoimmune diseases, such as Behcet's disease and systemic lupus erythematosus (Leffler et al., 2012; Safi et al., 2018). Consistent with previous studies, a higher NET formation indicates a higher pro-inflammatory status in the affected tissues (Vorobjeva and Pinegin, 2014; Dicker et al., 2018). To our knowledge, we are the first to report an effect of environmental temperature increase on the formation of NETs in EAU. During dissection, we found that the spleens of EAU mice kept at a high ambient temperature were smaller and lighter. However, according to former research on inflammation, animals with severer inflammation would have larger spleens. We suppose that the high ambient temperature may affect the spleen volume of EAU mice via hormonal alterations, but there is not enough research supporting this speculation at present (Leceta and Zapata, 1985) and this hypothesis awaits further investigation.

Previous studies have suggested that the intermediates α-ketoglutaric acid, fumaric acid and succinic acid of the aerobic

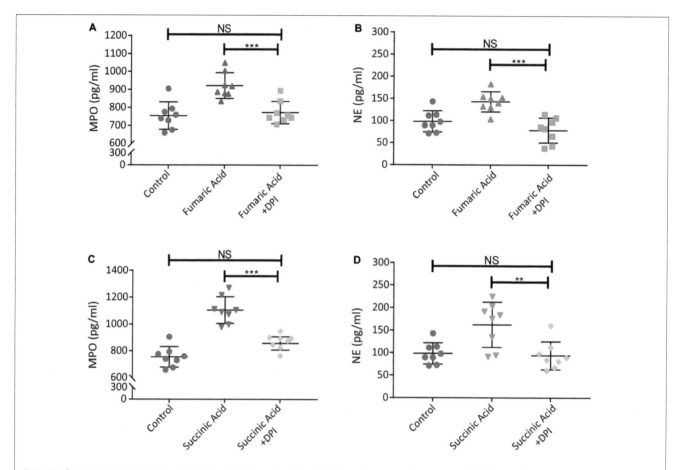

FIGURE 6 | Fumaric acid or succinic acid can induce NET formation via the NADPH oxidase-dependent pathway. **(A,B)** Neutrophils from normal mice were pretreated with DPI followed by the stimulation of fumaric acid. Quantification of MPO and NE in the supernatants of neutrophils. **(C,D)** Neutrophils from normal mice were pretreated with DPI followed by the stimulation of succinic acid. Quantification of MPO and NE in the supernatants of neutrophils (n = 8/group; mean ± SD; ***p < 0.001, **p < 0.01; Differences were accessed by one-way ANOVA test).

respiration-related TCA cycle were increased in plasma from animals kept at a high ambient temperature (Shi and Wang, 2016; Nonaka et al., 2018). Succinic acid can induce higher frequencies of helper T cells by amplifying the antigen presentation of monocytes through succinate receptor 1, but failed to activate T cells by itself (Rubic et al., 2008; Saraiva et al., 2018). These data are consistent with the results of the animal or cell studies we present here. Interestingly, fumaric acid or succinic acid accumulation may also enhance the TCA cycle, accelerating ROS production (Sudarshan et al., 2009; Ren et al., 2014). Previous studies indicate that the presence of ROS (NADPH oxidase-dependent) contributes to M1 polarization in macrophages and is also an important activator of NET formation (Branzk and Papayannopoulos, 2013; Chouchani et al., 2014; Vorobjeva and Pinegin, 2014; Dabrowska et al., 2016; Ko et al., 2018; Rendra et al., 2019). Our data showed that both fumaric acid and succinic acid can significantly increase the formation of NETs. Meanwhile, DPI could successfully inhibit fumaric acid or succinic acid from inducing NET formation. Therefore, we confirmed that increased NET formation induced by fumaric acid or succinic acid was NADPH oxidase-dependent. These data suggest a possible causality between a high temperature and NET

production, although further studies are needed to confirm these observations and to exclude other possible mechanisms of action.

Our study has several limitations. First, to observe possible effects on intraocular inflammation more clearly, we used a mild EAU model in this study, which is different from our earlier research on EAU mice (Huang et al., 2018, 2020). Second, due to a limited availability of experimental equipment, we only investigated the EAU development at only two levels of ambient temperature and did not measure the influence on the immune system of EAU mice prior to or after immunization at more time periods of heat stress. Since the majority of previous studies on EAU used 6–8 weeks old female mice or rats, we used a similar approach, but further study is needed to investigate whether our conclusions can be extrapolated to older mice and whether the same findings will also be seen in male animals (Agarwal et al., 2012). Third, the MPO staining in retinal tissues was too light to reliably quantify the differences. More sensitive techniques are necessary to address this issue. Finally, we assumed that energy metabolism was probably the most relevant target influenced by temperature, but other pathways or systemic effects may of course also be affected by temperature changes. A further limitation is that among the 17 differentially expressed metabolites detected, we only concentrated on the role of fumaric acid, succinic acid and NADPH oxidase, but other mechanisms cannot be excluded and deserve further study.

In conclusion, this study indicates that an increased ambient temperature is a risk factor for the development of uveitis. An increase in the ambient temperature was shown to upregulate the frequencies of Th1 and Th17 cells as well as the formation of NETs. The effect on neutrophils was probably mediated via the NADPH oxidase-dependent pathway. This study is the first to illustrate that a high ambient temperature has an effect on an autoimmune model of ocular inflammation and these findings may provide potential targets for the design of anti-inflammatory therapies and will hopefully promote policies to mitigate the burden of disease caused by global warming.

ETHICS STATEMENT

The animal study was reviewed and approved by the Animal Care and Use Committee of The First Affiliated Hospital of Chongqing Medical University.

AUTHOR CONTRIBUTIONS

PY and SP conceived the idea and designed the experiments. SP and HT performed all the experiments. SP, HT, and RC analyzed the data. QW contributed to FCM test and immunofluorescence. YZ, LC, and HL contributed to animal modeling. SP and HT wrote the manuscript. CZ and QC contributed to experimental equipment. PY, GS, and AK interpreted the data and revised the manuscript. All authors contributed to the article and approved the submitted version.

REFERENCES

Agarwal, R. K., Silver, P. B., and Caspi, R. R. (2012). Rodent models of experimental autoimmune uveitis. *Methods Mol. Biol.* 900, 443–469. doi: 10.1007/978-1-60761-720-4_22

Balkarli, A., Kucuk, A., Babur, H., and Erbasan, F. (2016). Neutrophil/lymphocyte ratio and mean platelet volume in Behcet's disease. *Eur. Rev. Med. Pharmacol. Sci.* 20, 3045–3050.

Branzk, N., and Papayannopoulos, V. (2013). Molecular mechanisms regulating NETosis in infection and disease. *Semin. Immunopathol.* 35, 513–530. doi: 10.1007/s00281-013-0384-6

Burke, M., González, F., Baylis, P., Heft-Neal, S., Baysan, C., Basu, S., et al. (2018). Higher temperatures increase suicide rates in the United States and Mexico. *Nat. Clim. Chang.* 8, 723–729. doi: 10.1038/s41558-018-0222-x

Chang, R., Chen, L., Su, G., Du, L., Qin, Y., Xu, J., et al. (2020). Identification of Ribosomal Protein S4, Y-linked 1 as a cyclosporin a plus corticosteroid resistance gene. *J. Autoimmun.* 112:102465. doi: 10.1016/j.jaut.2020.102465

Chang, R., Yi, S., Tan, X., Huang, Y., Wang, Q., Su, G., et al. (2018). MicroRNA-20a-5p suppresses IL-17 production by targeting OSM and CCL1 in patients with Vogt-Koyanagi-Harada disease. *Br. J. Ophthalmol.* 102, 282–290. doi: 10.1136/bjophthalmol-2017-311079

Chiu, Z. K., Lim, L. L., Rogers, S. L., and Hall, A. J. (2020). Patterns of vitamin d levels and exposures in active and inactive noninfectious uveitis patients. *Ophthalmology* 127, 230–237. doi: 10.1016/j.ophtha.2019.06.030

Chouchani, E. T., Pell, V. R., Gaude, E., Aksentijevic, D., Sundier, S. Y., Robb, E. L., et al. (2014). Ischaemic accumulation of succinate controls reperfusion injury through mitochondrial ROS. *Nature* 515, 431–435. doi: 10.1038/nature13909

Dabrowska, D., Jablonska, E., Garley, M., Ratajczak-Wrona, W., and Iwaniuk, A. (2016). New aspects of the biology of neutrophil extracellular traps. *Scand. J. Immunol.* 84, 317–322. doi: 10.1111/sji.12494

Dicker, A. J., Crichton, M. L., Pumphrey, E. G., Cassidy, A. J., Suarez-Cuartin, G., Sibila, O., et al. (2018). Neutrophil extracellular traps are associated with disease severity and microbiota diversity in patients with chronic obstructive pulmonary disease. *J. Allergy Clin. Immunol.* 141, 117–127. doi: 10.1016/j.jaci.2017.04.022

Gao, X., Colicino, E., Shen, J., Kioumourtzoglou, M. A., Just, A. C., Nwanaji-Enwerem, J. C., et al. (2019). Impacts of air pollution, temperature, and relative humidity on leukocyte distribution: an epigenetic perspective. *Environ. Int.* 126, 395–405. doi: 10.1016/j.envint.2019.02.053

Giles, D. A., Ramkhelawon, B., Donelan, E. M., Stankiewicz, T. E., Hutchison, S. B., Mukherjee, R., et al. (2016). Modulation of ambient temperature promotes inflammation and initiates atherosclerosis in wild type C57BL/6 mice. *Mol. Metab.* 5, 1121–1130. doi: 10.1016/j.molmet.2016.09.008

Hoffmann, J. H. O., Schaekel, K., Hartl, D., Enk, A. H., and Hadaschik, E. N. (2018). Dimethyl fumarate modulates neutrophil extracellular trap formation in a glutathione- and superoxide-dependent manner. *Br. J. Dermatol.* 178, 207–214. doi: 10.1111/bjd.15839

Huang, X., Yi, S., Hu, J., Du, Z., Wang, Q., Ye, Z., et al. (2020). Analysis of the role of palmitoleic acid in acute anterior uveitis. *Int. Immunopharmacol.* 84:106552. doi: 10.1016/j.intimp.2020.106552

Huang, Y., He, J., Liang, H., Hu, K., Jiang, S., Yang, L., et al. (2018). Aryl hydrocarbon receptor regulates apoptosis and inflammation in a murine model of experimental autoimmune uveitis. *Front. Immunol.* 9:1713. doi: 10.3389/fimmu.2018.01713

Huo, C., Xiao, C., She, R., Liu, T., Tian, J., Dong, H., et al. (2019). Chronic heat stress negatively affects the immune functions of both spleens and intestinal mucosal system in pigs through the inhibition of apoptosis. *Microb. Pathog.* 136:103672. doi: 10.1016/j.micpath.2019.103672

Ko, C. W., Counihan, D., Wu, J., Hatzoglou, M., Puchowicz, M. A., and Croniger, C. M. (2018). Macrophages with a deletion of the phosphoenolpyruvate carboxykinase 1 (Pck1) gene have a more proinflammatory phenotype. *J. Biol. Chem.* 293, 3399–3409. doi: 10.1074/jbc.M117.819136

Koch, F., Thom, U., Albrecht, E., Weikard, R., Nolte, W., Kuhla, B., et al. (2019). Heat stress directly impairs gut integrity and recruits distinct immune cell populations into the bovine intestine. *Proc. Natl. Acad. Sci. U.S.A.* 116, 10333–10338. doi: 10.1073/pnas.1820130116

Kokolus, K. M., Capitano, M. L., Lee, C. T., Eng, J. W., Waight, J. D., Hylander, B. L., et al. (2013). Baseline tumor growth and immune control in laboratory mice are significantly influenced by subthermoneutral housing temperature. *Proc. Natl. Acad. Sci. U.S.A.* 110, 20176–20181. doi: 10.1073/pnas.1304291110

Leceta, J., and Zapata, A. (1985). Seasonal changes in the thymus and spleen of the turtle, Mauremys caspica. A morphometrical, light microscopical study. *Dev. Comp. Immunol.* 9, 653–668. doi: 10.1016/0145-305x(85)90030-8

Leffler, J., Martin, M., Gullstrand, B., Tyden, H., Lood, C., Truedsson, L., et al. (2012). Neutrophil extracellular traps that are not degraded in systemic lupus erythematosus activate complement exacerbating the disease. *J. Immunol.* 188, 3522–3531. doi: 10.4049/jimmunol.1102404

Lewis, S. M., Williams, A., and Eisenbarth, S. C. (2019). Structure and function of the immune system in the spleen. *Sci. Immunol.* 4:eaau6085. doi: 10.1126/sciimmunol.aau6085

Mattapallil, M. J., Silver, P. B., Cortes, L. M., St.Leger, A. J., Jittayasothorn, Y., Kielczewski, J. L., et al. (2015). Characterization of a new epitope of IRBP that induces moderate to severe uveoretinitis in mice with H-2bHaplotype. *Invest. Opthalmol. Visu. Sci.* 56:5439. doi: 10.1167/iovs.15-17280

Meng, X., Fang, S., Zhang, Z., Wang, Y., You, C., Zhang, J., et al. (2017). Preventive effect of chrysin on experimental autoimmune uveitis triggered by injection of human IRBP peptide 1-20 in mice. *Cell. Mol. Immunol.* 14, 702–711. doi: 10.1038/cmi.2015.107

Merida, S., Palacios, E., Navea, A., and Bosch-Morell, F. (2015). Macrophages and uveitis in experimental animal models. *Mediators Inflamm.* 2015:671417. doi: 10.1155/2015/671417

Mills, E., and O'Neill, L. A. (2014). Succinate: a metabolic signal in inflammation. *Trends Cell Biol.* 24, 313–320. doi: 10.1016/j.tcb.2013.11.008

Moriyama, M., and Ichinohe, T. (2019). High ambient temperature dampens adaptive immune responses to influenza a virus infection. *Proc. Natl. Acad. Sci. U.S.A.* 116, 3118–3125. doi: 10.1073/pnas.1815029116

Nonaka, K., Une, S., Komatsu, M., Yamaji, R., and Akiyama, J. (2018). Heat stress prevents the decrease in succinate dehydrogenase activity in the extensor digitorum longus of streptozotocin-induced diabetic rats. *Physiol. Res.* 67, 117–126. doi: 10.33549/physiolres.933617

Ren, J. G., Seth, P., Clish, C. B., Lorkiewicz, P. K., Higashi, R. M., Lane, A. N., et al. (2014). Knockdown of malic enzyme 2 suppresses lung tumor growth, induces differentiation and impacts PI3K/AKT signaling. *Sci. Rep.* 4:5414. doi: 10.1038/srep05414

Rendra, E., Riabov, V., Mossel, D. M., Sevastyanova, T., Harmsen, M. C., and Kzhyshkowska, J. (2019). Reactive oxygen species (ROS) in macrophage activation and function in diabetes. *Immunobiology.* 224, 242–253. doi: 10.1016/j.imbio.2018.11.010

Rubic, T., Lametschwandtner, G., Jost, S., Hinteregger, S., Kund, J., Carballido-Perrig, N., et al. (2008). Triggering the succinate receptor GPR91 on dendritic cells enhances immunity. *Nat. Immunol.* 9, 1261–1269. doi: 10.1038/ni.1657

Safi, R., Kallas, R., Bardawil, T., Mehanna, C. J., Abbas, O., Hamam, R., et al. (2018). Neutrophils contribute to vasculitis by increased release of neutrophil extracellular traps in Behcet's disease. *J. Dermatol. Sci.* 92, 143–150. doi: 10.1016/j.jdermsci.2018.08.010

Saraiva, A. L., Veras, F. P., Peres, R. S., Talbot, J., de Lima, K. A., Luiz, J. P., et al. (2018). Succinate receptor deficiency attenuates arthritis by reducing dendritic cell traffic and expansion of Th17 cells in the lymph nodes. *FASEB J.* fj201800285. doi: 10.1096/fj.201800285 [Epub ahead of print].

Shi, Y., and Wang, D. (2016). Implication of metabolomic profiles to wide thermoneutral zone in Mongolian gerbils (*Meriones unguiculatus*). *Integr. Zool.* 11, 282–294. doi: 10.1111/1749-4877.12179

Slawinska, A., Hsieh, J. C., Schmidt, C. J., and Lamont, S. J. (2016). Heat stress and lipopolysaccharide stimulation of chicken macrophage-like cell line activates expression of distinct sets of genes. *PLoS One.* 11:e0164575. doi: 10.1371/journal.pone.0164575

Sudarshan, S., Sourbier, C., Kong, H.-S., Block, K., Romero, V. A. V., Yang, Y., et al. (2009). Fumarate hydratase deficiency in renal cancer induces glycolytic addiction and hypoxia-inducible transcription factor 1α stabilization by glucose-dependent generation of reactive oxygen species. *Mol. Cell. Biol.* 29, 4080–4090. doi: 10.1128/mcb.00483-09

Tan, H., Pan, S., Zhong, Z., Shi, J., Liao, W., Su, G., et al. (2020). Association between temperature changes and uveitis onset in mainland China. *Br. J. Ophthalmol.* doi: 10.1136/bjophthalmol-2020-317007 [Epub ahead of print].

Tian Xiao, Y., Ganeshan, K., Hong, C., Nguyen Khoa, D., Qiu, Y., Kim, J., et al. (2016). Thermoneutral housing accelerates metabolic inflammation to potentiate atherosclerosis but not insulin resistance. *Cell Metab.* 23, 165–178. doi: 10.1016/j.cmet.2015.10.003

Tomiyama, C., Watanabe, M., Honma, T., Inada, A., Hayakawa, T., Ryufuku, M., et al. (2015). The effect of repetitive mild hyperthermia on body temperature, the autonomic nervous system, and innate and adaptive immunity. *Biomed Res.* 36, 135–142. doi: 10.2220/biomedres.36.135

Van den Broeck, W., Derore, A., and Simoens, P. (2006). Anatomy and nomenclature of murine lymph nodes: descriptive study and nomenclatory standardization in BALB/cAnNCrl mice. *J. Immunol. Methods* 312, 12–19. doi: 10.1016/j.jim.2006.01.022

Vorobjeva, N. V., and Pinegin, B. V. (2014). Neutrophil extracellular traps: mechanisms of formation and role in health and disease. *Biochem. (Mosc).* 79, 1286–1296. doi: 10.1134/s0006297914120025

Wang, J., Xue, X., Liu, Q., Zhang, S., Peng, M., Zhou, J., et al. (2019). Effects of duration of thermal stress on growth performance, serum oxidative stress indices, the expression and localization of ABCG2 and mitochondria ROS

production of skeletal muscle, small intestine and immune organs in broilers. *J. Therm. Biol.* 85:102420. doi: 10.1016/j.jtherbio.2019.102420

Wang, L., Zhou, X., Yin, Y., Mai, Y., Wang, D., and Zhang, X. (2019). Hyperglycemia induces neutrophil extracellular traps formation through an nadph oxidase-dependent pathway in diabetic retinopathy. *Front. Immunol.* 9:3076. doi: 10.3389/fimmu.2018.03076

Wang, Y., Wang, W., Wang, N., Tall, A. R., and Tabas, I. (2017). Mitochondrial oxidative stress promotes atherosclerosis and neutrophil extracellular traps in aged mice. *Arterioscler. Thromb. Vasc. Biol.* 37, e99–e107. doi: 10.1161/atvbaha.117.309580

Yang, P., Zhang, Z., Zhou, H., Li, B., Huang, X., Gao, Y., et al. (2005). Clinical patterns and characteristics of uveitis in a tertiary center for uveitis in China. *Curr. Eye Res.* 30, 943–948. doi: 10.1080/02713680500263606

Yuen, B. G., Tham, V. M., Browne, E. N., Weinrib, R., Borkar, D. S., Parker, J. V., et al. (2015). Association between smoking and uveitis: results from the pacific ocular inflammation study. *Ophthalmology* 122, 1257–1261. doi: 10.1016/j.ophtha.2015.02.034

Zhou, Q., Hou, S., Liang, L., Li, X., Tan, X., Wei, L., et al. (2014). MicroRNA-146a and Ets-1 gene polymorphisms in ocular Behcet's disease and Vogt-Koyanagi-Harada syndrome. *Ann. Rheum. Dis.* 73, 170–176. doi: 10.1136/annrheumdis-2012-201627

6

Automatic Artery/Vein Classification using a Vessel-Constraint Network for Multicenter Fundus Images

Jingfei Hu[1,2,3,4], Hua Wang[1,2,3,4], Zhaohui Cao[2], Guang Wu[2], Jost B. Jonas[5,6],
Ya Xing Wang[5]* and Jicong Zhang[1,2,3,4,7]*

[1] School of Biological Science and Medical Engineering, Beihang University, Beijing, China, [2] Hefei Innovation Research
Institute, Beihang University, Hefei, China, [3] Beijing Advanced Innovation Centre for Biomedical Engineering, Beihang
University, Beijing, China, [4] School of Biomedical Engineering, Anhui Medical University, Hefei, China, [5] Beijing Institute of
Ophthalmology, Beijing Tongren Hospital, Capital Medical University, Beijing Ophthalmology and Visual Sciences Key
Laboratory, Beijing, China, [6] Department of Ophthalmology, Medical Faculty Mannheim of the Ruprecht-Karls-University
Heidelberg, Mannheim, Germany, [7] Beijing Advanced Innovation Centre for Big Data-Based Precision Medicine, Beihang
University, Beijing, China

Correspondence:
Jicong Zhang
jicongzhang@buaa.edu.cn
Ya Xing Wang
yaxingw@gmail.com

Retinal blood vessel morphological abnormalities are generally associated with cardiovascular, cerebrovascular, and systemic diseases, automatic artery/vein (A/V) classification is particularly important for medical image analysis and clinical decision making. However, the current method still has some limitations in A/V classification, especially the blood vessel edge and end error problems caused by the single scale and the blurred boundary of the A/V. To alleviate these problems, in this work, we propose a vessel-constraint network (VC-Net) that utilizes the information of vessel distribution and edge to enhance A/V classification, which is a high-precision A/V classification model based on data fusion. Particularly, the VC-Net introduces a vessel-constraint (VC) module that combines local and global vessel information to generate a weight map to constrain the A/V features, which suppresses the background-prone features and enhances the edge and end features of blood vessels. In addition, the VC-Net employs a multiscale feature (MSF) module to extract blood vessel information with different scales to improve the feature extraction capability and robustness of the model. And the VC-Net can get vessel segmentation results simultaneously. The proposed method is tested on publicly available fundus image datasets with different scales, namely, DRIVE, LES, and HRF, and validated on two newly created multicenter datasets: Tongren and Kailuan. We achieve a balance accuracy of 0.9554 and F1 scores of 0.7616 and 0.7971 for the arteries and veins, respectively, on the DRIVE dataset. The experimental results prove that the proposed model achieves competitive performance in A/V classification and vessel segmentation tasks compared with state-of-the-art methods. Finally, we test the Kailuan dataset with other trained fusion datasets, the results also show good robustness. To promote research in this area, the Tongren dataset and source code will be made publicly available. The dataset and code will be made available at https://github.com/huawang123/VC-Net.

Keywords: vessel constraint, artery/vein classification, vessel segmentation, multi-center, data fusion

INTRODUCTION

Retinal blood vessels have attracted widespread research efforts as these vessels represent the only internal human vascular structures that can be observed noninvasively. Retinal vessel abnormalities reflect the cumulative damage caused by chronic diseases such diabetes and hypertension and represent an important risk indicator for many systemic and cardiovascular diseases (Wong et al., 2004). And the artery/vein (A/V) may be affected differently by variations in disease types and progression. For example, artery narrowing is mostly associated with arterial hypertension, whereas vein widening is related to increased brain pressure, stroke, and similar cardiovascular diseases. Hence, accurate image-based analysis and evaluation methods for the morphological evaluation of A/V changes might give an early insight and a deeper understanding of the pathophysiology of such diseases. The A/V caliber ratio (Wong et al., 2004) has been used as a predictor for cardiovascular diseases. Current clinical methods for retinal vessel segmentation and A/V classification mainly rely on manual segmentation. However, due to the high complexity and diversity of vessel structures, manual segmentation brings inevitable shortcomings, including being time-consuming and laborious, having inter-rater variability and subjectivity, and having lower efficiency and accuracy. Thus, automatic methods for A/V classification and vessel segmentation are highly desirable in clinical settings. The advantages and disadvantages of current clinical methods and automatic methods are shown in **Figure 1**.

In recent years, several automated techniques have been proposed for retinal A/V classification (Ishikawa et al., 2005; Fraz et al., 2012a; Orlando et al., 2017). These techniques may be categorized into graph-based (Dashtbozorg et al., 2014; Joshi et al., 2014; Estrada et al., 2015; Hu et al., 2015; Pellegrini et al., 2018; Srinidhi et al., 2019) and feature-based (Niemeijer et al., 2009; Zamperini et al., 2012; Mirsharif et al., 2013; Xu et al., 2017; Huang et al., 2018a,b) techniques. Yet, in graph-based approaches, difficulties may be encountered when some vascular regions cannot be segmented, and hence, vessel segments cannot be reliably linked (Welikala et al., 2017). Besides, for feature-based techniques, most recent studies use a two-stage approach for retinal A/V classification. Vessels are firstly segmented from the background; next, the segmented vessels are categorized into arteries and veins by using purely handcrafted features in feature-based methods or by merging edge information in graph-based methods. However, the two-stage approach suffers from the heavy dependence of the A/V classification outcomes on vessel segmentation accuracy. In fact, if the accuracy of blood vessel segmentation is low in the first stage, the A/V classification results will not be good either in the second stage.

With the development of deep learning, many convolutional neural network-based methods have been proposed for joint vessel segmentation and A/V classification. Xu et al. (2018) adopted an improved fully convolutional network (FCN) architecture to segment retinal arteries and veins simultaneously. This method enabled end-to-end multilabel segmentation of color fundus images. AlBadawi and Fraz (2018) proposed an FCN architecture with an encoder–decoder structure for

pixel-based A/V categorization. Meyer et al. (2018) also adopted the FCN architecture for A/V classification and demonstrated high performance on major vessels with thicknesses of more than three pixels. Hemelings et al. (2019) proposed a novel FCN-based U-Net architecture for simultaneous blood vessel semantic segmentation and A/V discrimination. Ma et al. (2019) proposed an enhanced deep architecture with a spatial activation mechanism for joint vessel segmentation and A/V identification. Li et al. (2020) made a highly confident prediction about the peripheral vessels by taking the structural information among vessels into account with post-processing.

However, automatic vessel segmentation and A/V classification are still considered difficult tasks due to the following challenges:

(1) The multiscale structure of blood vessels is easily overlooked. These methods focus on large-scale structures such as thick blood vessels, but the performance is poor for small-scale structures such as the edge and the end of thick blood vessels, as shown in **Figure 2D**.

(2) There is extreme imbalance between positive samples (blood vessels) and negative samples (non-vessel areas) in retinal fundus images, where blood vessels account for only 15% of the whole image. Correspondingly, the proportion of arteries and veins is only about 7.5% each. As a result, directly classifying the pixels of the retinal image as background, artery, and vein pixels is very challenging.

(3) Distinguishing between arteries and veins can be highly confusing. The results of the aforementioned methods still show poor localization performance between arteries and veins; for example, the same blood vessel may be half recognized as an artery and half as a vein, as shown in **Figure 2B**.

(4) The choroid is similar to blood vessels and is easy to misclassify.

Besides, most of these existing methods are only validated on specific datasets. However, in clinical applications, the performance would underperform when tested on datasets with a different image resolution, imaging equipment, and population. For example, when generalizing a trained model to datasets with different center scales, the performance of the model usually deteriorates. The characteristic differences of retinal fundus images among different scales will also influence the segmentation results. One possible solution to this problem is labeling some samples of the new dataset to fine-tune the pre-trained model, but this process is expensive and time-consuming.

In order to alleviate these challenges, in this work, we introduce a novel convolutional neural network for joint A/V classification and vessel segmentation in retinal fundus images, named the vessel-constraint network (VC-Net). Firstly, in order to alleviate challenge (1), the VC-Net employs a vessel-constraint (VC) module to enhance the microvessels and the edge of thick vessels by using Gaussian kernel function probability maps to enhance the feature weights of the blood vessel edge area. And the multiscale feature (MSF) module is proposed to extract and express blood vessel features at different scales in the encoder.

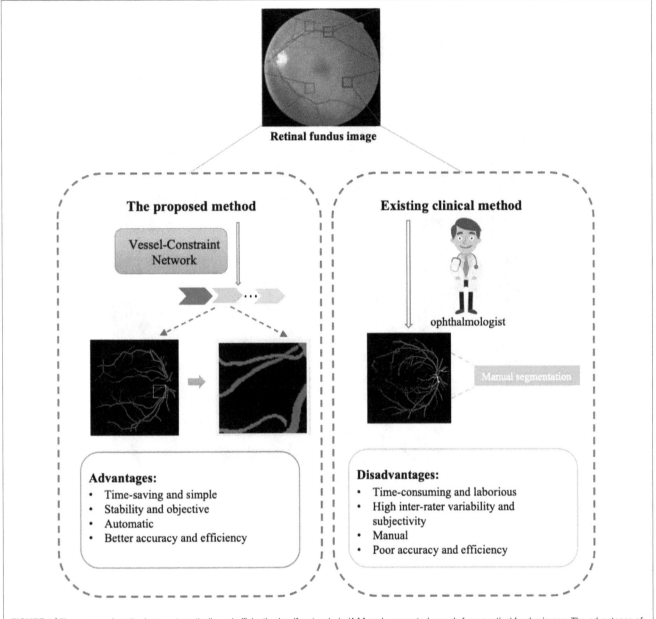

FIGURE 1 | The proposed method can automatically and efficiently classify artery/vein (A/V) and segmented vessels from a retinal fundus image. The advantages of this method are its great help to ophthalmologists compared with existing clinical methods.

Secondly, in order to alleviate challenges (2)–(4), the VC module combines the global and local vessel information to generate a weight map to constrain the A/V features, which suppresses the background features. Not only can this alleviate the imbalance of positive and negative samples, but this also pays more attention to the features of arteries and veins to achieve better A/V classification performance.

The key contributions of this study can be highlighted as follows:

- For the first time, we propose a VC-Net that uses vessel probability information to constrain A/V and enhance learning of discriminative A/V features. In addition, the VC-Net can also get blood vessel segmentation results simultaneously.

- The newly designed VC module is powerful in A/V feature extraction. The VC module is used to capture the distribution information of vessels as a weight to constrain the A/V features, which suppresses background-prone features to pay more attention to vessel features. Data fusion (DF) alleviates well the problem of imbalance between positive and negative samples and helps us learn more discriminative A/V features. At the same time, the VC module enhances the microvessels and the edge of thick vessels by using Gaussian kernel function probability maps to improve the feature weights of the blood vessel edge area.

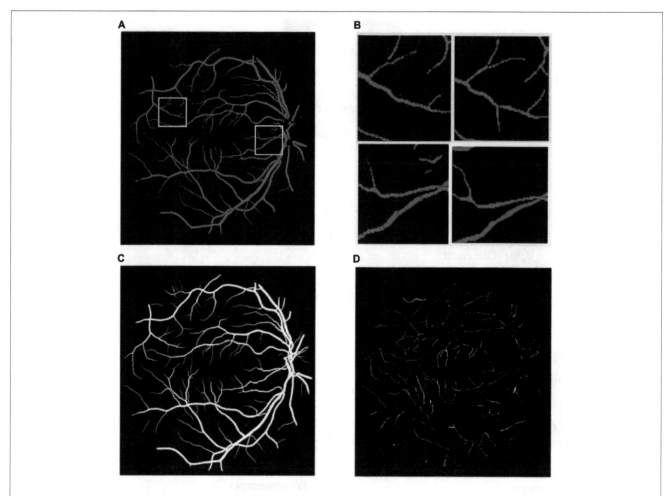

FIGURE 2 | Illustration of the challenges in classifying retinal blood vessels. The results shown in the figure are from U-Net. **(A)** The results map of artery and vein, **(B)** two regions of interest in panel **(A)** are magnified. Left is prediction and right is ground truth, **(C)** the probabilities of vessel, and **(D)** the vessel errors compared with ground truth.

- The MSF module of multiscale DF is proposed to extract and express blood vessel features at different scales in the encoder, where the diameters of the main vessels and microvessels vary greatly. The DF training strategy is applied to improve the robustness of the model by fusing information from datasets with different scales.
- We publicly released the Tongren dataset with ground truth annotation. The lack of retinal fundus image data with annotated label impedes further exploration of retinal vessel-related researches such as vessel segmentation and A/V classification in the deep-learning community. Therefore, we established a dataset to promote these studies with a detailed data description in the experimental setup section of this paper.

The rest of this paper is organized as follows. Firstly, we present the details of our proposed methodology in Section "Materials and Methods". Then, the descriptions of the datasets and the experimental details are described in Section "Experimental Setup". Next, our experimental results

are presented in Section "Results". Finally, the discussions and conclusions follow in Section "Discussion and Conclusion."

MATERIALS AND METHODS

The design details of the VC-Net are shown in **Figure 3**. Firstly, we propose a VC module to capture the DF feature of the distribution and edge information of the vessel and enhance the microvessel and the edge of thick vessels. Then the distribution and enhanced information are utilized as weights to activate the A/V features and enforce the A/V classification module to focus more on vessels and help us learn more discriminative A/V features, for extremely unbalanced vessel and background. In addition, we used the MSF module to extract blood vessel features at different scales for varied diameters of the main vessels and microvessels.

VC Module

In a retinal fundus image, blood vessels typically account for about 15% of the full image. Consequently, the area proportion

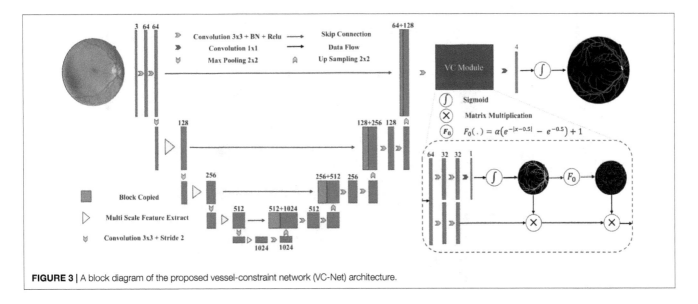

FIGURE 3 | A block diagram of the proposed vessel-constraint network (VC-Net) architecture.

of the arteries and veins is only about 7.5% each. Hence, directly classifying the retinal image pixels into background, artery, vein, and undecided pixels is a significant challenge task due to the high-class imbalance and the scarcity of training samples. To alleviate this problem, we designed a VC module at the end of the framework to enhance A/V classification.

The VC module combines the local and global vessel information to generate a weight map to constrain the A/V features, which suppresses the background-prone features to pay more attention to vessel features. In this way, it can alleviate the problem of severe imbalance between positive and negative samples. At the same time, we introduced Gaussian kernel function probability maps to improve feature weights of microvessels and the blood vessel edge area, thereby enhancing the feature representation of microvessels and the edge of thick vessels. The Gaussian activation function of the VC module is defined as

$$F(x) = \alpha \left(e^{-|x-0.5|} - e^{-0.5} \right) + 1$$

Where x belongs to the probability map of the whole blood vessel segmentation, with values between 0 and 1, and α is a fixed parameter (set to 1 in this experiment).

The function $F(x)$ further focuses on local vessel information, such as vascular boundaries and microvascular areas. Based on experimental observations and earlier studies, the probability of misclassifying vessel pixels is essentially concentrated around 0.5. These misclassified pixels come either from the vessel-background boundary or the microvascular areas whose features are not obvious and difficult to distinguish from the background. The background and thick vessel pixels have a value near 0 or 1.

Through the function $F(x)$, the activation weight value of a pixel with a probability close to 0.5 was increased to $[\alpha(1 - e^{-0.5}) + 1]$, while the activation weight values of the background and main thick vessels were set close to 1. The activation function constrains the activation weight value to be within $[1, \alpha(1 - e^{-0.5}) + 1]$. Note that $F(0.5 + x_1), x_1 \in [0, 0.5]$.

Multiscale Feature

As shown in **Figure 4**, the scale of blood vessels varies greatly in retinal fundus images. On the one hand, the average artery diameter is generally slightly smaller than the average vein diameter. On the other hand, the average diameter for the main blood vessels is much larger than that of the capillaries.

Therefore, we use the capabilities of the pre-trained Res2Net (Gao et al., 2019) model to learn and understand the retinal vessel image features at different scales in the encoder stage. Instead of extracting features using 3×3 filter groups as in the ResNet (He et al., 2016) bottleneck block (**Figure 5A**), smaller filter groups connected in a hierarchical residual-type manner are used (**Figure 5B**). After the 1×1 convolutional stage, the features are split into k subsets, where the ith subset is denoted by x_i, where $i \in \{1, 2, ..., k\}$. While all subsets have the same spatial size, the channel count for each subset is $1/k$ times that of the input feature map. Each subset x_i (except for x_1) has a 3×3 convolutional filter $F_i()$. Thus, the filter output y_i can be written as

$$y_i = \begin{cases} x_i & i = 1; \\ F_i(x_i) & i = 2; \\ F_i((x_i; y_{i-1})) & 2 < i \leq k. \end{cases}$$

Each 3×3 convolutional operator $F_i()$ might get information from all feature subsets $\{x_j, j \leq i\}$. When a feature subset x_j is processed by a 3×3 convolutional operator, the output result may have an enlarged receptive field compared to x_j.

Here, the scale dimension k is used as a control parameter. A larger k value enables learning features with larger receptive field sizes, with insignificant computation and memory overheads due to concatenation.

Loss Function

We employ an end-to-end deep-learning scheme as our underlying framework. The A/V loss is quantified by the

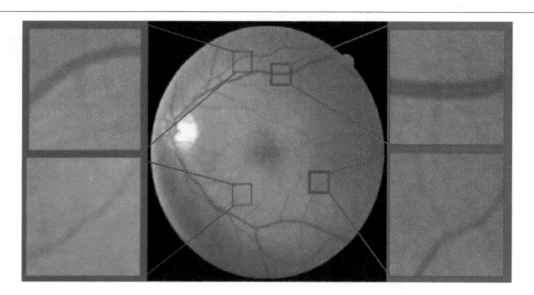

FIGURE 4 | Arteries and veins of different scales in the retinal fundus images. *Top left* a major artery. *Top right* a major vein. *Bottom left* a minor artery. *Bottom right* a minor vein.

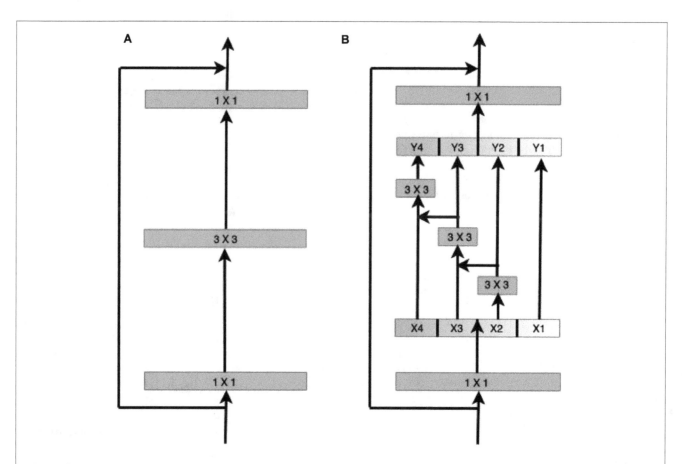

FIGURE 5 | Comparison of the ResNet and Res2Net blocks (with a scale dimension of *k* = 4). **(A)** The conventional ResNet building block in CNN architectures. **(B)** The multi-scale feature (MSF) module of Res2Net uses a group of 3 × 3 filters.

commonly used cross-entropy loss function

$$L\_AV_{ce} = -\frac{1}{n}\sum_{i=1}^{n}\left(y_i\log\left(y_i'\right) + (1 - y_i)\log\left(1 - y_i'\right)\right)$$

While the vessel segmentation loss is quantified by the binary cross-entropy

$$L\_V_{bce} = -\frac{1}{n}\sum_{c=0}^{1}\sum_{i=1}^{n} y_i\log\left(y_i'\right)$$

Where n denotes the number of pixels in the input image, y' is the predicted output probability of a foreground pixel, y is the ground-truth pixel label, and c denotes the cth class of the output. The total loss is defined as

$$\text{Loss} = \gamma * L\_AV_{ce} + \delta * L\_V_{bce} + \beta * \|W\|_2^2$$

Where $\gamma = 0.6$, $\delta = 0.4$, and $\delta + \gamma = 1$. We use L_2 regularization with a weight of $\beta = 0.0002$.

EXPERIMENTAL SETUP

In this section, we describe the used retinal image datasets, the evaluation metrics for retinal vessel segmentation and A/V classification, and the VC-Net training details.

Datasets

In this work, we evaluated our approach and assessed its clinical applicability on five retinal fundus image datasets of different scales. Three datasets are publicly available while the other two were collected by authors. In order to validate the generalization performance and robustness of our method by DF experiments, we specifically annotated two multiscale datasets. An overview of these datasets is given in **Table 1**.

DRIVE

Our model was firstly trained and tested on the publicly available DRIVE database (Hu et al., 2013). This database contains 40 color retinal fundus images with image dimensions of 584 × 565 pixels. These images were evenly divided into training and test sets with 20 images in each set. Pixel-wise labeling is provided for vessel segmentation and A/V classification.

LES

The LES dataset (Orlando et al., 2018) contains 22 images with a 30° field of view (FOV) and a resolution of 1,444 × 1,620 pixels for 21 images and a 45° FOV and a resolution of 1,958 × 2,196 pixels for one image. The images are equally divided into training and test sets with 11 images in each set.

HRF

The HRF dataset (Odstrcilik et al., 2013) contains 45 images equally divided among three categories, namely, healthy subjects, patients with diabetic retinopathy, and patients with glaucoma. Images were captured with an FOV of 60° and a pixel resolution of 3,304 × 2,336. Only one ground-truth segmentation map is available for each image. For each category, five images are used for training and the rest are used for testing.

Tongren

The Tongren clinical dataset contains 30 representative retinal fundus images with a 45° FOV and a resolution of 1,888 × 2,816 pixels, within which 20 images were normal and 10 images were of moderate cataract or retinal diseases including glaucoma, age-related macular degeneration, and retinal vein occlusion. An approval was obtained from the Ethics Committee of Beijing Tongren Hospital. The ocular fundus had been taken with a fundus camera (CR6-45NM camera, Canon Inc., Ota, Tokyo, Japan). These images were labeled by two experienced ophthalmologists with the ITK-SNAP toolkit (Yushkevich et al., 2006). For each category, half of the images are used for training, and the rest are used for testing.

Kailuan

The Kailuan database contains 30 images which were collected from participants of the community-based Kailuan Cohort Study (Jiang et al., 2015). These images have different sizes. The minimum, average, and maximum heights are 1,588, 1,902, and 2,112. The minimum, average, and maximum widths are 1,586, 1,901, and 2,112. We used 15 images for training and the rest for testing. Also, these images were labeled by experienced ophthalmologists with the ITK-SNAP toolkit (Yushkevich et al., 2006).

The binary ground-truth segmentation maps for the DRIVE, LES, and HRF images are publicly available. For the Tongren and Kailuan images, we have manually created FOV masks using methods similar to those of Soares et al. (2006), **Figure 6** shows samples of Tongren and Kailuan datasets.

Evaluation Metrics

The retinal vessel segmentation outcomes of the proposed method were compared against those of other reference methods using several metrics, namely, sensitivity (SE), specificity (SP), accuracy (ACC), the area under the ROC curve (AUC), and the F1 score (F1). The binary segmentation maps were generated through thresholding the probability maps with a 0.5 threshold.

For A/V classification, five performance evaluation metrics were adopted. We interpret arteries as positives and veins as negatives. The A/V sensitivity (SE_{AV}) and specificity (SP_{AV})

TABLE 1 | Overview of datasets used for artery/vein (A/V) classification and vessel segmentation.

Datasets	# images	Resolution
DRIVE (Hu et al., 2013)	40	584 × 565
LES (Orlando et al., 2018)	22	1,444 × 1,620, 1,958 × 2,196
HRF (Odstrcilik et al., 2013)	45	3,304 × 2,336
Tongren	30	1,888 × 2,816
Kailuan	30	(1,588–2,112) × (1,586–2,112)

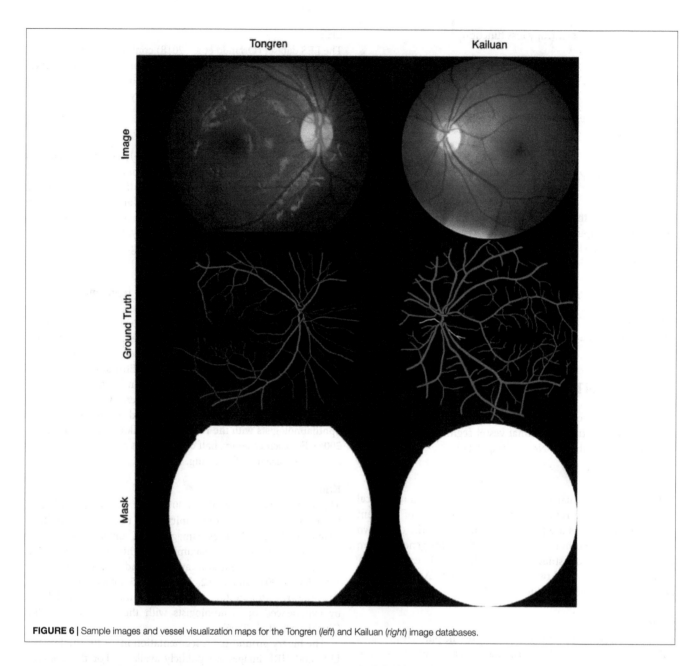

FIGURE 6 | Sample images and vessel visualization maps for the Tongren (*left*) and Kailuan (*right*) image databases.

reflect the model capability for correctly detecting arteries and veins, respectively. The balance accuracy (BACC) quantifies the overall performance of the model. These metrics are defined as follows.

$$SE_{AV} = \frac{TP}{TP + FN}$$

$$SP_{AV} = \frac{TN}{TN + FP}$$

$$BACC = \frac{SE_{AV} + SP_{AV}}{2}$$

Where TP is the count of the correctly classified artery pixels, TN is the count of the correctly classified vein pixels, FP is the count

of the vein pixels misclassified as artery pixels, and FN is the count of the artery pixels misclassified as vein pixels.

In addition, we compute the F1 score for arteries ($F1_A$) and the F1 score for veins ($F1_V$) when arteries and veins represent the relevant samples, respectively. The optimal value for each of these metrics is 1. Computations were restricted to pixels within the FOV.

Network Training Details

Few training samples are available in each of the five databases and are hence insufficient for handling model complexity. To alleviate this problem, several data augmentation strategies (Fraz et al., 2012b; Maninis et al., 2016; Feng et al., 2017; Oliveira et al., 2018; Guo et al., 2019) have been explored, including image scaling with different scale factors and image rotation by different angles. As no prior knowledge is available on the appropriate patch size selection, patches with a size of 512 × 512 were randomly picked from the retinal images and used for network training. For each test image, ordered patches were collected, and the final segmentation and classification outcomes were found by stitching together the associated patch predictions. A stochastic gradient descent algorithm with momentum was employed for optimizing model parameters with a maximum of 4,000 iterations. The learning rate was initially set to 0.001 and then cut in half every 1,500 iterations. Method implementations were carried out using a PyTorch backend the NVIDIA CUDA® Deep Neural Network library (cuDNN 9.0), and an Intel® Xeon® Gold 6148 CPU with a processor of 2.40 GHz, a RAM of 256 GB, and an Ubuntu 16.04 operating system.

RESULTS

In this section, we introduce the results of the experiment. Firstly, we conduct a series of ablation studies to systematically analyze the effectiveness of each component of the proposed network and its impacts on overall segmentation performance. Then, we apply our method to the aforementioned datasets and compare it with state-of-the-art methods. Finally, we verify the effectiveness of the DF strategy to address the challenges in new datasets.

Ablation Studies

Detailed ablation studies have been conducted to evaluate the contribution of each module of the proposed VC-Net architecture. These modules include the basic U-Net module, the MSF in the encoder, and the VC module for A/V classification. In **Table 2**, the first two methods apply direct recognition of retinal fundus images into background, artery, vein, and undecided pixels. Based on the recognition results, vessel segmentation indicators are calculated. The proposed method was used for vessel segmentation and A/V classification simultaneously; performance indices were calculated accordingly.

As shown in **Table 2**, the A/V classification results have been significantly improved with the addition of MSF. The MSF can extract and express the vessel features with different scales in the encoder to solve the varying diameters of the main vessels and microvessels. Remarkably, the blood vessel classification performance has been further improved to a certain extent by using the VC module; our results show that we achieved 0.9483, 0.9327, 0.9547, 0.7428, and 0.7880 on BACC, SE_{AV}, SP_{AV}, $F1_A$,

and $F1_V$, respectively. The VC module can suppress background-prone features to pay more attention to vessel features; it alleviates well the problem of positive and negative sample imbalance and helps us learn more discriminative A/V features. At the same time, the VC module can enhance the feature representation of microvessels and the edge of thick vessels. More importantly, from **Table 2**, we can see that the combination of U-Net, MSF, and VC modules achieves the best results with a BACC of 0.9542, SE_{AV} of 0.9351, SP_{AV} of 0.9732, $F1_A$ of 0.7605, and $F1_V$ of 0.7971. Therefore, the ablation study demonstrates the effectiveness of the proposed modules.

As shown in **Figure 7**, we visualized the A/V classification results for different modules of the proposed VC-Net architecture. In particular, results for four regions of interest were highlighted and magnified. We can see that A/V classification results of the U-Net are poor, where arteries and veins are seriously confused, and that there are many misclassifications at the edges and ends of blood vessels. With the introduction of MSF, the A/V classification results have been improved, but there is still the problem of arteries and veins being confused near the crossing and branching points of blood vessels. Obviously, in comparison with other models, we proposed the VC-Net as it achieves better A/V classification results both locally and globally. The above analysis proves that our model certainly improves the overall A/V classification performance.

As we can see, the VC-Net model outperformed other methods based on performance metrics and visualization results. In addition, we also explored the influence of varying the α parameter values on the VC-Net model performance. Specifically, we trained the model from scratch with different α values, ranging from 0.4 to 1.6. The results are shown in **Table 3**. For A/V classification, the BACC, SE_{AV}, $F1_A$, and $F1_V$ metrics increased with the decrease in α. Nevertheless, the increase between α = 0.4 and α = 0.6 was very small, and there was even a small decrease in $F1_A$ and $F1_V$. For vessel segmentation, α approaches 1.0–1.4, and the indicators show good performance. Therefore, the α value should be adjusted according to different scenarios. If a larger SE_{AV} value is desired, the α value can be appropriately reduced to train a model from scratch.

After training the VC-Net model, we varied the α values in the trained model to test the model performance on the test dataset. The results are shown in **Table 4**. Obviously, with the decrease of α, most indicators are increased except SE, F1, and $F1_V$. As a bonus and as SE is increased with α, the effectiveness of the VC model is verified from the side. When a model has been trained, if a larger indicator for A/V classification is needed, α can be appropriately reduced. And if a lager SE is needed, α can be appropriately increased.

Comparison With Existing Methods on the DRIVE Dataset

We compared the VC-Net performance with that of other state-of-the-art methods on the DRIVE dataset for vessel segmentation and A/V classification tasks. **Table 5** summarizes the vessel segmentation comparison results. As seen, the proposed VC-Net shows superior segmentation performance in terms of AUC

TABLE 2 | Results of the ablation study for A/V classification (α = 1.0).

Methods			A/V classification				
U-Net	MSF	VC	BACC	SE_{AV}	SP_{AV}	$F1_A$	$F1_V$
✓	×	×	0.9118	0.8950	0.9287	0.7089	0.7586
✓	✓	×	0.9481	0.9251	0.9711	0.7433	0.7861
✓	×	✓	0.9483	0.9327	0.9547	0.7428	0.7880
✓	✓	✓	**0.9542**	**0.9351**	**0.9732**	**0.7605**	**0.7971**

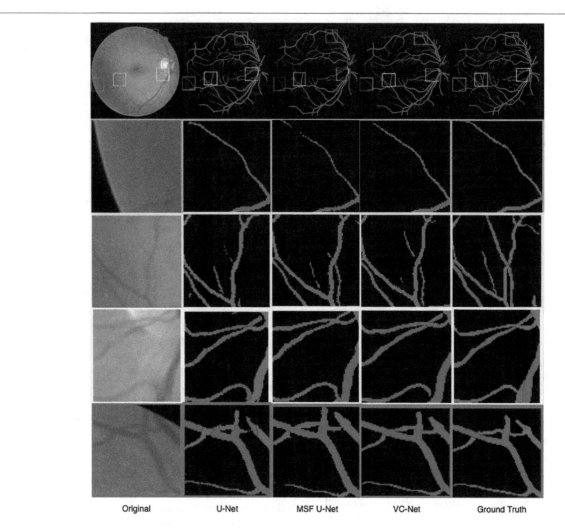

FIGURE 7 | Retinal fundus images and vessel maps for different modules. Four regions of interest are highlighted and magnified in rows 2–5.

TABLE 3 | The effect of α on vessel segmentation and classification training (VC-Net model training from scratch).

α	Segmentations					A/V classification				
	ACC	SE	SP	AUC	F1	BACC	SE_{AV}	SP_{AV}	$F1_A$	$F1_V$
0.4	0.9566	0.8302	0.9755	0.9799	0.8290	**0.9570**	**0.9405**	0.9735	0.7633	0.7988
0.6	0.9565	0.8311	0.9752	0.9801	0.8287	0.9568	0.9397	0.9740	**0.7634**	**0.7989**
0.8	0.9565	0.8305	0.9753	0.9803	0.8286	0.9563	0.9385	0.9740	0.7622	0.7985
1.0	**0.9570**	0.8258	**0.9766**	0.9812	**0.8296**	0.9542	0.9351	0.9732	0.7605	0.7971
1.2	0.9568	0.8288	0.9759	0.9804	0.8294	0.9535	0.9357	0.9714	0.7616	0.7954
1.4	0.9557	**0.8475**	0.9720	**0.9814**	0.8290	0.9540	0.9352	0.9728	0.7607	0.7963
1.6	0.9565	0.8261	0.9763	0.9811	0.8289	0.9564	0.9354	**0.9773**	0.7595	0.7963

and F1. In **Table 6**, the existing methods are evaluated for the classification performance on the segmented vessels only. On the contrary, we evaluated the VC-Net performance on all A/V ground-truth pixels. This evaluation is more challenging than that on the segmented vessels, since the identification of major vessels is an easier task if the capillary vessels are not segmented. The comparison with existing methods under the same criteria shows superior performance of our model, which achieves a BACC of 0.9554, SE_{AV} of 0.9360, SP_{AV} of 0.9748, $F1_A$ of 0.7616, and $F1_V$ of 0.7964. Indeed, our model surpasses the current best A/V classification method due to the introduction of the VC module.

TABLE 4 | The effect of α on vessel segmentation and classification testing (the VC-Net model has been trained).

α	Segmentations				A/V classification				
	ACC	SE	SP	F1	BACC	SE_{AV}	SP_{AV}	$F1_A$	$F1_V$
0.4	0.9574	0.7848	**0.9830**	0.8236	**0.9554**	**0.9360**	**0.9748**	**0.7616**	0.7964
0.6	**0.9575**	0.8015	0.9807	0.8270	0.9549	0.9356	0.9742	0.7615	0.7968
0.8	0.9573	0.8148	0.9786	0.8287	0.9545	0.9354	0.9737	0.7612	0.7970
1.0	0.9570	0.8258	0.9766	0.8296	0.9542	0.9351	0.9732	0.7605	0.7971
1.2	0.9566	0.8351	0.9748	**0.8299**	0.9539	0.9349	0.9729	0.7599	**0.7973**
1.4	0.9562	0.8429	0.9732	0.8298	0.9536	0.9348	0.9725	0.7587	0.7970
1.6	0.9557	**0.8496**	0.9716	0.8293	0.9535	0.9346	0.9723	0.7573	0.7966

TABLE 5 | Vessel segmentation results of vessel-constraint network (VC-Net) and other existing methods on the DRIVE dataset.

Methods	ACC	SE	SP	AUC	F1
U-Net (Ronneberger et al., 2015)	0.9541	**0.8319**	0.9713	0.9750	0.8162
DDNet (Mou et al., 2019a)	0.9594	0.8126	0.9788	0.9796	N/A
AC_Net (Ma et al., 2019)	0.9570	0.7916	0.9811	0.9810	N/A
CS-Net (Mou et al., 2019b)	**0.9632**	0.8170	**0.9854**	0.9798	N/A
CE-Net (Gu et al., 2019)	0.9545	0.8309	0.9747	0.9779	N/A
RU-Net (Alom et al., 2018)	0.9556	0.7792	0.9813	0.9784	0.8171
BTS-UNet (Guo et al., 2019)	0.9551	0.7800	0.9806	0.9796	0.8208
DE-UNet (Wang et al., 2019)	0.9567	0.7940	0.9816	0.9772	0.8270
VC-Net (α = 1)	0.9570	0.8258	0.9766	**0.9812**	**0.8296**

N/A, not available.

TABLE 6 | Artery/vein (A/V) classification results of VC-Net and other existing methods on the DRIVE dataset.

Methods	BACC	SE_{AV}	SP_{AV}	$F1_A$	$F1_V$
Dashtbozorg et al., 2014	0.8740	0.9000	0.8400	N/A	N/A
Estrada et al., 2015	0.9350	0.9300	0.9410	N/A	N/A
U-Net (Ronneberger et al., 2015)	0.9122	0.9145	0.9083	0.7089	0.7586
Xu et al., 2017	0.9230	0.9290	0.9150	N/A	N/A
DOS (Zhao et al., 2018)	N/A	0.9190	0.9150	N/A	N/A
AC_Net (Ma et al., 2019)	0.9450	0.9340	0.9550	N/A	N/A
VC-Net (α = 1)	0.9542	0.9351	0.9732	0.7605	**0.7971**
VC-Net (α = 0.4)	**0.9554**	**0.9360**	**0.9748**	**0.7616**	0.7964

In particular, for **Table 6**, it is noteworthy that VC-Net has outperformed existing methods in terms of all metrics in identifying arteries and veins. This performance superiority is mainly due to the fact that the vessel activation map not only enhanced the vascular boundaries and microvessels but also strengthened the main thick vessels, suppressed the background, and hence enabled the model to learn more vessel features. Besides, the vessel activation map eliminated the imbalance between the background and the blood vessel samples to a certain extent.

Comparison With Existing Methods on Other Datasets

The proposed VC-Net was also compared with existing methods on two other public datasets and two collected datasets. For vessel segmentation, the results on the LES and HRF public datasets are shown in **Table 7**. Clearly, VC-Net achieved significantly better

TABLE 7 | Performance comparison for different vessel segmentation methods on the LES and HRF datasets.

Datasets	Methods	Vessel segmentation				
		ACC	SE	SP	AUC	F1
LES	FC-CRF (Orlando et al., 2017)	N/A	0.7874	0.9584	0.9359	0.7158
	Jloss (Yan et al., 2018)	0.9400	0.7900	0.9600	N/A	N/A
	VC-Net (α = 1)	0.9722	0.8504	0.9840	0.9821	0.8417
HRF	DNN (Samuel and Veeramalai, 2019)	0.8531	**0.8655**	0.8523	0.9665	N/A
	UA_VA (Galdran et al., 2019)	0.9100	0.8500	0.9100	0.9400	0.6200
	MF-Net (Odstrcilik et al., 2013)	0.9494	0.7741	0.9669	0.9670	0.7316
	FCN-TL (Jiang et al., 2018)	0.9662	0.7686	0.9826	0.9770	N/A
	VC-Net (α = 1)	0.9663	0.7903	**0.9843**	0.9806	0.8101

TABLE 8 | Performance comparison of different A/V classification methods on the LES and HRF datasets.

Datasets	Methods	A/V classification				
		BACC	SE$_{AV}$	SP$_{AV}$	F1$_A$	F1$_V$
LES	UA_VA (Galdran et al., 2019)	0.8600	0.8800	0.8500	N/A	N/A
	VC-Net (α = 1)	**0.9446**	**0.9425**	**0.9467**	**0.7635**	**0.7988**
HRF	**VC-Net (α = 1)**	**0.9646**	**0.9588**	**0.9704**	**0.7389**	**0.7839**

results with an ACC of 0.9663, SP of 0.9843, AUC of 0.9806, and F1 of 0.8101 in the HRF-AV dataset.

The A/V classification outcomes are shown in **Table 8**. It can be seen that all indicators have been significantly improved compared to those in UA_VA (Galdran et al., 2019) on the LES dataset. In particular, the BACC, SE$_{AV}$, and SP$_{AV}$ metrics increased by 9.84, 7.10, and 11.38%, respectively. Moreover, the VC-Net also showed excellent performance on the HRF dataset

with a BACC of 0.9646. The above results once again demonstrate the excellent performance of VC-Net.

In addition, we tested the VC-Net performance for blood vessel segmentation and A/V classification on the two collected Tongren and Kailuan datasets. The results are shown in **Table 9**. For the Tongren dataset, there were significant improvements compared with the previous methods. Specifically, the ACC, BACC, F1$_A$, and F1$_V$ metrics for VC-Net were improved by 0.39, 4.41, 6.43, and 7.44%, respectively, in comparison with the basic U-Net method. And the VC-Net achieved better results with an SP of 0.9767, F1 of 0.7974, F1$_A$ of 0.7221, and F1$_V$ of 0.7741 on the Kailuan dataset. The experimental results demonstrate that our method achieves competitive performance for A/V classification and vessel segmentation.

Segmentation Results of Challenging Images

Sample images from the above-mentioned five databases and the corresponding predicted and ground-truth vessel maps are

TABLE 9 | Vessel segmentation and A/V classification performance of different methods on the Tongren and Kailuan datasets (α = 1).

Datasets	Methods	Segmentations					A/V classification				
		ACC	SE	SP	AUC	F1	BACC	SE$_{AV}$	SP$_{AV}$	F1$_A$	F1$_V$
Tongren	U-Net (Ronneberger et al., 2015)	0.9637	**0.8283**	0.9752	0.9813	0.7798	0.9068	0.9138	0.9018	0.6903	0.7208
	S-UNet (Hu et al., 2019)	0.9652	0.7822	0.9830	**0.9824**	0.7994	N/A	N/A	N/A	N/A	N/A
	VC-Net	**0.9675**	0.7705	**0.9863**	0.9819	**0.8048**	**0.9468**	**0.9421**	**0.9516**	**0.7347**	**0.7744**
Kailuan	VC-Net	**0.9516**	**0.7961**	**0.9767**	**0.9766**	**0.7974**	**0.9442**	**0.9413**	**0.9472**	**0.7221**	**0.7741**

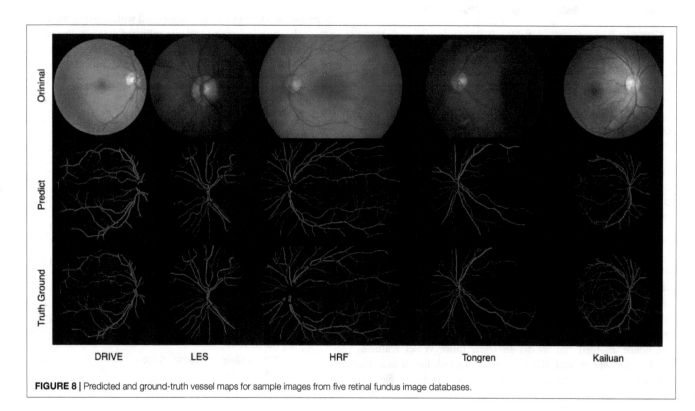

FIGURE 8 | Predicted and ground-truth vessel maps for sample images from five retinal fundus image databases.

TABLE 10 | The model is trained under the selected training dataset and tested under the Kailuan dataset with multiscale.

Training datasets			A/V classification				
DRIVE	LES	HRF	BACC	SE_{AV}	SP_{AV}	$F1_A$	$F1_V$
✓	✗	✗	0.6086	0.4721	0.7451	0.2052	0.2870
✗	✓	✗	0.8776	0.8942	0.8610	0.6273	0.6803
✗	✗	✓	0.9251	0.8876	**0.9626**	0.6504	0.7375
✓	✓	✓	**0.9412**	**0.9297**	0.9562	**0.6790**	**0.7449**

shown in **Figure 8**. Accurate segmentation of challenging images proves the effectiveness of our method. For the DRIVE and HRF datasets, both the overall and local vessel segmentation and A/V classification results are excellent with considerable continuity. Good results were achieved also on the other datasets, although the local results are not as well as those of the DRIVE and HRF datasets. Due to computational limitations, only patch-level networks can be trained on large-scale datasets, and hence, the results can be inferior to whole-image networks.

Evaluation Results on Unseen Datasets With Multiscale DF

Data fusion is a fundamental step to deal with the new data problem. To improve the robustness of the proposed model, DF from datasets with different scales could enrich the amount of training data and data distribution and could be validated on a new dataset with multiscale. We define this training strategy as DF training.

The first three rows of **Table 10** were only trained on the DRIVE, LES, or HRF datasets and tested on the Kailuan dataset. Finally, the three datasets combined and shuffled the images. The fused data are used as the training dataset and tested under the Kailuan dataset. It can be seen that the best results have been achieved on most indicators on the Kailuan dataset after DF. As a bonus, the DF training can enhance the robustness of the model, and it is more suitable for testing on new datasets.

DISCUSSION AND CONCLUSION

In this paper, we propose a VC network that utilizes information of vessel distribution and edge to enhance A/V classification. The proposed VC module combines local and global vessel information to generate a more reasonable weight map to constrain the A/V features, which suppresses the background-prone features and enhances the edge and end features of blood vessels. Meanwhile, we used an MSF module to obtain multiscale vessel features, such as the main thick vessels, vascular boundaries, and microvascular regions. Our method achieves better blood vessel segmentation and A/V classification performance. More importantly, we adopt the DF strategy to improve the robustness and generalization ability of the proposed model.

The VC-Net model demonstrates the effectiveness on multiscale and multicenter datasets. It outperforms existing methods and achieves state-of-the-art results for A/V classification and vessel segmentation on three public datasets. And the proposed model was tested on multicenter datasets: Tongren and Kailuan; the results indicate the superior generalization capability of the network. In addition, this model shows better performance on datasets with different resolutions. The visualized vessel maps reflect the importance of the MSF extraction module in our model and the excellent overall control of the global and detailed features by the VC module. In particular, to promote the development of this field, we collected two retinal fundus image datasets (Tongren and Kailuan), which labeled the arteries and veins with the ITK-SNAP toolkit, and we will be releasing the Tongren dataset.

One of the limitations of our work is that large-scale fundus images cannot be accommodated by the network; such images should be reduced to patches of a reasonable size to facilitate the training and testing processes. This patch-based approach distorts the global view of capillaries and large vessels. The other limitation is that computational resources are highly demanding. Therefore, we hope to use our work as a basis to further analyze the performance of vessel segmentation and A/V classification algorithms for large-scale fundus images and improve the utilization of computational resources.

In the future, we will deploy our algorithm to mobile terminals and develop an automatic retinal blood vessel analysis system, which is more conducive to clinicians' understanding and use of this algorithm and promotes the diagnosis of ophthalmology and systemic diseases.

AUTHOR CONTRIBUTIONS

JH: formal analysis, investigation, methodology, software, validation, and writing–original draft. HW: investigation, software, validation, and writing–original draft. ZC and GW: investigation and revise manuscript. JJ: supervision. YW: resources and supervision. JZ: funding acquisition, project administration, resources, and supervision. All authors contributed to the article and approved the submitted version.

REFERENCES

AlBadawi, S., and Fraz, M. M. (2018). "Arterioles and venules classification in retinal images using fully convolutional deep neural network," in *Proceedings of the International Conference Image Analysis and Recognition, Póvoa de Varzim, Portuga*, (Cham: Springer), 659–668. doi: 10.1007/978-3-319-93000-8_75

Alom, M. Z., Hasan, M., Yakopcic, C., Taha, T. M., and Asari, V. K. (2018). Recurrent residual convolutional neural network based on u-net (r2u-net) for medical image segmentation. *arXiv* [Preprint] arXiv:1802.06955,

Dashtbozorg, B., Mendonça, A. M., and Campilho, A. (2014). An automatic graph-based approach for artery/vein classification in retinal images. *IEEE Trans. Image Process.* 23, 1073–1083. doi: 10.1109/TIP.2013.2263809

Estrada, R., Allingham, M. J., Mettu, P. S., Cousins, S. W., Tomasi, C., and Farsiu, S. (2015). Retinal artery-vein classification via topology estimation. *IEEE Trans. Med. Imaging* 34, 2518–2534. doi: 10.1109/TMI.2015.2443117

Feng, Z., Yang, J., and Yao, L. (2017). "Patch-based fully convolutional neural network with skip connections for retinal blood vessel segmentation," in *Proceedings of the 2017 IEEE International Conference on Image Processing (ICIP)*, (Beijing: IEEE), 1742–1746. doi: 10.1109/ICIP.2017.8296580

Fraz, M. M., Remagnino, P., Hoppe, A., Uyyanonvara, B., Rudnicka, A. R., Owen, C. G., et al. (2012a). Blood vessel segmentation methodologies in retinal images–a survey. *Comput. Methods Programs Biomed.* 108, 407–433.

Fraz, M. M., Remagnino, P., Hoppe, A., Uyyanonvara, B., Rudnicka, A. R., Owen, C. G., et al. (2012b). An ensemble classification-based approach applied to retinal blood vessel segmentation. *IEEE Trans. Biomed. Eng.* 59, 2538–2548. doi: 10.1109/TBME.2012.2205687

Galdran, A., Meyer, M., Costa, P., and Campilho, A. (2019). "Uncertainty-aware artery/Vein classification on retinal images," in *Proceedings of the 2019 IEEE 16th International Symposium on Biomedical Imaging (ISBI 2019)*, (Venice: IEEE), 556–560. doi: 10.1109/ISBI.2019.8759380

Gao, S., Cheng, M. M., Zhao, K., Zhang, X. Y., Yang, M. H., and Torr, P. H. (2019). Res2net: a new multi-scale backbone architecture. *IEEE Trans. Pattern Anal. Mach. Intell.* 43, 652–662. doi: 10.1109/TPAMI.2019.2938758

Gu, Z., Cheng, J., Fu, H., Zhou, K., Hao, H., Zhao, Y., et al. (2019). CE-Net: context encoder network for 2D medical image segmentation. *IEEE Trans. Med. Imaging* 38, 2281–2292. doi: 10.1109/TMI.2019.2903562

Guo, S., Wang, K., Kang, H., Zhang, Y., Gao, Y., and Li, T. (2019). BTS-DSN: Deeply supervised neural network with short connections for retinal vessel segmentation. *Int. J. Med. Inf.* 126, 105–113. doi: 10.1016/j.ijmedinf.2019.03.015

He, K., Zhang, X., Ren, S., and Sun, J. (2016). "Deep residual learning for image recognition," in *Proceedings of the IEEE Conference on Computer Vision and Pattern Recognition*, (Las Vegas, NV: IEEE), 770–778.

Hemelings, R., Elen, B., Stalmans, I., Van Keer, K., De Boever, P., and Blaschko, M. B. (2019). Artery-vein segmentation in fundus images using a fully convolutional network. *Comput. Med. Imaging Graph.* 76:101636. doi: 10.1016/j.compmedimag.2019.05.004

Hu, J., Wang, H., Gao, S., Bao, M., Liu, T., Wang, Y., et al. (2019). S-UNet: a bridge-style U-Net framework with a saliency mechanism for retinal vessel segmentation. *IEEE Access* 7, 174167–174177. doi: 10.1109/ACCESS.2019.2940476

Hu, Q., Abràmoff, M. D., and Garvin, M. K. (2013). "Automated separation of binary overlapping trees in low-contrast color retinal images," in *Proceedings of the International Conference on Medical Image Computing and Computer-Assisted Intervention*, (Berlin: Springer), 436–443. doi: 10.1007/978-3-642-40763-5_54

Hu, Q., Abràmoff, M. D., and Garvin, M. K. (2015). Automated construction of arterial and venous trees in retinal images. *J. Med. Imaging* 2:044001. doi: 10.1117/1.JMI.2.4.044001

Huang, F., Dashtbozorg, B., Tan, T., and ter Haar Romeny, B. M. (2018a). Retinal artery/vein classification using genetic-search feature selection. *Comput. Methods Programs Biomed.* 161, 197–207. doi: 10.1016/j.cmpb.2018.04.016

Huang, F., Dashtbozorg, B., and ter Haar Romeny, B. M. (2018b). Artery/vein classification using reflection features in retina fundus images. *Mach. Vis. Appl.* 29, 23–34. doi: 10.1007/s00138-017-0867-x

Ishikawa, H., Geiger, D., and Cole, R. (2005). "Finding tree structures by grouping symmetries," in *Proceedings of the 10th IEEE International Conference on Computer Vision (ICCV'05) Volume 1*, Vol. 2, (Beijing: IEEE), 1132–1139. doi: 10.1109/ICCV.2005.100

Jiang, X., Liu, X., Wu, S., Zhang, G. Q., Peng, M., Wu, Y., et al. (2015). Metabolic syndrome is associated with and predicted by resting heart rate: a cross-sectional and longitudinal study. *Heart* 101, 44–49. doi: 10.1136/heartjnl-2014-305685

Jiang, Z., Zhang, H., Wang, Y., and Ko, S. B. (2018). Retinal blood vessel segmentation using fully convolutional network with transfer learning. *Comput. Med. Imaging Graph.* 68, 1–15. doi: 10.1016/j.compmedimag.2018.04.005

Joshi, V. S., Reinhardt, J. M., Garvin, M. K., and Abramoff, M. D. (2014). Automated method for identification and artery-venous classification of vessel trees in retinal vessel networks. *PLoS One* 9:e88061. doi: 10.1371/journal.pone.0088061

Li, L., Verma, M., Nakashima, Y., Kawasaki, R., and Nagahara, H. (2020). "Joint learning of vessel segmentation and Artery/Vein classification with post-processing," in *Proceedings of the International Conference on Medical Imaging with Deep Learning*, (Montréal, QC: MIDL).

Ma, W., Yu, S., Ma, K., Wang, J., Ding, X., and Zheng, Y. (2019). "Multi-task neural networks with spatial activation for retinal vessel segmentation and artery/vein classification," in *Proceedings of the International Conference on Medical Image Computing and Computer-Assisted Intervention, Shenzhen, China*, (Cham: Springer), 769–778. doi: 10.1007/978-3-030-32239-7_85

Maninis, K. K., Pont-Tuset, J., Arbeláez, P., and Van Gool, L. (2016). "Deep retinal image understanding," in *Proceedings of the International Conference on Medical Image Computing and Computer-Assisted Intervention, Athens, Greece*, (Cham: Springer), 140–148. doi: 10.1007/978-3-319-46723-8_17

Meyer, M. I., Galdran, A., Costa, P., Mendonça, A. M., and Campilho, A. (2018). ". Deep convolutional artery/vein classification of retinal vessels," in *Proceedings of the International Conference Image Analysis and Recognition, Póvoa de Varzim, Portugal*, (Cham: Springer), 622–630. doi: 10.1007/978-3-319-93000-8_71

Mirsharif, Q., Tajeripour, F., and Pourreza, H. (2013). Automated characterization of blood vessels as arteries and veins in retinal images. *Comput. Med. Imaging Graph.* 37, 607–617. doi: 10.1016/j.compmedimag.2013.06.003

Mou, L., Chen, L., Cheng, J., Gu, Z., Zhao, Y., and Liu, J. (2019a). Dense dilated network with probability regularized walk for vessel detection. *IEEE Trans. Med. Imaging.* 39, 1392–1403. doi: 10.1109/TMI.2019.2950051

Mou, L., Zhao, Y., Chen, L., Cheng, J., Gu, Z., Hao, H., et al. (2019b). "CS-Net: channel and spatial attention network for curvilinear structure segmentation," in *Proceedings of the International Conference on Medical Image Computing and Computer-Assisted Intervention, Shenzhen, China*, (Cham: Springer), 721–730. doi: 10.1007/978-3-030-32239-7_80

Niemeijer, M., van Ginneken, B., and Abràmoff, M. D. (2009). "Automatic classification of retinal vessels into arteries and veins," in *Proceedings of the SPIE 7260, Medical Imaging 2009: Computer-Aided Diagnosis*, Vol. 7260, (Lake Buena Vista, FL: SPIE), 72601F. doi: 10.1117/12.813826

Odstrcilik, J., Kolar, R., Budai, A., Hornegger, J., Jan, J., Gazarek, J., et al. (2013). Retinal vessel segmentation by improved matched filtering: evaluation on a new high-resolution fundus image database. *IET Image Process.* 7, 373–383. doi: 10.1049/iet-ipr.2012.0455

Oliveira, A., Pereira, S., and Silva, C. A. (2018). Retinal vessel segmentation based on fully convolutional neural networks. *Expert Syst. Appl.* 112, 229–242. doi: 10.1016/j.eswa.2018.06.034

Orlando, J. I., Breda, J. B., Van Keer, K., Blaschko, M. B., Blanco, P. J., and Bulant, C. A. (2018). "Towards a glaucoma risk index based on simulated hemodynamics from fundus images," in *Proceedings of the International Conference on Medical Image Computing and Computer-Assisted Intervention, Granada, Spain*, (Cham: Springer), 65–73. doi: 10.1007/978-3-030-00934-2_8

Orlando, J. I., Prokofyeva, E., and Blaschko, M. B. (2017). A discriminatively trained fully connected conditional random field model for blood vessel segmentation in fundus images. *IEEE Trans. Biomed. Eng.* 64, 16–27. doi: 10.1109/TBME.2016.2535311

Pellegrini, E., Robertson, G., MacGillivray, T., van Hemert, J., Houston, G., and Trucco, E. (2018). A graph cut approach to artery/vein classification in ultra-widefield scanning laser ophthalmoscopy. *IEEE Trans. Med. Imaging* 37, 516–526. doi: 10.1109/TMI.2017.2762963

Ronneberger, O., Fischer, P., and Brox, T. (2015). "U-net: Convolutional networks for biomedical image segmentation," in *Proceedings of the International Conference on Medical Image Computing and Computer-Assisted Intervention, Munich, Germany*, (Cham: Springer), 234–241. doi: 10.1007/978-3-319-24574-4_28

Samuel, P. M., and Veeramalai, T. (2019). Multilevel and multiscale deep neural network for retinal blood vessel segmentation. *Symmetry* 11:946. doi: 10.3390/sym11070946

Soares, J. V., Leandro, J. J., Cesar, R. M., Jelinek, H. F., and Cree, M. J. (2006). Retinal vessel segmentation using the 2-D Gabor wavelet and supervised classification. *IEEE Trans. Med. Imaging* 25, 1214–1222. doi: 10.1109/TMI.2006.879967

Srinidhi, C. L., Aparna, P., and Rajan, J. (2019). Automated method for retinal artery/vein separation via graph search metaheuristic approach. *IEEE Trans. Image Process.* 28, 2705–2718. doi: 10.1109/TIP.2018.2889534

Wang, B., Qiu, S., and He, H. (2019). "Dual encoding U-Net for retinal vessel segmentation," in *International Conference on Medical Image Computing and Computer-Assisted Intervention, Shenzhen, China*, (Cham: Springer), 84–92. doi: 10.1007/978-3-030-32239-7_10

Welikala, R. A., Foster, P. J., Whincup, P. H., Rudnicka, A. R., Owen, C. G., Strachan, D. P., et al. (2017). Automated arteriole and venule classification using deep learning for retinal images from the UK Biobank cohort. *Comput. Biol. Med.* 90, 23–32. doi: 10.1016/j.compbiomed.2017.09.005

Wong, T. Y., Klein, R., Sharrett, A. R., Duncan, B. B., Couper, D. J., Klein, B. E., et al. (2004). Retinal arteriolar diameter and risk for hypertension. *Ann. Intern. Med.* 140, 248–255. doi: 10.7326/0003-4819-140-4-200402170-00006

Xu, X., Ding, W., Abràmoff, M. D., and Cao, R. (2017). An improved arteriovenous classification method for the early diagnostics of various diseases in retinal image. *Comput. Methods Programs Biomed.* 141, 3–9. doi: 10.1016/j.cmpb.2017.01.007

Xu, X., Wang, R., Lv, P., Gao, B., Li, C., Tian, Z., et al. (2018). Simultaneous arteriole and venule segmentation with domain-specific loss function on a new public database. *Biom. Opt. Express* 9, 3153–3166. doi: 10.1364/BOE.9.003153

Yan, Z., Yang, X., and Cheng, K. T. (2018). Joint segment-level and pixel-wise losses for deep learning based retinal vessel segmentation. *IEEE Trans. Biomed. Eng.* 65, 1912–1923. doi: 10.1109/TBME.2018.2828137

Yushkevich, P. A., Piven, J., Hazlett, H. C., Smith, R. G., Ho, S., Gee, J. C., et al. (2006). User-guided 3D active contour segmentation of anatomical structures: significantly improved efficiency and reliability. *Neuroimage* 31, 1116–1128. doi: 10.1016/j.neuroimage.2006.01.015

Zamperini, A., Giachetti, A., Trucco, E., and Chin, K. S. (2012). "Effective features for artery-vein classification in digital fundus images," in *Proceedings of the 2012 25th IEEE International Symposium on Computer-Based Medical Systems (CBMS)*, (Rome: IEEE), 1–6. doi: 10.1109/CBMS.2012.6266336

Zhao, Y., Xie, J., Su, P., Zheng, Y., Liu, Y., Cheng, J., et al. (2018). "Retinal artery and vein classification via dominant sets clustering-based vascular topology estimation," in *International Conference on Medical Image Computing and Computer-Assisted Intervention, Granada, Spain*, (Cham: Springer), 56–64. doi: 10.1007/978-3-030-00934-2_7

7

Role of Junctional Adhesion Molecule-C in the Regulation of Inner Endothelial Blood-Retinal Barrier Function

Xu Hou[1]*, Hong-Jun Du[1], Jian Zhou[1], Dan Hu[1], Yu-Sheng Wang[1] and Xuri Li[2]*

[1] Department of Ophthalmology, Eye Institute of Chinese PLA, Xijing Hospital, Fourth Military Medical University, Xi'an, China,
[2] State Key Laboratory of Ophthalmology, Zhongshan Ophthalmic Center, Sun Yat-sen University, Guangzhou, China

*Correspondence:
Xu Hou
hxfmmu@163.com
orcid.org/0000-0002-2781-7219
Xuri Li
lixr6@mail.sysu.edu.cn

Although JAM-C is abundantly expressed in the retinae and upregulated in choroidal neovascularization (CNV), it remains thus far poorly understood whether it plays a role in the blood-retinal barrier, which is critical to maintain the normal functions of the eye. Here, we report that JAM-C is highly expressed in retinal capillary endothelial cells (RCECs), and VEGF or PDGF-C treatment induced JAM-C translocation from the cytoplasm to the cytomembrane. Moreover, JAM-C knockdown in RCECs inhibited the adhesion and transmigration of macrophages from wet age-related macular degeneration (wAMD) patients to and through RCECs, whereas JAM-C overexpression in RCECs increased the adhesion and transmigration of macrophages from both wAMD patients and healthy controls. Importantly, the JAM-C overexpression-induced transmigration of macrophages from wAMD patients was abolished by the administration of the protein kinase C (PKC) inhibitor GF109203X. Of note, we found that the serum levels of soluble JAM-C were more than twofold higher in wAMD patients than in healthy controls. Mechanistically, we show that JAM-C overexpression or knockdown in RCECs decreased or increased cytosolic Ca^{2+} concentrations, respectively. Our findings suggest that the dynamic translocation of JAM-C induced by vasoactive molecules might be one of the mechanisms underlying inner endothelial BRB malfunction, and inhibition of JAM-C or PKC in RCECs may help maintain the normal function of the inner BRB. In addition, increased serum soluble JAM-C levels might serve as a molecular marker for wAMD, and modulating JAM-C activity may have potential therapeutic value for the treatment of BRB malfunction-related ocular diseases.

Keywords: junctional adhesion molecule-C, blood-retinal barrier, retinal capillary endothelial cell, vascular endothelial growth factor, platelet-derived growth factor-C

INTRODUCTION

A healthy blood-retinal barrier (BRB) serves to balance the circulation of molecules and to maintain a homeostatic environment for the normal function of the neural retina (Hudson and Campbell, 2019). The inner and outer BRBs are formed by retinal capillary endothelial cells (RCECs) and retinal pigment epithelial cells (RPECs) in collaboration with Bruch's membrane and the choriocapillaris (Liu and Liu, 2019). Breakdown of the BRB is a common feature of many ocular diseases, such as diabetic retinopathy, wet age-related macular degeneration (wAMD), retinal vein occlusions, uveitis, and other chronic retinal diseases, which, if uncontrolled, can lead to blindness (Klaassen et al., 2013). Three types of junction molecules have been identified in retinal cell junctions: tight junctions (TJs), adherens junctions, and gap junctions (Klaassen et al., 2013). These junctions are dynamic structures (Kowalczyk and Nanes, 2012; Solan and Lampe, 2018; Heinemann and Schuetz, 2019). Junction molecules cycle continuously between the plasma membrane and intracellular compartments. TJs are the apical type of junction and are essential for cell polarity, whereas adherens junctions and gap junctions are organized in a scattered lateral distribution (Garrido-Urbani et al., 2014). TJs are the main junction type in both RCECs and RPECs contributing to BRB function (Cunha-Vaz et al., 2011). However, their composition and architecture are quite different (Dejana, 2004). After the identification of TJ molecules, including zonula occludens (ZO) (Stevenson et al., 1986), occludin (Furuse et al., 1993), and claudins (Furuse et al., 1998), the junctional adhesion molecule (JAM) family was discovered, and their functions in TJ dynamics and leukocyte transmigration were elucidated (Garrido-Urbani et al., 2014).

As a member of the classical JAM family, JAM-C was found to be abundantly expressed in the neural retinae and RPECs (Daniele et al., 2007). In our previous study, JAM-C was detected primarily in the RPEC layer, the inner and outer segments, and the inner plexiform layer of the retina. Meanwhile, JAM-C expression was found to be upregulated in the choroid-RPEC complex with choroidal neovascularization (CNV), whereas no such change was found in the neural retina. JAM-C blockade has been shown to suppress CNV formation by inhibiting macrophage transmigration and by reducing RPEC malfunction (Hou et al., 2012). Different from other members of the JAM family, JAM-C has been shown to regulate leukocytes to exit the abluminal compartment by reverse transmigration (Woodfin et al., 2011). However, it remains thus far unclear whether JAM-C plays a role in the regulation of inner endothelial BRB function, particularly, in relationship to ocular diseases.

In this study, we examined JAM-C expression in cultured human RCECs, and observed that JAM-C translocated from the cytoplasm to cytomembrane after treatment with vascular endothelial growth factor (VEGF) or platelet-derived growth factor-C (PDGF-C), two growth factors known to be critical for the function and morphology of the vascular system. Moreover, cytosolic Ca^{2+} concentrations in RCECs and the infiltration ability of macrophages from wAMD patients and healthy controls were investigated to verify the potential effect of JAM-C on the inner BRB. Importantly, we found that serum soluble JAM-C levels increased in wAMD patients, indicating a potential possibility of using soluble JAM-C as a biomarker for wAMD.

MATERIALS AND METHODS

Human RCECs and Macrophages
Primary human RCECs were purchased from the Type Culture Collection of the Chinese Academy of Sciences (Shanghai, China)

and were cultured in endothelial cell medium (ScienCell, Shanghai, China) containing 10% fetal bovine serum (FBS) at 37°C in a 5% CO_2 incubator. Cells of the third to fifth passages were used in all experiments.

All patients included in this study signed informed consent and the study was approved by the ethical and academic boards of Xijing Hospital of the Fourth Military Medical University. All procedures used conformed to the tenets of the Declaration of Helsinki. Peripheral blood monocytes from age- and gender-matched healthy adult donors and wAMD patients were isolated using a published method (Hou et al., 2012). Briefly, peripheral blood monocytes were isolated from leukopheresed buffy coat fractions after density gradient centrifugation using an aqueous medium (Amersham Biosciences, Piscataway, NJ) according to the manufacturer's protocol. Anti-human CD14 microbeads (Miltenyi Biotec, Cambridge, MA) were used for positive selection/purification of monocytes using a magnetic cell separation instrument (AutoMACS; Miltenyi Biotec, Gaithersburg, MD). The purity of the $CD14^+$ cell population was higher than 90%. Complete medium (Biosource, Rockville, MD) consisting of RPMI 1640 supplemented with penicillin (100 U/mL), streptomycin (100 U/mL), L-glutamine (2 mM), and 10% FBS was used for monocyte culture. The cells were cultured in the presence of macrophage-colony stimulating factor (PeproTech, Rocky Hill, NJ) for 6 days for differentiation into macrophages.

Immunofluorescence
Human RCECs were cultured on chamber slides in 4-well plates to approximately 90% confluence in serum-free medium overnight before experiments. The cells were then treated with PDGF-C (125 ng/mL, Sino Biological Inc., Beijing, China) or VEGF (10 ng/mL, Sino Biological Inc., Beijing, China) for 1 hr. The slides were then washed, fixed in 4% paraformaldehyde for 10 min, and permeabilized with 0.1% Triton X-100 in phosphate-buffered saline (PBS) for 5 min. The slides were blocked with 1% bovine serum albumin and 5% goat serum in PBS at room temperature for 1 hr. After incubation with rat anti-JAM-C (CRAM-18 F26) and rabbit anti-ZO1 (ab59720) (Abcam, Shanghai, China) antibodies and secondary antibodies (Alexa Fluor 488 and Alexa Fluor 594, Yeasen, Shanghai, China). The slides were washed and mounted in medium (DAPI Fluoromount G; SouthernBiotech, Birmingham, AL). A negative control staining followed the same protocol except that the anti-JAM-C or anti-ZO1 antibodies. Fluorescence images were captured using a laser scanning microscope (Leica Microsystems, Wetzlar, Germany).

Western Blot
Human RCECs in 6-well plates were treated with VEGF (10 ng/mL) or PDGF-C (125, 250 ng/mL) for 1 hr. After washing with PBS, the cells were lysed using a protein extraction kit (Beyotime, Shanghai, China). Equal amounts of protein were electrophoresed in 10% sodium dodecyl sulfate-polyacrylamide gels and transferred onto polyvinylidene difluoride membranes. The membranes were probed with a rabbit anti-JAM-C antibody (Abcam, Shanghai, China). An anti-rabbit horseradish

peroxidase-conjugated antibody (Pierce, Rockford, IL) was used as a secondary antibody. An enhanced chemiluminescence kit (SuperSignal Pico ECL; Pierce, Rockford, IL) was used to detect the signal using an imaging system (LAS-3000 Imager; Fujifilm, Tokyo, Japan). Densitometric quantification of the bands was performed using the ImageJ program (NIH, United States).

Lentiviral Vectors and Cell Transfection

For JAM-C knockdown, the lentiviral vector U6-MCS-Ubiquitin-Cherry-IRES-puromycin (GV298) encoding a JAM-C-RNAi sequence and the control lentiviral vector were purchased from Genechem Technology (Shanghai, China). Three different targeting sequences for JAM-C knockdown were used: 5′-TGAACATTGGCGGAATTAT-3′, 5′-AATCCCAGATTTCGCAATT-3′, and 5′-GCAGGAG ATGGAAGTCTAT-3′. Knockdown efficiencies were evaluated by quantitative reverse-transcription (RT-q) PCR and Western blot. The lentiviral vector with the highest knockdown efficiency was used for experiments.

For JAM-C overexpression, the lentiviral vector Ubi-MCS-3FLAG-SV40-puromycin (GV341) encoding human JAM-C and the control lentiviral vector (GV341-JAM-C) were purchased from Genechem Technology. Human RCECs were infected with GV341-JAM-C or control vector. JAM-C expression was assessed by RT-qPCR and Western blot.

RT-qPCR

Total cellular RNA was isolated using TRIzol reagent (Takara, Dalian, China). A One-Step RT-PCR kit from Takara was used following the manufacturer's instruction. The forward and reverse primers used for *JAM-C* were: 5′-GAGACTCAGCCCTTTATCGC-3′ and 5′-CCTTCGGCACTCTACAGACA-3′, and for ACTB: 5′- TGGACTTCGAGCAAGAGATG-3′ and 5′- GAAGGA AGGCTGGAAGAGTG-3′. SYBR Green PCR Master Mix (Applied Biosystems, Foster City, CA) was used for qPCRs. PCR products were analyzed by electrophoresis (Bio-Rad, Hercules, CA). mRNA levels were normalized to β-actin mRNA. Each experiment was repeated three times.

Flow Cytometry

Human RCECs were treated with VEGF (10 ng/mL) or PDGF-C (125 ng/mL) for 1 hr. After treatment with Fluo-3 (Invitrogen, Carlsbad, CA) in 1% working solution at 37°C for 30 min, the cells were washed three times with Ca^{2+}-free PBS and resuspended in PBS at 1×10^6 cells/mL. Cytosolic Ca^{2+} concentrations were detected by flow cytometry at an excitation wavelength of 488 nm and an emission wavelength of 530 nm (BD Biosciences, San Jose, CA). Cells not treated with Fluo-3 served as controls.

Enzyme-Linked Immunosorbent Assay (ELISA)

Soluble JAM-C protein levels in the serum of wAMD patients ($n = 10$) and healthy controls were determined using a human JAM-C ELISA kit from USCN Life Science Inc. (Wuhan, China).

The absorbance at 450 nm was measured using an ELX-800 Microplate Reader (BioTek Instruments Inc., Winooski, VT).

Macrophage Adhesion and Transwell Migration Assays

Macrophage adhesion assays were performed as described previously (Zhou et al., 2018). Briefly, human RCECs were cultured to confluence in 96-well plates. After treatment with lipopolysaccharide (LPS) for 4 h, macrophages from wAMD patients were added into 96-well plates (10^5/well) containing the RCEC monolayers and incubated for 1 h. After washing with PBS, the cells were imaged using an inverted microscope and adhered macrophages were counted in five random fields.

Macrophage Transwell migration assays were performed as described previously (Zhou et al., 2018). Briefly, human RCECs were cultured to confluence on the upper layer of a permeable membrane coated with collagen (Sigma-Aldrich, St. Louis, MO). Then, 600 μL of RPMI medium containing 50 ng/mL monocyte chemotactic protein-1 (MCP-1) (R&D Systems, Minneapolis, MN) was added to the lower chamber, and LPS-treated macrophages (4×10^5/well) were placed on the upper layer and allowed to migrate for 4 h. The macrophages that had migrated across the membrane to the lower chamber were stained with a 0.5% solution of gentian violet for 5 min and were counted in 5 random fields under a microscope. For protein kinase C (PKC) inhibition, confluent RCECs were pretreated with 1 μM GF109203X (Merck-Calbiochem, Darmstadt, Germany) for 2 h before MCP-1 was added to the lower chamber.

Statistical Analysis

Data are represented as the mean ± standard error of the mean and were analyzed using analysis of variance assuming equal variances. $P < 0.05$ was considered statistically significant. All experiments were conducted in triplicate.

RESULTS

JAM-C Is Expressed in Human RCECs

To investigate the potential role of JAM-C in RCECs, we checked whether these cells express JAM-C. Double immunostaining showed that JAM-C was expressed in RCECs and co-localized with ZO-1 (**Figure 1A**), an important TJ molecule critical for normal inner BRB function (Deissler et al., 2020). These results suggested a potential role of JAM-C in human RCECs.

VEGF and PDGF-C Induce Translocation of JAM-C

Under pathological conditions, such as inflammation, ischemia, or neovascularization, TJ molecules function to adjust the endothelial barrier status (Campbell and Humphries, 2012). Thus, we used VEGF and PDGF-C, two important angiogenic factors (Hou et al., 2010), to stimulate RCECs and investigated JAM-C expression in different cellular compartments, including whole-cell lysate, cytomembrane, and cytoplasm. JAM-C expression was detected in the whole-cell

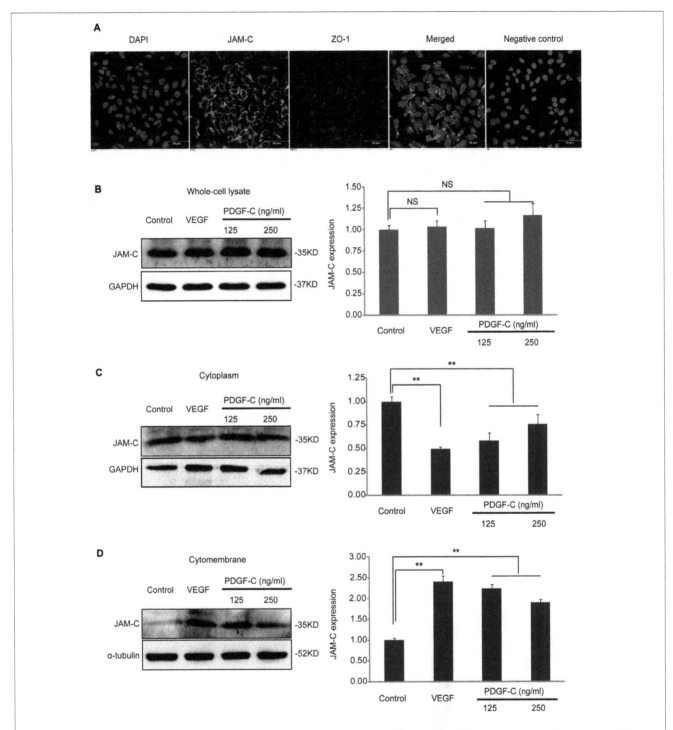

FIGURE 1 | JAM-C expression and translocation in human RCECs. **(A)** JAM-C expression in cultured human RCECs is shown by immunofluorescence staining (blue: DAPI, green: JAM-C, red: ZO-1, scale bar: 50 μm). JAM-C co-localized with ZO-1 in RCECs. A negative control staining without the primary antibody against JAM-C or ZO-1 showed no staining. **(B)** Cultured human RCECs were treated with VEGF (10 ng/mL) or PDGF-C (125, 250 ng/mL) for 1 h. JAM-C protein in the whole-cell lysate was similar as shown by Western blot. **(C)** In the cytoplasmic fraction, JAM-C protein levels decreased after VEGF or PDGF-C protein treatment. **(D)** In the cytomembrane fraction, JAM-C protein levels increased after VEGF or PDGF-C treatment. The dynamic changes in JAM-C translocation induced by PDGF-C were dose-dependent. **P < 0.01, NS, not significant.

lysate, and JAM-C protein levels were similar after VEGF or PDGF-C treatment (**Figure 1B**). However, in the cytoplasm fraction, JAM-C protein levels decreased after VEGF or

PDGF-C treatment (P < 0.01, **Figure 1C**). In contrast, in the cytomembrane fraction, JAM-C protein levels increased after VEGF or PDGF-C treatment, with (P < 0.01, **Figure 1D**).

Together, these data demonstrated that VEGF and PDGF-C stimulation induces translocation of JAM-C from cytoplasm to cytomembrane, indicating a potential role of JAM-C in VEGF- or PDGF-C-related effects.

JAM-C Knockdown and Overexpression in RCECs

To evaluate the role of JAM-C in RCECs, we conducted loss- and gain-of-function analyses using JAM-C knockdown and overexpression, respectively. For JAM-C knockdown, three different siRNAs were cloned into a lentiviral vector and transfected into RCECs. Knockdown efficiency at the mRNA level was verified by RT-qPCR, which showed that the second siRNA construct reduced JAM-C mRNA expression to about 12% of the basal level (**Figure 2A**). Western blot analysis also showed that the second siRNA was the most effective and the reduced JAM-C

protein level to about 25% of the basal level (**Figures 2B,C**). Thus, RCECs transfected with the second siRNA construct were used in subsequent loss-of-function experiments.

For gain of function assay, a lentiviral vector expressing human *JAM-C* was transfected into RCECs. RT-qPCR revealed an approximately 4.3-fold increase in JAM-C mRNA expression (**Figure 2A**), and Western blot showed an approximately 1.5-fold increase in the JAM-C protein level (**Figures 2B,C**). RCECs overexpressing JAM-C were used in subsequent experiments.

JAM-C Decreases Cytosolic Ca^{2+} Concentrations in RCECs

It is known that vasoactive molecules stimulate their receptors on endothelial cells to initiate signaling that increases cytosolic Ca^{2+}, and Ca^{2+} activation disrupts TJs (Vandenbroucke et al., 2008). Therefore, we used VEGF

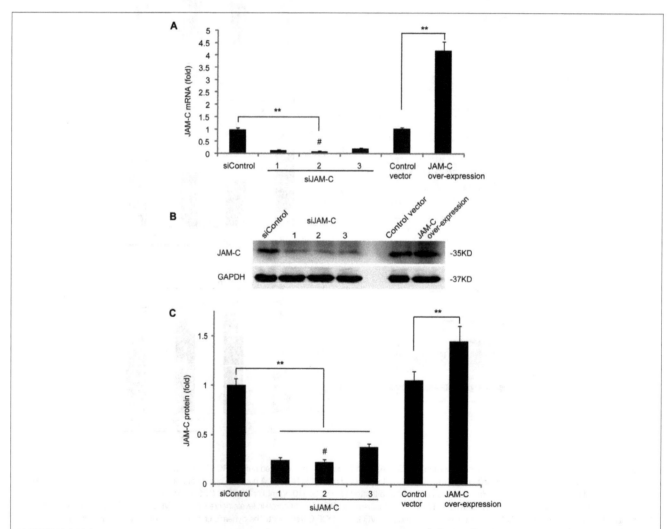

FIGURE 2 | JAM-C overexpression and knockdown in human RCECs. **(A)** Three different siRNAs for JAM-C knockdown were cloned into lentiviral vectors and transfected into RCECs. Knockdown efficiency was verified by RT-qPCR. The second siRNA construct most effectively reduced JAM-C mRNA expression to about 12%. For gain-of-function analysis, human *JAM-C* was cloned into a lentiviral vector and transfected into RCECs. RT-qPCR showed an approximately 4.3-fold increase of JAM-C transcripts. **(B,C)** For loss-of-function analysis, Western blot showed that the second siRNA construct was the most efficient and reduced JAM-C protein level to about 25%. For gain-of-function analysis, Western blot showed an approximately 1.5-fold increase of JAM-C protein in RCECs overexpressing human *JAM-C*. **P < 0.01. #: Used for subsequent experiments.

and PDGF-C to stimulate RCECs and found that cytosolic Ca^{2+} increased in endothelial cells (**Figure 3A**). We further investigated the potential role of JAM-C in the regulation of Ca^{2+} activation. Regardless of VEGF or PDGF-C treatment, overexpression and knockdown of JAM-C in RCECs decreased and markedly increased cytosolic Ca^{2+} concentrations, respectively (**Figure 3B**), indicating that increased endothelial Ca^{2+} levels could be reversed through JAM-C overexpression to "strengthen" TJs. However, VEGF and PDGF-C treatment did not increase Ca^{2+} influx in endothelial cells after JAM-C knockdown, suggesting that Ca^{2+} activation induced by VEGF and PDGF-C may require JAM-C, an essential molecule of TJs.

Inhibition of JAM-C in RCECs Decreases Macrophage Adhesion to RCECs

Macrophage adhesion to vascular endothelial cells is critical for their activation and infiltration in immune or inflammatory diseases (Futosi et al., 2013). To investigate the potential role of JAM-C in the regulation of inner BRB function, we investigated the adhesion ability of macrophages derived from wAMD patients or healthy controls to RCECs after JAM-C knockdown (siJAM-C). We found that the mean numbers of macrophages from healthy controls adhered to RCECs treated with siJAM-C were 59.4 ± 81.2 per field in the siJAM-C group and were 61.6 ± 9.3 per field in the siControl group with no statistical difference (**Figures 4A,B**). The mean numbers of macrophages from wAMD patients adhered to RCECs treated with siJAM-C were 81.2 ± 3.7 in the siJAM-C group and were 145.8 ± 9.3 in the siControl group (*P* < 0.01, **Figures 4A,B**), demonstrating that JAM-C knockdown inhibited the adhesion of macrophages from wAMD patients, but not of those from healthy controls. Moreover, the adhesion ability of macrophages from wAMD patients in both the siJAM-C and siControl groups increased compared to that of macrophages from healthy controls

(**Figure 4B**). These data suggest that the enhanced adhesion of macrophages in wAMD could be reduced by targeting JAM-C without affecting healthy macrophages.

Overexpression of JAM-C in RCECs Increases Macrophage Adhesion to Them

Using RCECs overexpressing JAM-C, we found that the mean numbers of macrophages from healthy controls adhered to RCECs were 57.8 ± 8.0 in the control group and were 85.6 ± 6.5 in the JAM-C overexpression group (*P* < 0.01, **Figures 4C,D**). The mean numbers of macrophages from wAMD patients adhered to RCECs were 159.6 ± 4.2 in the control group and were 170.2 ± 9.0 in the JAM-C overexpression group (*P* < 0.05, **Figures 4C,D**). These findings showed that JAM-C overexpression increased the adhesion of macrophages from both wAMD patients and healthy controls. In addition, the adhesion ability of macrophages from wAMD patients in both the control and JAM-C overexpression groups increased compared to that of macrophages from healthy controls (**Figure 4D**). Thus, increased JAM-C expression in vascular endothelial cells may impair inner BRB function by facilitating macrophage adhesion.

JAM-C Knockdown/Overexpression in RCECs Decreases/Increases Macrophage Transmigration Through RCECs

JAM-C-induced increase of macrophage transmigration through retinal pigment epithelium, the structure of the outer BRB, contributes to CNV (Hou et al., 2012). To verify the potential role of JAM-C in the regulation of macrophage transmigration through the inner BRB, we investigated the transmigration ability of macrophages from wAMD patients and healthy

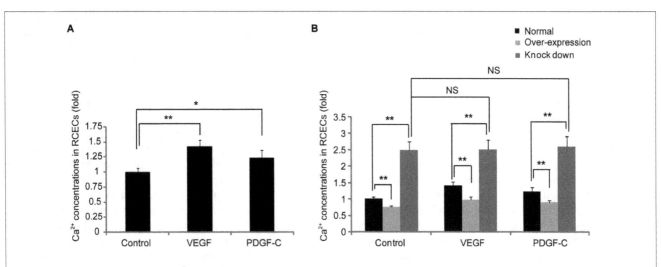

FIGURE 3 | JAM-C decreases cytosolic Ca^{2+} concentrations in human RCECs. Cultured human RCECs were treated with VEGF (10 ng/mL) or PDGF-C (125 ng/mL) for 1 h. Cytosolic Ca^{2+} concentrations were detected by flow cytometry. **(A)** VEGF and PDGF-C increased cytosolic Ca^{2+} concentrations in RCECs. **(B)** JAM-C overexpression decreased cytosolic Ca^{2+} concentrations, whereas JAM-C knockdown increased Ca^{2+} concentrations in RCECs. VEGF and PDGF-C did not increase calcium influx in RCECs after JAM-C knockdown. *P < 0.05, **P < 0.01, NS, not significant.

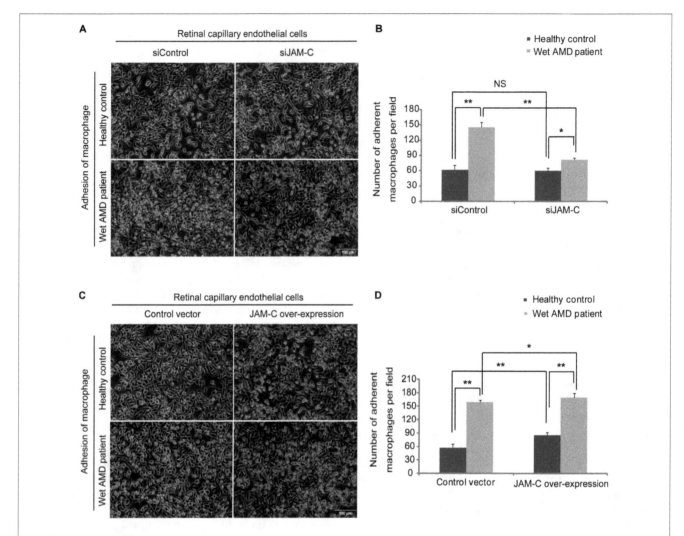

FIGURE 4 | JAM-C regulates macrophage adhesion to human RCECs. Macrophages from wAMD patients or healthy controls were added to culture plate wells containing a confluent monolayer of human RCECs, and the plates were incubated for 1 h. After washing the wells with PBS, adherent cells in five random fields were counted. Adherent macrophages were identified based on the cell size and morphology. **(A,B)** JAM-C knockdown in RCECs inhibits the adhesion of macrophages (small and round in shape) from wAMD patients to RCECs, but not those from healthy controls. The adhesion ability of macrophages from wAMD patients in both the siControl and siJAM-C groups increased compared to that of macrophages from healthy controls. **(C,D)** JAM-C overexpression increased the adhesion of macrophages from both wAMD patients and healthy controls. The adhesion ability of macrophages from wAMD patients in both the control and JAM-C overexpression groups increased compared to those from healthy controls. Scale bar: 100 μm, *P < 0.05, **P < 0.01, NS, not significant.

controls through monolayers of RCECs after JAM-C knockdown. The mean numbers of macrophages from healthy controls transmigrated through an RCEC monolayer were 12 ± 1.6 per field in the siControl group and were 12.4 ± 2.1 per field in the siJAM-C group (**Figures 5A,B**) with no statistical difference. The mean numbers of macrophages from wAMD patients transmigrated through an RCEC monolayer were 32.8 ± 3.7 in the siControl group and were 21.8 ± 2.6 in the siJAM-C group (P < 0.01, **Figures 5A,B**), indicating that JAM-C knockdown inhibited the transmigration of macrophages from wAMD patients, but not of those from healthy controls. In addition, the transmigration ability of macrophages from wAMD patients in both the siControl and siJAM-C groups increased compared to that of macrophages from healthy controls (**Figure 5B**). These data thus suggest that JAM-C targeting to inhibit macrophage

transmigration may be useful for wAMD treatment without affecting healthy macrophages.

Using RCECs overexpressing JAM-C, we found that the mean numbers of macrophages from healthy controls transmigrated through an RCEC monolayer were 14.6 ± 2.4 in the control group and were 19.6 ± 2.3 in the JAM-C overexpression group (P < 0.01, **Figures 5C,D**). The mean numbers of macrophages from wAMD patients transmigrated through an RCEC monolayer were 33.4 ± 3.1 in the control group and were 49.4 ± 6.2 in the JAM-C overexpression group (P < 0.01, **Figures 5C,D**). These findings indicated that JAM-C overexpression increased the transmigration of macrophages from both wAMD patients and healthy controls. The transmigration ability of macrophages from wAMD patients in both the control and JAM-C overexpression groups increased

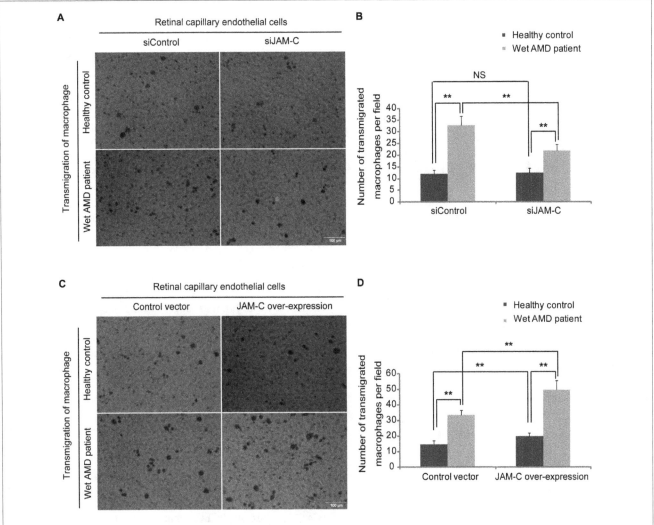

FIGURE 5 | JAM-C regulates macrophage transmigration through human RCECs. RCECs were cultured to confluence on the upper layer of a permeable membrane, and then macrophages were placed on the upper chamber and allowed to migrate through the RCEC monolayer to the lower chamber for 4 hr. Transmigrated macrophages were counted in five random fields. **(A,B)** JAM-C knockdown inhibited the transmigration of macrophages from wAMD patients, but not those from healthy controls. The transmigration of macrophages from wAMD patients in both the siControl and siJAM-C groups increased compared to those from healthy controls. **(C,D)** JAM-C overexpression increased the transmigration of macrophages from both wAMD patients and healthy controls. The transmigration of macrophages from wAMD patients in both the control and JAM-C overexpression groups increased compared to those from healthy controls. Scale bar: 100 μm, **P < 0.01, NS, not significant.

compared to that of macrophages from healthy controls (**Figure 5D**). These findings indicate that increased JAM-C expression may exacerbate macrophage infiltration and lead to a breakdown of the inner BRB in wAMD.

Inhibition of PKC in RCECs Decreases Transmigration of Macrophages From wAMD Patients

It has been shown that the translocation of JAMs is, at least in part, regulated by the PKC pathway (Sarelius and Glading, 2015). To investigate whether the increased transmigration of macrophages from wAMD patients promoted by JAM-C could be inhibited by PKC suppression, we treated RCECs with the PKC inhibitor GF109203X, and found that the transmigration of

macrophages from wAMD patients decreased for both JAM-C-overexpressing and control RCECs after GF109203X treatment ($P < 0.01$, **Figure 6**). Compared with the control cells without GF109203X treatment, JAM-C-overexpressing RCECs treated with GF109203X did not increase macrophage transmigration (**Figure 6**). Thus, the increased macrophage transmigration induced by JAM-C overexpression in RCECs was suppressed by PKC inhibition, suggesting that JAM-C regulates inflammatory cell infiltration at least in part via the PKC pathway.

Soluble JAM-C Levels Are Elevated in the Sera of wAMD Patients

Increased soluble JAM-C levels have been shown to be related to vascular inflammatory diseases (Manetti et al., 2013). To investigate whether soluble JAM-C is involved in wAMD, we

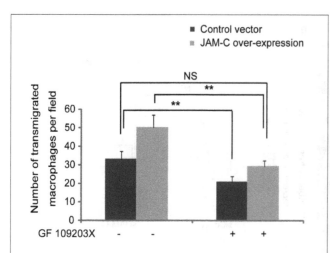

FIGURE 6 | Inhibition of PKC decreases the transmigration of macrophages from wAMD patients. An RCEC monolayer was pretreated with 1 μM of GF109203X for 2 hr. Macrophages from wAMD patients were then added and allowed to migrate for 4 h. Transmigrated macrophages were stained with a 0.5% gentian violet for 5 min and counted in five random fields. After GF109203X treatment, macrophage transmigration decreased in both JAM-C overexpressing and control RCECs. Compared with the control group without GF109203X treatment, JAM-C overexpressing RCECs treated with GF109203X did not induce any increase in macrophage transmigration. **P < 0.01, NS, not significant.

TABLE 1 | Clinical information of all patients and soluble JAM-C levels.

Patient	Age (years)	Gender (Male/Female)	Soluble JAM-C (pg/mL)
1	69	M	1393.9
2	55	M	1189.3
3	71	M	1006.7
4	66	F	1286.2
5	65	F	1085.3
6	77	M	1228.7
7	82	F	1259.7
8	63	F	1193.2
9	72	F	1353.4
10	76	M	1236.5
Average	69.6 ± 7.8		1223.3 ± 115.2

measured soluble JAM-C levels in the sera of wAMD patients (**Table 1**) and healthy controls by ELISA. We found that the mean concentration of soluble JAM-C in the control group was 475.8 ± 77.9 pg/mL, and was 1223.3 ± 115.2 pg/mL in the sera of wAMD patients ($P < 0.05$, $n = 10$). These findings indicate that increased soluble JAM-C levels in the serum might be able to serve as a biomarker for wAMD.

DISCUSSION

JAMs are a family of transmembrane proteins that play vital roles in the regulation of TJ dynamics. The roles of JAM-C in the development of the retinal structure (Daniele et al., 2007; Li et al., 2018), revascularization of the hypoxic retina (Economopoulou et al., 2015), RPEC BRB formation (Economopoulou et al.,

2009) and CNV (Hou et al., 2012) suggest its potential as a therapeutic target in the management of various retinal diseases. In this work, we found that JAM-C is expressed in RCECs and regulates the inner endothelial BRB function through its dynamic changes in cellular distribution. Increased JAM-C expression in human RCECs may lead to loss of retinal homeostasis by promoting macrophage infiltration, which can be inhibited by PKC inhibitor treatment.

The translocation of JAM-C upon stimulation with vasoactive molecules, such as VEGF, in macrovascular endothelial cells is different from that in microvascular endothelial cells. In the former, JAM-C is constitutively located at the interendothelial contacts and its localization is not affected by stimulation with vasoactive molecules, whereas in the latter, JAM-C is recruited from the cytoplasm to the cell-cell contacts after vasoactive molecule stimulation (Orlova et al., 2006). Accordingly, we found that RCECs showed a similar pattern as other microvascular endothelial cells, and total JAM-C did not change upon stimulation with VEGF or PDGF-C. Additionally, we also found that PDGF-C-induced JAM-C translocation in RCECs is dose-dependent. Our findings suggest that vasoactive molecules might serve as a switch to activate JAM-C in retinal diseases.

As an essential second messenger of endothelial cells, calcium plays a critical role in regulating barrier function and inflammation. And increased cytosolic Ca^{2+} levels can induce tight junction disassembly, increased permeability (Filippini et al., 2019; Dalal et al., 2020), and angiogenesis (Wong and Yao, 2011). VEGF has been shown to induce cytosolic Ca^{2+} elevation in retinal endothelial cells (Hiroishi et al., 2007). PDGF family molecules are potent angiogenic and survival factors (Kumar and Li, 2018). PDGF-BB can affect the integrity of the retinal microvasculature by modulating the intracellular calcium homeostasis of pericytes (Knorr et al., 1995). In this work, we showed that PDGF-C induced an increase of cytosolic Ca^{2+} in human RCECs, supporting a role of PDGF-C in pathological angiogenesis reported previously (Hou et al., 2010). Overexpression of JAM-C in RCECs decreased cytosolic Ca^{2+} levels regardless of PDGF-C treatment. However, after JAM-C knockdown, cytosolic Ca^{2+} markedly increased and treatment with vasoactive molecules did not further increase calcium influx. These data indicate that JAM-C knockdown may increase cytosolic Ca^{2+} more effectively than vasoactive molecules. Collectively, our data suggest that JAM-C is responsible for the maintenance of a dynamic Ca^{2+} balance, which may play an essential role in RCEC barrier function. Currently, how PDGF-C and JAM-C affect cytosolic Ca^{2+} is unclear. VEGF has been shown to induce entry of calcium into endothelial cells via multiple mechanisms, including by regulating calcium ions channel protein (Faehling et al., 2001; Kim et al., 2008; Li et al., 2015). PDGF-C could regulate cytosolic Ca^{2+} level by affecting calcium ions channel protein as well, which remains to be verified. It has also been shown that JAM-A malfunction reduces ATP levels in the mitochondrion and leads to Ca^{2+} overload in sperm (Aravindan et al., 2012). In this work, we found Ca^{2+} accumulation in RCECs after JAM-C knockdown, suggesting that JAM-C might use a similar mechanism to regulate Ca^{2+} in retinal vascular endothelial cells. However, further studies are needed to address this.

Besides its expression in the endothelial cells of TJs, JAM-C exists in a soluble form in human serum and the supernatant of cultured human microvascular endothelial cells (Rabquer et al., 2010). It has been suggested that soluble JAM-C mediates pathological angiogenesis (Rabquer et al., 2010). Serum soluble JAM-C levels increase in sepsis, and blockade of JAM-C can reduce the number of pro-inflammatory neutrophils (Hirano et al., 2018). We found that the mean serum soluble JAM-C concentration in wAMD patients was more than twofold of that of healthy controls. These data are consistent with the finding that increased soluble JAM-C levels correlate with vascular damage (Manetti et al., 2013). Thus, soluble JAM-C levels might be able to serve as a biomarker for pathological neovascular ocular diseases, such as wAMD.

JAM-C has been shown to play a critical role in endothelial permeability and neutrophil transmigration (Hu et al., 2020). Targeting JAM-C may have therapeutic usage in suppressing inflammation (Palmer et al., 2007; Shagdarsuren et al., 2009; Hirano et al., 2018), angiogenesis, and tumor growth (Lamagna et al., 2005) by inhibiting the infiltration of macrophages. Recruited macrophages outside or inside of the BRBs can profoundly influence retinal homeostasis (McMenamin et al., 2019). Both JAM-C and macrophage-1 antigen (Mac1) are expressed in leukocytes, and endothelial cells bind to their ligands for macrophage transmigration during inflammation and angiogenesis (Arrate et al., 2001; Bradfield et al., 2007). Previously, we found that JAM-C blockade inhibits macrophage transmigration to maintain normal RPEC barrier function (Hou et al., 2012). To investigate the role of JAM-C in the regulation of inner BRB function, we overexpressed JAM-C in cultured RCECs and found that the adhesion and transmigration of macrophages were increased. However, knockdown of JAM-C in RCECs did not significantly inhibit the adhesion and transmigration of macrophages from healthy controls, suggesting that under normal conditions, JAM-C in the inner BRB cells may not evidently affect TJ homeostasis. We subsequently investigated macrophages from wAMD patients and found marked increase of adhesion and transmigration of them. Moreover, JAM-C knockdown in RCECs suppressed the adhesion and transmigration of macrophages from wAMD patients. PKCs are serine/threonine kinases (Newton and Johnson, 1998), and JAM phosphorylation by PKC may affect its function and localization (Ozaki et al., 2000). We also found that the increased transmigration of macrophages from wAMD patients could be blocked by pretreatment of RCECs with GF109203X, a PKC inhibitor, indicating that PKC may be involved in the regulation of macrophage transmigration.

In conclusion, our data demonstrated that the dynamic translocation of JAM-C in RCECs and the activation of macrophages induced by vasoactive molecules affect inner endothelial BRB function, and JAM-C upregulation may contribute to the development of wAMD. Although further studies are required to fully clarify the role of JAM-C in ocular pathologies, our findings on the role of JAM-C in the regulation of inner endothelial BRB function may provide a potential therapeutic target for the treatment of BRB malfunction-related ocular diseases.

ETHICS STATEMENT

The studies involving human participants were reviewed and approved by the ethical and academic boards of Xijing Hospital of the Fourth Military Medical University. The patients/participants provided their written informed consent to participate in this study. Written informed consent was obtained from the individual(s) for the publication of any potentially identifiable images or data included in this article.

AUTHOR CONTRIBUTIONS

XH and XL designed the research and wrote the manuscript. XH, H-JD, JZ, DH, and Y-SW performed the experiments. XH, DH, and XL analyzed the data. All authors contributed to the article and approved the submitted version.

ACKNOWLEDGMENTS

We thank Dr. Fan Zhang (NHLBI, NIH, United States) for editorial assistance.

REFERENCES

Arrate, M. P., Rodriguez, J. M., Tran, T. M., Brock, T. A., and Cunningham, S. A. (2001). Cloning of human junctional adhesion molecule 3 (JAM3) and its identification as the JAM2 counter-receptor. J. Biol. Chem. 276, 45826–45832. doi: 10.1074/jbc.m105972200

Aravindan, R. G., Fomin, V. P., Naik, U. P., Modelski, M. J., Naik, M. U., Galileo, D. S., et al. (2012). CASK interacts with PMCA4b and JAM-A on the mouse sperm flagellum to regulate Ca2+ homeostasis and motility. J. Cell Physiol. 227, 3138–3150.

Bradfield, P. F., Nourshargh, S., Aurrand-Lions, M., and Imhof, B. A. (2007). JAM family and related proteins in leukocyte migration (Vestweber series). Arterioscler. Thromb. Vasc. Biol. 27, 2104–2112. doi: 10.1161/atvbaha.107.147694

Campbell, M., and Humphries, P. (2012). The blood-retina barrier: tight junctions and barrier modulation. Adv. Exp. Med. Biol. 763, 70–84. doi: 10.1007/978-1-4614-4711-5_3

Cunha-Vaz, J., Bernardes, R., and Lobo, C. (2011). Blood-retinal barrier. Eur. J. Ophthalmol. 21, S3–S9.

Dalal, P. J., Muller, W. A., and Sullivan, D. P. (2020). Endothelial Cell Calcium Signaling during Barrier Function and Inflammation. Am. J. Pathol. 190, 535–542. doi: 10.1016/j.ajpath.2019.11.004

Daniele, L. L., Adams, R. H., Durante, D. E., Pugh, E. N. Jr., and Philp, N. J. (2007). Novel distribution of junctional adhesion molecule-C in the neural retina and retinal pigment epithelium. *J. Comp. Neurol.* 505, 166–176. doi: 10.1002/cne.21489

Deissler, H. L., Stutzer, J. N., Lang, G. K., Grisanti, S., Lang, G. E., and Ranjbar, M. (2020). VEGF receptor 2 inhibitor nintedanib completely reverts VEGF-A165-induced disturbances of barriers formed by retinal endothelial cells or long-term cultivated ARPE-19 cells. *Exp. Eye Res.* 194:108004. doi: 10.1016/j.exer.2020.108004

Dejana, E. (2004). Endothelial cell-cell junctions: happy together. *Nat. Rev. Mol. Cell Biol.* 5, 261–270. doi: 10.1038/nrm1357

Economopoulou, M., Avramovic, N., Klotzsche-Von Ameln, A., Korovina, I., Sprott, D., Samus, M., et al. (2015). Endothelial-specific deficiency of Junctional Adhesion Molecule-C promotes vessel normalisation in proliferative retinopathy. *Thromb. Haemost.* 114, 1241–1249. doi: 10.1160/th15-01-0 051

Economopoulou, M., Hammer, J., Wang, F., Fariss, R., Maminishkis, A., and Miller, S. S. (2009). Expression, localization, and function of junctional adhesion molecule-C (JAM-C) in human retinal pigment epithelium. *Invest. Ophthalmol. Vis. Sci.* 50, 1454–1463. doi: 10.1167/iovs.08-2129

Faehling, M., Koch, E. D., Raithel, J., Trischler, G., and Waltenberger, J. (2001). Vascular endothelial growth factor-A activates Ca^{2+} -activated K^+ channels in human endothelial cells in culture. *Int. J. Biochem. Cell Biol.* 33, 337–346.

Filippini, A., D'amore, A., and D'alessio, A. (2019). Calcium Mobilization in Endothelial Cell Functions. *Int. J. Mol. Sci.* 20:4525. doi: 10.3390/ijms20184 525

Furuse, M., Hirase, T., Itoh, M., Nagafuchi, A., Yonemura, S., and Tsukita, S. (1993). Occludin: a novel integral membrane protein localizing at tight junctions. *J. Cell Biol.* 123, 1777–1788. doi: 10.1083/jcb.123.6.1777

Furuse, M., Sasaki, H., Fujimoto, K., and Tsukita, S. (1998). A single gene product, claudin-1 or -2, reconstitutes tight junction strands and recruits occludin in fibroblasts. *J. Cell Biol.* 143, 391–401. doi: 10.1083/jcb.143.2.391

Futosi, K., Fodor, S., and Mocsai, A. (2013). Reprint of Neutrophil cell surface receptors and their intracellular signal transduction pathways. *Int. Immunopharmacol.* 17, 1185–1197. doi: 10.1016/j.intimp.2013.11.010

Garrido-Urbani, S., Bradfield, P. F., and Imhof, B. A. (2014). Tight junction dynamics: the role of junctional adhesion molecules (JAMs). *Cell Tissue Res.* 355, 701–715. doi: 10.1007/s00441-014-1820-1

Heinemann, U., and Schuetz, A. (2019). Structural Features of Tight-Junction Proteins. *Int. J. Mol. Sci.* 20:6620. doi: 10.3390/ijms20236020

Hirano, Y., Ode, Y., Ochani, M., Wang, P., and Aziz, M. (2018). Targeting junctional adhesion molecule-C ameliorates sepsis-induced acute lung injury by decreasing CXCR4(+) aged neutrophils. *J. Leukoc. Biol.* 104, 1159–1171. doi: 10.1002/jlb.3a0218-050r

Hiroishi, G., Murata, T., and Ishibashi, T. (2007). Effect of thiazolidinedione on the proliferation of bovine retinal endothelial cells stimulated by vascular endothelial cell growth factor. *Jpn J. Ophthalmol.* 51, 21–26. doi: 10.1007/ s10384-006-0385-2

Hou, X., Hu, D., Wang, Y. S., Tang, Z. S., Zhang, F., Chavakis, T., et al. (2012). Targeting of junctional adhesion molecule-C inhibits experimental choroidal neovascularization. *Invest. Ophthalmol. Vis. Sci.* 53, 1584–1591. doi: 10.1167/ iovs.11-9005

Hou, X., Kumar, A., Lee, C., Wang, B., Arjunan, P., Dong, L., et al. (2010). PDGF-CC blockade inhibits pathological angiogenesis by acting on multiple cellular and molecular targets. *Proc. Natl. Acad. Sci. U. S. A.* 107, 12216–12221. doi: 10.1073/pnas.1004143107

Hu, W., Xu, B., Zhang, J., Kou, C., Liu, J., Wang, Q., et al. (2020). Exosomal miR-146a-5p from Treponema pallidum-stimulated macrophages reduces endothelial cells permeability and monocyte transendothelial migration by targeting JAM-C. *Exp. Cell Res.* 388:111823. doi: 10.1016/j.yexcr.2020.111 823

Hudson, N., and Campbell, M. (2019). Inner Blood-Retinal Barrier Regulation in Retinopathies. *Adv. Exp. Med. Biol.* 1185, 329–333. doi: 10.1007/978-3-030-27378-1_54

Kim, B. W., Choi, M., Kim, Y. S., Park, H., Lee, H. R., Yun, C. O., et al. (2008). Vascular endothelial growth factor (VEGF) signaling regulates hippocampal neurons by elevation of intracellular calcium and activation of calcium/calmodulin protein kinase II and mammalian target of rapamycin. *Cell Signal* 20, 714–725.

Klaassen, I., Van Noorden, C. J., and Schlingemann, R. O. (2013). Molecular basis of the inner blood-retinal barrier and its breakdown in diabetic macular edema and other pathological conditions. *Prog. Retin. Eye Res.* 34, 19–48. doi: 10.1016/ j.preteyeres.2013.02.001

Knorr, M., Hahn, B., Wunderlich, K., Hoppe, J., and Steuhl, K. P. (1995). [PDGF-induced effect on cytosolic free calcium concentration of cultured retinal pericytes]. *Ophthalmologe* 92, 692–697.

Kowalczyk, A. P., and Nanes, B. A. (2012). Adherens junction turnover: regulating adhesion through cadherin endocytosis, degradation, and recycling. *Subcell. Biochem.* 60, 197–222. doi: 10.1007/978-94-007-4186-7_9

Kumar, A., and Li, X. (2018). PDGF-C and PDGF-D in ocular diseases. *Mol. Aspects Med.* 62, 33–43. doi: 10.1016/j.mam.2017.10.002

Lamagna, C., Hodivala-Dilke, K. M., Imhof, B. A., and Aurrand-Lions, M. (2005). Antibody against junctional adhesion molecule-C inhibits angiogenesis and tumor growth. *Cancer Res.* 65, 5703–5710. doi: 10.1158/0008-5472.can-04-4012

Li, J., Bruns, A. F., Hou, B., Rode, B., Webster, P. J., Bailey, M. A., et al. (2015). Orai3 surface accumulation and calcium entry evoked by vascular endothelial growth factor. *Arterioscler. Thromb. Vasc. Biol.* 35, 1987–1994.

Li, Y., Zhang, F., Lu, W., and Li, X. (2018). Neuronal Expression of Junctional Adhesion Molecule-C is Essential for Retinal Thickness and Photoreceptor Survival. *Curr. Mol. Med.* 17, 497–508. doi: 10.2174/ 1566524018666180212144500

Liu, L., and Liu, X. (2019). Roles of Drug Transporters in Blood-Retinal Barrier. *Adv. Exp. Med. Biol.* 1141, 467–504. doi: 10.1007/978-981-13-7647-4_10

Manetti, M., Guiducci, S., Romano, E., Rosa, I., Ceccarelli, C., Mello, T., et al. (2013). Differential expression of junctional adhesion molecules in different stages of systemic sclerosis. *Arthritis Rheum* 65, 247–257. doi: 10.1002/art. 37712

McMenamin, P. G., Saban, D. R., and Dando, S. J. (2019). Immune cells in the retina and choroid: two different tissue environments that require different defenses and surveillance. *Prog. Retin. Eye Res.* 70, 85–98. doi: 10.1016/j.preteyeres.2018. 12.002

Newton, A. C., and Johnson, J. E. (1998). Protein kinase C: a paradigm for regulation of protein function by two membrane-targeting modules. *Biochim. Biophys. Acta* 1376, 155–172. doi: 10.1016/s0304-4157(98)00003-3

Orlova, V. V., Economopoulou, M., Lupu, F., Santoso, S., and Chavakis, T. (2006). Junctional adhesion molecule-C regulates vascular endothelial permeability by modulating VE-cadherin-mediated cell-cell contacts. *J. Exp. Med.* 203, 2703–2714. doi: 10.1084/jem.20051730

Ozaki, H., Ishii, K., Arai, H., Horiuchi, H., Kawamoto, T., Suzuki, H., et al. (2000). Junctional adhesion molecule (JAM) is phosphorylated by protein kinase C upon platelet activation. *Biochem. Biophys. Res. Commun.* 276, 873–878. doi: 10.1006/bbrc.2000.3574

Palmer, G., Busso, N., Aurrand-Lions, M., Talabot-Ayer, D., Chobaz-Peclat, V., Zimmerli, C., et al. (2007). Expression and function of junctional adhesion molecule-C in human and experimental arthritis. *Arthritis Res. Ther.* 9:R65.

Rabquer, B. J., Amin, M. A., Teegala, N., Shaheen, M. K., Tsou, P. S., Ruth, J. H., et al. (2010). Junctional adhesion molecule-C is a soluble mediator of angiogenesis. *J. Immunol.* 185, 1777–1785. doi: 10.4049/jimmunol.1000556

Sarelius, I. H., and Glading, A. J. (2015). Control of vascular permeability by adhesion molecules. *Tissue Barriers* 3:e985954. doi: 10.4161/21688370.2014. 985954

Shagdarsuren, E., Djalali-Talab, Y., Aurrand-Lions, M., Bidzhekov, K., Liehn, E. A., Imhof, B. A., et al. (2009). Importance of junctional adhesion molecule-C for neointimal hyperplasia and monocyte recruitment in atherosclerosis-prone mice-brief report. *Arterioscler. Thromb. Vasc. Biol.* 29, 1161–1163. doi: 10.1161/ atvbaha.109.187898

Solan, J. L., and Lampe, P. D. (2018). Spatio-temporal regulation of connexin43 phosphorylation and gap junction dynamics. *Biochim. Biophys. Acta Biomembr.* 1860, 83–90. doi: 10.1016/j.bbamem.2017.04.008

Stevenson, B. R., Siliciano, J. D., Mooseker, M. S., and Goodenough, D. A. (1986). Identification of ZO-1: a high molecular weight polypeptide associated with the tight junction (zonula occludens) in a variety of epithelia. *J. Cell Biol.* 103, 755–766. doi: 10.1083/jcb.103.3.755

Vandenbroucke, E., Mehta, D., Minshall, R., and Malik, A. B. (2008). Regulation of endothelial junctional permeability. *Ann. N. Y. Acad. Sci.* 1123, 134–145. doi: 10.1196/annals.1420.016

Wong, C. O., and Yao, X. (2011). TRP channels in vascular endothelial cells. *Adv. Exp. Med. Biol.* 704, 759–780. doi: 10.1007/978-94-007-026 5-3_40

Woodfin, A., Voisin, M. B., Beyrau, M., Colom, B., Caille, D., Diapouli, F. M., et al. (2011). The junctional adhesion molecule JAM-C regulates polarized transendothelial migration of neutrophils in vivo. *Nat. Immunol.* 12, 761–769. doi: 10.1038/ni.2062

Zhou, J., Bai, W., Liu, Q., Cui, J., and Zhang, W. (2018). Intermittent Hypoxia Enhances THP-1 Monocyte Adhesion and Chemotaxis and Promotes M1 Macrophage Polarization via RAGE. *Biomed. Res. Int.* 2018:1650456.

8

Mitophagy Protects the Retina against Anti-Vascular Endothelial Growth Factor Therapy-Driven Hypoxia *via* Hypoxia-Inducible Factor-1α Signaling

Yimeng Sun[1], Feng Wen[1], Chun Yan[1], Lishi Su[1], Jiawen Luo[1], Wei Chi[1]* and Shaochong Zhang[1,2]*

[1] State Key Laboratory of Ophthalmology, Zhongshan Ophthalmic Center, Sun Yat-sen University, Guangzhou, China,
[2] Shenzhen Key Laboratory of Ophthalmology, Shenzhen Eye Hospital, Jinan University, Shenzhen, China

*Correspondence:
Wei Chi
chiwei@mail.sysu.edu.cn
Shaochong Zhang
zhangshaochong@gzzoc.com

Anti-VEGF drugs are first-line treatments for retinal neovascular diseases, but these anti-angiogenic agents may also aggravate retinal damage by inducing hypoxia. Mitophagy can protect against hypoxia by maintaining mitochondrial quality, thereby sustaining metabolic homeostasis and reducing reactive oxygen species (ROS) generation. Here we report that the anti-VEGF agent bevacizumab upregulated the hypoxic cell marker HIF-1α in photoreceptors, Müller cells, and vascular endothelial cells of oxygen-induced retinopathy (OIR) model mice, as well as in hypoxic cultured 661W photoreceptors, MIO-MI Müller cells, and human vascular endothelial cells. Bevacizumab also increased expression of mitophagy-related proteins, and mitophagosome formation both *in vivo* and *in vitro*, but did not influence cellular ROS production or apoptosis rate. The HIF-1α inhibitor LW6 blocked mitophagy, augmented ROS production, and triggered apoptosis. Induction of HIF-1α and mitophagy were associated with upregulation of BCL2/adenovirus E1B 19-kDa protein-interacting protein 3 (BNIP3) and FUN14 domain containing 1 (FUNDC1), and overexpression of these proteins in culture reversed the effects of HIF-1α inhibition. These findings suggest that bevacizumab does induce retinal hypoxia, but that concomitant activation of the HIF-1α-BNIP3/FUNDC1 signaling pathway also induces mitophagy, which can mitigate the deleterious effects by reducing oxidative stress secondary. Promoting HIF-1α-BNIP3/FUNDC1-mediated mitophagy may enhance the safety of anti-VEGF therapy for retinal neovascular diseases and indicate new explanation and possible new target of the anti-VEGF therapy with suboptimal effect.

Keywords: mitophagy, bevacizumab, anti-VEGF, retina, hypoxia, retinal neovascular disease

INTRODUCTION

Retinal neovascularization (RNV) is a pathophysiological feature common to several retinal diseases, including retinopathy of prematurity (ROP), proliferative diabetic retinopathy (PDR), and retinal vein occlusion (RVO). ROP is the leading cause of blindness in childhood and DR is the leading cause in working-age adults. It is estimated that 230 million people worldwide are current living with RNV diseases, and prevalence is predicted to increase due to rising rates of diabetes (Fierson, 2018; Wong et al., 2018; Flaxel et al., 2020).

Vascular endothelial growth factor (VEGF) signaling is the predominant mechanism for pathological retinal neovascularization (Pierce et al., 1995; Campochiaro and Hackett, 2003; Campochiaro, 2015), so VEGF is the principal target of anti-angiogenic RNV treatments such as ranibizumab, aflibercept, and bevacizumab (Aiello et al., 1995; Campochiaro and Akhlaq, 2020). While these anti-VEGF drugs have shown promising efficacy in treating neovascularization of retinal tissue, many challenges remain. Numerous studies have demonstrated that VEGF is necessary for the survival of retinal and choroidal cells and that these pro-survival effects are independent of angiogenesis (Nishijima et al., 2007; Brockington et al., 2010). Accordingly, anti-VEGF drugs may compromise the *in vivo* requirement for VEGF and damage retina or choroidal cells. Indeed, approximately one-fifth of patients in the CATT trial developed geographic atrophy of the choriocapillaris and retinal pigmental epithelium (RPE) within 2 years after treatment (Grunwald et al., 2014), and Rofagha et al. (2013) reported that some treated eyes developed macular atrophy involving the foveal region. Studies investigating the direct ocular toxicity of anti-VEGF drugs by exposing cultured RPE and choroidal cells such as ARPE-19 cells to increasing concentrations of these compounds have not detected cellular apoptosis or toxicity within the therapeutic range (Malik et al., 2014). However, the pathogenic processes associated with RNV disease and treatment may be absent in culture systems consisting of a single cell type. For instance, cultured cell monolayers are usually well oxygenated. Consequently, further exploration is required to assess anti-VEGF toxicity in pathological contexts. In addition, a substantial proportion of patients do not respond optimally to these agents. In one trial, 41% of patients receiving aflibercept, 64% receiving bevacizumab, and 52% receiving ranibizumab for diabetic macular edema did not respond optimally and required focal/grid laser photocoagulation (Wells et al., 2016). These observations also suggest that effective therapy requires the suppression of pathological processes in addition to VEGF-A–VEGF receptor (VEGFR) signaling.

The hypoxia associated with anti-VEGF therapy may actually influence the clinical response. For instance, use of these agents for cancer chemotherapy increases tumor hypoxia *via* a hypoxia-inducible factor-1α (HIF-1α) signaling pathway (Miyazaki et al., 2014; Shi et al., 2017; Ueda et al., 2017; de Almeida et al., 2020). However, other studies have reported a decrease in tumor hypoxia (Lee et al., 2000; Dings et al., 2007; Myers et al., 2010). Further, the effects of anti-VEGF treatment for RNV diseases on retinal and cellular oxygenation status are largely uninvestigated.

Many hypoxic responses, including VEGF-dependent compensatory neovascularization, are mediated by a family of dimeric transcription factors termed hypoxia-inducible factors (HIFs). Cellular stressors including hypoxia also induce autophagy, a mechanism for degrading and recycling cellular components to maintain homeostasis (Manalo et al., 2005;

Elvidge et al., 2006; Glick et al., 2010; Mazure and Pouysségur, 2010). Autophagy can be highly selective for specific cellular components and conditions (Manalo et al., 2005). For instance, selective autophagic degradation of damaged mitochondria inside lysosomes (termed mitophagy) is considered essential for the maintenance of metabolic homeostasis and the prevention of pathological processes initiated by mitochondrial dysfunction such as oxidative stress and apoptosis. Thus, excessive or insufficient mitophagy may lead to cell death, especially under stress (Wallace, 1999; Li et al., 2001; Galluzzi et al., 2012). Reactive oxygen species (ROS) are the byproduct of mitochondrial oxidative phosphorylation. ROS are generated at low levels by functional mitochondria and at an enhanced rate by damaged mitochondria and during reperfusion following hypoxia. Clearance of damaged mitochondria by mitophagy can prevent excessive ROS production and ensuing apoptotic cell death (Li et al., 2015). Mitophagy is regulated by both receptor-dependent and receptor-independent pathways. The BCL2 and adenovirus E1B 19kDa-interacting protein 3 (BNIP3) and FUN14 domain containing 1 (FUNDC1) are two important receptors in a recently described hypoxia-induced mitophagy pathway. These proteins localize on the outer mitochondrial membrane and interact with the autophagy-associated protein microtubule-associated protein 1 light chain 3 (LC3). Upon binding, an autophagic bilayer membrane envelope the mitochondrion to form an autophagosome, which then fuses with a lysosome to form an autophagolysosome within which the mitochondrion is degraded (Zhang et al., 2008; Liu et al., 2012; Ney, 2015).

Collectively, these findings suggest that anti-VEGF drugs may induce mitophagy *via* an HIF1-α pathway. However, potential effects on retina and therapeutic response are unknown. Here we examined the effects of the anti-VEGF drug bevacizumab on mitophagy in oxygen-induced retinopathy (OIR) model mouse retina as well as in cultured 661W photoreceptors, MIO-MI Müller cells, and human vascular endothelial cells (HUVECs) under hypoxia. We further investigate the functions of HIF-1α, BNIP3, and FUNDC1 on bevacizumab-induced changes in retinal cell oxidative stress, mitophagy, and survival.

MATERIALS AND METHODS

Ethics Statement

Pregnant female wild type C57BL/6J mice were purchased from the Laboratory Animal Center of Southern Medical University (Guangzhou, China), and raised in the Experimental Animal Center of Zhongshan Ophthalmic Center, Sun Yat-sen University, under specific pathogen-free conditions. All procedures involving animals were conducted strictly in accordance with the Association for Research in Vision and Ophthalmology (ARVO) Statement for the use of Animals in Ophthalmic and Vision Research. All animal experiments were formally reviewed and approved by the Animal Care and Ethics Committee of the Zhongshan Ophthalmic Center (Approval number: 2020-023). All efforts were made to ensure the welfare and alleviate the suffering of animals.

Cell Culture and Hypoxia Model

Human umbilical vein endothelial cells were obtained from the American Type Culture Collection (ATCC, #CRL-1730), while the 661W photoreceptor cell line was generously provided by Dr. Muayyad Al-Ubaidi (University of Oklahoma, Oklahoma City, OK, United States). The human Moorfield/Institute of Ophthalmology-Müller 1 (MIO-M1) cell line was established and characterized previously by Dr. Astrid Limb and colleagues (University College London, London, United Kingdom) (Limb et al., 2002). Cells were grown in Dulbecco's Modified Eagle's Medium F12 (DMEM/F12) supplemented with 10% fetal bovine serum (FBS) and 1% antibiotic mixture (penicillin and streptomycin) at 37°C in a humidified incubator under a 5% CO_2 atmosphere. To mimic hypoxic conditions *in vitro*, cells were cultivated in serum-free DMEM in a portable three-gas controlled incubator (Smartor 118) under 5% CO_2 and 1% O_2 for 12 h at 37°C prior to harvesting.

Transfections and Drug Treatments

BNIP3-overexpression plasmid and FUNDC1-overexpression plasmid were purchased from GeneCopoeia (United States). Briefly, human BNIP3 cDNA was cloned from NM_004052.4, mouse BNIP3 cDNA from NM_00976, human FUNDC1 from NM_173794, and mouse FUNDC1 cDNA from NM_028058. The resultant fragments were inserted into the OmickLink™ Expression Vector pEZ-M02. Cultured 661W photoreceptors, Müller cells, and HUVECs were plated (1×10^6 cell/6 well) in DMEM + FBS. The medium was then exchanged for Opti-MEM (Gibco) with Lipofectamine and 5 μg of the BNIP3- and FUNDC1-overexpression plasmids for 48 h using Lipofectamine 3000 (GLPBIO, United States, GK20006) under normal culture conditions. The HIF-1α inhibitor LW6 was purchased from (GLPBIO, United States, GC32724) and dissolved in dimethyl sulfoxide (DMSO) to a final concentration of 10 mM for cell application. Similarly, chloroquine (CQ) (GLPBIO, United States, G6423) was dissolved in DMSO to a final concentration of 10 mM. All these solutions were stored at −20°C before use. Subgroups of cells were incubated with 0.625 mg/mL bevacizumab (Avastin®, Roche, Switzerland), 0.5 mg/mL aflibercept (Eylea®, Bayer, Germany), or 0.125 mg/mL ranibizumab (Lucentis®, Novartis, Switzerland) as indicated. When combined with bevacizumab, LW6 and CQ were used at 25 μM.

Western Blotting

Cells were harvested following treatment and cellular proteins isolated using standard procedures. Proteins were fractionated by SDS-PAGE and transferred to polyvinylidene difluoride membranes (Millipore, Billerica, MA, United States). Membranes were blocked with 5% skim milk for 60 min and then incubated with the following primary antibodies overnight at 4°C: anti-HIF-1α (1:1000, ABclonal, China, A11945), anti-LC3B (1:1000, Abcam, United Kingdom, ab48394), anti-BNIP3 (1:500, ABclonal, China, A5683), anti-FUNDC1 (1:500, ABclonal, China, A16318), anti-P62 (1:10000, Abcam, United Kingdom, ab109012), and anti-β-actin (1:10000, Bioss,

China, bs-0061R). Blotted membranes were then incubated with 1:10000 horseradish peroxidase (HRP)-conjugated goat anti-rabbit secondary antibody (bs-0295G-HRP), and target bands visualized using an enhanced chemiluminescence detection system. Band intensities were calculated from gray scale images using ImageJ (Version 1.51). Target protein band intensities were normalized to β-actin band intensity (the gel-loading control). The ratio of cytosolic inactive LC3 (LC3-I) to lipidated LC3 (LC3-II) was calculated as an index of autophagic activation.

Detection of Mitophagosome Formation by Laser Confocal Imaging

The Ad-HBmTur-Mito and Ad-LC3-GFP viral vectors (Hanbio, Shanghai, China) were used to directly detect mitophagosome formation by fluorescence confocal imaging. Briefly, cells were seeded on 35 mm glass-bottom dishes (NEST, China), allowed to be infected with virus for 8 h. The culture medium was then exchanged for fresh medium and cells incubated for 48–72 h before the indicated treatments (hypoxia and drug exposure). Treated cells were fixed with 4% paraformaldehyde and counterstained with 4, 6-diamidino-2-phenylindole dilactate (DAPI) (Solarbio, China, C0065). Confocal images of mitophagosomes were acquired using a confocal microscope (SP8 Leica, Germany).

Immunofluorescence

Cells treated as indicated were fixed in 4% paraformaldehyde, permeabilized with 0.05% Triton X-100 for 15 min, blocked in 3% bovine serum albumin (BSA) for 1 h, then incubated overnight at 4°C with primary antibodies against BNIP3 (Abcam, United Kingdom, ab10433, 1:100) and FUNDC1 (Abcam, United Kingdom, ab224722, 1:100). Labeled cells were then incubated with Alexa Flour 594-conjugated goat secondary antibodies (1:200 BIOSS, China, bs-0295P-AF594 and bs-0296P-AF594) for 1 h at room temperature. Finally, cells were counterstained with DAPI, washed three times with PBS, and photographed using an inverted fluorescence microscope (Olympus FV1000, Olympus, Japan). At least three randomly chosen visual fields were photographed and analyzed for each sample. For double-stained retina tissue immunofluorescence, paraffin-embedded 4 μm sections were deparaffinized, dehydrated in gradient alcohol, heated in 20 min for antigen repair, then incubated with antibodies against LC3 (1:100, Abcam, United Kingdom, ab48394), HIF-1α (1:200, Abcam, United Kingdom, ab1), BNIP3 (1:100, Abcam, United Kingdom, ab10433), FUNDC1 (1:100, Abcam, United Kingdom, ab224722), CD31 (1:100, ABclonal, China, A4900), Rhodopsin (1:100, Abcam, United Kingdom, ab98887), and (or) Glutamine Synthetase (1:100, Abcam, United Kingdom, ab228590) overnight at 4°C. Immunolabeled retinal samples were incubated with Goat Anti-Rabbit IgG (HRP) (1:4000, Abcam, United Kingdom, ab205718) for 45 min and FITC-TSA-conjugated antibodies for 10 min. For incubation with the secondary primary antibody, sections were incubated in primary antibody rabbit overnight at 4°C followed by washing and incubation with Alexa Fluor®594 donkey anti-rabbit IgG (H + L) (A21207, Life Technologies, Germany). DAPI was used to counterstain cell nuclei. Images were captured using a confocal microscope (SP8, Leica, Germany).

Cell Viability Assay

Cell viability was determined using a CCK-8 assay (GLPBIO, United States). This assay based on the conversion of the tetrazolium salt WST-8 by viable mitochondria to water-soluble WST-8 formazan. Briefly, cells were seeded in 96-well plates and treated as described. Cells were then incubated with 10 μL CCK-8 solution at 37°C for 2.5 h and the absorbance recorded at 450 nm as an estimate of viable cell number using a microplate reader (BioTek SynergyH1 microplate reader, United States).

Measurement of Mitochondrial Membrane Potential (ΔΨm)

Changes in the mitochondrial membrane potential (ΔΨm) were measured by JC-1 staining (Solarbio, China). Cells were cultured on 35-mm glass-bottom dishes (NEST, China). Following the indicated treatments, cells were washed with PBS, incubated with 1 mL JC-1 working solution for 30 min at 37°C in the dark, and washed twice with JC-1 staining buffer.

The wavelength at excitation/emission 525/590 nm was used to assess JC-1 aggregates, and at excitation/emission 488/525 nm was used to assess JC-1 monomers under confocal microscopy (SP8, Leica, Germany) as an indicator of ΔΨm, with green emission indicative of relative depolarization.

Measurement of Intracellular Reactive Oxygen Species

Intracellular ROS levels were measured using a fluorescent ROS Assay Kit (Solarbio, China). Cells were seeded in 6-well plates and incubated in 1 ml serum-free DMEM/F12 containing 1:1,000 dichloro-dihydro-fluorescein diacetate (DCFH-DA) for 20 min at 37°C under 5% CO_2 as directed by the manufacturer. Cells were then washed three times in serum-free medium, deplated using trypsin, centrifuged at $600 \times g$ for 4 min, and washed again with PBS. The fluorescence change due to ROS oxidation of DCFH-DA to DCFH was measured using a Fortessa X-20 flow cytometer (BD, United States) and analyzed using FlowJo (FlowJo, Ashland, OR, United States).

TdT-Mediated dUTP Nick-End Labeling Staining for Apoptosis

Paraffin-embedded retinal sections were deparaffinized in dimethylbenzene, dehydrated in graded ethanol, incubated with proteinase K for antigen retrieval, washed three times in PBS, and then stained by using a TdT-mediated dUTP Nick-End Labeling (TUNEL) kit (Roche, Switzerland) followed by DAPI counterstaining of cell nuclei using an inverted fluorescence microscope (Olympus FV1000, Olympus, Japan).

Oxygen-Induced Retinopathy Model

The C57/BL6J mice used to establish the OIR model were generated from pregnant females and reared by the Laboratory Animal Center of Southern Medical University (Guangzhou, China). The day of birth was defined as postnatal day (P0). At P7, both male and female neonatal mice and their nursing mothers were exposed to 75% oxygen for 5 days, followed by another 5 days of exposure to a normoxic environment prior to sacrifice at P17. Chloroquine (10 mg/kg) was given 1 h prior to bevacizumab vitreous injection and then every 24 h until sacrifice.

Vitreous Injection

On P12, mice were anesthetized by 3% isoflurane followed by 2% isoflurane during drug injections. Eyes were first dilated with 1% tropicamide and treated with 0.5% proparacaine hydrochloride as a topical anesthetic (Alcaine, Alcon, United States). Mice then received intravitreal injection of bevacizumab (1 μL), LW6 (0.3 μL), or both (1 μL + 0.3 μL) under a stereomicroscope (Hamilton, United States) using a 33-gauge Hamilton syringe (Hamilton, United States).

Detection of Tissue Hypoxia

To determine whether bevacizumab injection aggravates hypoxia in OIR model, the Hypoxyprobe Plus Kit (Hypoxyprobe Inc., Burlington, MA, United States) was used. 1 h before mice were euthanized, 60 mg pimonidazole hydrochloride per kg body weight was injected into the peritoneal cavities of mice. Retinal sections obtained from paraffin-embedded retinas were prepared as described above. Sets of sections were deparaffinized using xylene and then hydrated with decreasing concentrations of ethanol. Slides were then washed with PBS with 0.5% Tween 20, incubated for 10 min in 3% hydrogen peroxide at room temperature, and followed by another PBS with a 0.5% Tween 20 wash. Epitope unmasking was accomplished by incubating the sections in boiling 10 mM citrate buffer (pH 6.0) for 10 min. Anti-pimonidazole mouse monoclonal antibody, FITC-Mab1(1:50, Hypoxyprobe-1 Plus Kit, Hypoxyprobe Inc., Burlington, United States) was used as primary antibody with incubation overnight, and HRP linked to rabbit anti-FITC (1:50, Hypoxyprobe-1 Plus Kit, Hypoxyprobe Inc., Burlington, United States) was used as the secondary antibody for 30 min at room temperature according to the kit protocol. Immunohistochemical staining was performed with DAB (Chemicon International, United States, 71895) and were counterstained with hematoxylin (Solarbio, China, G1140). Images were acquired under Olympus FV1000 microscope (Olympus, Japan).

Transmission Electron Microscopy

Eyes were excised at P17, fixed for 24 h in 4% glutaraldehyde, post-fixed in 1% osmium tetroxide, dehydrated in gradient ethanol, paraffin-embedded, and cut into 80 nm sections using an ultra-microtome. Sections were stained with uranyl acetate and lead citrate, followed by observation under transmission electron microscopy (TEM).

Statistical Analysis

All data are expressed as mean ± SD and all statistical analyses were conducted using GraphPad Prism software (Version 5.0, United States). Group means were compared by one-way analysis of variance followed by *post hoc* Turkey's tests for pair-wise comparisons. A $P < 0.05$ (two-tailed) was considered statistically significant for all tests.

RESULTS

Bevacizumab Upregulated Hypoxia-Inducible Factor-1α Expression and Autophagic Markers in Cultured Photoreceptors, Müller Cells, and Vascular Endothelial Cells Under Hypoxia

We examined whether bevacizumab increased HIF-1α and mitophagy in 661W cells, MIO-M1 cells, and HUVEC cells. HIF-1α was upregulated in all three cell types following bevacizumab treatment under 1% O_2 hypoxia as measured by western blotting. Further, all cells exhibited an increased LC3-II/LC3-I ratio and downregulation of P62 (SQSTM1), consistent with induction of autophagy (**Figures 1A–C**). Moreover, cells transfected with Ad-GFP-LC3 and Ad-HBmTur-Mito showed enhanced colocalization of LC3 and Mitotracker following bevacizumab treatment under hypoxia condition but no changes after bevacizumab under normoxia condition, indicating an elevated rate of mitophagosome formation under hypoxia (**Figures 1D–F**).

Bevacizumab Exacerbated Hypoxia and Increased Hypoxia-Inducible Factor-1α Expression and Autophagy in Photoreceptors, Müller Cells, and Vascular Endothelial Cells of Oxygen-Induced Retinopathy Model Retina

We then established an OIR model using the protocol described in **Figure 2A**. To explore whether bevacizumab exacerbates hypoxia in OIR model, we use Hypoxyprobe detected by immunohistochemistry to assess the hypoxic condition of retina. There is no positive staining in wide type mice retinal section which prove the specificity of the probe. The average color intensity of hypoxic areas (brown-stained retinal tissue) showed in retinas of the OIR mouse treated with bevacizumab is increased compared that in OIR model (**Figure 2B**). TEM was employed to further investigate whether mitophagy was occured in OIR combined with bevacizumab treatment. Mitophagy is a dynamic process and we get the static "snapshots" of different stage of mitophagy in OIR model injected with bevacizumab. In **Figure 2C**, compared with normal mitochondria in the retina of wide type mice (lower right), Upper left showed that mitochondria is engulfed by autophagosome at early stage. We observed that mitochondria degraded in upper right and normal morphology of mitochondria totally disappeared

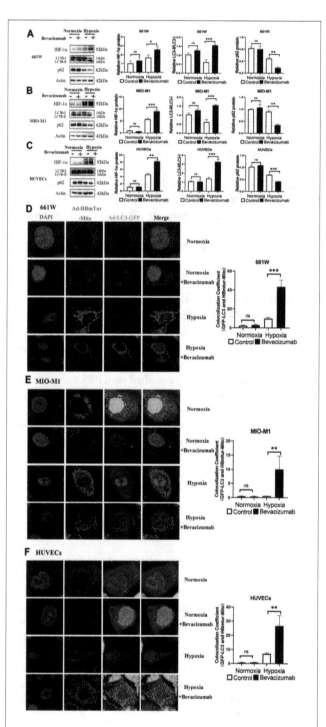

FIGURE 1 | Bevacizumab exacerbated hypoxia and induces mitophagy in cultured photoreceptors, Müller cells, and vascular endothelial cells. **(A–C)** Representative western blots and densitometric results showing significant upregulation of HIF-1α and autophagy-related proteins LC3 and downregulation of P62 in hypoxic 661W photoreceptors, MIO-M1 Müller cells, and human umbilical vascular endothelial cells (HUVECs) following bevacizumab treatment compared with that in normoxia condition. **(D–F)** Representative immunofluorescence images and quantification showing that bevacizumab induced mitophagosome formation under hypoxia as indicated by LC3B and Mitotracker colocalization but no changes after bevacizumab treatment under normoxia. Bar: 10 μm. ns: no significance, *$P < 0.05$, **$P < 0.01$, ***$P < 0.001$.

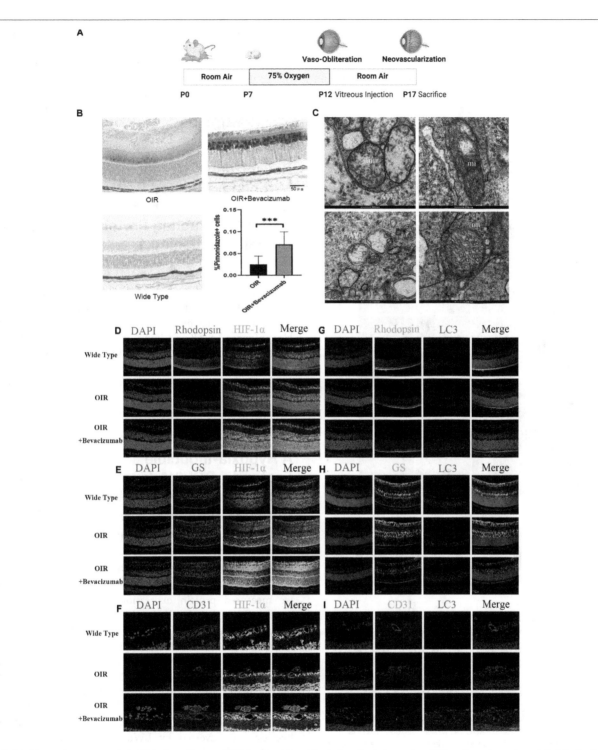

FIGURE 2 | Bevacizumab exacerbated hypoxia and increased HIF-1α expression and autophagy in photoreceptors, Müller cells, and vascular endothelial cells of OIR model retina. **(A)** A time line schematic of oxygen-induced retinopathy (OIR) modeling. **(B)** Pimonidazole staining images and quantification showed more serious hypoxia within the retinal tissue after injected with bevacizumab in OIR mice. Bar = 50 μm. **(C)** Representative transmission electron microscopy (TEM) images depicting mitochondria, mitophagosomes, and mitolysosomes. In OIR mouse treated with bevacizumab, autophagosomes, referred as initial autophagic vacuoles (Avi) have double membrane contain mitochondria (mi) (upper left). Late and Degenerative autophagic vacuoles (Avd) have mitochondria at various stages of degradation (upper right and lower left), which have different morphology of mitochondria with normal mitochondria (lower right). Bar = 200 nm. **(D–F)** Representative dual immunofluorescence images showing HIF-1α accumulation in photoreceptors (rhodopsin-positive), Müller cells (glutamine synthetase-positive) and vascular endothelial cells (CD31-positive) following intravitreal injection of bevacizumab. Bar = 50 μm. **(G–I)** Representative dual immunofluorescence images showing LC3 upregulation in photoreceptors, Müller cells, and vascular endothelial cells following intravitreal injection of bevacizumab. Bar = 50 μm. ns: no significance, *P < 0.05, **P < 0.01, ***P < 0.001.

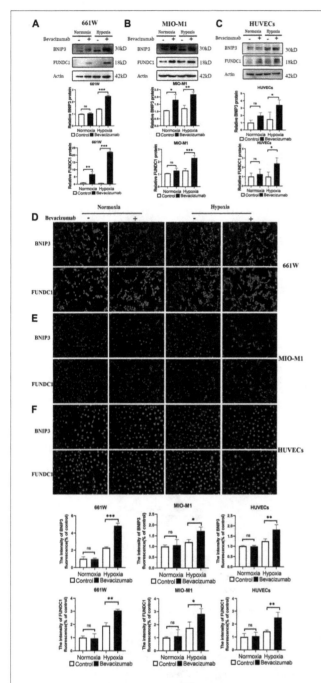

FIGURE 3 | Mitophagy-related proteins BNIP3 and FUNDC1 were upregulated by bevacizumab treatment. **(A–C)** Representative western blot images and densitometric results showing upregulation of BNIP3 and FUNDC1 in 661W photoreceptors, MIO-M1 Müller cells, and HUVECs following bevacizumab treatment under hypoxia which was more significant compared to normoxia. **(D–F)** Representative immunofluorescence images and quantification confirming that bevacizumab upregulated BNIP3 and FUNDC1 in 661W photoreceptors, MIO-M1 Müller cells, and HUVECs especially under hypoxia. Bar: 100 μm. ns: no significance, *P < 0.05, **P < 0.01, ***P < 0.001.

marker rhodopsin, the Müller cell marker glutamine synthetase, or the vascular endothelial cells marker CD31 (**Figures 2D–F**). As shown in confocal images, HIF-1α immunoexpression was increased in all three cell types after intravitreal injection of 1 μL (per eye) 25 mg/mL bevacizumab (Avastin®). Similarly, co-staining for LC3-B and one of the aforementioned markers indicated increased autophagy in all three cell types (**Figures 2G–I**).

Bevacizumab Upregulated the Mitophagy-Related Proteins BCL2/Adenovirus E1B 19-kDa Protein-Interacting Protein 3 and FUN14 Domain Containing 1

BCL2/adenovirus E1B 19-kDa protein-interacting protein 3 and FUNDC1 mediate ischemia-induced mitophagy by interacting with and recruiting LC3 to mitochondria. We examined whether BNIP3 and FUNDC1 participate in bevacizumab-induced mitophagy by measuring protein expression by western blot (**Figures 3A–C**) and immunofluorescence (**Figures 3D–F**). Both methods revealed that BNIP3 and FUNDC1 protein levels were significantly upregulated following bevacizumab treatment of cultured cells especially under hypoxia. These findings suggest that BNIP3 and FUNDC1 are potential downstream regulators of HIF-1α-mediated mitophagy.

A Hypoxia-Inducible Factor-1α-BCL2/Adenovirus E1B 19-kDa Protein-Interacting Protein 3/FUN14 Domain Containing 1 Signaling Pathway Mediated Bevacizumab-Induced Mitophagy

To examine whether bevacizumab-induced mitophagy induction is dependent on HIF-1α, BNIP3, and FUNDC1 upregulation, we measured protein expression levels in retinal cells co-treated with bevacizumab plus the HIF-1α inhibitor LW6 under hypoxia. As expected, HIF-1α expression was reduced by LW6. Consistent with a central role for HIF-1α/BNIP3/FUNDC1 signaling in bevacizumab-induced mitophagy, LW6 cotreatment also reduced the protein levels of BNIP3 and FUNDC1, decreased the LC3-II/LC3-I ratio, and upregulated P62 (**Figures 4A–C**). Further, the increased colocalization of Ad-GFP-LC3 and Ad-HBmTur-Mito following bevacizumab treatment under hypoxia was reversed by LW6 (**Figures 4D–F**). Therefore, inhibition of HIF-1α blocked both downstream BNIP3/FUNDC1 signaling and mitophagy. Conversely, transfection with BNIP3 and FUNDC1 overexpression plasmids reversed the inhibitory effect of LW6 on mitophagy-related proteins (**Figures 4G–I**). Moreover, co-injection of LW6 with bevacizumab reversed the elevations in LC3-B, HIF-1α, BNIP3, and FUNDC1 in OIR model (**Figures 5A–C**). These findings suggest that the HIF-1α-BNIP3/FUNDC1 signaling pathway mediates bevacizumab-induced mitophagy.

in lower left. Then we examined cell type-specific changes in oxygenation status induced by intravitreal bevacizumab injection by co-staining for HIF-1α and the photoreceptor

Hypoxia-Inducible Factor-1α-BCL2/Adenovirus E1B 19-kDa Protein-Interacting Protein 3/FUN14 Domain Containing 1-Mediated Mitophagy Prevented Reactive Oxygen Species Accumulation and Reactive Oxygen Species-Induced Apoptosis Under Bevacizumab-Induced Hypoxia

To examine if HIF-1α-BNIP3/FUNDC1-induced mitophagy can improve mitochondrial function under hypoxia, intracellular ROS production, cell viability, and apoptosis rate were measured in cultured hypoxic 661W, MIO-M1, and HUVEC cells were treated with bevacizumab or CQ alone or bevacizumab plus the mitophagy inhibitor CQ. The CCK-8 assay indicated that bevacizumab or CQ alone did not reduce the number of viable 661W photoreceptors, Müller cells, or HUVECs. However, addition of CQ did reduce the number of viable cells in the presence of bevacizumab, suggesting that HIF-1α mediated mitophagy promotes cell survival (**Figures 6A–C**). Cells stained with JC-1 emitted strong red fluorescence following vehicle or bevacizumab treatment, indicating well preserved ΔΨm polarization (a prerequisite for efficient oxidative phosphorylation), while cells stained with JC-1 and treated with bevacizumab in combination with CQ showed greater green fluorescence emission, which indicates ΔΨm depolarization (**Figures 6D–F**). Depolarization of the mitochondrial membrane is also a seminal early event in apoptosis, and TUNEL staining demonstrated that intravitreal injection of bevacizumab plus intraperitoneal CQ injection enhanced apoptotic cell numbers compared to bevacizumab injection only (**Figure 5D**). Further, inhibition of mitophagy increased intracellular ROS levels in cultured cells during bevacizumab treatment compared to bevacizumab treatment alone as measured by DCFH-DA staining and flow cytometry (**Figures 6G–I**). Similar results were obtained in OIR mice. Intravitreal injection of bevacizumab plus CQ injection enhanced ROS production, while bevacizumab injection alone had no detectable effect on intracellular ROS (**Figure 5E**). Thus, despite exacerbation of hypoxia, bevacizumab did not induce oxidative stress or apoptosis if HIF-1α-mediated mitophagy was maintained, suggesting that HIF-1α-mediated mitophagy normally serves to protect retinal cells against hypoxic damage from bevacizumab.

Other Anti-Vascular Endothelial Growth Factor Agents Have Similar Effects on Cell Viability

Several anti-VEGF agents have been approved for therapeutic use, so we also investigated the effects of two additional drugs, ranibizumab (Lucentis®), and aflibercept (Eylea®). Neither agent induced measurable cytotoxicity when applied alone to hypoxic cultured retinal cells as indicated by CCK-8 assay. However, cell viability was reduced by addition of mitophagy inhibitors (**Figures 7A–F**). Thus, HIF-1α-dependent mitophagy is broadly

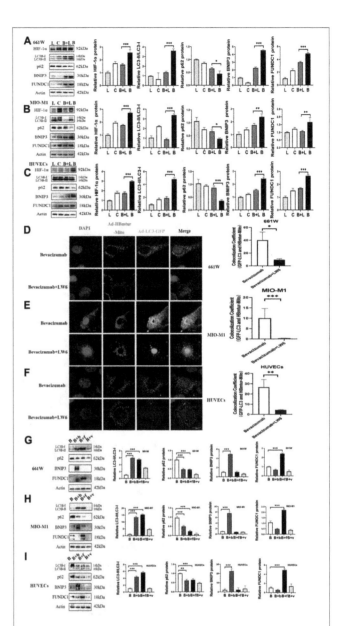

FIGURE 4 | A HIF-1α-BNIP3/FUNDC1 signaling pathway mediated bevacizumab-induced mitophagy under hypoxia. **(A–C)** Representative western blot images and densitometric results showing that the upregulation of BNIP3, FUNDC1, and LC3-II/LC3-I ratio, and the downregulation of P62 following bevacizumab were reversed by the HIF-1α inhibitor LW6 under hypoxia. L, LW6; C, Control; B + L, Bevacizumab + LW6; B, Bevacizumab. **(D–F)** Representative immunofluorescence images and quantification showing that HIF-1α inhibition by LW6 decreased mitophagosome formation as indicated by reduced LC3B/Mitotracker colocalization under hypoxia. Bar: 10 μm. **(G–I)** Representative western blot images and densitometric results showing that transfection with BNIP3 or FUNDC1 overexpression plasmids reversed the inhibitory effect of LW6 on mitophagy-related protein expression. B: Bevacizumab; B + b: Bevacizumab + BNIP3 overexpression plasmid, B + f, Bevacizumab + FUNDC1 overexpression plasmid, B + v, Bevacizumab + plasmid vector. ns: no significance, *P < 0.05, **P < 0.01, ***P < 0.001.

protective against retinal damage from anti-VEGF drug-induced hypoxia. These findings are summarized by a schematic diagram (**Figure 7G**). Anti-VEGF treatment can exacerbate retinal

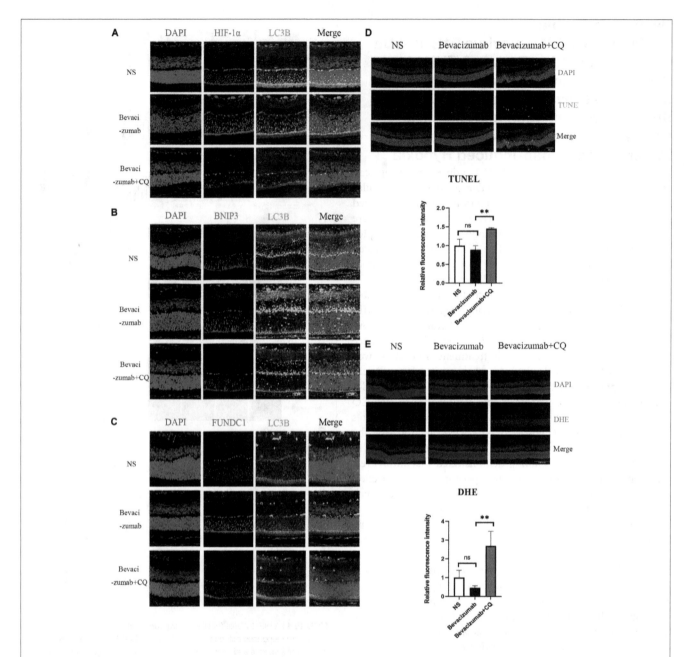

FIGURE 5 | Hypoxia-inducible factor-BNIP3/FUNDC1-mediated mitophagy prevented bevacizumab-induced ROS accumulation and ROS-induced apoptosis in OIR mouse retina: **(A–C)** OIR mice received intravitreal injection of bevacizumab alone or bevacizumab plus LW6, Representative immunofluorescence images showing LC3 co-staining with HIF, BNIP3, or FUNDC1 in retina of OIR model. **(D)** OIR mice received intravitreal injection of bevacizumab alone or bevacizumab plus CQ injection, Representative TUNEL staining imaging that CQ suppressed mitophagy and promotes apoptosis in bevacizumab-treated retina. Bar = 100 µm. **(E)** Representative fluorescence images showing that CQ interfered with mitophagy and promotes ROS production in bevacizumab-treated retina. Bar:100 µm. ns: no significance, $^*P < 0.05$, $^{**}P < 0.01$, $^{***}P < 0.001$.

hypoxia but also induces HIF-1α/BNIP3/FUNDC1-mediated mitophagy, which sustains mitochondrial function and thereby reduces oxidative stress and apoptosis (**Figure 7G**).

DISCUSSION

In this study, we examined if the efficacy and safety of anti-VEGF drugs for RNV diseases are limited by induction of

hypoxia. While intravitreal bevacizumab did indeed exacerbate hypoxia in the mouse retina and enhance the hypoxic responses of cultured retinal cells, we also found that these responses were accompanied by elevated mitophagy and that this concomitant mitophagy acted to preserve mitochondrial function and reduce apoptosis. Further investigations showed that mitophagy induction was dependent on activation of the HIF-1α-BNIP3/FUNDC1 signaling pathway and that inhibition of HIF-1α and mitophagy increased oxidative

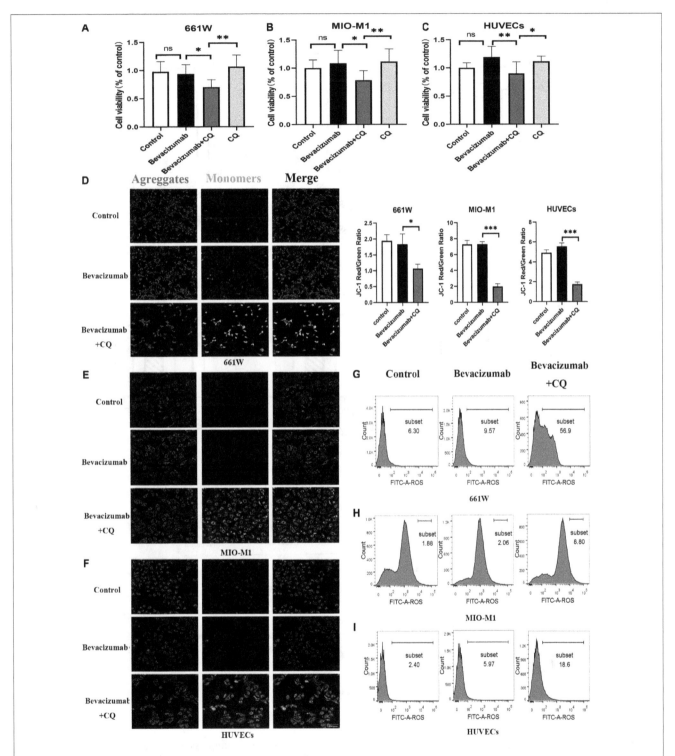

FIGURE 6 | Hypoxia-inducible factor-1α-mediated mitophagy prevented bevacizumab-induced ROS accumulation and apoptosis *in vitro*: Cultured 661W photoreceptors, MIO-M1 Müller cells, and HUVECs were treated with bevacizumab or CQ alone, bevacizumab plus autophagy inhibitor CQ under hypoxia **(A–C)** cell viability was analyzed by CCK-8. **(D–F)** Mitochondrial membrane potential was analyzed by JC-1 staing. Bar: 200 μm. **(G–I)** ROS was analyzed by DCFH-DA staining and flow cytometry. ns: no significance, *$P < 0.05$, **$P < 0.01$, ***$P < 0.001$.

stress and apoptosis in response to bevacizumab. Thus, mitophagy acts as a vital protective mechanism during bevacizumab treatment.

Expression of HIF-1α was increased in photoreceptors, Müller cells, and vascular endothelia cells exposed to bevacizumab as evidenced by western blotting of lysates from cultured

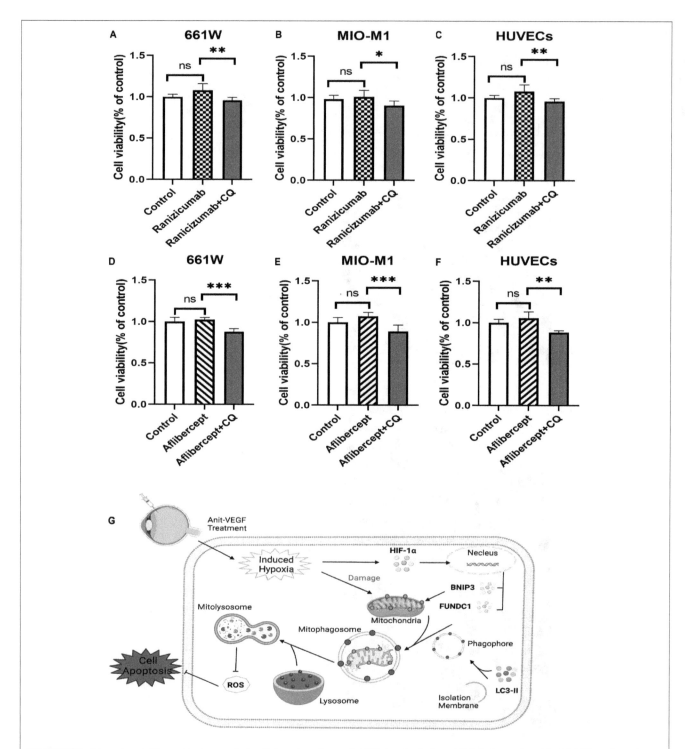

FIGURE 7 | Ranibizumab and aflibercept had same effects with bevacizumab on cell viability in cells of retina. 661W photoreceptors, MIO-M1 Müller cells, and HUVECs were treated with ranibizumab and aflibercept alone or in combination with CQ. **(A–F)** Cell viability was analyzed by CCK-8 assay. **(G)** Schematic diagram illustrating that anti-VEGF treatment can exacerbate hypoxia but also induce HIF-1α/cBNIP3/FUNDC1-mediated mitophagy to reduce ROS production and apoptosis, thereby maintaining cell viability. ns: no significance, *$P < 0.05$, **$P < 0.01$, ***$P < 0.001$.

661W photoreceptors, MIO-M1 Müller cells, and HUVECs. It was noteworthy that these changes were not detected under normoxia but was notably induced by hypoxia. These findings were further verified by co-immunostaining for HIF-1α and cell-specific markers in OIR model, an *in vivo* model of hypoxia-induced ocular neovascularization. Increased levels of HIF-1α can indirectly reflect enhanced hypoxia exposure in bevacizumab treated cells and tissue in retina. We then use Hypoxyprobe to provide direct support for this. Pimonidazole hydrochloride (HP-1) is reductively activated in hypoxic tissue and forms stable adducts with thiol (sulphydryl) groups in proteins, peptides and amino acids. The images showed more serious hypoxia within the retinal tissue after injected with bevacizumab in OIR mice. Thus, bevacizumab appears to enhance retinal hypoxia, in according with previous suggestions that bevacizumab may induce local retinal hypoxia and alter photoreceptor function (Schraermeyer and Julien, 2012). Hypoxia is a critical driver of pathological neovascularization, and HIF-1α is a hypoxia-sensing transcription factor controlling the expression of hypoxia-inducible genes. Thus, bevacizumab may amplify the responses of retinal cells to hypoxia. Similarly, several studies have reported that anti-VEGF therapy increased tumor hypoxia. Neovascularization is a compensatory process meant to restore oxygen homeostasis and promote recovery from hypoxic damage, and blocking the formation of new blood vessels may increase intra-tumor hypoxia, which is the rationale for anti-VEGF therapy in cancer patients. Meyer et al. (2009) also found that bevacizumab could activate platelet FcRIIa in monkeys, resulting in platelet aggregation, degranulation, and thrombosis. Thus, bevacizumab may promote tissue hypoxia through multiple pathways.

Transcription factor HIF-1α is implicated in the regulation of many physiological and pathological processes, including angiogenesis, apoptosis, proteolysis, metabolism, cell survival, cell migration, and tumor invasion (Dayan et al., 2006; Pouysségur et al., 2006) as well as autophagy (Tracy et al., 2007). Autophagy or "self-eating" by lysosomes was first observed in the 1950s (Yang and Klionsky, 2010) and is now considered an ubiquitous stress response that facilitates the removal of dysfunctional or superfluous cellular components and the recycling of base elements for both biosynthesis and energy generation (Levine and Kroemer, 2019). Autophagy has long been considered a non-selective process but it is now known that some organelles, such as mitochondria and endoplasmic reticulum, can be selectively targeted by the autophagic machinery (Zaffagnini and Martens, 2016). Mitochondria are the main sites of aerobic respiration and so are highly sensitive to cellular oxygen levels. If oxygen levels become unstable, mitochondrial ATP generation may be reduced and ROS generation increased, which can induce local damage. Under these conditions, mitophagy may mitigate oxidative stress and downstream pathology by removing damaged mitochondria (Kim et al., 2007), while insufficient or excessive mitophagy could lead to further damage and cell death. In our models, mitophagy appeared to protect against hypoxia induced by anti-VEGF treatment (Shintani and Klionsky, 2004). Cell viability, mitochondrial membrane potential, and apoptosis assays indicated that bevacizumab had little deleterious effect on retinal cells, even under hypoxia. However, inhibition of mitophagy reduced cell viability, depolarized the mitochondrial membrane potential, and increased apoptosis rate.

We then investigated the mechanisms linking bevacizumab treatment to mitophagy and mitophagy to cellular protection. Reactive oxygen species (ROS), including superoxide, hydroxyl radical, nitric oxide, hydrogen peroxide, and singlet oxygen, are generated directly by the mitochondrial electron transport chain driving oxidative phosphorylation and by various downstream reactions. Damaged mitochondria release more ROS (Oyewole and Birch-Machin, 2015), while mitophagy may prevent ROS generation and ensuing oxidative stress by removing damaged mitochondria (Wang, 2001; Dan Dunn et al., 2015). Indeed, inhibition of HIF-1α- mediated mitophagy resulted in higher ROS generation during bevacizumab exposure, suggesting that mitophagy is necessary for the maintenance of mitochondrial quality. Mitophagy is classically mediated by the PINK-PARKIN pathway (Kitada et al., 1998) but several additional receptor-mediated mitophagy pathways have been described. Mitophagy receptors such as Atg32, BNIP3, and FUNDC1 are localized to the outer mitochondrial membrane and have the classic tetrapeptide sequence allowing interactions with LC3 (Liu et al., 2014). In addition to changes in mitochondrial function, hypoxia is known to trigger autophagy (Bursch et al., 2008) and several independent studies have demonstrated that BNIP3 and FUNDC1 are necessary for induction (Chourasia et al., 2015; O'Sullivan et al., 2015; Li et al., 2019; Livingston et al., 2019). BNIP3 was first identified as a Bcl-2-interacting molecule that regulates apoptotic death and programmed necrosis but also contains a typical LIR motif for interaction with the autophagy-targeting protein LC3. FUN14 domain-containing 1 (FUNDC1), a three transmembrane domain protein localized on the outer mitochondrial membrane with an N-terminus domain exposed to the cytosol, also processes a LIR motif allowing interaction with LC3 (Hanna et al., 2012). Bevacizumab treatment upregulated BNIP3 and FUNDC1 in addition to HIF-1α, while pharmacological inhibition of HIF-1α reversed BNIP3 and FUNDC1 upregulation and concomitantly decreased the expression of other mitophagy-related proteins. Conversely, BNIP3 or FUNDC1 overexpression plasmids reversed the downregulation of mitophagy-related proteins by HIF-1α inhibition. These findings strongly suggest that HIF-1α induced mitophagy via receptors BNIP3 and FUNDC1.

In contrast to previous studies on the cellular effects of anti-VEGF drugs, we examined in vitro cellular responses under hypoxia to better approximate the clinical condition and combined culture experiments with examination of OIR mice, a well-accepted in vivo angiogenesis model. Müller cells are the principal glial cell type in retina and provide essential structural support as well as trophic and metabolic support to neurons and photoreceptors. In addition, Müller cells protect neurons from exposure to excess neurotransmitters by regulating the extracellular concentration through uptake mechanisms (Reichenbach and Bringmann, 2013). Photoreceptors are the primary sites of light transduction and provide primary outputs to bipolar and horizontal cells, which in turn active ganglion cells, the primary output cells. Photoreceptors have high metabolic demands that thus require efficient delivery of nutrients and oxygen from retinal vessels (Lamb, 2013). Therefore, it is expecting that cellular functions would be markedly disrupted by anti-VEGF drug-induced hypoxia. However, bevacizumab had no deleterious effects on photoreceptors or Müller cells under hypoxia but did induce oxidative stress and apoptosis under mitophagy inhibition. Inhibition of mitophagy also suppressed

HUVECs viability. Thus, mitophagy in HUVECs is an adaptive response that hampers the efficacy of anti-VEGF drugs to suppress angiogenesis. Strategies to inhibit mitophagy in vascular endothelial cells while promoting mitophagy in photoreceptors, Müller cells, and neurons may therefore optimize therapeutic efficacy and safety.

Finally, we also report that two additional anti-VEGF drugs, ranibizumab and aflibercept, did not influence cell viability under hypoxia conditions, while inhibition of mitophagy reduced cell viability. Thus, concomitant mitophagy appears to be a common protective mechanism under anti-VEGF treatment.

In summary, the present study demonstrates that photoreceptors, Müller cells, and vascular endothelial cells are not adversely affected by anti-VEGF agents even under hypoxia due to concomitant activation of HIF-1α-BNIP3/FUNDC1-mitophagy. The regulation of mitophagy in specific retinal cell types may be a useful strategy to optimize the therapeutic efficacy and safety of anti-VEGF drugs.

ETHICS STATEMENT

The animal study was reviewed and approved by Animal Care and Ethics Committee of the Zhongshan Ophthalmic Center (Approval number: 2020-023).

AUTHOR CONTRIBUTIONS

SZ, WC and YS contributed to the study concept and design. YS, LS, and JL contributed to the experimental and technical support. YS and CY contributed to the acquisition, analysis, or interpretation of data. WC and YS contributed to the drafting of the manuscript and statistical analysis. WC, FW, and YS contributed to the critical revision of the manuscript for important intellectual content. All authors contributed to the article and approved the submitted version.

REFERENCES

Aiello, L. P., Pierce, E. A., Foley, E. D., Takagi, H., Chen, H., Riddle, L., et al. (1995). Suppression of retinal neovascularization *in vivo* by inhibition of vascular endothelial growth factor (VEGF) using soluble VEGF-receptor chimeric proteins. *Proc. Natl. Acad. Sci. U. S. A.* 92, 10457–10461.

Brockington, A., Heath, P. R., Holden, H., Kasher, P., Bender, F. L. P., Claes, F., et al. (2010). Downregulation of genes with a function in axon outgrowth and synapse formation in motor neurones of the VEGFdelta/delta mouse model of amyotrophic lateral sclerosis. *BMC Genomics* 11:203. doi: 10.1186/1471-2164-11-203

Bursch, W., Karwan, A., Mayer, M., Dornetshuber, J., Fröhwein, U., Schulte-Hermann, R., et al. (2008). Cell death and autophagy: cytokines, drugs, and nutritional factors. *Toxicology* 254, 147–157. doi: 10.1016/j.tox.2008.07.048

Campochiaro, P. A. (2015). Molecular pathogenesis of retinal and choroidal vascular diseases. *Prog. Retin. Eye Res.* 49, 67–81. doi: 10.1016/j.preteyeres.2015.06.002

Campochiaro, P. A., and Akhlaq, A. (2020). Sustained suppression of VEGF for treatment of retinal/choroidal vascular diseases. *Prog. Retin. Eye Res.* 83:100921. doi: 10.1016/j.preteyeres.2020.100921

Campochiaro, P. A., and Hackett, S. F. (2003). Ocular neovascularization: a valuable model system. *Oncogene* 22, 6537–6548.

Chourasia, A. H., Tracy, K., Frankenberger, C., Boland, M. L., Sharifi, M. N., Drake, L. E., et al. (2015). Mitophagy defects arising from BNip3 loss promote mammary tumor progression to metastasis. *EMBO Rep.* 16, 1145–1163. doi: 10.15252/embr.201540759

Dan Dunn, J., Alvarez, L. A., Zhang, X., and Soldati, T. (2015). Reactive oxygen species and mitochondria: a nexus of cellular homeostasis. *Redox Biol.* 6, 472–485. doi: 10.1016/j.redox.2015.09.005

Dayan, F., Roux, D., Brahimi-Horn, M. C., Pouyssegur, J., and Mazure, N. M. (2006). The oxygen sensor factor-inhibiting hypoxia-inducible factor-1 controls expression of distinct genes through the bifunctional transcriptional character of hypoxia-inducible factor-1alpha. *Cancer Res.* 66, 3688–3698.

de Almeida, P. E., Mak, J., Hernandez, G., Jesudason, R., Herault, A., Javinal, V., et al. (2020). Anti-VEGF treatment enhances CD8 T-cell antitumor activity by amplifying hypoxia. *Cancer Immunol. Res.* 8, 806–818. doi: 10.1158/2326-6066.CIR-19-0360

Dings, R. P. M., Loren, M., Heun, H., McNiel, E., Griffioen, A. W., Mayo, K. H., et al. (2007). Scheduling of radiation with angiogenesis inhibitors anginex and Avastin improves therapeutic outcome via vessel normalization. *Clin. Cancer Res.* 13, 3395–3402.

Elvidge, G. P., Glenny, L., Appelhoff, R. J., Ratcliffe, P. J., Ragoussis, J., and Gleadle, J. M. (2006). Concordant regulation of gene expression by hypoxia and 2-oxoglutarate-dependent dioxygenase inhibition: the role of HIF-1alpha, HIF-2alpha, and other pathways. *J. Biol. Chem.* 281, 15215–15226.

Fierson, W. M. (2018). Screening examination of premature infants for retinopathy of prematurity. *Pediatrics* 142:e20183061. doi: 10.1542/peds.2018-3061

Flaxel, C. J., Adelman, R. A., Bailey, S. T., Fawzi, A., Lim, J. I., Vemulakonda, G. A., et al. (2020). Retinal vein occlusions preferred practice pattern®. *Ophthalmology* 127, P288–P320. doi: 10.1016/j.ophtha.2019.09.029

Galluzzi, L., Kepp, O., Trojel-Hansen, C., and Kroemer, G. (2012). Mitochondrial control of cellular life, stress, and death. *Circ. Res.* 111, 1198–1207. doi: 10.1161/CIRCRESAHA.112.268946

Glick, D., Barth, S., and Macleod, K. F. (2010). Autophagy: cellular and molecular mechanisms. *J. Pathol.* 221, 3–12. doi: 10.1002/path.2697

Grunwald, J. E., Daniel, E., Huang, J., Ying, G.-S., Maguire, M. G., Toth, C. A., et al. (2014). Risk of geographic atrophy in the comparison of age-related macular degeneration treatments trials. *Ophthalmology* 121, 150–161. doi: 10.1016/j.ophtha.2013.08.015

Hanna, R. A., Quinsay, M. N., Orogo, A. M., Giang, K., Rikka, S., and Gustafsson, ÅB. (2012). Microtubule-associated protein 1 light chain 3 (LC3) interacts with Bnip3 protein to selectively remove endoplasmic reticulum and mitochondria via autophagy. *J. Biol. Chem.* 287, 19094–19104. doi: 10.1074/jbc.M111.322933

Kim, I., Rodriguez-Enriquez, S., and Lemasters, J. J. (2007). Selective degradation of mitochondria by mitophagy. *Arch. Biochem. Biophys.* 462, 245–253.

Kitada, T., Asakawa, S., Hattori, N., Matsumine, H., Yamamura, Y., Minoshima, S., et al. (1998). Mutations in the parkin gene cause autosomal recessive juvenile parkinsonism. *Nature* 392, 605–608.

Lamb, T. D. (2013). Evolution of phototransduction, vertebrate photoreceptors and retina. *Prog. Retin. Eye Res.* 36, 25–119. doi: 10.1016/j.preteyeres.2013.06.001

Lee, C. G., Heijn, M., di Tomaso, E., Griffon-Etienne, G., Ancukiewicz, M., Koike, C., et al. (2000). Anti-vascular endothelial growth factor treatment augments tumor radiation response under normoxic or hypoxic conditions. *Cancer Res.* 60, 5565–5570.

Levine, B., and Kroemer, G. (2019). Biological functions of autophagy genes: a disease perspective. *Cell* 176(1–2), 11–42. doi: 10.1016/j.cell.2018.09.048

Li, L., Tan, J., Miao, Y., Lei, P., and Zhang, Q. (2015). ROS and autophagy: interactions and molecular regulatory mechanisms. *Cell. Mol. Neurobiol.* 35, 615–621. doi: 10.1007/s10571-015-0166-x

Li, L. Y., Luo, X., and Wang, X. (2001). Endonuclease G is an apoptotic DNase when released from mitochondria. *Nature* 412, 95–99.

Li, W., Li, Y., Siraj, S., Jin, H., Fan, Y., Yang, X., et al. (2019). FUN14 domain-containing 1-mediated mitophagy suppresses hepatocarcinogenesis by inhibition of inflammasome activation in mice. *Hepatology* 69, 604–621. doi: 10.1002/hep.30191

Limb, G. A., Salt, T. E., Munro, P. M. G., Moss, S. E., and Khaw, P. T. (2002). *In vitro* characterization of a spontaneously immortalized human Müller cell line (MIO-M1). *Invest. Ophthalmol. Vis. Sci.* 43, 864–869.

Liu, L., Feng, D., Chen, G., Chen, M., Zheng, Q., Song, P., et al. (2012). Mitochondrial outer-membrane protein FUNDC1 mediates hypoxia-induced mitophagy in mammalian cells. *Nat. Cell Biol.* 14, 177–185. doi: 10.1038/ncb2422

Liu, L., Sakakibara, K., Chen, Q., and Okamoto, K. (2014). Receptor-mediated mitophagy in yeast and mammalian systems. *Cell Res.* 24, 787–795. doi: 10.1038/cr.2014.75

Livingston, M. J., Wang, J., Zhou, J., Wu, G., Ganley, I. G., Hill, J. A., et al. (2019). Clearance of damaged mitochondria via mitophagy is important to the protective effect of ischemic preconditioning in kidneys. *Autophagy* 15, 2142–2162. doi: 10.1080/15548627.2019.1615822

Malik, D., Tarek, M., Caceres del Carpio, J., Ramirez, C., Boyer, D., Kenney, M. C., et al. (2014). Safety profiles of anti-VEGF drugs: bevacizumab, ranibizumab, aflibercept and ziv-aflibercept on human retinal pigment epithelium cells in culture. *Br. J. Ophthalmol.* 98 Suppl 1, i11–i16. doi: 10.1136/bjophthalmol-2014-305302

Manalo, D. J., Rowan, A., Lavoie, T., Natarajan, L., Kelly, B. D., Ye, S. Q., et al. (2005). Transcriptional regulation of vascular endothelial cell responses to hypoxia by HIF-1. *Blood* 105, 659–669.

Meyer, T., Robles-Carrillo, L., Robson, T., Langer, F., Desai, H., Davila, M., et al. (2009). Bevacizumab immune complexes activate platelets and induce thrombosis in FCGR2A transgenic mice. *J. Thromb. Haemost.* 7, 171–181. doi: 10.1111/j.1538-7836.2008.03212

Mazure, N. M., and Pouysségur, J. (2010). Hypoxia-induced autophagy: cell death or cell survival? *Curr. Opin. Cell Biol.* 22, 177–180. doi: 10.1016/j.ceb.2009.11.015

Miyazaki, S., Kikuchi, H., Iino, I., Uehara, T., Setoguchi, T., Fujita, T., et al. (2014). Anti-VEGF antibody therapy induces tumor hypoxia and stanniocalcin 2 expression and potentiates growth of human colon cancer xenografts. *Int. J. Cancer* 135, 295–307. doi: 10.1002/ijc.28686

Myers, A. L., Williams, R. F., Ng, C. Y., Hartwich, J. E., and Davidoff, A. M. (2010). Bevacizumab-induced tumor vessel remodeling in rhabdomyosarcoma xenografts increases the effectiveness of adjuvant ionizing radiation. *J. Pediatr. Surg.* 45, 1080–1085. doi: 10.1016/j.jpedsurg.2010.02.068

Ney, P. A. (2015). Mitochondrial autophagy: origins, significance, and role of BNIP3 and NIX. *Biochim. Biophys. Acta* 1853(10 Pt B), 2775–2783. doi: 10.1016/j.bbamcr.2015.02.022

Nishijima, K., Ng, Y.-S., Zhong, L., Bradley, J., Schubert, W., Jo, N., et al. (2007). Vascular endothelial growth factor-A is a survival factor for retinal neurons and a critical neuroprotectant during the adaptive response to ischemic injury. *Am. J. Pathol.* 171, 53–67.

O'Sullivan, T. E., Johnson, L. R., Kang, H. H., and Sun, J. C. (2015). BNIP3- and BNIP3L-mediated mitophagy promotes the generation of natural killer cell memory. *Immunity* 43, 331–342. doi: 10.1016/j.immuni.2015.07.012

Oyewole, A. O., and Birch-Machin, M. A. (2015). Mitochondria-targeted antioxidants. *FASEB J.* 29, 4766–4771. doi: 10.1096/fj.15-275404

Pierce, E. A., Avery, R. L., Foley, E. D., Aiello, L. P., and Smith, L. E. (1995). Vascular endothelial growth factor/vascular permeability factor expression in a mouse model of retinal neovascularization. *Proc. Natl. Acad. Sci. U. S. A.* 92, 905–909.

Pouysségur, J., Dayan, F., and Mazure, N. M. (2006). Hypoxia signalling in cancer and approaches to enforce tumour regression. *Nature* 441, 437–443.

Reichenbach, A., and Bringmann, A. (2013). New functions of Müller cells. *Glia* 61, 651–678. doi: 10.1002/glia.22477

Rofagha, S., Bhisitkul, R. B., Boyer, D. S., Sadda, S. R., and Zhang, K. (2013). SEVEN-UP study group. Seven-year outcomes in ranibizumab-treated patients in ANCHOR, MARINA, and HORIZON: a multicenter cohort study (SEVEN-UP). *Ophthalmology* 120, 2292–2299. doi: 10.1016/j.ophtha.2013.03.046

Schraermeyer, U., and Julien, S. (2012). Formation of immune complexes and thrombotic microangiopathy after intravitreal injection of bevacizumab in the primate eye. *Graefes Arch. Clin. Exp. Ophthalmol.* 250, 1303–1313. doi: 10.1007/s00417-012-2055-z

Shi, Y., Oeh, J., Hitz, A., Hedehus, M., Eastham-Anderson, J., Peale, F. V., et al. (2017). Monitoring and targeting anti-VEGF induced hypoxia within the viable tumor by F-MRI and multispectral analysis. *Neoplasia* 19, 950–959. doi: 10.1016/j.neo.2017.07.010

Shintani, T., and Klionsky, D. J. (2004). Autophagy in health and disease: a double-edged sword. *Science* 306, 990–995.

Tracy, K., Dibling, B. C., Spike, B. T., Knabb, J. R., Schumacker, P., and Macleod, K. F. (2007). BNIP3 is an RB/E2F target gene required for hypoxia-induced autophagy. *Mol. Cell. Biol.* 27, 6229–6242.

Ueda, S., Saeki, T., Osaki, A., Yamane, T., and Kuji, I. (2017). Bevacizumab induces acute hypoxia and cancer progression in patients with refractory breast cancer: multimodal functional imaging and multiplex cytokine analysis. *Clin. Cancer Res.* 23, 5769–5778. doi: 10.1158/1078-0432.CCR-17-0874

Wallace, D. C. (1999). Mitochondrial diseases in man and mouse. *Science* 283, 1482–1488.

Wang, X. (2001). The expanding role of mitochondria in apoptosis. *Genes Dev.* 15, 2922–2933.

Wells, J. A., Glassman, A. R., Ayala, A. R., Jampol, L. M., Bressler, N. M., Bressler, S. B., et al. (2016). Aflibercept, Bevacizumab, or Ranibizumab for diabetic macular edema: two-year results from a comparative effectiveness randomized clinical trial. *Ophthalmology* 123, 1351–1359. doi: 10.1016/j.ophtha.2016.02.022

Wong, T. Y., Sun, J., Kawasaki, R., Ruamviboonsuk, P., Gupta, N., Lansingh, V. C., et al. (2018). Guidelines on diabetic eye care: the international council of ophthalmology recommendations for screening, follow-up, referral, and treatment based on resource settings. *Ophthalmology* 125, 1608–1622. doi: 10.1016/j.ophtha.2018.04.007

Yang, Z., and Klionsky, D. J. (2010). Eaten alive: a history of macroautophagy. *Nat. Cell Biol.* 12, 814–822. doi: 10.1038/ncb0910-814

Zaffagnini, G., and Martens, S. (2016). Mechanisms of selective autophagy. *J. Mol. Biol.* 428(9 Pt A), 1714–1724. doi: 10.1016/j.jmb.2016.02.004

Zhang, H., Bosch-Marce, M., Shimoda, L. A., Tan, Y. S., Baek, J. H., Wesley, J. B., et al. (2008). Mitochondrial autophagy is an HIF-1-dependent adaptive metabolic response to hypoxia. *J. Biol. Chem.* 283, 10892–10903. doi: 10.1074/jbc.M800102200

9

Metabolite Changes in the Aqueous Humor of Patients with Retinal Vein Occlusion Macular Edema

Xiaojing Xiong[1], Xu Chen[1], Huafeng Ma[1], Zheng Zheng[1], Yazhu Yang[1], Zhu Chen[1], Zixi Zhou[1], Jiaxin Pu[1], Qingwei Chen[2] and Minming Zheng[1]*

[1]Department of Ophthalmology, Second Affiliated Hospital of Chongqing Medical University, Chongqing, China, [2]Department of general practice, Second Affiliated Hospital of Chongqing Medical University, Chongqing, China

*Correspondence:
Minming Zheng
381393002@qq.com

Macular edema (ME) is the main cause of visual impairment in patients with retinal vein occlusion (RVO). The degree of ME affects the prognosis of RVO patients, while it lacks objective laboratory biomarkers. We aimed to compare aqueous humor samples from 28 patients with retinal vein occlusion macular edema (RVO-ME) to 27 age- and sex-matched controls by ultra-high-performance liquid chromatography equipped with quadrupole time-of-flight mass spectrometry, so as to identify the key biomarkers and to increase the understanding of the mechanism of RVO-ME at the molecular level. Through univariate and multivariate statistical analyses, we identified 60 metabolites between RVO-ME patients and controls and 40 differential metabolites in mild RVO-ME [300 μm ≤ central retinal thickness (CRT) < 400 μm] patients compared with severe RVO-ME (CRT ≥ 400 μm). Pathway enrichment analysis showed that valine, leucine, and isoleucine biosynthesis; ascorbate and aldarate metabolism; and pantothenate and coenzyme A biosynthesis were significantly altered in RVO-ME in comparison with controls. Compared with mild RVO-ME, degradation and biosynthesis of valine, leucine, and isoleucine; histidine metabolism; beta-alanine metabolism; and pantothenate and coenzyme A biosynthesis were significantly changed in severe RVO-ME. Furthermore, the receiver operating characteristic (ROC) curve analysis revealed that adenosine, threonic acid, pyruvic acid, and pyro-L-glutaminyl-L-glutamine could differentiate RVO-ME from controls with an area under the curve (AUC) of >0.813. Urocanic acid, diethanolamine, 8-butanoylneosolaniol, niacinamide, paraldehyde, phytosphingosine, 4-aminobutyraldehyde, dihydrolipoate, and 1-(beta-D-ribofuranosyl)-1,4-dihydronicotinamide had an AUC of >0.848 for distinguishing mild RVO-ME from severe RVO-ME. Our study expanded the understanding of metabolomic changes in RVO-ME, which could help us to have a good understanding of the pathogenesis of RVO-ME.

Keywords: retinal vein occlusion, macular edema, macular central thickness, aqueous humor, metabolomics analysis

INTRODUCTION

Retinal vein occlusion (RVO) is the major cause of vision loss by retinal vascular diseases. Classified by the location of obstruction, RVO can be differentiated into central retinal vein occlusion (CRVO) and branch retinal vein occlusion (BRVO). Known risk factors for RVO include hypertension, atherosclerosis, hyperlipidemia, diabetes, thrombosis, and other inflammatory and myeloproliferative diseases (Petr, 2014; Balaratnasingam et al., 2016). Clinical presentations of RVO include retinal hemorrhage, tortuous retinal veins, optic nerve swelling, and macular edema (ME) (Querques et al., 2013). Among them, the most common cause of vision loss in RVO is ME. Studies have shown that central retinal thickness (CRT) was closely related to visual acuity and prognosis (Eng and Leng, 2020). Although the diagnosis of retinal vein occlusion macular edema (RVO-ME) was undoubted, the initial pathogenesis and following pathophysiology of RVO-ME remained controversial.

Abundant metabolomics studies have been carried out in animal models or humans under pathophysiological conditions to identify the most important metabolites in various ophthalmic diseases by analyzing blood or intraocular fluid samples (Deng et al., 2020). Aqueous humor (AH) provides nutrition for the surrounding avascular cornea and lens and discharges the metabolic waste from the eyes to the venous blood. The metabonomic information of AH could directly reflect the physiological state of the eyes (Haines et al., 2018). Recent studies using liquid chromatography–mass spectrometry (LC-MS) have also identified almost 250 metabolites belonging to 47 metabolic pathways in AH (Karolina et al., 2017). Additionally, wet age-related macular degeneration (Han et al., 2020), diabetic retinopathy (Pietrowska et al., 2018), severe myopia (Ji et al., 2017), primary open-angle glaucoma (Buisset et al., 2019), and primary congenital glaucoma (Breda et al., 2020) were also found to be associated with metabolomic signatures in the aqueous humor. However, AH metabolism of RVO-ME has not been reported yet.

The aims of the current study were to identify differential metabolites in the RVO-ME compared with controls, to screen biomarkers from these differential metabolites, and to identify potential biomarkers that could differentiate patients between mild RVO-ME (mRVO-ME) (300 μm ≤ CRT < 400 μm) and severe RVO-ME (sRVO-ME) (CRT ≥ 400 μm) (Kim et al., 2020) (**Figure 1**).

METHODS

Sample Collection

The study was conducted in accordance with the requirements of the Ethics Committee of The Second Affiliated Hospital of Chongqing Medical University, which approved the study (2020405). The study follows the principles of the Helsinki Declaration. All aqueous humor samples from patients with RVO-ME ($n = 28$) and the age- and sex-matched control group ($n = 27$) were collected from ophthalmology department of the Second Affiliated Hospital of Chongqing Medical

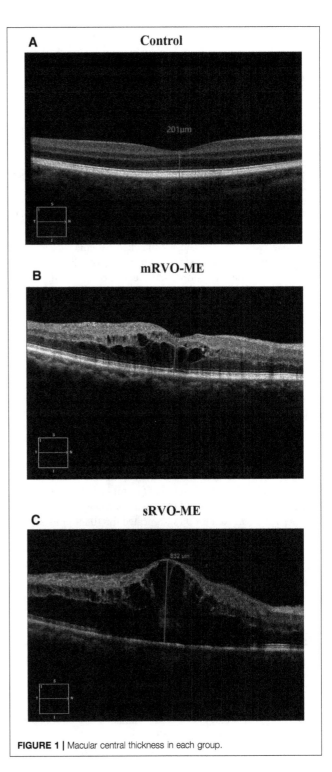

FIGURE 1 | Macular central thickness in each group.

University, from October 2020 to March 2021. All participants were informed and signed the informed consent.

Cataract grading had been assessed using the Lens Opacities Cataract Classification System III (LOCS III) (Chylack et al., 1993). LOCS III of both the RVO group and the control group were N2C2P2. The diagnosis of RVO was made using the International Classification of Diseases, Ninth Revision,

Clinical Modification (ICD-9-CM). CRVO was defined as ICD-9 362.35 and BRVO as ICD-9 362.36 (Kupka, 1978). The inclusion criteria for RVO-ME were as follows: 1) age ≥18 years, 2) diagnosis within 1 year, and 3) CRT ≥ 300 μm. Exclusion criteria included the following: 1) age-related macular degeneration; 2) diabetic retinopathy; 3) previous intravitreal injection of anti-vascular endothelial growth factor or steroids; 4) previous intraocular surgery; 5) previous retinal photocoagulation; 6) glaucoma, including neovascular glaucoma; 7) iris redness and anterior chamber hemorrhage; 8) vitreous hemorrhage and other vitreoretinal disease; 9) cerebrovascular accident or myocardial infarction in the past 3 months; and 10) any kind of eye drops has been used within 3 months prior to sample collection. Samples of the control group were collected from age- and sex-matched patients who received aqueous humor samples before cataract surgery. All subjects and controls were not using hormonal medication.

Sample Preparation

AH samples were taken by puncture after surface anesthesia and disinfection. Approximately 200 μl of aqueous humor was collected. The AH samples were immediately transferred to dust-free Eppendorf tubes, centrifuged twice at 4°C and 16,000×g for 15 min, and then the supernatants were collected in cryogenic vials. Finally, the supernatant was collected and quickly stored at−80°C until metabolomics analysis.

For metabolomics analysis, ultra-high-performance liquid chromatography equipped with quadrupole time-of-flight mass spectrometry (UHPLC-Q-TOF/MS) analysis has been carried out. To an EP tube, 50 μl of sample was transferred. After the addition of 200 μl of extract solution (acetonitrile/methanol = 1:1, containing isotopically labelled internal standard mixture), the samples were vortexed for 30 s, sonicated for 10 min in ice water bath, and incubated for 1 h at −40°C to precipitate proteins. Then, the samples proceeded to centrifugation at 12,000 rpm [RCF = 13,800 (×g), R = 8.6 cm] for 15 min at 4°C. The resulting supernatant was transferred to a fresh glass vial for analysis. The quality control (QC) sample was prepared by mixing an equal aliquot of the supernatants from all of the samples.

Metabolomics Analysis

LC-MS/MS analysis was performed using an UHPLC system (Vanquish, Thermo Fisher Scientific) with a UPLC BEH Amide column (2.1 mm × 100 mm, 1.7 μm) coupled to Q Exactive HFX mass spectrometer (Orbitrap MS, Thermo) by Shanghai Biotree Biomedical Technology Co., Ltd., China. The mobile phase consisted of 25 mmol/l ammonium acetate and 25 ammonia hydroxide in water (pH = 9.75) (A) and acetonitrile (B). The auto-sampler temperature was 4°C, and the injection volume was 3 μl.

The QE HFX mass spectrometer was used for its ability to acquire MS/MS spectra on information-dependent acquisition (IDA) mode in the control of the acquisition software (Xcalibur, Thermo). In this mode, the acquisition software continuously evaluated the full-scan MS spectrum. The ESI source conditions were set as follows: sheath gas flow rate at 30 Arb, Aux gas flow rate at 25 Arb, capillary temperature 350°C, full MS resolution at 60,000, MS/MS resolution at 7,500, collision energy at 10/30/60 in NCE mode, and spray voltage at 3.6 kV (positive) or −3.2 kV (negative), respectively.

Data Processing

The raw data was converted to the mzXML format using ProteoWizard and processed with an in-house program, which was developed using R and based on XCMS, for peak detection, extraction, alignment, and integration. Then, an in-house MS2 database (BiotreeDB) was applied in metabolite annotation. The cutoff for annotation was set at 0.3.

Then, we performed principal component analysis (PCA) and partial least squares discriminant analysis (PLS-DA) by using SIMCA version 16.0.2 (Umetrics AB, Sweden) to obtain an overview of metabolomics data. The contribution of each metabolite was calculated according to the PLS-DA model and expressed as variable importance in the prediction (VIP) score. In order to evaluate the significance of metabolites, the metabolites with a VIP score >1 were analyzed by Student's t-test. The categories of metabolites were defined by using the Human Metabolome Database (HMDB) (https://hmdb.ca/).

Bioinformatics Analysis

Volcano plots were made using GraphPad Prism V.7.0.0. Meanwhile, we calculated the Euclidean distance matrix for the quantitative value of differential metabolites and clustered the differential metabolites by complete linkage method. Then, we mapped authoritative metabolite databases such as KEGG and PubChem through differential metabolites. After obtaining the matching information of differential metabolites, we searched the pathway database of the corresponding species Homo sapiens (human) and conducted an enrichment analysis and a topological analysis to find the most critical pathways that are most related to differential metabolites.

Receiver Operating Characteristic Curve Analysis

To identify potential diagnostic biomarkers, a receiver operating characteristic (ROC) curve analysis was used to assess the diagnostic potential of differential metabolites, and the area under the curve (AUC) was calculated.

Statistical Analysis

SPSS 22.0 was used to analyze the data. The results were expressed as mean ± standard deviation (SD) of continuous variables. The normality was tested by Shapiro–Wilk test. Student's t-test, ANOVA, Fisher's exact test, and Pearson chi square test were used. A p value <0.05 was considered statistically significant.

RESULTS

Clinical Characteristics of Participants

To investigate the metabolic profile of aqueous humor in RVO-ME, we enrolled 27 age- and sex-matched controls and 28 RVO-ME patients (11 mRVO-ME, 300 μm ≤ CRT < 400 μm,

TABLE 1 | Demographic and clinical characteristics of participants.

	RVO-ME (28)		Control (27)	p value[a]
	mRVO-ME (11)	sRVO-ME (17)		
Gender (male/female)	5/6	8/9	12/15	0.986
Age (years), median	70 ± 8.35	70.12 ± 8.03	70.33 ± 8.06	0.992
BMI (kg/m^2)	23.2 ± 1.73	23.3 ± 1.82	22.88 ± 2.03	0.753
Hypertension (yes/no)	3/8	13/4	19/8	0.907
Diabetes (yes/no)	2/9	3/14	4/23	0.956
Coronary heart disease (yes/no)	2/9	3/14	5/22	0.997
Hyperlipidemia (yes/no)	4/7	6/11	9/18	0.981

RVO-ME, retinal vein occlusion macular edema; mRVO-ME, mild retinal vein occlusion macular edema; sRVO-ME, severe retinal vein occlusion macular edema.
[a]P-value was calculated by Student's t-test.

17 sRVO-ME, CRT $\geq$ 400 µm) for untargeted metabolomics analysis. There was no significant difference in age, gender, hypertension, coronary heart disease, and diabetes mellitus among the groups (**Table 1**).

AH Metabolism Analysis

In order to identify the metabolism of aqueous humor, untargeted metabolomics analysis was applied. The results showed that the method had good reproducibility, and only slight changes of the spectral peaks of the QC samples were found (**Supplementary Figure S1**). A total of 4,945 signals were identified by peak alignment, missing value reconstruction, and data normalization. After Pareto scaling the data, PCA models displayed that QC samples were closely clustered (**Supplementary Figure S2**), which also indicated the high repeatability of the method and the reliability of the data. In order to visualize and identify the most prominent metabolic differences among the various groups, PLS-DA was performed. Using median coordinates for the training sets, the scatter plot of the latent variables of the PLS-DA models showed good discrimination for comparisons between RVO-ME versus controls and mRVO-ME versus sRVO-ME (**Figure 2**).

Differentially Expressed Metabolites Between Groups

A total of 60 differential metabolites were found in RVO-ME when compared with controls and 40 differential metabolites in mRVO-ME compared with sRVO-ME (VIP > 1 and $p < 0.05$), including amino acids, carboxylic acids, fatty acid purine, pyrimidine, and so on (**Table 2**). Volcano plots (**Figure 3**), heat plot, and hierarchical cluster analysis (**Figure 4**) were used to investigate variation tendencies for the differential metabolites. Twenty-two metabolites were significantly elevated and 38 metabolites were significantly decreased in RVO-ME compared to controls. We also found 30 increased metabolites and 20 decreased metabolites when comparing mRVO-ME with sRVO-ME.

Pathway Analysis of Differential Aqueous Metabolites

MetaboAnalyst was applied to compare metabolic disturbances in RVO-ME versus controls and mRVO-ME versus sRVO-ME

(**Table 3**). When comparing RVO-ME patients with controls, a total of three differential pathways were found, namely, valine, leucine, and isoleucine biosynthesis; pantothenate and coenzyme A (CoA) biosynthesis; and ascorbate and aldarate metabolism. Valine, leucine, and isoleucine biosynthesis; pantothenate and CoA biosynthesis; beta-alanine metabolism; histidine metabolism; and valine, leucine, and isoleucine degradation were altered in sRVO-ME when compared to mRVO-ME (**Figure 5**).

ROC Curve Analysis

Further screening of the metabolic indicators was conducted by ROC analysis (**Figure 6**). As shown in **Figure 6A**, threonic acid, pyro-L-glutaminyl-L-glutamine, adenosine, and pyruvic acid had an AUC $\geq$ 0.813 for distinguishing RVO-ME from controls. When comparing sRVO-ME with mRVO-ME patients, the ROC analysis showed that nine metabolites had an AUC $\geq$ 0.848, including urocanic acid, 1-(beta-D-ribofuranosyl)-1,4-dihydronicotinamide, phytosphingosine, niacinamide, 8-butanoylneosolaniol, dihydrolipoate, paraldehyde, 4-aminobutyraldehyde, and diethanolamine (**Figure 6B**).

DISCUSSION

In the present study, we explored the metabolomic changes in AH of patients with RVO-ME disease. To the best of our knowledge, this is the first time that UHPC-Q-TOF/MS was used to analyze the discrepancy of AH metabolomics in RVO-ME versus controls and mRVO-ME versus sRVO-ME. After correction, 60 and 40 metabolites were differentially expressed in RVO-ME versus controls and mRVO-ME versus sRVO-ME, respectively. Notably, amino acids were the most abundant differential metabolite category. Also, significant alterations were noted in several metabolic pathways. Interestingly, we found that pantothenate and CoA biosynthesis and valine, leucine, and isoleucine biosynthesis were significantly altered both in RVO-ME versus controls and mRVO-ME versus sRVO-ME. Additionally, ROC curves were also performed to assess the metabolites of AH, which could best distinguish RVO-ME from the controls and mRVO-ME from sRVO-ME.

Previous studies have revealed that intraocular angiogenic factors and inflammatory cytokines play pivotal roles in the

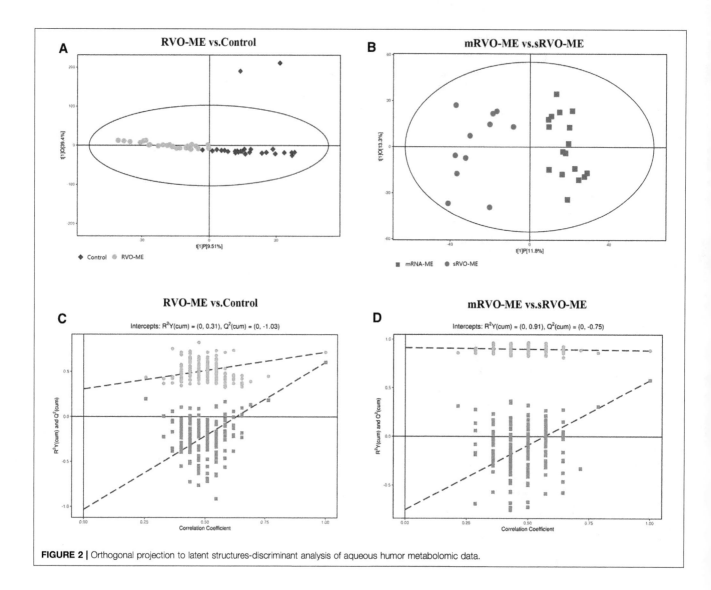

FIGURE 2 | Orthogonal projection to latent structures-discriminant analysis of aqueous humor metabolomic data.

occurrence and progression of ocular complications in patients with RVO (An et al., 2021; Yong et al., 1007). In the current study, many inflammation-related metabolites have also been found in RVO-ME when compared with controls. Adenosine is an endogenous purine nucleoside, which is widely distributed in the body and interacts with G-protein-coupled receptors (Sebastião and Ribeiro, 2009; Santiago et al., 2020). Under the stress conditions of tissue ischemia, hypoxia, and inflammatory response, the concentration of extracellular adenosine increased exponentially. Previous studies have shown that adenosine or its analogues could raise intraocular angiogenic factors and inflammatory cytokines, such as vascular endothelial growth factor, insulin-like growth factor-1, basic fibroblast growth factor, interleukin-8, and angiogenin-2 (Feoktistov et al., 2003; Haskó and Pacher, 2012). Luo et al. (2019) found that adenosine attenuated the inflammatory response of human endothelial cells through negative regulation of Toll-like receptor MyD88 signal. Haas et al. (2011) showed that adenosine could induce a reduction of Toll-like receptor4 expression at the surface of

human macrophages, resulting in a robust inhibition of TNF-α production. In this study, compared with the controls, the level of adenosine in RVO-ME increased, which suggests that RVO-ME was associated with inflammatory process, to some extent. In addition, adenosine also regulates vascular tension and thus blood flow. Adenosine, acting predominantly at $A_{2A}R$, induced the production of NO, which causes vasodilation of retinal vessels (Riis-Vestergaard et al., 2014; Riis-Vestergaard and Bek, 2015). We speculated that the decrease of $A_{2A}R$ also resulted in the increase of free adenosine, which might play a crucial role in RVO vascular occlusion. Threonic acid, also known as threonate, is a central signaling hub in ascorbate–aldarate pathway (Wang et al., 2019). We detected an abnormal expression of threonine and ascorbate and aldarate metabolism in RVO-ME. As shown by the experiment of corneal neovascularization in a rodent model, ascorbic acid might inhibit angiogenesis, which was regarded as a vital event of RVO (Ashino et al., 2003). In our present study, we also found that adenosine and threonic acid could act as a potential

TABLE 2 | Identified differential metabolites.

Metabolites	RVO-ME vs. control			mRVO-ME vs. sRVO-ME			Category
	VIP	FC	p value	VIP	FC	p value[a]	
Ketoleucine	1.158	0.80	0.034	1.86	0.68	0.012	Amino acids
Cis-4-Hydroxy-D-proline	1.71	0.70	0.030	1.43	0.89	0.022	Amino acids
8-Butanoylneosolaniol	1.66	7.98	0.008	2.38	10.97	0.007	Fatty acid
Dihydrouracil	1.87	0.74	0.004	1.47	0.88	0.030	Pyrimidones
L-trans-4-methyl-2-pyrrolidinecarboxylic acid	1.06	2.04	0.033	1.06	2.04	0.033	Amino acids
D-mannose	1.17	1.36	0.030	1.17	1.36	0.030	Carbohydrate
Dihydrolipoate	2.18	1.72	0.004	2.48	2.52	0.003	Fatty acids
1-(beta-D-ribofuranosyl)-1,4-dihydronicotinamide	1.51	0.49	0.010	1.70	0.75	0.002	Carbohydrate
D-1-amino-2-pyrrolidinecarboxylic acid	1.18	1.39	0.001	1.15	0.79	0.034	Amino acids
Sec-butylamine	1.15	0.57	0.043	/	/	/	Monoalkyl amines
Adenosine	1.92	2.20	0.000	/	/	/	Purine
Aucubin	1.22	2.36	0.000	/	/	/	Iridoid o-glycosides
Pyruvic acid	2.01	0.38	0.001	/	/	/	Amino acids
1-Methylhypoxanthine	1.70	0.44	0.007	/	/	/	Purine
4-Dodecylbenzenesulfonic acid	1.12	1.65	0.039	/	/	/	Benzenesulfonic acids
2-Keto-3-deoxy-D-gluconic acid	1.98	1.41	0.000	/	/	/	Amino acids
4-Guanidinobutanoic acid	1.37	0.77	0.000	/	/	/	Amino acids
Pyro-L-glutaminyl-L-glutamine	2.33	40.20	0.005	/	/	/	Amino acids
Dipropyl disulfide	1.49	0.54	0.006	/	/	/	Dialkyldisulfides
N-Acetylhistidine	1.57	1.64	0.000	/	/	/	Histidine
3-Methyluridine	1.43	0.88	0.029	/	/	/	Pyrimidine
Thymine	1.88	0.80	0.002	/	/	/	Pyrimidine
Pyrimidine	1.23	0.61	0.008	/	/	/	Pyrimidine
(+)-Setoclavine	1.38	2.29	0.000	/	/	/	Clavines
L-Methionine	1.47	0.56	0.009	/	/	/	Amino acids
1H-indole-3-carboxaldehyde	1.43	0.66	0.008	/	/	/	Indoles
Citraconic acid	1.94	1.90	0.001	/	/	/	Fatty acids
3,4-Dihydro-4-[(5-methyl-2-furanyl)methylene]-2H-pyrrole	1.33	6.99	0.026	/	/	/	Heteroaromatic
PC(22:2 (13Z,16Z)/16:1 (9Z))	1.91	0.13	0.011	/	/	/	Cholines
Threonic acid	2.22	2.18	0.000	/			Sugar acids
Trimethylaminoacetone	1.07	0.71	0.020	/	/	/	Amino acids
Squamolone	1.61	0.78	0.000	/	/	/	Pyrrolidine carboxamides
SM(d18:1/18:1 (9Z))	1.80	0.17	0.007	/	/	/	Phosphosphingolipids
PC[22:5 (4Z,7Z,10Z,13Z,16Z)/16:0]	1.98	0.12	0.004	/	/	/	Phosphatidylcholines
2,3-Dihydro-5-(3-hydroxypropanoyl)-1H-pyrrolizine	1.58	7.47	0.020	/	/	/	Pyrrolizines
SM(d18:1/24:1 (15Z))	1.70	0.14	0.005	/	/	/	Phosphatidylcholines
PC(22:4 (7Z,10Z,13Z,16Z)/16:0)	1.63	0.17	0.003	/	/	/	Phosphatidylcholines
Cystathionine ketimine	1.23	1.43	0.046	/	/	/	Amino acids
Beta-D-galactose	1.73	1.45	0.001	/	/	/	Hexoses
L-Hexanoylcarnitine	1.72	0.33	0.010	/	/	/	Carnitines
apo-[(3-methylcrotonoyl-CoA:carbon-dioxide ligase (ADP-forming)]	1.73	0.33	0.034	/	/	/	Carboximidic acids
Vinylacetylglycine	1.16	0.64	0.009	/	/	/	Amino acids
2-Methoxy-3-methylpyrazine	1.78	0.43	0.024	/	/	/	Methoxypyrazines
PC[18:3 (6Z,9Z,12Z)/18:1 (11Z)]	1.62	0.16	0.006	/	/	/	Cholines
4-Butyloxazole	2.01	0.42	0.001	/	/	/	Oxazoles
PC(20:4 (8Z,11Z,14Z,17Z)/P-18:0)	1.87	0.21	0.014	/	/	/	Cholines
Perillic acid	1.31	0.20	0.034	/	/	/	Menthane monoterpenoids
PC(18:2 (9Z,12Z)/18:0)	1.43	0.14	0.013	/	/	/	Phosphatidylcholines
PC(20:2 (11Z,14Z)/14:0)	1.54	0.12	0.012	/	/	/	Phosphatidylcholines
PC(22:2 (13Z,16Z)/14:0)	1.47	0.15	0.029	/	/	/	Phosphatidylcholines
Linamarin	1.62	0.51	0.004	/	/	/	Cyanogenic glycosides
Lycoperoside	1.94	11.14	0.049	/	/	/	Steroidal saponins
SM(d16:1/24:1 (15Z))	1.84	0.21	0.003	/	/	/	Cholines
Halosulfuron-methyl	1.87	0.34	0.002	/	/	/	Carboxylic acids
SM(d18:1/22:0)	2.08	0.15	0.004	/	/	/	Cholines
Lucidenic acid F	1.31	2.12	0.032	/	/	/	Triterpenoids
Aminofructose 6-phosphate	1.24	1.42	0.001	/	/	/	Triterpenoids
LysoPC(18:2 (9Z,12Z))	2.21	12.57	0.010	/	/	/	Phosphocholines
2′,4′,6′-Trihydroxyacetophenone	1.35	0.44	0.047	/	/	/	Alkyl-phenylketones
L-Norleucine	/	/	/	1.26	0.78	0.019	Amino acids
3,3,5-triiodo-L-thyronine-beta-D-glucuronoside	/	/	/	1.44	0.78	0.010	Steroid glucuronide conjugates
L-Valine	/	/	/	1.14	0.86	0.026	Amino acid
Niacinamide	/	/	/	2.16	6.78	0.003	Nicotinamide

(Continued on following page)

TABLE 2 | (*Continued*) Identified differential metabolites.

Metabolites	RVO-ME vs. control			mRVO-ME vs. sRVO-ME			Category
	VIP	FC	*p* value	VIP	FC	*p* value[a]	
Foeniculoside VII	/	/	/	2.56	17.16	0.012	Terpene glycosides
Piperidine	/	/	/	1.38	0.80	0.013	Piperidines
Urocanic acid	/	/	/	1.39	7.10	0.010	Carboxylic acids
Prolylglycine	/	/	/	1.29	0.28	0.012	Dipeptides
Diethanolamine	/	/	/	2.58	4.47	0.004	1,2-Aminoalcohols
Isopropylpyrazine	/	/	/	1.51	0.74	0.008	Pyrazines
Phytosphingosine	/	/	/	2.14	7.99	0.032	1,3-Aminoalcohols
Saccharin	/	/	/	2.41	12.29	0.008	Benzothiazoles
8-Butanoylneosolaniol	/	/	/	2.38	10.97	0.007	Fatty acid
5-Oxo-2(5H)-isoxazolepropanenitrile	/	/	/	2.54	11.22	0.010	Isoxazoles
Pyrrolidine	/	/	/	1.13	0.87	0.030	Amino acids
D-Fructosazine	/	/	/	2.42	4.42	0.004	Pyrazines
Paraldehyde	/	/	/	2.49	6.48	0.007	Trioxanes
1-(beta-D-ribofuranosyl)-1,4-dihydronicotinamide	/	/	/	1.70	0.75	0.002	Glycosylamines
5-Amino-3-oxohexanoate	/	/	/	1.07	2.10	0.049	Medium-chain keto acids
D-1-amino-2-pyrrolidinecarboxylic acid	/	/	/	1.15	0.79	0.034	Amino acids
2-(Methylthio)-3H-phenoxazin-3-one	/	/	/	2.00	0.40	0.003	Phenoxazines
Ribothymidine	/	/	/	1.87	0.41	0.006	Pyrimidine nucleosides
Adipic acid	/	/	/	2.42	2.99	0.012	Fatty acids
L-Agaridoxin	/	/	/	1.51	0.58	0.019	Amino acids
N-Acetyl-L-alanine	/	/	/	1.27	0.38	0.008	Amino acids
4-Aminobutyraldehyde	/	/	/	2.49	2.93	0.007	Alpha-hydrogen aldehydes
N-Acetylserine	/	/	/	1.38	0.72	0.013	Amino acids
3-Furoic acid	/	/	/	2.03	0.36	0.042	Furoic acids
1-Methylhistamine	/	/	/	1.10	0.74	0.032	2-Arylethylamines
Acetoin	/	/	/	1.74	2.75	0.035	Acyloins
N-acetyldopamine	/	/	/	1.66	0.45	0.001	Catechols
LysoPE (0:0/22:2 (13Z,16Z))	/	/	/	2.39	34.45	0.017	Phosphoethanolamines
LysoPC(18:2 (9Z,12Z))	/	/	/	2.43	9.26	0.019	Phosphocholines
Tylosin	/	/	/	2.55	82.48	0.045	Aminoglycosides

RVO-ME, retinal vein occlusion macular edema; mRVO-ME, mild retinal vein occlusion macular edema; sRVO-ME, severe retinal vein occlusion macular edema; VIP, variable importance in the projection; FC, fold change.
[a]*P-value was calculated by Student's t-test.*

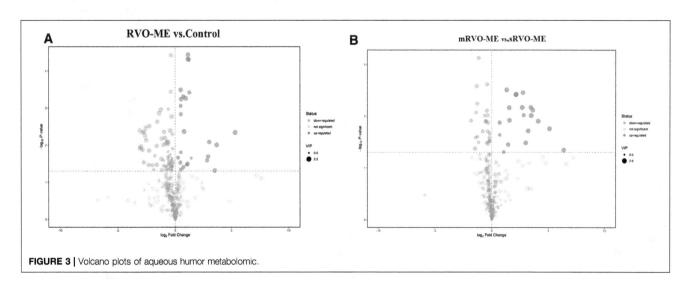

FIGURE 3 | Volcano plots of aqueous humor metabolomic.

biomarker to distinguish RVO-ME from the controls according to ROC analysis. Therefore, we hold the view that adenosine and threonic acid may play a crucial role in RVO-ME.

When compared with mRVO-ME, we found that the level of D-mannose decreased in sRVO-ME. D-mannose is a natural C-2 epimer of glucose, which can be transported to

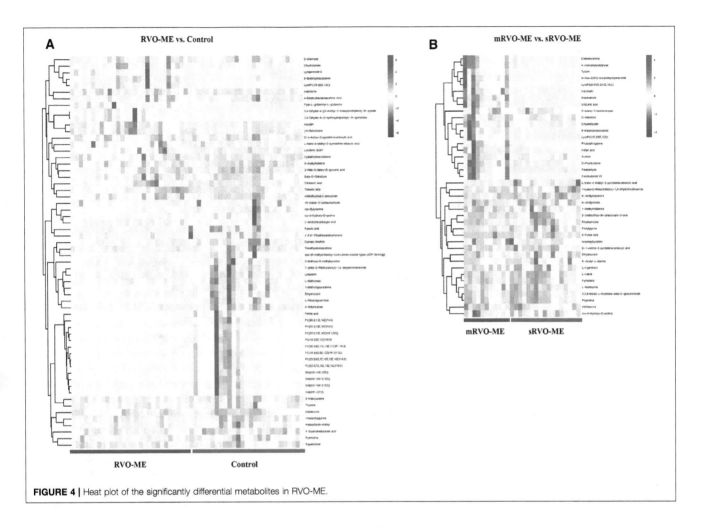

FIGURE 4 | Heat plot of the significantly differential metabolites in RVO-ME.

TABLE 3 | The significantly altered pathways in RVO-ME.

Pathway	RVO-ME vs. controls		sRVO-ME vs. mRVO-ME	
	p value[a]	Metabolites	p value[a]	Metanolites
Valine, leucine, and isoleucine biosynthesis	<0.001	Pyruvic acid; citraconic acid; 4-methyl-2-oxopentanoate	0.016	L-valine; 4-methyl-2-oxopentanoate
Pantothenate and CoA biosynthesis	0.016	Dihydrouracil; pyruvic acid	0.016	Dihydrouracil; L-valine
Ascorbate and aldarate metabolism	0.043	Pyruvic acid; threonic acid	–	–
Beta-alanine metabolism	–	–	0.018	4-Aminobutyraldehyde; dihydrouracil
Valine, leucine, and isoleucine degradation	–	–	0.035	L-valine; M-4-methyl-2-oxopentanoate
Histidine metabolism	–	–	0.042	Urocanic acid; 1-methylhistamine

RVO-ME, retinal vein occlusion macular edema; mRVO-ME, mild retinal vein occlusion macular edema; sRVO-ME, severe retinal vein occlusion macular edema.
[a]*P-value was calculated by Student's t-test.*

mammalian cells through the plasma membrane to promote the diffusion of glucose transporter (GLUT). Rehak et al. (2010) found that IL-1 was rapidly and strongly up-regulated in the retina and retinal pigment epithelium (to levels 80 times higher than controls) in RVO-ME, whereas D-mannose can inhibit macrophage IL-1 (Torretta et al., 2020) and delay the development of osteoarthritis *in vivo* by enhancing autophagy activated by the AMPK pathway (Lin et al., 2021). Consequently, we considered that D-mannose

supplementation may be a meaningful treatment for macular edema caused by RVO.

Oxidative stress played a momentous role in the occurrence and prognosis of RVO-ME (Chen et al., 2018; Hwang et al., 2020); accordingly, related metabolic abnormalities were also found in our study. Many amino acids expressed differently in our study were also involved in oxidative stress response, such as glycine (Knebel et al., 2012), histidine (Nasri et al., 2020), methionine (Demerchi et al., 2021), N-acetylserine (Kim et al., 2019),

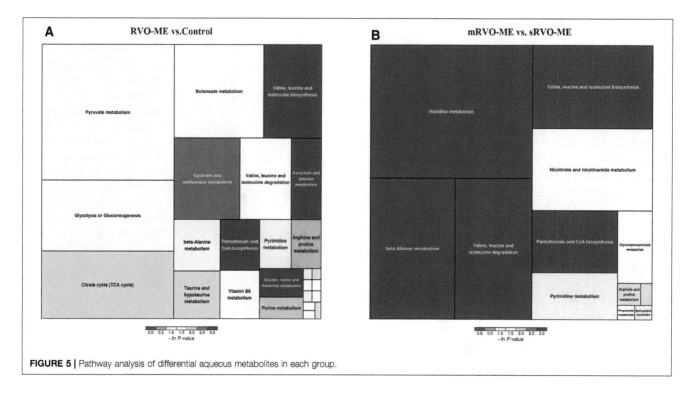

FIGURE 5 | Pathway analysis of differential aqueous metabolites in each group.

urocanic acid (Jauhonen et al., 2011), cis-4-hydroxy-D-proline (Aswani et al., 2019), et al. We also detected a significant metabolite in nucleotide metabolism: nicotinamide (NAM). NAM, the amide of vitamin B3 and precursor for nicotinamide adenine dinucleotide (NAD+), has a strong antioxidant property and can effectively reduce the damage to cells caused by reactive oxygen species (ROS) during oxidative stress (Mejía et al., 2017). Compared with mRVO-ME, the level of NAM in sRVO-ME was decreased. In addition, the AUC of NAM was found to be 0.848 in the ROC analysis, which could serve as a potential biomarker for differentiation between sRVO-ME and mRVO-ME. We believe that the degree and prognosis of RVO-ME are closely related to oxidative stress response. NAM may become an important prognostic biomarker for the treatment of RVO-ME.

Another interesting finding from our study was that the pantothenate (PA) and CoA biosynthesis and valine, leucine, and isoleucine biosynthesis pathways showed a difference in mRVO-ME versus sRVO-ME and RVO-ME versus controls, respectively. Therefore, we speculated that these two metabolic pathways were not only correlated to the occurrence of RVO-ME but also affected the severity of RVO macular edema. Studies had reported that these two metabolic pathways were associated to oxidative stress. PA can regulate cell membrane CoA synthesis and protect endothelial function from enhanced oxidative stress (Demirci et al., 2014). Many studies had also confirmed that this metabolic pathway was abnormal in a variety of diseases, like diabetic kidney disease (Tao et al., 2020), neurodegeneration (Zizioli et al., 2015), Vogt–Koyanagi–Harada (Xu et al., 2021), et al. Valine, leucine, and isoleucine, namely, branched-chain amino acids (BCAAs), which could over-induce oxidative processes and up-regulate proinflammatory factors (Zhenyukh

et al., 2017), are unable to be synthesized by animals. Hence, a variety of pathological changes, such as maple syrup urine disease (MSUD) (Xu et al., 2020), type 2 diabetes (Zeng et al., 2019), and cancer (Peng et al., 2020; Sivanand and Vander Heiden, 2020) could be detected when there is a disorder in BCAA metabolism. Nevertheless, the molecular mechanisms of BCAAs involved in the pathogenesis of RVO-ME-inducing retinopathy remain unknown, thus warranting future research.

We recognized the limitations of our research. Firstly, the sample size of patients was small, due to the difficulty in collecting AH sample from patients and controls. Secondly, obtaining AH samples for the diagnosis of RVO-ME or judgment of severity and prognosis of macular edema is not so practical to perform due to the invasive nature of the procedure. Subsequent studies will recruit more participants and combine serum or urine sample analysis to strengthen the results. Thirdly, owing to geographical limitations, our research was limited to the Chinese Han population. We look forward to get the results of other ethnic samples from other researchers. Last but not the least, further research is needed to shed more light on the exact role of these metabolites and relevant metabolic pathways in the pathogenesis of RVO-ME.

In conclusion, to our knowledge, this study is the first one to provide a comprehensive understanding of the metabolomics of AH in patients with RVO-ME. The results showed that a series of complex and serious metabolic disorders occurred in AH in patients with RVO-ME. Furthermore, we also found significant differences in metabolites between mild macular edema and severe macular edema in RVO-ME patients. Significantly, intraocular angiogenic factors, inflammatory mechanisms, and oxidative stress response may play a prominent role in the occurrence and development of RVO-ME. The above-mentioned results may elucidate the metabolic

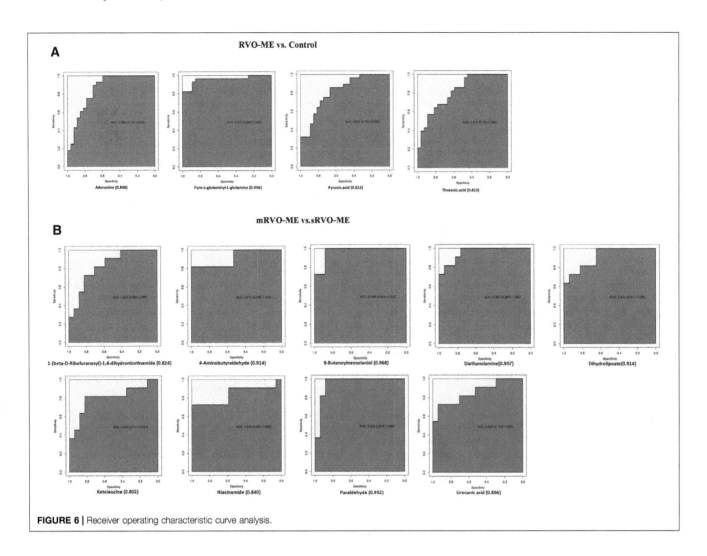

FIGURE 6 | Receiver operating characteristic curve analysis.

biomarkers for the prognosis and novel therapeutic strategies to prevent or delay the development of RVO-ME.

ETHICS STATEMENT

The studies involving human participants were reviewed and approved by the Ethics Committee of the Second Affiliated Hospital of Chongqing Medical University. The patients/participants provided their written informed consent to participate in this study.

AUTHOR CONTRIBUTIONS

XX and MZ conceived the idea and designed the study. XX, MZ, HM, ZZ, YY, ZC, and XC contributed to collecting the aqueous humor and clinical data. XX, JP, and ZX performed the experiments. MZ and QC analyzed the data. XX wrote the manuscript. MZ and XC reviewed the data interpretation and edited the manuscript. All authors contributed to the article and approved the submitted version.

ACKNOWLEDGMENTS

The authors thank all participants in this study. The authors also would like to thank the technical support of the BIOTREE company in Shanghai, China.

REFERENCES

An, Y., Park, S. P., and Kim, Y. K. (2021). Aqueous Humor Inflammatory Cytokine Levels and Choroidal Thickness in Patients with Macular Edema Associated with branch Retinal Vein Occlusion. *Int. Ophthalmol.*, 1–12. doi:10.1007/s10792-021-01798-x

Ashino, H., Shimamura, M., Nakajima, H., Dombou, M., Kawanaka, S., Oikawa, T., et al. (2003). Novel Function of Ascorbic Acid as an Angiostatic Factor. *Angiogenesis* 6 (4), 259–269. doi:10.1023/b:agen.0000029390.09354.f8

Aswani, V., Rajsheel, P., Bapatla, R. B., Sunil, B., and Raghavendra, A. S. (2019). Oxidative Stress Induced in Chloroplasts or Mitochondria Promotes Proline Accumulation in Leaves of Pea (Pisum Sativum): Another Example of Chloroplast-Mitochondria Interactions. *Protoplasma* 256 (2), 449–457. doi:10.1007/s00709-018-1306-1

Balaratnasingam, C., Inoue, M., Ahn, S., Mccann, J., Dhrami-Gavazi, E., Yannuzzi, L. A., et al. (2016). Visual Acuity Is Correlated with the Area of the Foveal

Avascular Zone in Diabetic Retinopathy and Retinal Vein Occlusion. *Ophthalmology* 123, 2352–2367. doi:10.1016/j.ophtha.2016.07.008

Breda, J. B., Sava, A. C., Himmelreich, U., Somers, A., and Stalmans, I. (2020). Metabolomic Profiling Of Aqueous Humor from Glaucoma Patients - The Metabolomics in Surgical Ophthalmological Patients (Miso) Study. *Experi. Eye Res.* 201 (1), 108268. doi:10.1016/j.exer.2020.108268

Buisset, A., Gohier, P., Leruez, S., Muller, J., Amati-Bonneau, P., Lenaers, G., et al. (2019). Metabolomic Profiling of Aqueous Humor in Glaucoma Points to Taurine and Spermine Deficiency: Findings from the Eye-D Study. *J. Proteome Res.* doi:10.1021/acs.jproteome.8b00915

Chen, K. H., Hsiang, E. L., Hsu, M. Y., Chou, Y. C., Lin, T. C., Chang, Y. L., et al. (2018). Elevation of Serum Oxidative Stress in Patients with Retina Vein Occlusions. *Acta Ophthalmol.* 97 (2), e290. doi:10.1111/aos.13892

Chylack, L. T., Wolfe, J. K., Singer, D. M., Leske, M. C., Bullimore, M. A., Bailey, I. L., et al. (1993). The Lens Opacities Classification System III. *Arch. Ophthalmol.* 111 (6), 831–836. doi:10.1001/archopht.1993.01090060119035

Demerchi, S. A., King, N., Mcfarlane, J. R., and Moens, P. D. J. (2021). Effect of Methionine Feeding on Oxidative Stress, Intracellular Calcium and Contractility in Cardiomyocytes Isolated from Male and Female Rats. *Mol. Cel Biochem* 476 (5), 2039–2045. doi:10.1007/s11010-020-04011-2

Demirci, B., Demir, O., Dost, T., and Birincioglu, M. (2014). Protective Effect of Vitamin B5 (Dexpanthenol) on Cardiovascular Damage Induced by Streptozocin in Rats. *Bratisl Lek Listy* 115 (4), 190–196. doi:10.4149/bll_2014_040

Deng, Y., Liang, Y., Lin, S., Wen, L., Li, J., Zhou, Y., et al. (2020). Design and Baseline Data of a Population-Based Metabonomics Study of Eye Diseases in Eastern China: the Yueqing Ocular Diseases Investigation. *Eye Vis.* 7, 8. doi:10.1186/s40662-019-0170-1

Eng, V. A., and Leng, T. (2020). Subthreshold Laser Therapy for Macular Oedema from branch Retinal Vein Occlusion: Focused Review. *Br. J. Ophthalmol.* 104 (9), 1184–1189. doi:10.1136/bjophthalmol-2019-315192

Feoktistov, I., Ryzhov, S., Goldstein, A. E., and Biaggioni, I. (2003). Mast Cell-Mediated Stimulation of Angiogenesis. *Circ. Res.* 92 (5), 485–492. doi:10.1161/01.res.0000061572.10929.2d

Haas, B., Leonard, F., Ernens, I., Rodius, S., Vausort, M., Rolland-Turner, M., et al. (2011). Adenosine Reduces Cell Surface Expression of Toll-like Receptor 4 and Inflammation in Response to Lipopolysaccharide and Matrix Products. *J. Cardiovasc. Trans. Res.* 4 (6), 790–800. doi:10.1007/s12265-011-9279-x

Haines, N. R., Manoharan, N., Olson, J. L., D'Alessandro, A., and Reisz, J. A. (2018). Metabolomics Analysis of Human Vitreous in Diabetic Retinopathy and Rhegmatogenous Retinal Detachment. *J. Proteome Res.* 17, 2421–2427. doi:10.1021/acs.jproteome.8b00169

Han, G., Wei, P., He, M., Teng, H., and Chu, Y. (2020). Metabolomic Profiling of the Aqueous Humor in Patients with Wet Age-Related Macular Degeneration Using UHPLC-MS/MS. *J. Proteome Res.* 19 (6), 2358–2366. doi:10.1021/acs.jproteome.0c00036

Haskó, G., and Pacher, P. (2012). Regulation of Macrophage Function by Adenosine. *Atvb* 32 (4), 865–869. doi:10.1161/atvbaha.111.226852

Hwang, D. K., Chang, Y. L., Lin, T. C., Peng, C. H., Chien, K. H., Tsai, C. Y., et al. (2020). Changes in the Systemic Expression of Sirtuin-1 and Oxidative Stress after Intravitreal Anti-vascular Endothelial Growth Factor in Patients with Retinal Vein Occlusion. *Biomolecules* 10 (10), 1414. doi:10.3390/biom10101414

Jauhonen, H. M., Kauppinen, A., Paimela, T., Laihia, J. K., Leino, L., Salminen, A., et al. (2011). Cis-urocanic Acid Inhibits SAPK/JNK Signaling Pathway in UV-B Exposed Human Corneal Epithelial Cells In Vitro. *Mol. Vis.* 17, 2311–2317.

Ji, Y., Rao, J., Rong, X., Lou, S., Zheng, Z., and Lu, Y. (2017). Metabolic Characterization of Human Aqueous Humor in Relation to High Myopia. *Exp. Eye Res.* 159, 147–155. doi:10.1016/j.exer.2017.03.004

Karolina, P., Anna, D. D., Paulina, S., Tomasz, K., Pawel, K., Malgorzata, W., et al. (2017). LC-MS-Based Metabolic Fingerprinting of Aqueous Humor. *J. Anal. Methods Chem.* 2017, 6745932. doi:10.1155/2017/6745932

Kim, K. Y., Hwang, S.-K., Park, S. Y., Kim, M. J., Jun, D. Y., and Kim, Y. H. (2019). l-Serine Protects Mouse Hippocampal Neuronal HT22 Cells against Oxidative Stress-Mediated Mitochondrial Damage and Apoptotic Cell Death. *Free Radic. Biol. Med.* 141, 447–460. doi:10.1016/j.freeradbiomed.2019.07.018

Kim, M., Park, Y. G., Jeon, S. H., Choi, S. Y., and Roh, Y. J. (2020). The Efficacy of Selective Retina Therapy for Diabetic Macular Edema Based on Pretreatment central Foveal Thickness. *Lasers Med. Sci.* 35 (8), 1781–1790. doi:10.1007/s10103-020-02984-6

Knebel, L. A., Zanatta, Â., Tonin, A. M., Grings, M., Alvorcem, L. d. M., Wajner, M., et al. (2012). 2-Methylbutyrylglycine Induces Lipid Oxidative Damage and Decreases the Antioxidant Defenses in Rat Brain. *Brain Res.* 1478, 74–82. doi:10.1016/j.brainres.2012.08.039

Kupka, K. (1978). International Classification of Diseases: Ninth Revision. *WHO Chron.* 32 (6), 219–225.

Lin, Z., Miao, J., Zhang, T., He, M., Zhou, X., Zhang, H., et al. (2021). D-Mannose Suppresses Osteoarthritis Development In Vivo and Delays IL-1β-induced Degeneration In Vitro by Enhancing Autophagy Activated via the AMPK Pathway. *Biomed. Pharmacother.* 135, 111199. doi:10.1016/j.biopha.2020.111199

Luo, X., Xiao, B., and Xiao, Z. (2019). Anti-Inflammatory Activity of Adenosine 5'-Trisphosphate in Lipopolysaccharide-Stimulated Human Umbilical Vein Endothelial Cells through Negative Regulation of Toll-like Receptor MyD88 Signaling. *DNA Cel Biol* 38 (12), 1557–1563. doi:10.1089/dna.2019.4773

Mejía, S., Gutman, L. B., Camarillo, C. O., Navarro, R. M., Becerra, M. S., Santana, L. D., et al. (2017). Nicotinamide Prevents Sweet Beverage-Induced Hepatic Steatosis in Rats by Regulating the G6PD, NADPH/NADP+ and GSH/GSSG Ratios and Reducing Oxidative and Inflammatory Stress. *Eur. J. Pharmacol.*, S0014299917306969.

Nasri, M., Mahdavifard, S., Babaeenezhad, E., Adibhesami, G., Nouryazdan, N., Veiskarami, S., et al. (2020). Ameliorative Effects of Histidine on Oxidative Stress, Tumor Necrosis Factor Alpha (TNF-α), and Renal Histological Alterations in Streptozotocin/nicotinamide-Induced Type 2 Diabetic Rats. *Iran J. Basic Med. Sci.* 23 (6), 714–723. doi:10.22038/ijbms.2020.38553.9148

Peng, H., Wang, Y., and Luo, W. (2020). Multifaceted Role of Branched-Chain Amino Acid Metabolism in Cancer. *Oncogene.* doi:10.1038/s41388-020-01480-z

Petr, K. (2014). Risk Factors for Central and Branch Retinal Vein Occlusion: A Meta-Analysis of Published Clinical Data. *J. Ophthalmol.* (4), 724780. doi:10.1155/2014/724780

Pietrowska, K., D Muchowska, D. A., Krasnicki, P., Bujalska, A., Samczuk, P., Parfieniuk, E., et al. (2018). An Exploratory LC-MS-based Metabolomics Study Reveals Differences in Aqueous Humor Composition between Diabetic and Non-diabetic Patients with Cataract. *Electrophoresis* 39 (9-10), 1233–1240. doi:10.1002/elps.201700411

Querques, G., Triolo, G., Casalino, G., García-Arumí, J., Badal, J., Zapata, M., et al. (2013). Retinal Venous Occlusions: Diagnosis and Choice of Treatments. *Ophthalmic Res.* 49 (4), 215–222. doi:10.1159/000346734

Rehak, M., Hollborn, M., Iandiev, I., Pannicke, T., Wiedemann, P., and Bringmann, A. (2010). Inflammatory Factors in Experimental Retinal Vein Occlusion. *Acta Ophthalmologica* 21 (s2), 0.

Riis-Vestergaard, M. J., and Bek, T. (2015). Purinergic Mechanisms and Prostaglandin E Receptors Involved in ATP-Induced Relaxation of Porcine Retinal Arterioles In Vitro. *Ophthalmic Res.* 54 (3), 135–142. doi:10.1159/000438905

Riis-Vestergaard, M. J., Misfeldt, M. W., and Bek, T. (2014). Dual Effects of Adenosine on the Tone of Porcine Retinal Arterioles In Vitro. *Invest. Ophthalmol. Vis. Sci.* 55 (3), 1630–1636. doi:10.1167/iovs.13-13428

Santiago, A. R., Madeira, M. H., Boia, R., Aires, I. D., Rodrigues-Neves, A. C., Santos, P. F., et al. (2020). Keep an Eye on Adenosine: Its Role in Retinal Inflammation. *Pharmacol. Ther.* 210, 107513. doi:10.1016/j.pharmthera.2020.107513

Sebastião, A. M., and Ribeiro, J. A. (2009). Adenosine Receptors and the central Nervous System. *Handbook Exp. Pharmacol.* 83 (3Suppl. 193), 471–534. doi:10.1007/978-3-540-89615-9_16

Sivanand, S., and Vander Heiden, M. G. (2020). Emerging Roles for Branched-Chain Amino Acid Metabolism in Cancer. *Cancer Cell* 37 (2), 147–156. doi:10.1016/j.ccell.2019.12.011

Tao, M. A., Tl, B., Px, A., Sheng, J. C., Wy, A., Pei, D. A., et al. (2020). UPLC-MS-based Urine Nontargeted Metabolic Profiling Identifies Dysregulation of Pantothenate and CoA Biosynthesis Pathway in Diabetic Kidney Disease - ScienceDirect. *Life Sci.* 258, 118160. doi:10.1016/j.lfs.2020.118160

Torretta, S., Scagliola, A., Ricci, L., Mainini, F., Di Marco, S., Cuccovillo, I., et al. (2020). D-mannose Suppresses Macrophage IL-1β Production. *Nat. Commun.* 11 (1), 6343. doi:10.1038/s41467-020-20164-6

Wang, H., Fang, J., Chen, F., Sun, Q., Xu, X., Lin, S. H., et al. (2019). Metabolomic Profile of Diabetic Retinopathy: a GC-TOFMS-Based Approach Using Vitreous and Aqueous Humor. *Acta Diabetol.* 57 (24), 41–51. doi:10.1007/s00592-019-01363-0

Xu, J., Jakher, Y., and Ahrens-Nicklas, R. C. (2020). Brain Branched-Chain Amino Acids in Maple Syrup Urine Disease: Implications for Neurological Disorders. *Int. J. Mol. Sci.* 21 (20), 7490. doi:10.3390/ijms21207490

Xu, J., Su, G., Huang, X., Chang, R., and Yang, P. (2021). Metabolomic Analysis of Aqueous Humor Identifies Aberrant Amino Acid and Fatty Acid Metabolism in Vogt-Koyanagi-Harada and Behcet's Disease. *Front. Immunol.* 12, 587393. doi:10.3389/fimmu.2021.587393

Yong, H., Qi, H., Yan, H., Wu, Q., and Zuo, L. The Correlation between Cytokine Levels in the Aqueous Humor and the Prognostic Value of Anti-vascular Endothelial Growth Factor Therapy for Treating Macular Edema Resulting from Retinal Vein Occlusion. *Graefe's Archive Clin. Exp. Ophthalmol.* 259 (11), 3243–3250. doi:10.1007/s00417-021-05211-2

Zeng, Y., Mtintsilana, A., Goedecke, J. H., Micklesfield, L. K., Olsson, T., and Chorell, E. (2019). Alterations in the Metabolism of Phospholipids, Bile Acids and Branched-Chain Amino Acids Predicts Development of Type 2 Diabetes in Black South African Women: a Prospective Cohort Study. *Metabolism* 95, 57–64. doi:10.1016/j.metabol.2019.04.001

Zhenyukh, O., Civantos, E., Ruiz-Ortega, M., Soledad Sánchez, M., Vázquez, C., Peiró, C., et al. (2017). High Concentration of Branched-Chain Amino Acids Promotes Oxidative Stress, Inflammation and Migration of Human Peripheral Blood Mononuclear Cells via mTORC1 Activation. *Free Radic. Biol. Med.* 104, 165–177. doi:10.1016/j.freeradbiomed.2017.01.009

Zizioli, D., Tiso, N., Guglielmi, A., Saraceno, C., Busolin, G., Giuliani, R., et al. (2015). Knock-down of Pantothenate Kinase 2 Severely Affects the Development of the Nervous and Vascular System in Zebrafish, Providing New Insights into PKAN Disease. *Neurobiol. Dis.* 85 (8), 35–48. doi:10.1016/j.nbd.2015.10.010

10

Abnormal Expression of YAP is Associated with Proliferation, Differentiation, Neutrophil Infiltration and Adverse Outcome in Patients with Nasal Inverted Papilloma

Tian Yuan[1,2†], Rui Zheng[1†], Xiang-min Zhou[3†], Peng Jin[3], Zhi-qun Huang[4], Xiao-xue Zi[3], Qing-wu Wu[1], Wei-hao Wang[1], Hui-yi Deng[1], Wei-feng Kong[1], Hui-jun Qiu[1], Sui-zi Zhou[5], Qian-min Chen[5], Yan-yi Tu[3], Tao Li[3], Jing Liu[2,6], Kai Sen Tan[2,6,7,8], Hsiao Hui Ong[2,6], Li Shi[3], Zhuang-gui Chen[9], Xue-kun Huang[1], Qin-tai Yang[1]* and De-yun Wang[2,6]*

[1] Department of Otolaryngology-Head and Neck Surgery, Department of Allergy, The Third Affiliated Hospital of Sun Yat-sen University, Guangzhou, China, [2] Department of Otolaryngology, Yong Loo Lin School of Medicine, National University of Singapore, Singapore, Singapore, [3] Department of Otolaryngology-Head and Neck Surgery, Shandong Provincial ENT Hospital, Cheeloo College of Medicine, Shandong University, Jinan, China, [4] Department of Otolaryngology-Head and Neck Surgery, The First Affiliated Hospital of Nanchang University, Nanchang, China, [5] Department of Otolaryngology, Zhujiang Hospital, Southern Medical University, Guangzhou, China, [6] NUHS Infectious Diseases Translational Research Program, Yong Loo Lin School of Medicine, National University of Singapore, Singapore, Singapore, [7] Department of Microbiology and Immunology, Yong Loo Lin School of Medicine, National University of Singapore, Singapore, Singapore, [8] Biosafety Level 3 Core Facility, Yong Loo Lin School of Medicine, National University Health System, National University of Singapore, Singapore, Singapore, [9] Department of Pediatrics, Department of Allergy, The Third Affiliated Hospital of Sun Yat-sen University, Guangzhou, China

*Correspondence:
Qin-tai Yang
yang.qt@163.com
De-yun Wang
entwdy@nus.edu.sg

† These authors have contributed equally to this work

Background: Nasal inverted papilloma (NIP) is a common benign tumor. Yes-associated protein (YAP) is the core effector molecule of the Hippo pathway, which regulates the proliferation and differentiation of airway epithelium. While its role in proliferation may be connected to NIP formation, no definitive association has been made between them.

Methods: We compared the difference of YAP expression and proliferation level between the control inferior turbinate, NP (nasal polyps), and NIP groups. In addition, we further used PCR, immunofluorescence, and immunohistochemistry to investigate YAP's role in the proliferation and differentiation of the nasal epithelium and inflammatory cell infiltration, correlating them with different grades of epithelial remodeling. We further used an IL-13 remodeling condition to investigate YAP's role in differentiation in an *in vitro* air-liquid interface (ALI) human nasal epithelial cell (hNECs) model. Finally, we also explored the correlation between YAP expression and clinical indicators of NIP.

Results: The expression of YAP/active YAP in the NIP group was significantly higher than that in the NP group and control group. Moreover, within the NIP group, the higher grade of epithelial remodeling was associated with higher YAP induced proliferation, leading to reduced ciliated cells and goblet cells. The finding was further verified using an IL-13 remodeling condition in differentiating ALI hNECs. Furthermore, YAP expression was positively correlated with proliferation and neutrophil infiltration in NIP. YAP expression was also significantly increased in NIP patients with adverse outcomes.

Conclusion: Abnormal expression of YAP/active YAP is associated with proliferation, differentiation, neutrophil infiltration, and adverse outcome in NIP and may present a novel target for diagnosis and intervention in NIP.

Keywords: nasal inverted papilloma, yes-associated protein, epithelial cells, proliferation, differentiation, neutrophils

INTRODUCTION

Nasal inverted papilloma (NIP) is a benign epithelial tumor growing in the nasal cavity and sinuses, characterized by their local invasiveness, recurrence, and malignant transformation (Katori et al., 2006; Sun et al., 2017). NIP grows as an extraneous polypoid with an endophytic (inverted) growth pattern. NIP can be formed from epithelial cells of different tissue origins, including squamous epithelium, respiratory epithelium, and transitional epithelium (Nielsen et al., 1991). At present, the etiology of NIP is unclear. Some researchers hold the view that NIP is a kind of tumor-derived from the Schneider's membrane; some think that NIP may be the result of an initial inflammatory response (Orlandi et al., 2002). Additionally, it was also found that HPV may be responsible for causing NIP's malignant transformation (Zhao R. W. et al., 2016). While NIP can be surgically treated, the disease is often easily misdiagnosed as a nasal polyp because of their similar clinical features (Paz Silva et al., 2015). However, compared with nasal polyps, NIP has a higher recurrence and malignancy rate. Many studies have found that the proliferation level of NIP is significantly higher than that of nasal polyps, which may be an important reason for the recurrence and malignant transformation of NIP (Mumbuc et al., 2007; Meng et al., 2014). Our previous research showed that inflammatory cells were identified as a significant cell population in NIP (Zhao L. et al., 2016), which supports the hypothesis that NIP formation is associated with inflammatory response (Orlandi et al., 2002). However, the mechanism of the high proliferation level and abnormal inflammatory cell infiltration in NIP is still unclear.

Yes-associated protein (YAP) is a transcriptional co-activator in the conserved Hippo pathway, which was shown to regulate cell proliferation, cell differentiation, and apoptosis (Yu et al., 2015). In airway epithelial stem cells, the Hippo pathway plays an important role in the self-renewal of stem cells and progenitor cells, as well as maintaining the balance between undifferentiated and differentiated cells. During the development of mouse lower airway, YAP can control the fate of lower airway epithelial progenitor cells and airway morphogenesis (Mahoney et al., 2014). In the mature lower airway of mice, YAP deletion leads to the loss of basal stem cells and uncontrolled differentiation. On the contrary, the overexpression of YAP strengthens the self-renewal and inhibits the differentiation of basal stem cells, resulting in epithelial proliferation and the formation of multi-layer undifferentiated cells (Zhao R. et al., 2014; Lange et al., 2015). In the nasal epithelium (upper airway), our team found

that the expression of YAP in nasal polyps was abnormal and was involved in the epithelial proliferation and tissue remodeling of nasal polyps (Deng et al., 2019). Furthermore, it was also found that the Hippo pathway plays a role in inflammation. For example, defects in MST1 (mammalian sterile 20-like kinase 1), an upstream factor of YAP, leads to the downregulation of neutrophils (Kurz et al., 2018), and the specific knockout of YAP in vascular endothelium will lead to an increase of neutrophil infiltration (Lv et al., 2018). Thus, YAP has been shown to affect the airway proliferation and inflammation, which may likely be associated with NIP pathogenesis. Therefore, the present study aims to investigate the relationship between YAP and proliferation, differentiation, and inflammation in NIP pathogenesis.

MATERIALS AND METHODS

Patients and Samples

Control subjects (inferior turbinate, IT), patients with nasal polyps (NP), and patients with NIP were recruited from the Qilu Hospital of Shandong University (Jinan, China) and 3rd Affiliated Hospital of Sun Yat-sen University (Guangzhou, China). Control samples were obtained from healthy inferior turbinate tissues of patients who underwent septal plastic surgery. The diagnosis of NP and NIP was confirmed and reported by a pathologist. Other types of nasal papilloma (exophytic and cylindrical cell papilloma) were excluded from the study. The nasal polyps group had no concurrent NIP. The samples of NP and NIP were from different individuals. For patients with recurrent NIP, they went through NIP surgery before specimen collection. All patients had not used any form of glucocorticosteroids or antibiotics within 3 months prior to specimen collection.

The NIP clinical stages I to IV was evaluated according to previous studies (Krouse, 2000). In addition, we further based the evaluation on the results of patients' computed tomography (CT) scans and endoscopic examination. History of recurrence was obtained with patient records and confirmed by outpatient and intraoperative endoscopic evidence of prior nasal surgery. Smokers were defined as current cigarette smokers who consume one or more packs of cigarettes a day, averaged over 1 year. Fresh specimens were fixed in formalin and preserved in RNAlater solution for histologic evaluation and detecting gene expression, respectively. Approval for this study was obtained from the institutional review boards of Qilu Hospital of Shandong

University (2019124 Jinan, China) and 3rd Affiliated Hospital of Sun Yat-sen University ([2016]2–40, Guangzhou, China). Each subject provided written informed consent before participation.

Remodeling Evaluation of NIP Epithelium

The NIP was graded into three categories based on comprehensive results of hematoxylin and eosin (HE)-staining and immunofluorescent staining, according to a previous study (Roh et al., 2004; **Figures 2A,E**). Grade I was defined as ciliated respiratory epithelium with underlying squamous metaplasia; Grade II as partially ciliated respiratory epithelium with luminal squamous metaplasia and increased prominence of inversion; and Grade III as almost complete absence of respiratory epithelium with dominant stratified squamous epithelium. For each NIP specimen, the grading of remodeling was based on the predominant remodeling present (>70% of the epithelium showing this feature).

RNA Extraction and Quantitative Real-Time Polymerase Chain Reaction

Total RNA was extracted from frozen nasal tissues in RNA later. Then, 1,000 ng of total RNA was reverse transcribed into cDNA using Maxima Reverse Transcriptase Kit (Thermo Fisher Scientific) according to manufacturer's protocol. The mRNA level was detected by SYBR green gene expression assays. Relative gene expression was calculated using the comparative $2^{-\Delta\Delta Ct}$ method normalized against the housekeeping gene [ribosomal protein L13a (RPL13A)]. The primers sequences were as follows: YAP forward (5′-AATTGAGAACAATGACGACC-3′), YAP reverse (5′-AGTATCACCTGTATCCATCTC-3′); Ki-67 forward (5′-ACGAGACGCCTGGTTACTATC-3′), Ki-67 reverse (5′-GCTCATCAATAACAGACCCATTTAC-3′); RPL13A forward (5′-GTCTGAAGCCTACAAGAAAG-3′), RPL13A reverse (5′-TGTCAATTTTCTTCTCCACG-3′).

Human Nasal Epithelial Cells Culture and IL-13 Treatment

Human nasal epithelial cells (hNECs) were developed from primary human nasal epithelial stem/progenitor cells (hNESPCs) (Li et al., 2014; Liu et al., 2018; Yuan et al., 2020), obtained from fresh healthy inferior turbinate mucosa. The hNESPCs were transplanted to an air-liquid interface (ALI) system to form a pseudostratified layer within 4 weeks. A detailed description of the hNEC culture method used is found in our previously published papers (Li et al., 2014; Liu et al., 2018; Yuan et al., 2020). To establish a remodeling condition *in vitro*, IL-13 (10 ng/mL, R&D System, Minneapolis, MN, United States) was added to the basal cell culture medium of the hNECs during their entire duration of differentiation.

Immunofluorescence Staining and Analysis

Protein expression of YAP (sc101199, Santa Cruz Biotechnology), active YAP (ab205270, Abcam), P63 (ab124762, Abcam), Ki-67 (ab15580, Abcam), β4-TUBULIN (ab179504, Abcam), and MUC5AC (sc20118, Santa Cruz Biotechnology) on paraffin tissue

sections were examined by immunofluorescence staining (IF). All the sections were blocked using 10% normal goat serum for 30 min at room temperature. They were then incubated with a primary antibody solution overnight at 4°C, followed by 1 h incubation with Alexa Fluor 488- or 594-conjugated secondary antibodies in the dark at room temperature. Cellular nuclei were visualized using 4′,6-diamidino-2-phenylindole (DAPI) (Life Technologies, Carlsbad, CA, United States). For negative controls, primary antibodies were substituted with the species- and subtype-matched antibodies at the same concentration. The slides were analyzed with fluorescent microscopy (Olympus IX51, Tokyo, Japan).

Images of YAP on tissue sections were captured at ×400 magnification with a fluorescence microscope (Olympus IX51, Tokyo, Japan). Fluorescence intensity was performed by YAP antibody (sc101199, Santa Cruz Biotechnology) and was analyzed using ImageJ software (National Institutes of Health, Bethesda, MD, United States) through calculating the raw mean fluorescence intensity (rMFI) in YAP IF staining and the mean autofluorescence intensity (MAI) in negative controls. YAP expression was measured by corrected mean fluorescence intensity (MFI), which was equal to rMFI minus MAI. Percentage of nuclear active YAP was performed using active YAP antibody (ab205270, Abcam). Nuclear active YAP (nuclear-aYAP) was only counted in the epithelium. For every sample, MFI and nuclear-aYAP were averaged from three images. Clinical characteristics of patients used in YAP MFI and qPCR were listed in **Table 1**. Patient characteristics used in calculating the percentage of nuclear active YAP were listed in **Supplementary Table 1**.

TABLE 1 | Clinical characteristics of patients.

Clinical parameters	Control (n = 10) No. (%)	NP (n = 20) No. (%)	NIP (n = 29) No. (%)
Age, year, median (1st and 3rd interquartile)	35 (20,50)	42 (29,52)	47 (39,55)
Gender			
Male	8 (80%)	15 (75%)	23 (79%)
Female	2 (20%)	5 (25%)	6 (21%)
Smoking			
Smoker	2 (20%)	4 (20%)	11 (38%)
Non-smoker	8 (80%)	16 (80%)	18 (62%)
Concurrent CRS			
Yes	–	–	9 (31%)
No	–	–	20 (69%)
Concurrent NP			
Yes	–	–	8 (28%)
No	–	–	21 (72%)
Krouse staging system			
Stage I	–	–	1 (3%)
Stage II	–	–	1 (3%)
Stage III	–	–	24 (83%)
Stage IV	–	–	3 (10%)

NIP, nasal inverted papilloma; CRS, chronic rhinosinusitis; NP, nasal polyps.

Immunohistochemistry Staining and Evaluation of Inflammatory Cells

Evaluation of inflammatory cells was examined by immunohistochemistry staining (IHC), except eosinophils were measured by HE–staining. The specific inflammatory cell markers were as follows: mouse monoclonal anti-human neutrophil elastase (clone NP57) (Dako, Glostrup, Denmark) for neutrophils, mouse monoclonal anti-human CD68 (clone KP1) (Abcam, Cambridge, United Kingdom) for macrophages, mouse monoclonal anti-human CD4 (clone 4B12) (Dako) for helper T cells, mouse monoclonal anti-human CD8 (clone C8/144B) (Thermo Scientific, Fremont, CA, United States) for cytotoxic T cells, and mouse monoclonal anti-human Foxp3 [clone, 236A/E7] (Abcam) for regulatory T cells.

Nasal inverted papilloma tissue was embedded in paraffin and sectioned at 4 μm with a Leica microtome (Leica, Wetzlar, Germany). Paraffin tissue sections were blocked using 10% normal goat serum for 30 min at room temperature. They were pretreated with Target Retrieval Buffer (Dako) and then incubated with a primary antibody solution overnight at 4°C. The next day the cellular markers were stained by using a modified horseradish peroxidase (HRP) technique with the DakoCytomation EnVision1System-HRP (Dako). Species- and subtype-matched antibodies were used as negative controls (Dako). The slides were then incubated with Dako EnVision + System-HRP (Dako) at room temperature for 30 min, after which the substrate diaminobenzidine was added for color development. All slides were counterstained with hematoxylin.

When evaluating inflammatory cells, we first used low magnification to locate the areas with the most severe infiltration of inflammatory cells. Then observed 3 high-power fields and counted at least 300 leukocytes. Epithelial cells, fibroblasts, glandular cells, and endothelial cells were excluded. Of the 3 fields, the proportion of each type of inflammatory cell is the ratio of all this type of cell to all leukocytes. For IF and IHC, two researchers evaluated the data independently, and the third researcher independently evaluated and solved any disagreement between the first two researchers.

Statistical Analysis

All data were analyzed using GraphPad Prism 8 (GraphPad Software, La Jolla, CA, United States). For comparison of differences between two groups, Mann–Whitney test and Wilcoxon matched-pairs signed rank test were applied. Kruskal–Wallis test was used to analyze differences between multiple groups. Correlation analysis was performed using the Spearman r test. A P-value of <0.05 was considered statistically significant.

RESULTS

YAP Is Overexpressed in Nasal Inverted Papilloma

We first evaluated YAP expression in control inferior turbinate (IT), nasal polyps (NP), and nasal inverted papilloma (NIP).

In immunofluorescence staining (IF), epithelial MFI of YAP (**Figures 1A,D**) and percentage of nuclear active YAP positive cells (nuclear-aYAP$^+$/DAPI) (**Figures 1B,E** and **Supplementary Figure 1**) in NIP was found to be higher than in IT and NP tissues. The same results could be observed at the mRNA level where YAP mRNA was increased in NIP compared to IT and NP (**Figure 1G**). Secondly, we examined the proliferation level of IT, NP, and NIP. We choose Ki-67, a widely recognized proliferation marker, co-stained with P63 to represent basal cells with proliferative ability. Thus, the ratio of Ki-67$^+$ cells to P63$^+$ cells (Ki-67/P63) would indicate the level of proliferation in the basal epithelium. Ki-67/P63 was increased in NIP compared with IT and NP (**Figures 1C,F** and **Supplementary Figure 2**), Ki-67/P63 in NP was also found to be higher than that in IT, congruent with our previous findings (Deng et al., 2019). The result of immunofluorescence staining was consistent with the PCR results. At the mRNA level, both NIP and NP showed increased Ki-67 expression, with NIP being higher than that of NP (**Figure 1H**). This trend of Ki-67 levels was consistent with YAP expression and indicated the correlation of high proliferation levels in NIP with YAP expression.

Higher YAP Expression Level Is Associated With Reduced Nasal Epithelial Differentiation in NIP

Based on a previous study, NIP can be further divided into three categories (Roh et al., 2004). The nasal epithelial remodeling was found to increase in severity from Grade I to Grade III accompanied by reduced nasal epithelial differentiation, and the representative HE and IF were shown in **Figures 2A,E**. The number and proportion of three types of NIP in this study were shown in **Table 2** and **Supplementary Table 1**. As there were not enough Grade I samples, we only compared Grade II to Grade III. In Grade III NIP, YAP mRNA level (**Figure 2F**), YAP MFI (**Figures 2B,H**), and percentage of nuclear active YAP positive cells (nuclear-aYAP$^+$/DAPI) (**Figures 2C,I**) were all significantly higher than that in Grade II.

In terms of proliferation, Grade III NIP has a higher level of Ki-67 than Grade II on both protein level (**Figures 2D,J**) and mRNA level (**Figure 2G**). We explored the relationship between YAP and proliferation in NIP. YAP MFI is positively correlated to Ki-67/P63 (**Figure 2K**). In terms of differentiation, ciliated cell ratio (β4-TUBULIN$^+$/DAPI) (**Figures 2E,M**) and goblet cell ratio (MUC5AC$^+$/DAPI) (**Figures 2E,L**) was decreased in Grade III compared with Grade II. While total YAP MFI was positively correlated with ciliated cell ratio in Grade II NIP (**Supplementary Figure 3A**), nuclear active YAP was found to be negatively correlated with ciliated cells ratio (**Figure 2N**). There was no significant difference between the goblet cell ratio and YAP MFI (**Supplementary Figure 3B**). For the goblet cell ratio, as the numbers are low in NIP groups, we did not explore its correlation with nuclear active YAP positive cells ratio. These results indicated that YAP may be involved in the severity of NIP via dysregulation of proliferation and differentiation of the nasal epithelium.

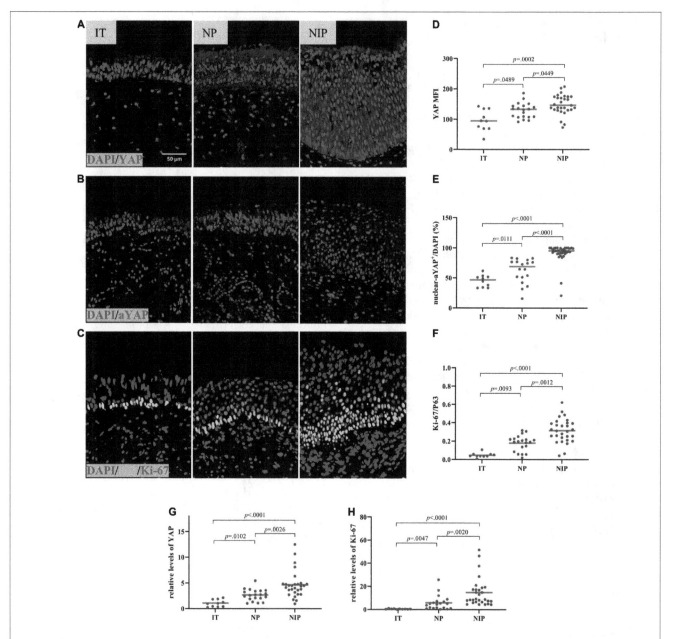

FIGURE 1 | YAP is overexpressed in nasal inverted papilloma. **(A,B)** Total YAP and active YAP IF staining in control IT, NP, and NIP tissues. **(C)** Ki-67 and P63 double IF staining in control IT, NP, and NIP tissues. **(D–F)** Semi-quantitative analysis of mean fluorescence intensity (MFI) stained for total YAP, percentage of nuclear active YAP positive cells (nuclear-aYAP$^+$/DAPI), ratio of Ki-67$^+$ cells to P63$^+$ cells (Ki-67/P63) on IF staining in control IT, NP, and NIP tissues. **(G,H)** The mRNA levels of YAP and Ki-67 in control IT, NP, and NIP tissues were quantified by RT-qPCR assays and relative expression of the target gene was normalized to $2^{-\Delta CT}$ with RPL13A. Multiple group comparison was using Kruskal–Wallis test. Red lines show median values. **(A–C)**, ×400 magnification, scale bar = 50 μm. **(D,F–H)**, n(IT) = 10, n(NP) = 20, n(NIP) = 29. **(E)**, n(IT) = 10, n(NP) = 18, n(NIP) = 36.

Active YAP Is Negatively Correlated With Ciliated Cells in hNESPCs Culture Model

A recent study has demonstrated that YAP/TAZ activity may be involved in the regulation of ciliogenesis (Kim et al., 2015). In order to explore the role of YAP during tissue remodeling processes in NIP, we used IL-13 on hNECs ALI cell culture. IL-13–mediated cellular remodeling of the human airway epithelium has been examined in multiple studies. IL-13 stimulation could

induce more MUC5AC-positive mucus cells and fewer ciliated cells during the process of airway epithelia cell differentiation (Atherton et al., 2003; Dellagrammaticas et al., 2008). After the maturation of the hNECs, we found that IL-13 could induce a 2.9-fold increase in percentage of nuclear active YAP positive cells (nuclear-aYAP$^+$/DAPI) (**Figures 3A–C**) while a 0.3-fold decrease in the ratio of ciliated cells (**Figures 3A,D**), albeit not statistically significant compared to untreated hNECs. The *in vitro* results were consistent with that of NIP Grade II and the trend

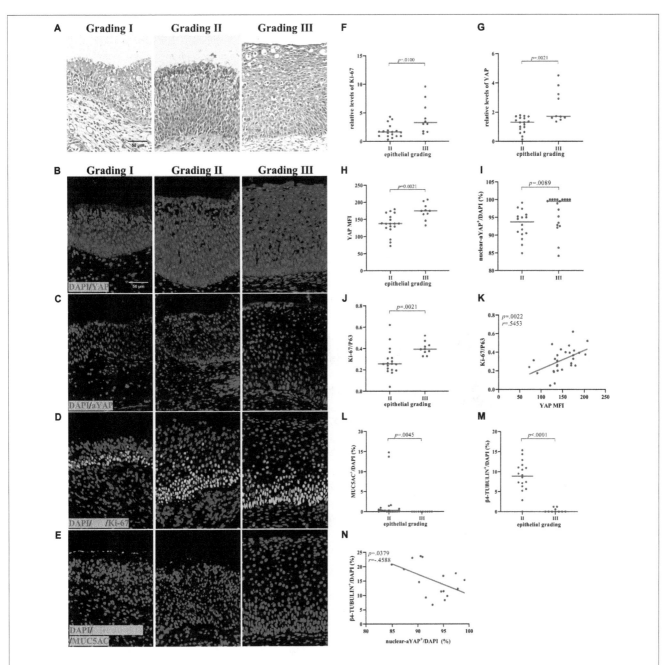

FIGURE 2 | Increased YAP levels are associated with proliferation and differentiation in NIP. **(A)** HE staining in different epithelial remodeling grade of NIP tissues. **(B,C)** Total YAP and active YAP IF staining in different epithelial remodeling grade of NIP tissues. **(D,E)** Ki-67 and P63, β4-TUBULIN, and MUC5AC double IF staining in different epithelial remodeling grade of NIP tissues. **(F,G)** The mRNA levels of YAP and Ki-67 in control IT, NP, and NIP tissues were quantified by RT-qPCR assays and relative expression of the target gene was normalized to $2^{-\Delta\ CT}$ with RPL13A. **(H–J,L,M)** Semi-quantitative analysis of mean fluorescence intensity (MFI) stained for total YAP, percentage of nuclear active YAP positive cells (nuclear-aYAP$^+$/DAPI), ratio of Ki-67$^+$ cells to P63$^+$ cells (Ki-67/P63), goblet cell ratio (MUC5AC$^+$/DAPI), ciliated cell ratio (β4-TUBULIN$^+$/DAPI) on IF staining in Grade II and Grade III of NIP tissues. **(K)** Correlation analysis between YAP MFI and Ki-67/P63 on IF staining in NIP tissues. **(N)** Correlation analysis between nuclear-aYAP$^+$/DAPI and β4-TUBULIN$^+$/DAPI on IF staining in Grade II NIP tissues. Two group difference was analyzed with Mann–Whitney test, and correlation analysis was performed using the Spearman r test. Red lines show median values. **(A–E)**, ×400 magnification, scale bar = 50 μm. **(F–H,J,L,M)**, n(Grade II) = 18, n(Grade III) = 10; **(I)**, n(Grade II) = 16, n(Grade III) = 19; **(K)**, n = 29; N, n = 16.

between Grade II and Grade III NIP, suggesting the inhibitory effect of functional YAP on cilia in NIP. However, using IL-13 treatment as model, accompanied with nuclear-aYAP$^+$/DAPI increasing, goblet cell ratio (MUC5AC$^+$/DAPI) had a 2.9-fold increase (**Figures 3B,E**). The observation was not consistent with

NIP tissue, potentially as IL-13 was unlikely the driver in NIP formation as compared to NP, or potentially due to the very low levels of MUC5AC$^+$ cells in NIP suggesting that the higher levels of nuclear active YAP may have suppress differentiation of all epithelial cells. Nevertheless, we established that nuclear active

TABLE 2 | Clinical characteristics of patients with NIP.

Epithelial remodeling grading	No. (%) (n = 29)
Grade I	1 (3%)
Grade II	18 (62%)
Grade III	10 (34%)

YAP plays a role in reducing the differentiation of basal cells into ciliated cells during tissue remodeling processes.

YAP Is Positively Correlated With Neutrophils in NIP Tissue

In our previous study, we have explored the characteristics of inflammatory cells in NIP (Zhao L. et al., 2016). In the present study, we investigated the relationship between YAP expression and inflammatory cells. The detailed inflammatory cell data was described in **Table 3**. We explored all the relationship

between inflammatory cells and YAP expression. Interestingly, even though no correlation between YAP mRNA level and neutrophils infiltration was observed (**Figure 4B**), we found that increased YAP protein is significantly correlated with increased neutrophils infiltration (**Figure 4A**), which implied that there was a connection between YAP and neutrophil infiltration. Neither YAP MFI nor YAP mRNA level had significant correlation with eosinophil count (**Figures 4C,D**), macrophage count (**Figures 4E,F**), CD4+ T cell count (**Figures 4G,H**), CD8+ T cell count (**Figures 4I,J**), CD4+/CD8+ ratio (**Figures 4K,L**), and FoxP3+ T-reg count (**Figures 4M,N**).

NIP With Adverse Outcomes Has a High Level of YAP Expression

When comparing YAP expression to NIP clinical data, we found that 15 had adverse outcomes, of which 15 (52%) had recurrence, and 3 (10%) underwent malignancy (**Table 4**). The results of immunofluorescence showed that the YAP MFI and percentage

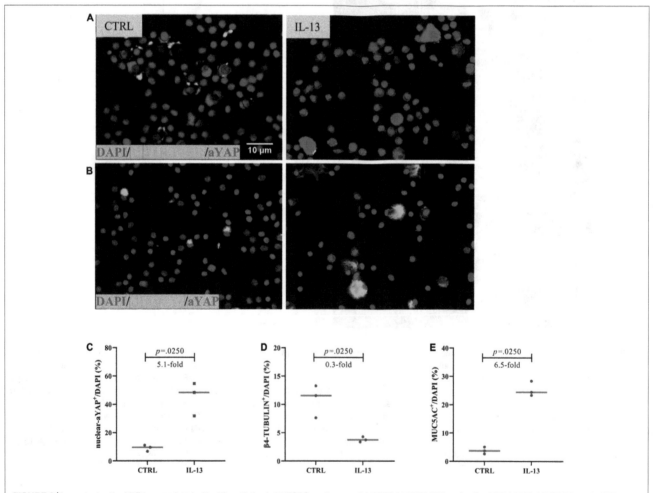

FIGURE 3 | Increased active YAP is associated with differentiation in hNESPCs culture model. **(A,B)** β4-TUBULIN and active YAP (aYAP), MUC5AC, and aYAP double IF staining in control and IL-13 treatment group. **(C–E)** Percentage of nuclear active YAP positive cells (nuclear-aYAP+/DAPI), ciliated cell ratio (β4-TUBULIN+/DAPI), goblet cell ratio (MUC5AC+/DAPI) on IF staining in control and IL-13 treatment group. Two group difference was analyzed with Wilcoxon matched-pairs signed rank test, and fold-change was shown. Red lines show median values. **(A,B)** ×800 magnification, scale bar = 10 μm. n(CTRL) = 3, n(IL-13) = 3.

TABLE 3 | Inflammatory or immune cell feature in NIP.

Inflammatory or immune cell count, median (1st, 3rd quartile)	
Eosinophil, %	4.85 (2.74, 11.11)
Neutrophil, %	57.14 (43.03, 69.56)
Macrophage, %	13.57 (8.24, 18.62)
CD4+T cell, %	14.49 (9.71, 18.29)
CD8+T cell, %	17.92 (8.52, 21.96)
CD4+/CD8+ ratio	0.77 (0.50, 1.36)
Regulator T cell (FoxP3+), %	1.28 (0.00, 2.50)

TABLE 4 | Clinical characteristics of patients with NIP.

Clinical parameters	No. (%) (n = 29)
Recurrent NIP	
Yes	15 (52%)
No	14 (48%)
Carcinogenesis	
Yes	3 (10%)
No	26 (90%)

of nuclear YAP+ cells (nuclear-aYAP+/DAPI) in patients with recurrence or malignancy were both significantly higher than that in patients without adverse outcomes (**Figures 5B,C**). However, while YAP mRNA level was increased in patients with adverse outcomes, no statistical significance was observed between the two groups (**Figure 5A**). There was no difference in YAP expression with respect to smoking status (**Figures 5D–F**).

DISCUSSION

Our study has demonstrated that the expression of YAP, a core effector of the Hippo pathway, and proliferation level in NIP were higher than those of the NP group and control group. At the same time, we identified the positive relationship between proliferation level and YAP expression in NIP. In addition, YAP was also found to be related to epithelial differentiation and neutrophil infiltration in NIP. Clinically, there was also a

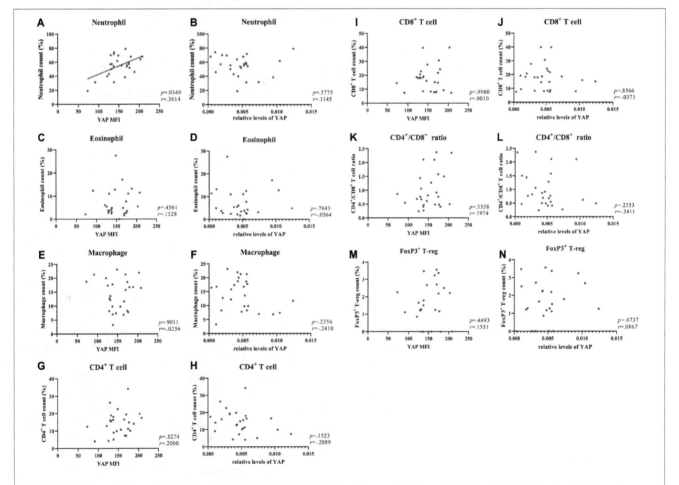

FIGURE 4 | YAP is positively correlated with neutrophils in NIP. **(A,C,E,G,I,K,M)** Correlation analysis between MFI stained for total YAP and neutrophil count, eosinophil count, macrophage count, CD4+ T cell count, CD8+ T cell count, CD4+/CD8+ ratio, FoxP3+ T-reg count in NIP. **(B,D,F,H,J,L,N)** Correlation between YAP mRNA level and neutrophil count, eosinophil count, macrophage count, CD4+ T cell count, CD8+ T cell count, CD4+/CD8+ ratio, FoxP3+ T-reg count in NIP. YAP mRNA level was quantified by RT-qPCR assays and relative expression of the target gene was normalized to $2^{-\Delta CT}$ with RPL13A. Correlation analysis was performed using the Spearman r test (n = 26).

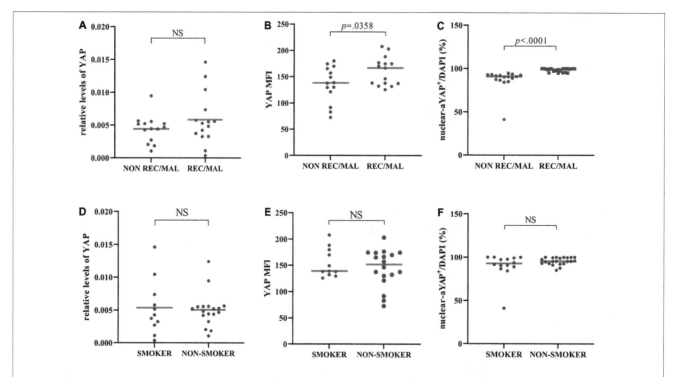

FIGURE 5 | NIP with adverse outcomes has a higher level of YAP expression. **(A–C)** YAP mRNA level, Semi-quantitative analysis of mean fluorescence intensity (MFI) stained for total YAP, percentage of nuclear active YAP positive cells (nuclear-aYAP$^+$/DAPI) in recurrence or malignancy (REC/MAL) status. **(D–F)** YAP mRNA level, YAP MFI, nuclear-aYAP$^+$/DAPI in smoking status. The mRNA levels of YAP were quantified by RT-qPCR assays and relative expression of the target gene was normalized to $2^{-\Delta\ CT}$ with RPL13A. Two group difference was analyzed with Mann–Whitney test. Red lines show median values. **(A,B)**, n(NON-REC/MAL) = 14, n(REC/MAL) = 15; **(C)**, n(NON-REC/MAL) = 16, n(REC/MAL) = 20; **(D,E)**, n(SMOKER) = 11, n(NON-SMOKER) = 18; **(F)**, n(SMOKER) = 14, n(NON-SMOKER) = 22.

correlation established between YAP and the adverse outcomes in NIP. Hence, further studies of YAP and the Hippo pathway in NIP may further explain its pathogenesis and may potentially serve as a target for treatment and prognostic marker for adverse outcomes.

The Hippo pathway, particularly its effector YAP, has been implicated in airway epithelial cell proliferation and differentiation (Zhao R. et al., 2014). In our previous study, we illustrated that YAP is involved in epithelial proliferation and remodeling in nasal polyps (Deng et al., 2019). In this study, we found that inverted papilloma similarly has increased YAP expression at levels higher than that of nasal polyp. YAP was found to be upregulated in NIP than that in healthy control and is positively correlated with the ratio of Ki-67 positive cells to basal cells. Because the ratio of Ki-67 positive cells to basal cells can represent cell proliferation, this result indicates that YAP was involved in the abnormal proliferation of NIP. Additionally, we also found that the severity of remodeling positively correlates with YAP expression. In our study, in both mRNA and protein levels, YAP expression was found to increase with grade, where Grade III levels were significantly higher than that of Grade II.

Yes-associated protein can also affect airway epithelium not only through promoting proliferation but also through affecting epithelial differentiation. In the mature lung airway of mice, the absence of YAP leads to an epithelial pattern of unlimited differentiation of airway epithelium. Conversely,

the overexpression of YAP resulted in an opposite pattern of epithelial with a multilayer of poorly differentiated basal cells (Zhao R. et al., 2014). In our previous article, we demonstrated that YAP contributes to epithelial remodeling in NP (Deng et al., 2019). In this study, compared to Grade II, Grade III NIP has a decreased proportion of ciliated and goblet cells but an increased epithelial YAP expression. Therefore, YAP may contribute inverted papilloma remodeling in at least two different ways: promoting proliferation and suppressing normal differentiation. Interestingly, we also found that in Grade II NIP, the proportion of ciliated cells is negatively related to percentage of nuclear active YAP positive cells, although it is positively associated with YAP MFI. Conversely, the lack of correlation between YAP and goblet cells levels indicate that YAP is more likely to play a role in suppression of ciliated cells formation but not goblet cells, which may involve other pathways. This is evidenced by our *in vitro* hNECs study with IL-13 treatment, where the proportion of ciliated cells and percentage of nuclear active YAP positive cells show opposite trends, which is consistent with Grade II NIP and between Grade II and Grade III NIP. For goblet cells differentiation, no significant association of nuclear active YAP was found in Grade II NIP, as goblet cells levels are very low in NIP. However, in our recently published paper (Yuan et al., 2020), YAP may play a double role in repressing ciliated cell differentiation while promoting goblet cell differentiation, which was not seen in NIP. The difference in the levels of nuclear active YAP may lead to the discrepancies between NP and NIP observation, which remained to be further explored if there are other pathways influencing the goblet cell differentiation. These results may suggest that in lower grade NIP, YAP may not be the only factor influencing NIP differentiation. Additionally, the differentiation mechanism of NIP is also complex and has not been clarified. Further study is needed to explain the function of YAP on differentiation in NIP or other nasal diseases.

Finally, the proliferation level of NIP was not only higher than normal nasal epithelium but also than nasal polyps (Mumbuc et al., 2007; Meng et al., 2014). Our study confirmed this and indicated that the NIP epithelium was likely populated with cells with high proliferative ability. The increased proliferation level may explain why NIP has a faster growth rate and hence a higher clinical recurrence rate. In addition, we found that although there are many layers of basal cells in the NIP epithelium, they still exist near the side of the basement membrane. This is true even in areas where squamous metaplasia is very severe. These results can explain at least partly why NIP has the characteristic of growing into a matrix. The special location of the proliferative cells may partially explain the special structure of NIP: where cells in the apical side of NIP epithelia do not proliferate significantly compared to the basal side. Further study is needed to confirm this observation.

In our previous study, we also found a significant increase in neutrophils in Chinese NIP patients (Zhao L. et al., 2016). Interestingly, YAP was found to be related to neutrophils in this study. Although PCR that represents both epithelial and subcutaneous tissues did not show a correlation with neutrophils, YAP MFI that represents the epithelial levels of YAP showed a significant positive correlation between YAP and neutrophil count. This result is consistent with the high neutrophil level of NIP and is supported by literature (Kurz et al., 2018; Lv et al., 2018). Because one of the characteristics of NIP is the significant increase of neutrophils (Zhao L. et al., 2016), YAP's regulation on neutrophils may at least partly contribute to the formation and development of NIP. This hypothesis would require further investigation. A small number of studies have shown that nicotine could up-regulate YAP expression in other tissue (Zhao Y. et al., 2014; Takahashi et al., 2020), but we did not detect difference of YAP expression between smoker and non-smoker in NIP. One reason may be that the influence of nicotine diluted by other factors affecting YAP; the other may be the difference of tissue. Further study is needed to explain the effect of nicotinic in nasal tissue.

The study, however, is not without its limitations. Firstly, some results were based on correlation analysis, and we did not further explore the mechanism of YAP function in NIP pathogenesis. Future experiments using gene-edited cell or animal models can be employed to investigate the mechanism in depth. Secondly, there were insufficient Grade I NIP samples for meaningful analysis of its association with YAP. In the future, more patients can be recruited to provide a more comprehensive elucidation of YAP expression in different grades of NIP. Finally, a part of our study, especially for those in tissues, only focused on total YAP expression, which includes both nuclear YAP and cytoplasmic YAP; only nuclear YAP is the functional form exerting its effect. This is due to the difficulty to clarify nuclear YAP in the tissue sections, and coupled with the lack of *in vivo* models, we were not able to further establish the mechanism between neutrophils infiltration and YAP in NIP. Further studies using *in vivo* animal models and YAP nuclear import blockers may be required for the investigation of YAP's effect on neutrophils infiltration.

In this study, YAP was abnormally increased in NIP patients with adverse outcomes. At the same time, with the increase of the grade of NIP epithelial remodeling, the levels of YAP became higher. These results suggest that YAP may be an important metric of NIP and should be incorporated in future clinical assessment, including the severity of the disease and the normal airway function of the epithelium. Since the inhibitor of YAP, Verteporfin, has been used in the clinical treatment of other diseases (Bakri and Kaiser, 2004), YAP may be explored as a therapeutic target for NIP to reverse or alleviate the adverse outcomes of NIP.

ETHICS STATEMENT

The studies involving human participants were reviewed and approved by the Institutional Review Boards of Qilu Hospital of Shandong University and 3rd Affiliated Hospital of Sun Yat-sen University. The patients/participants provided their written informed consent to participate in this study.

AUTHOR CONTRIBUTIONS

Q-TY, TY, X-MZ, RZ, and D-YW: study conception and design. PJ, Z-QH, LS, and JL: patient consent and enrollment. PJ, X-MZ, and X-XZ: surgery. TY, KST, HO, JL, S-ZZ, Q-MC, Q-WW, W-HW, and H-YD: acquisition of data or analysis and interpretation of data. W-FK, Y-YT, TL, H-JQ, X-KH, and Q-TY: quality control of the study. TY, Q-TY, and D-YW: drafting the article. All authors: involving in the study, revising the article critically for important intellectual content, and final approval of the version to be published.

ACKNOWLEDGMENTS

The authors would like to thank all the patients for their participation in this study, funding, and staff involved in the study from The Third Affiliated Hospital, Sun Yat-sen University.

REFERENCES

Atherton, H. C., Jones, G., and Danahay, H. (2003). IL-13-induced changes in the goblet cell density of human bronchial epithelial cell cultures: MAP kinase and phosphatidylinositol 3-kinase regulation. *Am. J. Physiol. Lung Cell. Mol. Physiol.* 285, L730–9.

Bakri, S. J., and Kaiser, P. K. (2004). Verteporfin ocular photodynamic therapy. *Expert Opin. Pharmacother.* 5, 195–203. doi: 10.1517/14656566.5.1.195

Dellagrammaticas, D., Lewis, S. C., Gough, M. J., and Collaborators, G. T. (2008). Is heparin reversal with protamine after carotid endarterectomy dangerous? *Eur. J. Vasc. Endovasc. Surg.* 36, 41–44. doi: 10.1016/j.ejvs.2008.01.021

Deng, H., Sun, Y., Wang, W., Li, M., Yuan, T., Kong, W., et al. (2019). The hippo pathway effector yes-associated protein promotes epithelial proliferation and remodeling in chronic rhinosinusitis with nasal polyps. *Allergy* 74, 731–742. doi: 10.1111/all.13647

Katori, H., Nozawa, A., and Tsukuda, M. (2006). Histopathological parameters of recurrence and malignant transformation in sinonasal inverted papilloma. *Acta Otolaryngol.* 126, 214–218. doi: 10.1080/00016480500312554

Kim, J., Jo, H., Hong, H., Kim, M. H., Kim, J. M., Lee, J. K., et al. (2015). Actin remodelling factors control ciliogenesis by regulating YAP/TAZ activity and vesicle trafficking. *Nat. Commun.* 6:6781.

Krouse, J. H. (2000). Development of a staging system for inverted papilloma. *Laryngoscope* 110, 965–968. doi: 10.1097/00005537-200006000-00015

Kurz, A. R. M., Catz, S. D., and Sperandio, M. (2018). Noncanonical hippo signalling in the regulation of leukocyte function. *Trends Immunol.* 39, 656–669. doi: 10.1016/j.it.2018.05.003

Lange, A. W., Sridharan, A., Xu, Y., Stripp, B. R., Perl, A. K., and Whitsett, J. A. (2015). Hippo/Yap signaling controls epithelial progenitor cell proliferation and differentiation in the embryonic and adult lung. *J. Mol. Cell Biol.* 7, 35–47. doi: 10.1093/jmcb/mju046

Li, Y. Y., Li, C. W., Chao, S. S., Yu, F. G., Yu, X. M., Liu, J., et al. (2014). Impairment of cilia architecture and ciliogenesis in hyperplastic nasal epithelium from nasal polyps. *J. Allergy Clin. Immunol.* 134, 1282–1292. doi: 10.1016/j.jaci.2014.07.038

Liu, J., Li, Y. Y., Andiappan, A. K., Yan, Y., Tan, K. S., Ong, H. H., et al. (2018). Role of IL-13Ralpha2 in modulating IL-13-induced MUC5AC and ciliary changes in healthy and CRSwNP mucosa. *Allergy* 73, 1673–1685. doi: 10.1111/all.13424

Lv, Y., Kim, K., Sheng, Y., Cho, J., Qian, Z., Zhao, Y. Y., et al. (2018). YAP controls endothelial activation and vascular inflammation through TRAF6. *Circ. Res.* 123, 43–56. doi: 10.1161/circresaha.118.313143

Mahoney, J. E., Mori, M., Szymaniak, A. D., Varelas, X., and Cardoso, W. V. (2014). The hippo pathway effector Yap controls patterning and differentiation of airway epithelial progenitors. *Dev. Cell* 30, 137–150. doi: 10.1016/j.devcel.2014.06.003

Meng, X., Wu, X., and Yuan, Y. (2014). [Significances of COX-2, p21, Ki-67 expression and HPV infection in nasal inverted papilloma]. *Lin Chung Er Bi Yan Hou Tou Jing Wai Ke Za Zhi* 28, 1823–1827.

Mumbuc, S., Karakok, M., Baglam, T., Karatas, E., Durucu, C., and Kibar, Y. (2007). Immunohistochemical analysis of PCNA, Ki67 and p53 in nasal polyposis and sinonasal inverted papillomas. *J. Int. Med. Res.* 35, 237–241. doi: 10.1177/147323000703500208

Nielsen, P. L., Buchwald, C., Nielsen, L. H., and Tos, M. (1991). Inverted papilloma of the nasal cavity: pathological aspects in a follow-up study. *Laryngoscope* 101, 1094–1101.

Orlandi, R. R., Rubin, A., Terrell, J. E., Anzai, Y., Bugdaj, M., and Lanza, D. C. (2002). Sinus inflammation associated with contralateral inverted papilloma. *Am. J. Rhinol.* 16, 91–95. doi: 10.1177/194589240201600204

Paz Silva, M., Pinto, J. M., Corey, J. P., Mhoon, E. E., Baroody, F. M., and Naclerio, R. M. (2015). Diagnostic algorithm for unilateral sinus disease: a 15-year retrospective review. *Int. Forum Allergy Rhinol.* 5, 590–596. doi: 10.1002/alr.21526

Roh, H. J., Procop, G. W., Batra, P. S., Citardi, M. J., and Lanza, D. C. (2004). Inflammation and the pathogenesis of inverted papilloma. *Am. J. Rhinol.* 18, 65–74. doi: 10.1177/194589240401800201

Sun, Q., An, L., Zheng, J., and Zhu, D. (2017). Advances in recurrence and malignant transformation of sinonasal inverted papillomas. *Oncol. Lett.* 13, 4585–4592. doi: 10.3892/ol.2017.6089

Takahashi, T., Shiraishi, A., and Osawa, M. (2020). Upregulated nicotinic ACh receptor signaling contributes to intestinal stem cell function through activation of Hippo and Notch signaling pathways. *Int. Immunopharmacol.* 88:106984. doi: 10.1016/j.intimp.2020.106984

Yu, F. X., Zhao, B., and Guan, K. L. (2015). Hippo pathway in organ size control, tissue homeostasis, and cancer. *Cell* 163, 811–828. doi: 10.1016/j.cell.2015.10.044

Yuan, T., Zheng, R., Liu, J., Tan, K. S., Huang, Z. Q., Zhou, X. M., et al. (2020). Role of yes-associated protein in interleukin-13 induced nasal remodeling of chronic rhinosinusitis with nasal polyps. *Allergy* 76, 600–604. doi: 10.1111/all.14699

Zhao, L., Li, C. W., Jin, P., Ng, C. L., Lin, Z. B., Li, Y. Y., et al. (2016). Histopathological features of sinonasal inverted papillomas in chinese patients. *Laryngoscope* 126, E141–7.

Zhao, R., Fallon, T. R., Saladi, S. V., Pardo-Saganta, A., Villoria, J., Mou, H., et al. (2014). Yap tunes airway epithelial size and architecture by regulating the identity, maintenance, and self-renewal of stem cells. *Dev. Cell* 30, 151–165. doi: 10.1016/j.devcel.2014.06.004

Zhao, R. W., Guo, Z. Q., and Zhang, R. X. (2016). Human papillomavirus infection and the malignant transformation of sinonasal inverted papilloma: a meta-analysis. *J. Clin. Virol.* 79, 36–43. doi: 10.1016/j.jcv.2016.04.001

Zhao, Y., Zhou, W., Xue, L., Zhang, W., and Zhan, Q. (2014). Nicotine activates YAP1 through nAChRs mediated signaling in esophageal squamous cell cancer (ESCC). *PLoS One* 9:e90836. doi: 10.1371/journal.pone.0090836

11

Exosome-Mediated Delivery of the Neuroprotective Peptide PACAP38 Promotes Retinal Ganglion Cell Survival and Axon Regeneration in Rats with Traumatic Optic Neuropathy

Tian Wang[1,2†], Yiming Li[1,2†], Miao Guo[1,2], Xue Dong[1,2,3], Mengyu Liao[1,2], Mei Du[2,3], Xiaohong Wang[2,3]*, Haifang Yin[4]* and Hua Yan[1]*

[1] Department of Ophthalmology, Tianjin Medical University General Hospital, Tianjin, China, [2] Laboratory of Molecular Ophthalmology, Tianjin Medical University, Tianjin, China, [3] Tianjin Key Laboratory of Inflammation Biology, Department of Pharmacology, School of Basic Medical Sciences, Tianjin Medical University, Tianjin, China, [4] Tianjin Key Laboratory of Cellular Homeostasis and Human Diseases, Department of Cell Biology, Tianjin Medical University, Tianjin, China

*Correspondence:
Xiaohong Wang
xiaohongwang@tmu.edu.cn
Haifang Yin
haifangyin@tmu.edu.cn
Hua Yan
zyyyanhua@tmu.edu.cn

†These authors have contributed equally to this work and share first authorship

Traumatic optic neuropathy (TON) refers to optic nerve damage caused by trauma, leading to partial or complete loss of vision. The primary treatment options, such as hormonal therapy and surgery, have limited efficacy. Pituitary adenylate cyclase-activating polypeptide 38 (PACAP38), a functional endogenous neuroprotective peptide, has emerged as a promising therapeutic agent. In this study, we used rat retinal ganglion cell (RGC) exosomes as nanosized vesicles for the delivery of PACAP38 loaded via the exosomal anchor peptide CP05 ($EXO_{PACAP38}$). $EXO_{PACAP38}$ showed greater uptake efficiency in vitro and in vivo than PACAP38. The results showed that $EXO_{PACAP38}$ significantly enhanced the RGC survival rate and retinal nerve fiber layer thickness in a rat TON model. Moreover, $EXO_{PACAP38}$ significantly promoted axon regeneration and optic nerve function after injury. These findings indicate that $EXO_{PACAP38}$ can be used as a treatment option and may have therapeutic implications for patients with TON.

Keywords: traumatic optic neuropathy, exosomes, PACAP38, axon regeneration, retina ganglion cell survival

INTRODUCTION

Traumatic optic neuropathy (TON) refers to optic nerve damage secondary to trauma, and leads to partial and complete loss of vision. TON is one of the most severe eye traumas, accounting for 0.5–5% of all craniocerebral traumas (Pirouzmand, 2012). Intraductal optic nerve injury is the most common cause of TON owing to the anatomical structure and physiological characteristics of the region (Ganguly and Barik, 2015). TON can result in axonal damage, leading to the gradual irreversible loss of retinal ganglion cells (RGCs) and, consequently, to permanent visual deficiency. Currently, no effective treatment is available for TON (Chaon and Lee, 2015; Singman et al., 2016; Yan et al., 2016). The clinical treatment options for TON include observation (conservative management), high-dose corticosteroid treatment, or surgery (optic canal decompression), which are based on studies on small patient cohorts (Goldberg and Steinsapir, 1996; Yu-Wai-Man and Griffiths, 2013; Yan et al., 2016; Yu et al., 2016; Kashkouli et al., 2017). In comparative nonrandomized studies on the treatment outcomes in patients with TON, the results showed no clear effect of either hormonal therapy or surgical treatment (Levin et al., 1999; Carta et al., 2003). Therefore, more effective therapies to restore the vision of patients with TON are urgently needed (Bastakis et al., 2019).

Pituitary adenylate cyclase-activating polypeptide (PACAP) is an endogenous neuropeptide originally identified in the hypothalamus of sheep, and was named after its ability to activate adenylate cyclase in rat pituitary cells (Miyata et al., 1989). PACAP, as a neurotransmitter, neuromodulator, or neurotrophic factor, plays an important role in neuronal development and regeneration, and may possess potent neuroprotective effects under pathophysiological conditions (White et al., 2010; Sherwood et al., 2016). It regulates various physiological processes through two different types of receptors: PACAP receptor type 1 (PAC1R) and vasoactive intestinal peptide/PACAP receptor (Rampelbergh et al., 1997). Previous studies have shown that PACAP and its receptors are widely distributed in brain tissues, and that PACAP plays a neuroprotective role in neurodegenerative diseases such as stroke (Matsumoto et al., 2016), traumatic brain injury (Toth et al., 2020), Alzheimer's disease (Han et al., 2014), and Parkinson's disease (Wang et al., 2008). Previous observations have revealed that PACAP is expressed in the ganglion cell layer (GCL) and in the body of amacrine and horizontal cells. Moreover, it was also found to be expressed in the nerve fiber layer (NFL) and inner plexiform layer (INL) of the rat retina (Atlasz et al., 2010). Endogenous PACAP has been reported to be involved in the development of neurodegeneration in optic nerve crush (ONC) injury, which closely mimics the axonal degeneration of RGCs and subsequent loss of RGCs in TON (Tang et al., 2011). PACAP and its receptor PAC1R are primarily expressed in the GCL, and their expression has been shown to undergo spatiotemporal changes in ONC rats. Intravitreal injections of PACAP38 have been shown to decrease the apoptosis of RGCs at 7 days after injury in ONC rats (Ye et al., 2019). However, PACAP38 has the drawbacks of insufficient uptake and need for repeated injections. Therefore, an efficient delivery system may be able to overcome this limitation.

Exosomes are membranous nanovesicles with a diameter of 50–150 nm that are secreted by various types of cells after the fusion of multiple vesicular bodies with the plasma membrane (Hessvik and Llorente, 2017). Exosomes are known to be intercellular messengers whose cargo, containing proteins, lipids, and nucleic acids, could be delivered into recipient cells (Colombo et al., 2014). In the retina, exosomes present multiple advantages over existing synthetic systems for the treatment of posterior ocular diseases through intravitreal injection. First, exosomes show low immunogenicity, which can avoid the vitreous opacity or secondary retinal damage caused by the hyperplastic membrane formed by proliferating cells (Kuriyan et al., 2017). Second, the phospholipid bilayer of exosomes may fuse with the target cell plasma membrane and bypass the endosomal-lysosomal pathway utilized by other synthetic

nanoparticles, which can activate the inflammasomes (Hornung et al., 2008; Tatischeff and Alfsen, 2011). Moreover, the size of exosomes might be beneficial for the treatment of TON, as studies have shown that only small particles (50–200 nm) could reach the retina after intravitreal injection, whereas micron-sized particles usually remain in the trabecular meshwork and vitreous cavity (Barza et al., 1987; Sakurai et al., 2001).

In this study, we aimed to investigate the feasibility of using exosomes derived from rat RGCs (EXOs) as an ideal system for the delivery of PACAP38 to the retina, to improve the barrier penetration capacity and stability of PACAP38. CP05 has been demonstrated to function as an exosomal anchor peptide by binding to the exosomal surface protein CD63, which is a tetraspanin present in large amounts on the exosome surface and has been used as an exosomal marker (Gao et al., 2018). By using this system, we have successfully loaded an anti-angiogenic peptide for ocular delivery to treat proliferative retinopathy (Dong et al., 2021). In this study, we aimed to load PACAP38 onto exosomes via CP05, and to evaluate whether this systemic EXO$_{PACAP38}$ can mediate effective neuroprotection and axon regeneration in TON rats.

MATERIALS AND METHODS

Exosome Isolation and Identification
The supernatants of RGC culture medium were collected in polypropylene centrifuge tubes and centrifuged at 300 g at 4°C for 10 min, aimed at removing the free cells. Then supernatants were transferred to fresh polypropylene tubes. It was centrifuged at 2,000 g at 4°C for 10 min to remove the cell debris and again at 10,000 g at 4°C for 30 min, aimed at further removing the cell particles. Next, the supernatants were filtered through a 0.22 mm filter to remove the particles larger than 200 nm and dead cells. Finally, it was ultracentrifuged at 100,000 g at 4°C for 70 min to collect the exosomes. The supernatants were discarded, and the pellets were resuspended to an appropriate concentration with 0.9% sodium chloride solution that has been centrifuged and stored at -80°C for further experiments.

Exosomal size distribution was detected and analyzed by by Nanosight NS300 (Malvern, UK) strictly following the manufacturer's instructions. The morphology of particles was examined using a transmission electron microscopy (TEM, HT7700; Hitachi, Tokyo, Japan). Biomarkers for exosomes including CD63(Cat#sc-5275, Santa Cruz, United States), CD81 (Cat#sc-166029, Santa Cruz, United States), CD9 (Cat#ab92726, abcam), Alix (Cat#2171, Cell Signaling Technology), and Cytochrome C (Cat#11940, Cell Signaling Technology, United States) were detected with Western blot analysis.

Cellular Uptake *in vitro*
To test the cellular uptake of EXO with PACAP38 and EXO$_{PACAP38}$, DiR-labeled exosomes (1 μg) were incubated with FITC-labeled CP05-PACAP38 (20 μM) or FITC-labeled PACAP38 (20 μM) at 4°C for 6 h. Isolated exosomes from rat RGCs were labeled with DiR (Invitrogen, United States).

Subsequently, peptides and exosomes mixture or peptide-exosome complexes were incubated with RGCs for 24 or 48 h. Cells were washed with cold phosphate-buffered saline (PBS) and fixed with 4% PFA for 30 min at RT and stained with DAPI. Images were obtained by confocal microscope (LSM800, Cari Zeiss, Germany). To compare peptide delivery efficiency, cells of each group were harvested and then analyzed with fluorescence-activated cell sorting (FACS, Verse, BD, United States).

Animals
8-week-old male Sprague-Dawley (SD) rats (weighing 180–200 g) were purchased from the Chinese Academy of Military Science (Beijing, China). All experimental procedures were approved by the Tianjin Medical University Animal Care and Use Committee.

Retinal Uptake *in vivo*
To test the distribution of PACAP38 and EXO$_{PACAP38}$ in the retina, PACAP38 and EXO$_{PACAP38}$ was administered intravitreally into SD rats. Rhodamine-labeled CP05-PACAP38 (20 μM) were incubated with EXO at 4°C for 6 h in saline solution (0.9% NaCl). Rhodamine-labeled PACAP38 (20 μM) or rhodamine-labeled EXO$_{PACAP38}$ (20 μM) was injected intravitreally. After 2 or 6 h, rats were sacrificed, and the eyeballs were harvested and fixed in 4% PFA for 1 h at 4°C. Afterward, eyeballs were enucleated in PBS and transferred to 30% sucrose/PBS at 4°C overnight and embedded in optimal cutting temperature compound (Sakura, Japan) and frozen. Serial 20 μm-thick sections were cut using a cryostat (CM1950, Leica, Germany). Cryosections were washed, then permeabilized and blocked in 5%BSA, 0.5% PBST (PBS with Triton X-100). Sections were incubated in rabbit anti-RBPMS antibody (1:200, Cat#ab152101, abcam) dissolved in 1% goat serum in 0.1% PBST overnight, then washed with PBS and incubated with anti-rabbit Alexa Fluor 594 (1:400; Cat #111-585-003, Jackson ImmunoResearch) and DAPI. Images were collected on a confocal microscope (LSM900, Carl Zeiss, Germany).

Optic Nerve Crush and Intraocular Injection
The rats were anesthetized with 5% isoflurane/1.5 liter per minute O$_2$ and maintained 3% throughout the procedure. The eye injection and ONC were performed as previously described (Mead and Tomarev, 2017). Briefly, the optic nerve was exposed intraorbitally by blunt dissection and crushed with reverse microscopic self-closing forceps (Dumont #N7, Roboz, Cat #RS-5027) for 10 s at a point~1.5 mm posterior to the optic disk. Extreme care was taken not to damage the ocular blood vessels. Control rats underwent the same procedures except for the ONC. For intravitreal injections, a Hamilton syringe needle (33G) was inserted into the peripheral retina, taking care to avoid damaging the lens. 4 μL of EXO, PACAP38, or EXO$_{PACAP38}$ (20 μM) were intravitreally injected after crush and 7 days after injury. Animals were sacrificed 7 days or 14 days after injury, and their retinae and optic nerves were harvested.

Quantification of RGC Survival
Eyeballs were dissected and fixed with PFA (4%) for 30 mins at room temperature. Wholemount retina eyecups were permeabilized with 1% PBST and blocked in 5% goat serum in 0.5% PBST. Next, the wholemount was incubated for 2 days on a shaker at 4°C in rabbit anti-RBPMS antibody (1:200, Cat#ab152101, abcam) dissolved in 1% goat serum in 0.1% PBST. After being washed five times by 0.1% PBST, the retinal wholemount was incubated with anti-rabbit Alexa Fluor 594 (1:400; Cat #111-585-003, Jackson ImmunoResearch) 2 h at room temperature, protect from light. Finally, after being washed six times with 0.1% Triton-X100 in PBS at room temperature, protect from light, and then flat mounted. Images of flat-mounted retinae were taken using a × 10 objective with tile scans with Z-stacks on a Zeiss LSM800 confocal microscope. Fiji software was used to count RBPMS$^+$ cells per retina from 12 fluorescence images taken at specific areas with one square millimeter, including four at 0.5 mm, four at 1.5 mm, and four at 2.5 mm from the optic nerve head, and overall RGCs survival was estimated.

Measurement of the Retinal Nerve Fiber Layer (RNFL) Thickness
Animals were administered intraperitoneal anesthesia with 10% chloral hydrate based on their body weight (300 mg/kg). Next, rats were given atropine eye drops to dilated pupils for 10 min, then surface anesthesia with Promethazine Hydrochloride Caine eye drops was applied to the target eye for 5 min. Finally, transparent eye gel is covered on the cornea of both eyes to keep the cornea moist. Optical coherence tomography (OCT) imaging and analyzing were performed on rats under above anesthesia pre-injury, 7 and 14 days after injury, before sacrifice and tissue collection. The images of the rat retina around the optic nerve head were captured and measured by a Phoenix Micron IV Retinal Imaging Microscope (United States). Its in-built software was used to segment the RNFL and quantify the thickness. Segmentation could be manually adjusted when necessary to prevent the inclusion of blood vessels populated by the RNFL.

Quantification of Axon Regeneration
Alexa Fluor®488-conjugated Cholera Toxin B (Cat#C34778, Thermo Fisher Scientific, Waltham, MA) was injected into the rat vitreous at 12 days after ONC surgery for anterograde labeling of the regenerated axons. Optic nerves were dissected and fixed with 4% paraformaldehyde in PBS overnight. The optic nerve was infiltrated in FocusClear^{TM} (CelExplorer, Hsinchu, Taiwan) for 6 h to make the tissue completely transparent. The whole nerve is then transferred into a small chamber built on the load glass slide aimed at providing enough space for the tissue and protecting it from squashed. Finally, the optic nerve in the chamber was coated in MountClear^{TM} mounting media (CelExplorer, Hsinchu, Taiwan), and the cover glass slide was coverslipped. Cleared optic nerve was imaged and analyzed with a confocal microscope by scanning each optical slice of different levels. A total of 7–15 optical slices were scanned for each optic nerve, and stacked optical images were captured at 10 μm intervals. The number of CTB-labeled regenerated axons at

specific distance from the injury site were measured in at least three optical sections from the individual cases and analyzed with the formula as described previously (Leon et al., 2000).

$$\sum \mathrm{ad} = \pi r^2 * \left[\frac{\text{Average number of axons}}{\text{mm width}} \right] / \text{Section thickness}$$

The virtual thickness of per optical slice imaged with confocal microscope was analyzed using the formula as described previously (Leon et al., 2000).

$$dz \cong \frac{0.64 * \lambda \mathrm{exc}}{n - \sqrt{n^2 - NA^2}}$$

We calculated that the thickness of an optical section was 4.6 μm, in which the excitation wavelength was 488 nm, the refractive index (n) of the cover glass slide was 1.517. Our numerical aperture (Na) was 0.45. As the optical section's virtual thickness was 4.6 μm, which is less than 10 μm intervals between the optical sections, single axons were not analyzed multiple times. For quantifying the number of axons at 0.5 mm from injury site, as there are very few axons observed in some cases, the optic nerve axons' counts were used as the evaluation index of regeneration.

Flash Visual Evoked Potentials (F-VEP) Recording

An RETI-port/scan 21 vision electrophysiological diagnostic apparatus (Roland Consult, German) was used, following the International Society for the Clinical Electrophysiology of Vision (ISCEV) standard electrophysiological studies. After 15 min of dark adaptation, Animals were administered intraperitoneal anesthesia with 10% chloral hydrate based on their body weight (300 mg/kg). F-VEP were recorded using silver needle electrodes, which were implanted under the skin in the middle of two ears. A reference electrode was implanted into the cheek of the recorded side, and the ground electrode was implanted into the tail of the rat. White flash stimuli were delivered at a frequency of 1.4 Hz, 250–500 ms for analysis, and superposition was conducted 100 times. Stable waveforms were recorded three times in each eye, and the contralateral eye was shaded with an eyeshade. The parameters observed were F-VEP latency (P2 wave response time, ms), N2-P2 amplitude (from N2 wave to P2 trough wave peak, mV). All parameter values were measured automatically by computer output, and the average of the three measurements was calculated.

Statistics

All data are expressed as means ± SEM. Statistical differences between control and experimental groups were analyzed by Prism. Both parametric (used for samples with a normal distribution) and nonparametric (performed for samples on a non-normal distribution) analyses were evaluated. Statistical comparison between at least three groups was analyzed with one-way analysis of variance (ANOVA). A value of $P < 0.05$ was considered significant.

RESULTS

Exosomes Mediate Efficient Uptake of PACAP38 *in vitro* and *in vivo*

To load PACAP38 on EXOs, we synthesized a chimeric peptide consisting of PACAP38 and CP05 and incubated it with EXOs for 4 h (**Figure 1A**). The FACS results showed that PACAP38 was efficiently loaded onto EXOs, with approximately 87.1% binding efficiency (**Figure 1B**). Consistent with previous reports (Gao et al., 2018), TEM showed a sauce-cup shape, with a size range of 30–150 nm (**Supplementary Figures 1A,B**). Exosome marker proteins, including Alix, CD63, CD81, and CD9 (Gao et al., 2018), were found to be expressed in EXOs, but not cytochrome C, a marker for mitochondria (**Supplementary Figure 1C**), indicating that there was no contamination of organelles. Notably, significantly increased fluorescence intensity was found in RGCs incubated with $EXO_{PACAP38}$, in which EXOs were labeled with DiR and PACAP38 was labeled with FITC, compared with RGCs treated with the mixture of EXOs and PACAP38 without CP05 (**Figure 1C**). Consistently, the FACS results showed up to 86.9% uptake in RGCs treated with $EXO_{PACAP38}$ (**Figure 1D**), indicating that EXOs mediate the efficient delivery of PACAP38 to RGCs.

To determine whether EXOs could have a similar impact *in vivo*, we intravitreally injected rhodamine-labeled PACAP38 or EXOs loaded with rhodamine-labeled PACAP38 (rhodamine-$EXO_{PACAP38}$) in rats (**Figure 1E**). The results showed that $EXO_{PACAP38}$ was preferentially taken up by RGCs over PACAP38 at 2 and 6 h after injection (**Figure 1F**). These data indicate that CP05 mediates the efficient loading of PACAP38 on EXOs, and EXOs promote the delivery of PACAP38 to RGCs *in vivo*.

$EXO_{PACAP38}$ Enhances the Survival of RGCs in TON Rats

To mimic the conditions of TON, we adopted a commonly used ONC injury rat model, which is characterized by axonal degeneration and subsequent loss of neurons dominated by RGCs (Tang et al., 2011; **Figure 2A**). Consistent with previous studies (Nadal-Nicolas et al., 2009, 2015; Galindo-Romero et al., 2013), a significant loss of RBPMS$^+$ RGCs was observed 7 days after injury (729 ± 28.96/mm^2 of the retina) and 14 days after injury (76.84 ± 7.63/mm^2 of the retina), compared with that in uninjured rats (2070.35 ± 54.42/mm^2 of the retina; **Supplementary Figure 1D**), indicating massive death of RGCs within 2 weeks after ONC in rats. We next investigated whether $EXO_{PACAP38}$ could prevent the progressive loss of RGCs in TON rats. We administered EXOs, PACAP, and $EXO_{PACAP38}$ into the retinas of TON rats and examined RBPMS$^+$ RGCs at 7 or 14 days after injury using the retinal whole-mount technique. Strikingly, significantly more RBPMS$^+$ RGCs were observed in $EXO_{PACAP38}$-treated rats, at about 1198.90 ± 28.06/mm^2 of the retina, whereas 729.00 ± 28.96, 1007.03 ± 28.96, and 949.69 ± 37.40/mm^2 were found in the untreated group, EXO-treated group, and PACAP38-treated group of TON rats at 7 days after injury (**Figures 2B,C**). Corroborating the data of day 7, significantly more RBPMS$^+$ RGCs were found

Exosome-Mediated Delivery of the Neuroprotective Peptide PACAP38 Promotes Retinal Ganglion Cell Survival...

123

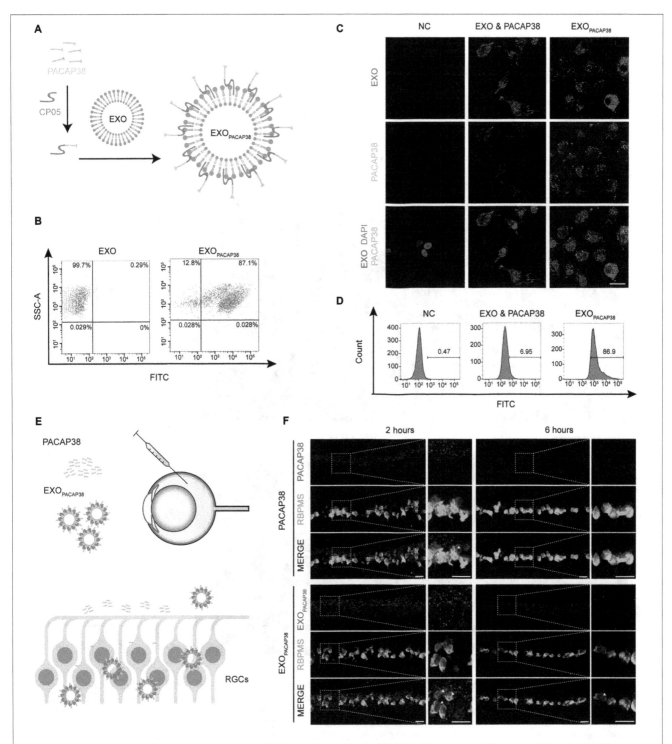

FIGURE 1 | Efficient uptake of EXO$_{PACAP38}$ *in vitro* and *in vivo*. **(A)** Scheme of preparing the PACAP38 delivery system, EXO$_{PACAP38}$. **(B)** Results of FACS assessing the binding efficiency of PACAP38 on EXOs via the exosome anchor peptide CP05. CP05 and PACAP38 form the chimera CP05-PACAP38 through a chemical method *in vitro*, and CP05-PACAP38 was labeled with FITC. **(C)** Representative fluorescence microscopic images showing the uptake of PACAP38 in RGCs. PACAP38 and CP05-PACAP38 were labeled with FITC, and the EXOs were labeled with DiR (scale bar = 20 μm). **(D)** Results of flow cytometry measuring the cellular uptake efficiency in RGCs in each group. **(E)** Scheme of PACAP38 and EXO$_{PACAP38}$ delivery after intravitreal injection. **(F)** Representative images of retinal sections showing the delivery efficiency of PACAP38 and EXO$_{PACAP38}$. The retinal sections are from animals at 2 and 6 h after injection, and counterstained with RBPMS (green) and DAPI (blue) (scale bar = 20 μm) (NC: normal control).

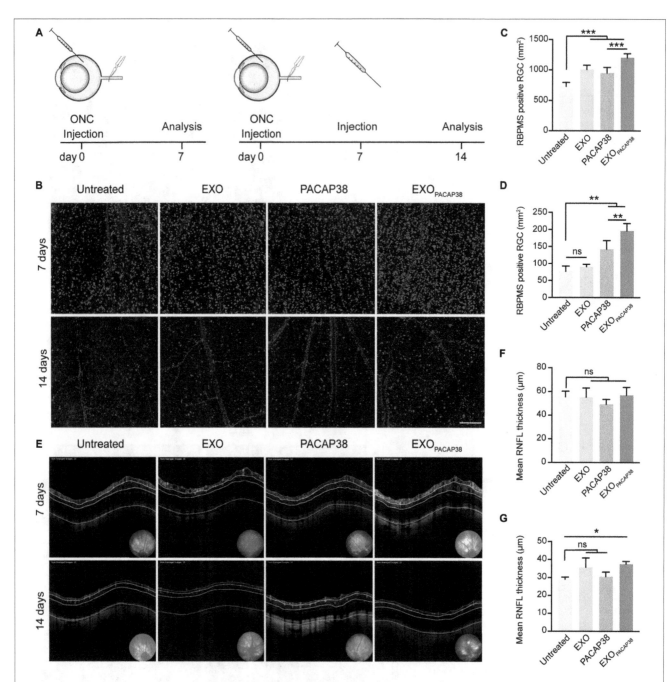

FIGURE 2 | Examination of the survival of RGCs in EXO*PACAP38*-treated rat retinas after ONC. **(A)** Experimental timeline. ONC was performed on rats followed by intravitreal injection of EXOs, PACAP38, and EXO*PACAP38*. After 7 days, some rats were sacrificed. The remaining rats were given a second injection and sacrificed at 14 days after injury. **(B)** Representative fluorescence images of RBPMS-labeled RGCs in a 1-mm^2 region of the retina at 7 and 14 days after injury, divided into the untreated, EXO-treated, PACAP38-treated, and EXO*PACAP38*-treated groups (scale bar = 200 μm). **(C)** Quantitative analysis of the number of RGCs at 7 days after injury (n = 4–5; values are mean ± SEM, one-way ANOVA, ***P < 0.001). **(D)** Quantitative analysis of the number of RGCs at 14 days after injury (n = 4; values are mean ± SEM, one-way ANOVA, **P < 0.01). **(E)** Representative OCT images showing the thickness of different layers of the retina within a range of 3,600 μm in circumference with the optic disc as the center (black circle) at 7 and 14 days after injury, divided into the untreated, EXO-treated, PACAP38-treated, and EXO*PACAP38*-treated groups. RNFL refers to the distance between the red and yellow lines. **(F)** Quantitative analysis of the mean RNFL thickness (μm) of rats at 7 days after injury (n = 3, values are mean ± SEM, one-way ANOVA). **(G)** Quantitative analysis of the mean RNFL thickness (μm) of rats at 14 days after injury (n = 3; values are mean ± SEM, one-way ANOVA, *P < 0.05).

in the EXO*PACAP38*-treated TON rats (195.63 ± 11.09/mm^2) than in the untreated, EXO-treated, and PACAP38-treated rats (76.84 ± 7.63, 90.48 ± 3.60, and 141.79 ± 12.77/mm^2, respectively) at 14 days after injury (**Figures 2B,D**). These data demonstrate that EXO*PACAP38* significantly promotes RGC survival at 7 and 14 days after injury.

EXO$_{PACAP38}$ Preserves the RNFL Thickness in TON Rats

The thickness of the RNFL is an important parameter for the axonal density of RGCs (Mead and Tomarev, 2017). To evaluate whether EXO$_{PACAP38}$ can preserve the thickness of the RNFL, we examined RNFL thickness using OCT, a noninvasive method for assessing degenerative changes in the converging axons of RGCs. The results showed a much less reduction in RNFL thickness in TON rats treated with EXO$_{PACAP38}$, with a thickness of 37.44 ± 0.90 μm, than in rats treated with EXOs (35.70 ± 2.99 μm), rats treated with PACAP38 (30.50 ± 1.48 μm), and untreated control rats (29.09 ± 0.69 μm) at 14 days after injury (**Figures 2E,F**). In contrast, the change in the RNFL thickness among the groups at 7 days after injury was minor (**Figures 2E,G**), suggesting that 14 days after injury is a better time point for subsequent experiments, which is consistent with previous reports (Mead and Tomarev, 2017). Altogether, these results demonstrate that EXO$_{PACAP38}$ can delay RNFL loss.

EXO$_{PACAP38}$ Promotes RGC Axon Regeneration in TON Rats

Cholera toxin subunit B (CTB) can be used to trace neurites including RGC axons in an antegrade or retrograde manner, and can be used as a marker for evaluating the damage and regeneration of RGC axons (Lanciego and Wouterlood, 2011; de Sousa et al., 2013; Duan et al., 2015). We examined axon regeneration with CTB-conjugated Alexa Fluor 488 in TON rats 14 days after injury (**Figure 3A**). Strikingly, much stronger fluorescence signals of CTB far from the crush site were detected in EXO$_{PACAP38}$-treated TON rats than in EXO- or PACAP38-treated rats. In contrast, there was no fluorescence signal of CTB far from the injury site in the untreated group (**Figure 3B**). A distance of 0.5 mm from the crush site was established as the optimal area for examining axon regeneration (Mak et al., 2020). A significant increase in the number of RGC axons (275.75 ± 88.12) was detected in the nerves (at least with a distance of 0.5 mm to the crush site) of TON rats treated with EXO$_{PACAP38}$ compared with rats treated with PACAP38 (117.00 ± 43.91), rats treated with EXOs (71.00 ± 24.05), or untreated control rats (9.50 ± 9.50) under identical conditions. Although we observed differences, only the EXO$_{PACAP38}$ group showed a statistically significantly enhanced axon regeneration compared with the untreated group (**Figure 3C**). These data demonstrate that EXO$_{PACAP38}$ significantly promotes axon regeneration at 14 days after injury.

EXO$_{PACAP38}$ Improves Optic Nerve Function in TON Rats

Changes in the functional properties of RGCs after ONC were tested by measuring the F-VEP. The amplitude and latency of the P2-wave are measures of optic nerve function (Chien et al., 2016). As expected, intravitreal injection of PACAP38 (2.62 ± 0.31 μV) or EXO$_{PACAP38}$ (4.7 ± 0.19 μV) improved the amplitude of the P2-wave at 7 days after injury compared with no treatment (2.72 ± 0.58 μV), whereas EXO treatment (2.37 ± 0.54 μV)

caused no difference. Furthermore, at 7 days after injury, the latency of the P2-wave was significantly decreased in TON rats. The latency of the P2-wave increased from 75.5 ± 1.55 to 119.5 ± 4.17 ms at 7 days after injury, whereas EXO$_{PACAP38}$ treatment preserved the P2 latency (86.75 ± 5.98 ms). Moreover, the EXO-treated group (100 ± 7 ms) and PACAP38-treated group (91.5 ± 7.35 ms) showed no significant difference from the untreated group (**Figures 4A–C**).

The results at 14 days after injury showed considerable similarities to those at 7 days. Intravitreal injection of EXO$_{PACAP38}$ significantly improved the amplitude of the P2-wave (4.99 ± 0.43 μV) at 14 days after injury, compared with no treatment (2.84 ± 0.41 μV), EXO treatment (3.69 ± 0.24 μV), and PACAP38 treatment (4.16 ± 0.06 μV). Notably, EXO$_{PACAP38}$ treatment significantly reduced the P2-wave latency (114.5 ± 8.68 ms) at 14 days after injury compared with PACAP38 treatment (168.5 ± 5.95 ms), EXO treatment (190.25 ± 19.75 ms), and no treatment (184.5 ± 15.76 ms) under identical conditions (**Figures 4D–F**). These results confirmed the potent effect of EXO$_{PACAP38}$ in improving optic nerve function in TON rats.

EXO$_{PACAP38}$ Does Not Elicit Any Detectable Adverse Effect in TON Rats

To investigate whether the administration of EXO$_{PACAP38}$ causes any toxicity to the retina and optic nerve, we examined the morphological and structural changes of the retina and optic nerve 14 days after injection. Hematoxylin and eosin (H&E) staining revealed the typical morphology of the cell layers in rats treated with EXO$_{PACAP38}$, rats treated with PBS, and negative controls (**Figure 5A**). OCT was used to examine the changes in retinal thickness in response to a stimulus, and the results showed no difference in the RNFL and whole retinal layer (**Figures 5B,D**). In addition, there was no change in the F-VEP response of the P2-wave amplitudes among the groups (**Figures 5C,E,F**). These results indicate that there were no drug-related adverse effects.

DISCUSSION

In this study, we demonstrated that EXOs could load PACAP38 via CP05 and efficiently transport this functional neuropeptide to the retina in a TON rat model. EXO$_{PACAP38}$ improved RGC survival and axon regeneration in response to injury. Importantly, EXOs improved the transport efficiency of the neuroprotective peptide by overcoming its shortcomings of low tissue penetration and short half-life. This study on ophthalmic peptide drug transport showed the capability of exosomes as carriers for efficiently supplementing the endogenous neuroprotective peptide PACAP38 for the treatment of TON. This study also further suggests the theoretical feasibility of using exosomes as a tool for the delivery of different types of neuropeptides that can effectively offset the complex pathological conditions of TON, as a combination therapy.

Notably, some studies have indicated the therapeutic potential of exosomes in several retinal disease models

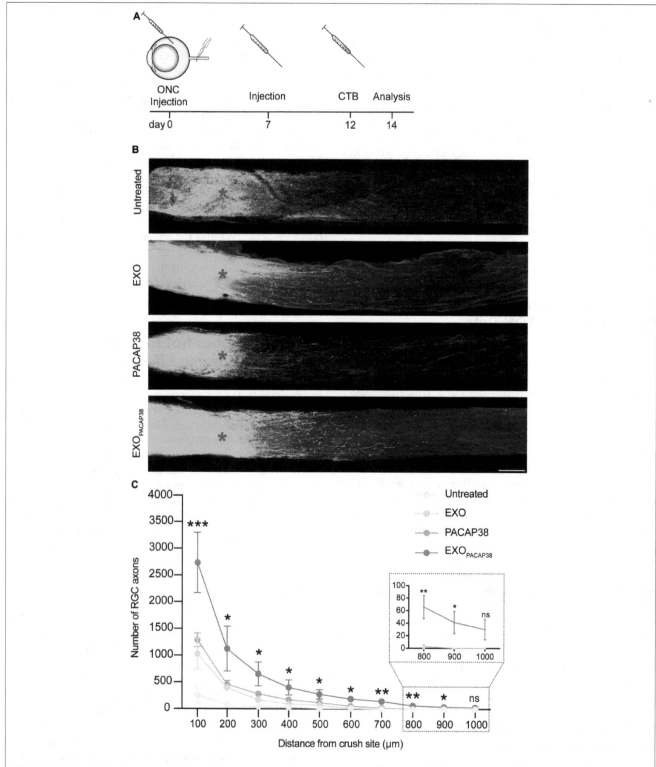

FIGURE 3 | Evaluation of optic nerve regeneration in EXO$_{PACAP38}$-treated rats after ONC. **(A)** Experimental timeline. ONC was performed on rats followed by intravitreal injection of EXOs, PACAP38, and EXO$_{PACAP38}$. After 7 days, the rats were given a second injection. Axons were traced with CTB-conjugated Alexa Fluor 488 at 2 days before animal sacrifice. **(B)** Laser scanning confocal microscope images showing the regeneration of optic nerve axons at 14 days after injury, divided into the untreated, EXO-treated, PACAP38-treated, and EXO$_{PACAP38}$-treated groups (scale bar = 100 μm). Optic nerve axons were traced using CTB. Asterisks indicate the ONC site. **(C)** Quantitative analysis of optic nerve axon number in the range of 100–1,000 μm from the crush site (red asterisks in B) (n = 4; one-way ANOVA on Tukey's multiple comparisons test,*P < 0.05, **P < 0.01, ***P < 0.001, relative to the untreated group).

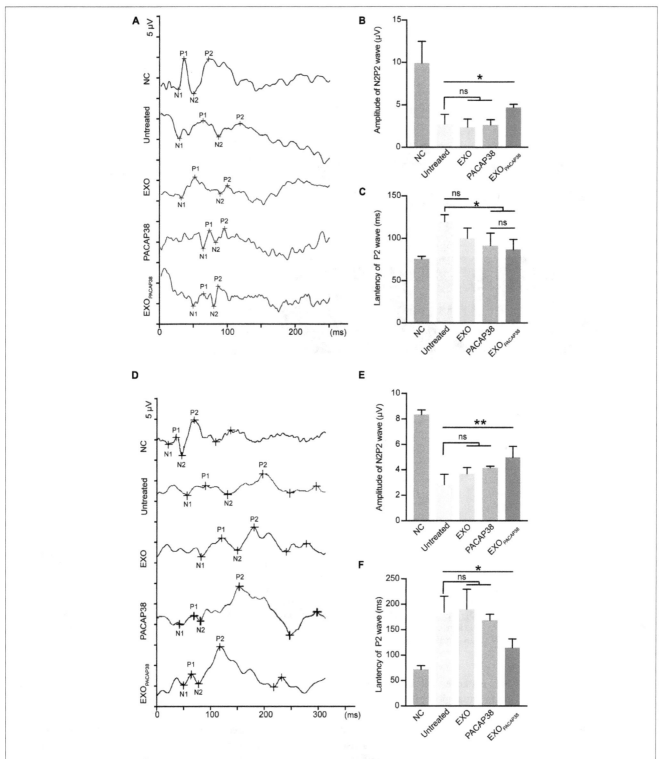

FIGURE 4 | Evaluation of visual function in EXO$_{PACAP38}$-treated rats after ONC. **(A)** F-VEP was recorded at 7 days after injury in normal controls; untreated group; and EXO-, PACAP38-, and EXO$_{PACAP38}$-treated groups. **(B)** Analysis of N2P2 wave at 7 days after injury ($n = 4$; values are mean ± SEM, one-way ANOVA, *$P < 0.05$). **(C)** Analysis of P2-wave latencies at 7 days after injury. No statistical significance in P2-wave amplitudes was observed at 7 days after injury in the EXO$_{PACAP38}$-treated group compared with the untreated group ($n = 4$; values are mean ± SEM, one-way ANOVA, *$P < 0.05$). **(D)** F-VEP was recorded at 14 days after injury in normal controls; untreated group; and EXO-, PACAP38-, and EXO$_{PACAP38}$-treated groups. **(E)** Analysis of N2P2 wave at 14 days after injury ($n = 4$; values are mean ± SEM, one-way ANOVA, **$P < 0.01$). **(F)** Analysis of P2-wave latencies at 14 days after injury. Significant improvement in P2-wave latencies was achieved at 14 days after injury in the EXO$_{PACAP38}$-treated group compared with the untreated group ($n = 4$; values are mean ± SEM, one-way ANOVA, *$P < 0.05$).

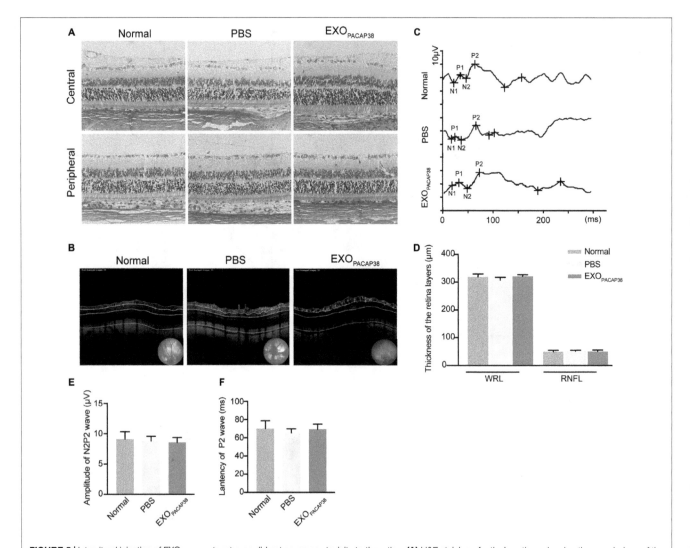

FIGURE 5 | Intravitreal injection of EXO$_{PACAP38}$ to rat eyes did not cause any toxicity to the retina. **(A)** H&E staining of retinal sections showing the morphology of the central (top) and peripheral (bottom) parts of retinal tissues in the normal control, vehicle (PBS)-treated, and EXO$_{PACAP38}$-treated groups. **(B)** Representative OCT images showing the thickness of different layers of the retina within a range of 3600 μm in circumference with the optic disc as the center (black circle) at 14 days after injury in the normal control, vehicle (PBS)-treated, and EXO$_{PACAP38}$-treated groups. RNFL refers to the distance between the red and yellow lines. The whole retinal layer (WRL) refers to the distance between red and blue lines. **(C)** Quantitative analysis of the mean thickness of the RNFL and WRL of rats at 14 days. No significance in the mean thickness of the RNFL or WRL was observed at 14 days among the normal control, PBS-treated, and EXO$_{PACAP38}$-treated groups (n = 3; values are mean ± SEM, one-way ANOVA). **(D)** F-VEP was recorded at 14 days in the normal control, PBS-treated, and EXO$_{PACAP38}$-treated groups. **(E,F)** EXO$_{PACAP38}$ did not induce F-VEP changes. No significant improvement in the amplitudes and latencies of the P2-wave was achieved at 14 days after injury among the normal control, PBS-treated, and EXO$_{PACAP38}$-treated groups (n = 4; values are mean ± SEM, one-way ANOVA).

(Mead and Tomarev, 2020). For instance, exosomes released from retinal astrocyte cells contain antiangiogenic proteins such as endostatin and pigment epithelium-derived factor, which may contribute to the inhibition of laser-induced choroidal neovascularization in mice (Hajrasouliha et al., 2013). It is also known that exosomes derived from mesenchymal stem cells are beneficial for RGCs after optic nerve injury. Both exosomes derived from bone marrow mesenchymal stem cells and exosomes derived from umbilical cord mesenchymal stem cells could promote RGC survival depending on their miRNA cargo (Mead and Tomarev, 2017; Pan et al., 2019). However, neither of the mesenchymal stem cell-derived exosomes specifically targets RGCs. In our study, we aimed to efficiently deliver

the neuroprotective peptide to RGCs. Several studies have demonstrated that autologous exosomes could be used as ideal vehicles for the delivery of therapeutic agents to parent cells, with a homing effect. It has been shown that drug-loaded glioma cell (GM)-derived exosomes inhibited the proliferation of parent GMs more than they inhibited heterologous GMs (Thakur et al., 2020). It has also been shown that cell-type tropism leads to "homing" of cancer cell-derived exosomes and their preferential uptake by the donor cancer cells and tumor-associated immune cells in solid tumors (Emam et al., 2019). At the same time, recent studies have shown that replacing lost or damaged RGCs with healthy RGCs or RGC precursors could facilitate the development and enhancement of connections to ganglion cells

Exosome-Mediated Delivery of the Neuroprotective Peptide PACAP38 Promotes Retinal Ganglion Cell Survival...

129

and optic nerve axons (Behtaj et al., 2020), and that healthy neuronal exosomes can regulate the development of neural circuits and have great potential to repair damaged brain cells (Sharma et al., 2019). Accordingly, we chose RGC-derived exosomes as delivery carriers in our study.

The neuroprotective and axogenic effects of PACAP have been proven in numerous animal models of neurological diseases, such as cerebral ischemia, Alzheimer's disease, and traumatic brain injury (Han et al., 2014; Matsumoto et al., 2016; Toth et al., 2020). In the retina, PACAP has been shown to attenuate RGC apoptosis. However, multiple intravitreal injections are required within a short time period (Ye et al., 2019). Therefore, loading the peptide to EXOs provides a better solution.

In our study, we observed that $EXO_{PACAP38}$ had a high affinity for RGCs in $vitro$ and in $vivo$. In the TON model, $EXO_{PACAP38}$ significantly enhanced RGC survival and preserved RNFL thickness. It is interesting that EXOs slightly rescued the loss of RGCs at first. We hypothesized that healthy neuronal exosomes might have the potential to rescue damaged neuronal cells, as previously discussed. In addition, RNFL thickness measurements showed no significant difference among groups until 14 days after injury, which might be explained by the acute responses to ONC injury including tissue edema, as reported in previous studies (Nagata et al., 2009; Li et al., 2020).

Axonal regeneration is essential to restore neuronal connectivity and to reestablish the function of the visual system. As in other parts of the central nervous system (CNS) in adult mammals, injured axons in the optic nerve do not spontaneously regenerate after injury (Williams et al., 2020). Previous studies have identified several crucial regulators of the intrinsic regenerative ability of RGCs using mouse genetics, transcriptomics, and viral vectors (Williams et al., 2020). For instance, genetic deletion of $KLF4$ in RGCs increased the number of regenerating axons at multiple distances from the injury site (Moore et al., 2009). Another study showed that manipulating the ectopic expression of $Oct4$ through the adeno-associated virus (AAV) system in mouse RGCs restores youthful DNA methylation patterns and transcriptomes and promotes axon regeneration after injury (Lu et al., 2020). Although the gene therapy strategy have achieved positive results in some clinical and preclinical settings, there are still potential risks such as immune responses and genomic changes (Mingozzi and High, 2013; Nguyen et al., 2021). Exosomes are natural products of the body that induce a low immune response and has a high safety profile. In the current study, we evaluated the axon regeneration effects of EXOs, PACAP38, and $EXO_{PACAP38}$.

The results showed that only $EXO_{PACAP38}$ promoted robust regeneration of axons and preserved the function of RGCs. PACAP has been demonstrated to promote peripheral nerve repair after injury (Woodley et al., 2019; Baskozos et al., 2020); however, it is dysfunctional in the CNS (Ye et al., 2019). These results indicate that this system may strengthen the biological function of the peptide. In a previous study, we successfully loaded two peptides with distinctive functions onto exosomes (Gao et al., 2018). Thus, further studies may be conducted to test whether better therapeutic outcomes can be achieved by loading more types of peptides with different biological functions using this delivery system.

In conclusion, we demonstrated that exosomes derived from rat RGCs can be employed as a new biological nano-drug-loading system for the neuroprotective peptide PACAP38. The connection complex, $EXO_{PACAP38}$, can mediate high-efficiency neuroprotection and has axon regeneration effects, providing an approach for future clinical translation.

ETHICS STATEMENT

The animal study was reviewed and approved by the Tianjin Medical University Animal Care and Use Committee.

AUTHOR CONTRIBUTIONS

TW, HFY, and HY designed the project. TW, YL, MG, XD, and ML performed the experiments. TW and YL analyzed the data and wrote the manuscript. MD, XW, HFY, and HY reviewed and edited the manuscript. All authors discussed the results and approved the submitted version.

SUPPLEMENTARY MATERIAL

Supplementary Figure 1 | Characterization of exosomes derived from rat RGCs. (A) Transmission electron microscopy image of the EXOs (scale bar = 100 nm). (B) Nanoparticle tracking analysis detection of the size distribution of EXOs. (C) Western blot detection showing the expression of exosomal biomarkers in EXOs. The total protein (20 or 40 µg) from RGC lysates or EXOs was loaded, and cytochrome C was used as an organelle marker. Sup: supernatant; RGC: referring to the RGC lysate. (D) Whole mount of an intact retina of 1 mm² (scale bar = 200 µm). (E) Quantitative analysis of the number of RGCs at 7 and 14 days after injury (dpi: days post injury; n = 3, values are mean ± SEM, one-way ANOVA, ***P < 0.01).

REFERENCES

Atlasz, T., Szabadfi, K., Kiss, P., Racz, B., Gallyas, F., Tamas, A., et al. (2010). Pituitary adenylate cyclase activating polypeptide in the retina: focus on the retinoprotective effects. $Ann.$ $N.$ $Y.$ $Acad.$ $Sci.$ 1200, 128–139. doi: 10.1111/j. 1749-6632.2010.05512.x

Barza, M., Stuart, M., and Szoka, F. (1987). Effect of size and lipid composition on the pharmacokinetics of intravitreal liposomes. $Invest.$ $Ophthalmol.$ $Vis.$ $Sci.$ 28, 893–900.

Baskozos, G., Sandy-Hindmarch, O., Clark, A., Windsor, K., Karlsson, P., Weir, G., et al. (2020). Molecular and cellular correlates of human nerve regeneration: ADCYAP1/PACAP enhance nerve outgrowth. $Brain$ 143, 2009–2026. doi: 10. 1093/brain/awaa163

Bastakis, G. G., Ktena, N., Karagogeos, D., and Savvaki, M. (2019). Models and treatments for traumatic optic neuropathy and demyelinating optic neuritis. $Dev.$ $Neurobiol.$ 79, 819–836. doi: 10.1002/dneu.22710

Behtaj, S., Öchsner, A., Anissimov, Y. G., and Rybachuk, M. (2020). Retinal tissue bioengineering, materials and methods for the treatment of glaucoma. *Tissue Eng. Regen. Med.* 17, 253–269. doi: 10.1007/s13770-020-00254-8

Carta, A., Ferrigno, L., Salvo, M., Bianchi-Marzoli, S., and Boschi, A. (2003). Visual prognosis after indirect traumatic optic neuropathy. *J. Neurol. Neurosurg. Psychiatry* 74, 246–248. doi: 10.1136/jnnp.74.2.246

Chaon, B. C., and Lee, M. S. (2015). Is there treatment for traumatic optic neuropathy? *Curr. Opin. Ophthalmol.* 26, 445–449. doi: 10.1097/ICU.0000000000000198

Chien, J. Y., Sheu, J. H., Wen, Z. H., Tsai, R. K., and Huang, S. P. (2016). Neuroprotective effect of 4-(Phenylsulfanyl)butan-2-one on optic nerve crush model in rats. *Exp. Eye Res.* 143, 148–157. doi: 10.1016/j.exer.2015.10.004

Colombo, M., Raposo, G., and Théry, C. (2014). Biogenesis, secretion, and intercellular interactions of exosomes and other extracellular vesicles. *Annu. Rev. Cell Dev. Biol.* 30, 255–289. doi: 10.1146/annurev-cellbio-101512-122326

de Sousa, T. B., de Santana, M. A., Silva Ade, M., Guzen, F. P., Oliveira, F. G., Cavalcante, J. C., et al. (2013). Mediodorsal thalamic nucleus receives a direct retinal input in marmoset monkey (*Callithrix jacchus*): a subunit B cholera toxin study. *Ann. Anat.* 195, 32–38. doi: 10.1016/j.aanat.2012.04.005

Dong, X., Lei, Y., Yu, Z., Wang, T., Liu, Y., Han, G., et al. (2021). Exosome-mediated delivery of an anti-angiogenic peptide inhibits pathological retinal angiogenesis. *Theranostics* 11, 5107–5126. doi: 10.7150/thno.54755

Duan, X., Qiao, M., Bei, F., Kim, I. J., He, Z., and Sanes, J. R. (2015). Subtype-specific regeneration of retinal ganglion cells following axotomy: effects of osteopontin and mTOR signaling. *Neuron* 85, 1244–1256. doi: 10.1016/j.neuron.2015.02.017

Emam, S. E., Abu Lila, A. S., Elsadek, N. E., Ando, H., Shimizu, T., Okuhira, K., et al. (2019). Cancer cell-type tropism is one of crucial determinants for the efficient systemic delivery of cancer cell-derived exosomes to tumor tissues. *Eur. J. Pharm. Biopharm.* 145, 27–34. doi: 10.1016/j.ejpb.2019.10.005

Galindo-Romero, C., Valiente-Soriano, F. J., Jimenez-Lopez, M., Garcia-Ayuso, D., Villegas-Perez, M. P., Vidal-Sanz, M., et al. (2013). Effect of brain-derived neurotrophic factor on mouse axotomized retinal ganglion cells and phagocytic microglia. *Invest. Ophthalmol. Vis. Sci.* 54, 974–985. doi: 10.1167/iovs.12-11207

Ganguly, N. C., and Barik, S. K. (2015). Traumatic optic neuropathy: a review. *Craniomaxillofac. Trauma Reconstr.* 8, 031–041. doi: 10.1055/s-0034-1393734

Gao, X., Ran, N., Dong, X., Zuo, B., Yang, R., Zhou, Q., et al. (2018). Anchor peptide captures, targets, and loads exosomes of diverse origins for diagnostics and therapy. *Sci. Transl. Med.* 10:eaat0195. doi: 10.1126/scitranslmed.aat0195

Goldberg, R. A., and Steinsapir, K. D. (1996). Extracranial optic canal decompression: indications and technique. *Ophthalmic Plast. Reconstr. Surg.* 12, 163–170. doi: 10.1097/00002341-199609000-00002

Hajrasouliha, A. R., Jiang, G., Lu, Q., Lu, H., Kaplan, H. J., Zhang, H.-G., et al. (2013). Exosomes from retinal astrocytes contain antiangiogenic components that inhibit laser-induced choroidal neovascularization. *J. Biol. Chem.* 288, 28058–28067. doi: 10.1074/jbc.M113.470765

Han, P., Liang, W., Baxter, L. C., Yin, J., Tang, Z., Beach, T. G., et al. (2014). Pituitary adenylate cyclase-activating polypeptide is reduced in Alzheimer disease. *Neurology* 82, 1724–1728. doi: 10.1212/wnl.0000000000000417

Hessvik, N. P., and Llorente, A. (2017). Current knowledge on exosome biogenesis and release. *Cell. Mol. Life Sci.* 75, 193–208. doi: 10.1007/s00018-017-2595-9

Hornung, V., Bauernfeind, F., Halle, A., Samstad, E. O., Kono, H., Rock, K. L., et al. (2008). Silica crystals and aluminum salts activate the NALP3 inflammasome through phagosomal destabilization. *Nat. Immunol.* 9, 847–856. doi: 10.1038/ni.1631

Kashkouli, M. B., Yousefi, S., Nojomi, M., Sanjari, M. S., Pakdel, F., Entezari, M., et al. (2017). Traumatic optic neuropathy treatment trial (TONTT): open label, phase 3, multicenter, semi-experimental trial. *Graefes Arch. Clin. Exp. Ophthalmol.* 256, 209–218. doi: 10.1007/s00417-017-3816-5

Kuriyan, A. E., Albini, T. A., Townsend, J. H., Rodriguez, M., Pandya, H. K., Leonard, R. E., et al. (2017). Vision loss after intravitreal injection of autologous "Stem Cells" for AMD. *N. Engl. J. Med.* 376, 1047–1053. doi: 10.1056/NEJMoa1609583

Lanciego, J. L., and Wouterlood, F. G. (2011). A half century of experimental neuroanatomical tracing. *J. Chem. Neuroanat.* 42, 157–183. doi: 10.1016/j.jchemneu.2011.07.001

Leon, S., Yin, Y., Nguyen, J., Irwin, N., and Benowitz, L. I. (2000). Lens injury stimulates axon regeneration in the mature rat optic nerve. *J. Neurosci.* 20, 4615–4626. doi: 10.1523/JNEUROSCI.20-12-04615.2000

Levin, L. A., Beck, R. W., Joseph, M. P., Seiff, S., and Kraker, R. (1999). The treatment of traumatic optic neuropathy–The International Optic Nerve Trauma Study. *Ophthalmol.* 106, 1268–1277. doi: 10.1016/s0161-6420(99)00707-1

Li, L., Huang, H., Fang, F., Liu, L., Sun, Y., and Hu, Y. (2020). Longitudinal morphological and functional assessment of RGC neurodegeneration after optic nerve crush in mouse. *Front. Cell. Neurosci.* 14:109. doi: 10.3389/fncel.2020.00109

Lu, Y., Brommer, B., Tian, X., Krishnan, A., Meer, M., Wang, C., et al. (2020). Reprogramming to recover youthful epigenetic information and restore vision. *Nature* 588, 124–129. doi: 10.1038/s41586-020-2975-4

Mak, H. K., Ng, S. H., Ren, T., Ye, C., and Leung, C. K. (2020). Impact of PTEN/SOCS3 deletion on amelioration of dendritic shrinkage of retinal ganglion cells after optic nerve injury. *Exp. Eye Res.* 192:107938. doi: 10.1016/j.exer.2020.107938

Matsumoto, M., Nakamachi, T., Watanabe, J., Sugiyama, K., Ohtaki, H., Murai, N., et al. (2016). Pituitary Adenylate Cyclase-Activating Polypeptide (PACAP) is involved in adult mouse hippocampal neurogenesis after stroke. *J. Mol. Neurosci.* 59, 270–279. doi: 10.1007/s12031-016-0731-x

Mead, B., and Tomarev, S. (2017). Bone marrow-derived mesenchymal stem cells-derived exosomes promote survival of retinal ganglion cells through miRNA-dependent mechanisms. *Stem Cells Transl. Med.* 6, 1273–1285. doi: 10.1002/sctm.16-0428

Mead, B., and Tomarev, S. (2020). Extracellular vesicle therapy for retinal diseases. *Prog. Retin. Eye Res.* 79:100849. doi: 10.1016/j.preteyeres.2020.100849

Mingozzi, F., and High, K. A. (2013). Immune responses to AAV vectors: overcoming barriers to successful gene therapy. *Blood* 122, 23–36. doi: 10.1182/blood-2013-01-306647

Miyata, A., Arimura, A., Dahl, R. R., Minamino, N., and Coy, D. H. (1989). Isolation of a novel 38 residue-hypothalamic polypeptide which stimulates adenylate cyclase in pituitary cells. *Biochem. Biophys. Res. Commun.* 164, 567–574. doi: 10.1016/0006-291x(89)91757-9

Moore, D. L., Blackmore, M. G., Hu, Y., Kaestner, K. H., Bixby, J. L., Lemmon, V. P., et al. (2009). KLF family members regulate intrinsic axon regeneration ability. *Science* 326, 298–301. doi: 10.1126/science.1175737

Nadal-Nicolas, F. M., Jimenez-Lopez, M., Sobrado-Calvo, P., Nieto-Lopez, L., Canovas-Martinez, I., Salinas-Navarro, M., et al. (2009). Brn3a as a marker of retinal ganglion cells: qualitative and quantitative time course studies in naive and optic nerve-injured retinas. *Invest. Ophthalmol. Vis. Sci.* 50, 3860–3868. doi: 10.1167/iovs.08-3267

Nadal-Nicolas, F. M., Sobrado-Calvo, P., Jimenez-Lopez, M., Vidal-Sanz, M., and Agudo-Barriuso, M. (2015). Long-term effect of optic nerve axotomy on the retinal ganglion cell layer. *Invest. Ophthalmol. Vis. Sci.* 56, 6095–6112. doi: 10.1167/iovs.15-17195

Nagata, A., Higashide, T., Ohkubo, S., Takeda, H., and Sugiyama, K. (2009). In vivo quantitative evaluation of the rat retinal nerve fiber layer with optical coherence tomography. *Invest. Ophthalmol. Vis. Sci.* 50, 2809–2815. doi: 10.1167/iovs.08-2764

Nguyen, G. N., Everett, J. K., Kafle, S., Roche, A. M., Raymond, H. E., Leiby, J., et al. (2021). A long-term study of AAV gene therapy in dogs with hemophilia A identifies clonal expansions of transduced liver cells. *Nat. Biotechnol.* 39, 47–55. doi: 10.1038/s41587-020-0741-7

Pan, D., Chang, X., Xu, M., Zhang, M., Zhang, S., Wang, Y., et al. (2019). UMSC-derived exosomes promote retinal ganglion cells survival in a rat model of optic nerve crush. *J. Chem. Neuroanat.* 96, 134–139. doi: 10.1016/j.jchemneu.2019.01.006

Pirouzmand, F. (2012). Epidemiological trends of traumatic optic nerve injuries in the largest Canadian adult trauma center. *J. Craniofac. Surg.* 23, 516–520. doi: 10.1097/SCS.0b013e31824cd4a7

Rampelbergh, J. V., Poloczek, P., François, I., Delporte, C., Winand, J., Robberecht, P., et al. (1997). The pituitary adenylate cyclase activating polypeptide (PACAP I) and VIP (PACAP II VIP1) receptors stimulate inositol phosphate synthesis in transfected CHO cells through interaction with different G proteins. *Biochim. Biophys. Acta* 1357, 249–255. doi: 10.1016/s0167-4889(97)00028-1

Sakurai, E., Ozeki, H., Kunou, N., and Ogura, Y. (2001). Effect of particle size of polymeric nanospheres on intravitreal kinetics. *Ophthalmic Res.* 33, 31–36. doi: 10.1159/000055638

Sharma, P., Mesci, P., Carromeu, C., McClatchy, D. R., Schiapparelli, L., Yates, J. R. III, et al. (2019). Exosomes regulate neurogenesis and circuit assembly. *Proc. Natl. Acad. Sci. U.S.A.* 116, 16086–16094. doi: 10.1073/pnas.1902513116

Sherwood, N. M., Krueckl, S. L., and McRory, J. E. (2016). The origin and function of the pituitary adenylate cyclase-activating polypeptide (PACAP)/glucagon superfamily*. *Endocrine Rev.* 6, 619–670. doi: 10.1210/edrv.21.6.0414

Singman, E. L., Daphalapurkar, N., White, H., Nguyen, T. D., Panghat, L., Chang, J., et al. (2016). Indirect traumatic optic neuropathy. *Mil. Med. Res.* 3:2. doi: 10.1186/s40779-016-0069-2

Tang, Z., Zhang, S., Lee, C., Kumar, A., Arjunan, P., Li, Y., et al. (2011). An optic nerve crush injury murine model to study retinal ganglion cell survival. *J. Vis. Exp.* 25:2685. doi: 10.3791/2685

Tatischeff, I., and Alfsen, A. (2011). A new biological strategy for drug delivery: eucaryotic cell-derived nanovesicles. *J. Biomater. Nanobiotechnol.* 2, 494–499. doi: 10.4236/jbnb.2011.225060

Thakur, A., Sidu, R. K., Zou, H., Alam, M. K., Yang, M., and Lee, Y. (2020). Inhibition of glioma cells' proliferation by doxorubicin-loaded exosomes via microfluidics. *Int. J. Nanomed.* 15, 8331–8343. doi: 10.2147/IJN.S263956

Toth, D., Tamas, A., and Reglodi, D. (2020). The neuroprotective and biomarker potential of PACAP in human traumatic brain injury. *Int. J. Mol. Sci.* 21:827. doi: 10.3390/ijms21030827

Wang, G., Pan, J., Tan, Y. Y., Sun, X. K., Zhang, Y. F., Zhou, H. Y., et al. (2008). Neuroprotective effects of PACAP27 in mice model of Parkinson's disease involved in the modulation of KATP subunits and D2 receptors in the striatum. *Neuropeptides* 42, 267–276. doi: 10.1016/j.npep.2008.03.002

White, C. M., Ji, S., Cai, H., Maudsley, S., and Martin, B. (2010). Therapeutic potential of vasoactive intestinal peptide and its receptors in neurological disorders. *CNS Neurol. Disord. Drug Targets* 9, 661–666. doi: 10.2174/187152710793361595

Williams, P., Benowitz, L., Goldberg, J., and He, Z. (2020). Axon regeneration in the mammalian optic nerve. *Annu. Rev. Vis. Sci.* 6, 195–213. doi: 10.1146/annurev-vision-022720-094953

Woodley, P., Min, Q., Li, Y., Mulvey, N., Parkinson, D., and Dun, X. (2019). Distinct VIP and PACAP functions in the distal nerve stump during peripheral nerve regeneration. *Front. Neurosci.* 13:1326. doi: 10.3389/fnins.2019.01326

Yan, W., Chen, Y., Qian, Z., Selva, D., Pelaez, D., Tu, Y., et al. (2016). Incidence of optic canal fracture in the traumatic optic neuropathy and its effect on the visual outcome. *Br. J. Ophthalmol.* 101, 261–267. doi: 10.1136/bjophthalmol-2015-308043

Ye, D., Shi, Y., Xu, Y., and Huang, J. (2019). PACAP attenuates optic nerve crush-induced retinal ganglion cell apoptosis via activation of the CREB-Bcl-2 pathway. *J. Mol. Neurosci.* 68, 475–484. doi: 10.1007/s12031-019-01309-9

Yu, B., Ma, Y., Tu, Y., and Wu, W. (2016). The outcome of endoscopic transethmosphenoid optic canal decompression for indirect traumatic optic neuropathy with no-light-perception. *BMC Ophthalmol.* 18:152. doi: 10.1186/s12886-018-0792-4

Yu-Wai-Man, P., and Griffiths, P. G. (2013). Surgery for traumatic optic neuropathy. *Cochrane Database Syst. Rev.* 6:CD005024. doi: 10.1002/14651858.CD005024.pub3

12

Validation of the Relationship Between Iris Color and Uveal Melanoma using Artificial Intelligence with Multiple Paths in a Large Chinese Population

Haihan Zhang[1†], Yueming Liu[1†], Kai Zhang[2], Shiqi Hui[1], Yu Feng[1], Jingting Luo[1], Yang Li[1]* and Wenbin Wei[1]*

[1] Beijing Tongren Eye Center, Beijing Key Laboratory of Intraocular Tumor Diagnosis and Treatment, Beijing Ophthalmology and Visual Sciences Key Lab, Medical Artificial Intelligence Research and Verification Key Laboratory of the Ministry of Industry and Information Technology, Beijing Tongren Hospital, Capital Medical University, Beijing, China, [2] SenseTime Group Ltd., Shanghai, China

*Correspondence:
Wenbin Wei
weiwenbintr@163.com
Yang Li
liyang_8151@126.com

[†] These authors have contributed equally to this work and share first authorship

Previous studies have shown that light iris color is a predisposing factor for the development of uveal melanoma (UM) in a population of Caucasian ancestry. However, in all these studies, a remarkably low percentage of patients have brown eyes, so we applied deep learning methods to investigate the correlation between iris color and the prevalence of UM in the Chinese population. All anterior segment photos were automatically segmented with U-NET, and only the iris regions were retained. Then the iris was analyzed with machine learning methods (random forests and convolutional neural networks) to obtain the corresponding iris color spectra (classification probability). We obtained satisfactory segmentation results with high consistency with those from experts. The iris color spectrum is consistent with the raters' view, but there is no significant correlation with UM incidence.

Keywords: uveal melanoma, iris color, artificial intelligence, machine learning, Chinese population

INTRODUCTION

Uveal melanoma (UM) is the most common primary intraocular malignancy in adults. In a study by Shields et al. (2009) of 8,033 UM patients, tumors were located in the iris in 285 cases (4%), the ciliary body in 492 cases (6%), and the choroid in 7,256 cases (90%). About half of patients eventually developed blood metastases, often on the liver. Most tumors can be treated by irradiation (e.g., radioactive plaque, proton beam), and larger tumors may require eye excision (Dogrusöz et al., 2017). The main goal of treatment is to locally control tumor growth and prevent tumor metastasis and spreading. There is currently no effective treatment for metastasis. Consequently, the vast majority of patients die in a short period (6–8 months) (Singh et al., 2005; Cerbone et al., 2014). UM is primarily diagnosed by clinical examination, including indirect ophthalmoscopy and ancillary examinations such as fluorescent angiography and ophthalmic ultrasound. However, many patients come to the doctor late because they have no symptoms. When patients have symptoms, they often suffer blurred vision, light patches (seeing flashes of light), visual field defects, etc., (Damato and Damato, 2012).

The annual incidence of UM is 6 per 1 million people (Boyle et al., 1983). Among a host of factors associated with an increased incidence of UM, ethnicity is the strongest risk factor for UM. UM is approximately 20–30 times more common in whites than in blacks and Asians. Among whites, light skin color and light iris color are established risk factors (Gallagher et al., 1985; Holly et al., 1990; Vajdic et al., 2002; Shah et al., 2005). In a meta-analysis of the association between host susceptibility factors and UM presented by Weis et al. (2006), the following statistically significant factors were revealed: light eye color (RR, 1.75), light skin color (RR, 1.80), and inability to tan (RR, 1.64). The increased incidence of UM in eyes with light iris (blue or gray) may be associated with a decrease in uveal melanin. Iris pigmentation has many physiological functions, including protection of the underlying tissues from ultraviolet radiation, and a protective role in various diseases (e.g., age-related macular degeneration, age-related cataract) (Cumming et al., 2000; Tomany et al., 2003). Lack of pigmentation leads to more light penetration into the uvea and less protection from ultraviolet radiation (UV), which increases the risk of UM (Egan et al., 1988; Singh and Topham, 2003). It has also been suggested (Houtzagers et al., 2020) that most UV rays are absorbed by the cornea, lens, and vitreous, while other wavelengths, such as visible light, penetrate the back of the eye and contribute to the production of toxic reactive oxygen species (ROS), thereby increasing the chance of malignant transformation of uveal melanocytes.

Although several studies from Canada, the United States, Germany, France, the Netherlands, and Australia have shown that UM is more prevalent in people with lighter iris color (Gallagher et al., 1985; Holly et al., 1990; Seddon et al., 1990; Pane and Hirst, 2000; Guénel et al., 2001; Stang et al., 2003; Schmidt-Pokrzywniak et al., 2009; Houtzagers et al., 2020), the proportion of patients with brown eyes in these studies is very low. Therefore, the relationship between iris color and the incidence of UM in the Asian population requires a closer examination. For the first time, we applied deep learning methods to retrospectively evaluate the iris color of the eyes with UM using the photos from Chinese patients, to investigate the correlation between iris color and the prevalence of UM in the East Asian population.

MATERIALS AND METHODS

Study Population

We randomly recruited patients with benign eye diseases admitted to Beijing Tongren Hospital between 2015 and 2020 as a control group. We excluded eyes with previous iris laser treatment, or under IOP-lowering medication, as these conditions may have changed the iris color or morphology in some eyes. We also excluded some eyes with iris depigmentation or corneal leucoma, which may affect our judgment of iris color. Our study included 778 UM patients and 2,239 nontumor patients, all of which have clearly recognizable anterior segment photos of both eyes. None of the patients received any treatment, including tumor resection, radiotherapy, and chemotherapy, before we took images of their anterior segments. According

to patients' medical records and clinical photos, all patients' iris colors were divided into five groups. **Table 1** shows the baseline characteristics of the study population. As shown in **Figure 1**, there is no significant difference in the ratio of males to females between the two groups. As shown in **Figure 2**, in both populations, eyes with an iris color rating of 3 or 4 were the most common. The mean age of UM patients was 48 years, and that of nontumor patients was 52 years. **Figure 3** shows the age distribution of the two groups of patients. **Figure 4** shows that 379 of the UM patients had tumors in the left eye and 399 in the right eye, with no significant difference in the affected eye. The detailed information of the included patients is shown in **Supplementary Tables 1, 2**.

Iris Color Grading

A retrospective assessment of iris color was performed by using anterior segment photos of UM patients and nontumor patients at their first visit to Beijing Tongren Hospital from 2015 to 2020. Color images of the iris of both eyes were taken using a slit lamp (DC3, Topcon Corporation, Tokyo, Japan) with a × 16

TABLE 1 | Baseline characteristics of the study population.

	UM (n = 778)		Normal (2,239)	
	n	**%**	**N**	**%**
Gender				
Male	396	0.51	879	0.39
Female	382	0.49	1360	0.61
Age				
Mean	48.0		52.0	
Iris Color	**1,556**		**4,478**	
①	85	0.055	212	0.047
②	248	0.159	687	0.153
③	620	0.398	1079	0.241
④	354	0.228	1636	0.365
⑤	249	0.160	864	0.193

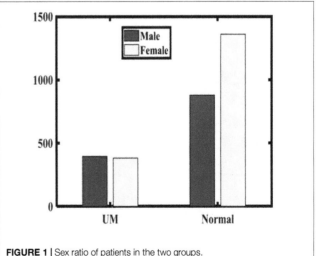

FIGURE 1 | Sex ratio of patients in the two groups.

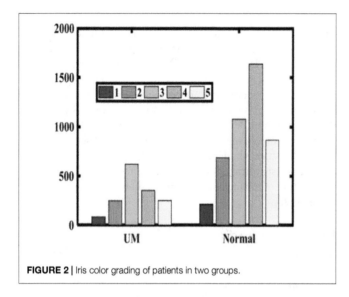

FIGURE 2 | Iris color grading of patients in two groups.

magnification, bandwidth (> 20 mm), height (14 mm), brightness at 30% of the brightest, and angle of 45°. Shot in a darkened room (20 lux), photos are saved in JPEG format (RGB 3120 × 4160) (ACDSee Photo Manager Version 11.0 Software View)[1].

The iris color-grading scheme in our study is the same as described in previous studies of Asians (Sidhartha et al., 2014a,b; Pan et al., 2018). The participants' demographic information and clinical diagnosis were masked, and the color of all iris photos was rated independently by two raters. We select a set of reference photos that best represent the changes observed in the study population. The iris is rated on a scale of 1–5 based on the overall color of the iris: 1 for the lightest color and 5 for the darkest. If a photograph is considered to be between two consecutive levels,

---

[1]https://www.acdsee.com/en/index/

the higher level is assigned. If the two raters' observations do not agree, a third person makes the judgment.

Our raters all have some medical background and general knowledge of ophthalmology.

Annotation Site Segmentation From Slit-Lamp Images

We applied U-NET (Ronneberger et al., 2015) to automatically extract iris zones and obtained the post-processed images which only contain iris sites. Then, the segmented mask results were used to detect connected zones and the largest zone was retained and the others were discarded, as demonstrated in **Figure 5**.

The architecture of U-NET is shown in **Figure 6**. The input and output are the slit-lamp image and mask image, respectively. U-NET can classify all pixels in images to corresponding classes. In the current research, we need to distinguish the pupil, iris, sclera, and eyelid. Then the iris was retained and the pixels in other parts were set as 0. The largest connected region in the slit-lamp image was extracted, and other small components in the iris part are discarded.

Iris Color Spectrum Extraction and Differentiation of UM Patients' Images

We used random forest (RF; Zhang et al., 2019; Lin et al., 2020) and convolutional neural network (CNN; Yang et al., 2019; Li et al., 2020; Zhang K. et al., 2020; Zhang Y. et al., 2020) to extract the iris color spectrum, which represents the iris color grading scores of five categories. Then the iris color spectrum was used as the descriptor to differentiate the nontumor patients from UM patients. RF and CNN received the color features and the segmented iris images, respectively. Color features (Shih and Liu, 2016; Wang et al., 2017; Zhang et al., 2018) were computed with RGB (red, green, blue), HSV (hue, saturation, value) (Hamuda et al., 2017), and YCbCr

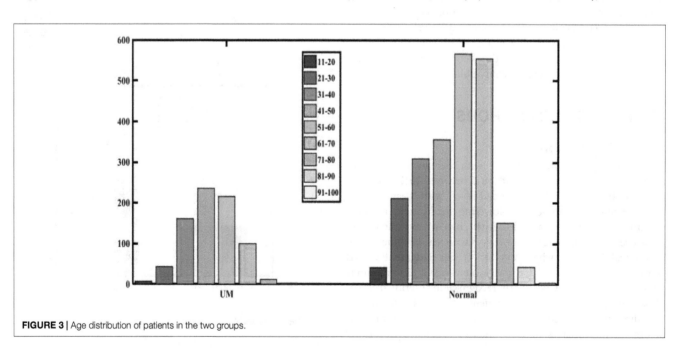

FIGURE 3 | Age distribution of patients in the two groups.

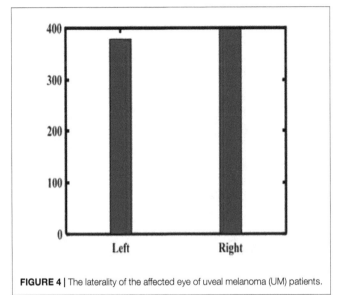

FIGURE 4 | The laterality of the affected eye of uveal melanoma (UM) patients.

Direct Identification of UM With Iris Images

The iris images were directly fed into CNN to test whether it can be used to identify the UM patients from normal persons. The subjects in the training, validation, and testing datasets are different to guarantee the fair evaluation of the relationship between the iris color and UM.

Statistical Analysis

All statistical analyses were performed using Python 3.7.3 (Wilmington, DE, United States) and MATLAB R2016a.[2] We used the accuracy, sensitivity, specificity, receiver-operating characteristic curve, and precision recall curve to assess the performance of the machine learning models. The area under the curve (AUC) was calculated.

(Noda and Niimi, 2007) color spaces. A total of 27 (three types of color space × three channels × three orders of momentum) features were summarized as the descriptor of the color of iris.

The random forest, a common machine learning algorithm, is shown in **Figure 7**. It consists of many decision trees, and each tree can iteratively split a dataset into subsets as a certain discipline (e.g., Gini index) to complete the classification or regression task. Finally, all trees vote for a specific sample to determine the predictive result.

RESULTS

The loss curve of the UM patient group and the segmentation results are shown in **Figure 8**. The performance is satisfactory. The iris color spectrum was consistent with the raters' view. Although the top 1 accuracy is not high, the overall trend is consistent. Because of the physiological limitation and subjectivity of human beings, this result is acceptable and it also verifies that the labels of all samples are objective.

The differentiation results are shown in **Figure 8**, which is not satisfactory and cannot be discerned by the iris color spectrum.

---

[2]https://www.mathworks.com/

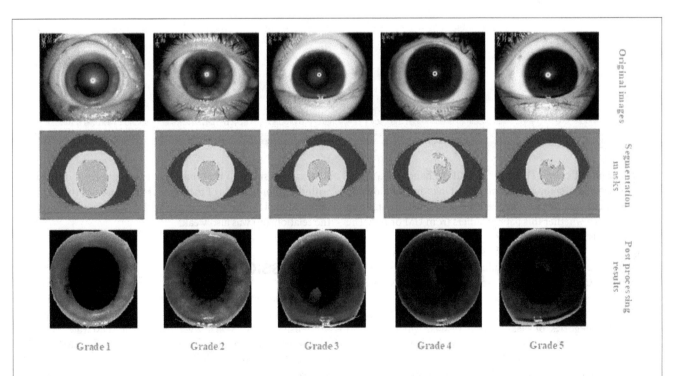

FIGURE 5 | The most representative photos in the current study population were selected as a reference for scoring and the corresponding segmentation results.

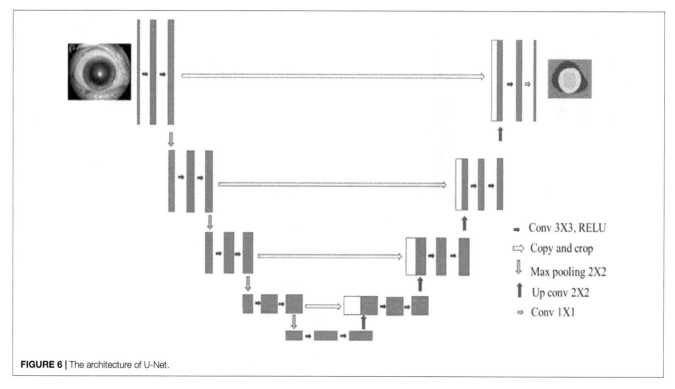

FIGURE 6 | The architecture of U-Net.

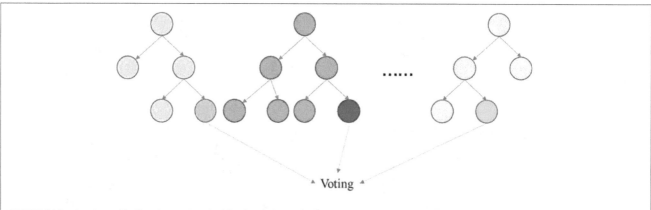

FIGURE 7 | Random forest. The iris color spectrum is defined as the vector in which the five probabilities ($[p_1, p_2, p_3, p_4, p_5]$) correspond to the five grades of the color of the iris.

The ROC and PR curves (Wang et al., 2017; Zhang et al., 2018) show that the iris color spectrum almost has no relationship with UM incidence. We also applied the segmented iris map to directly discern whether this patient suffers from UM or not. The performance is also not satisfactory.

Figures 9, 10 show the classification performance for evaluating the iris color, including RF and CNN, which distinguishes UM with the color spectrum of the iris and iris image. The results of the RF and CNN classification for iris color are in good agreement with our raters. A small number of different categories of classification results, which are also mainly in the adjacent categories of the raters' markup results, are shown in the red boxes in Figures 9, 10. Our results show no significant correlation between UM incidence and iris color in our population-based study, as demonstrated in Figure 11. The

ROS curves signified that machine learning cannot discern UM with the color features of the iris. Furthermore, we try to directly differentiate UM from the normal with the iris image using CNN, the relationship was also weak.

DISCUSSION

Uveal melanoma is an aggressive malignancy that originates from melanocytes in the eye and remains to have a poor prognosis with a 5-year overall survival (OS) rate of <50%. The prevalence in Asian populations is about (0.1–0.6)/1,000,000 (Hu et al., 2005; Stang et al., 2005; Park et al., 2015; Tomizuka et al., 2017), which is much lower than that in the non-Hispanic white population (Hu et al., 2005), the

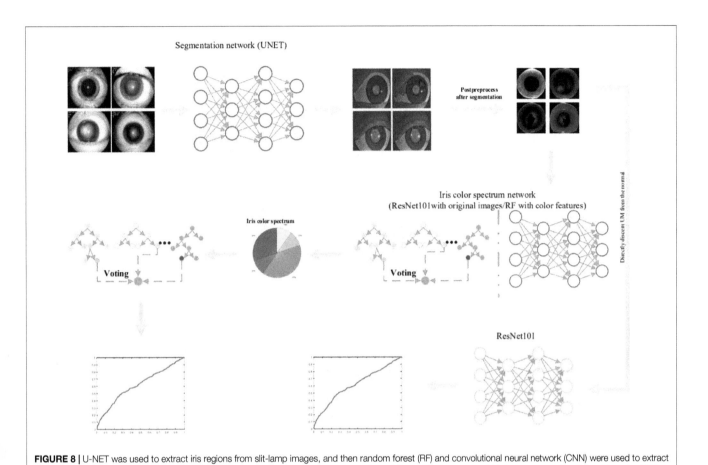

FIGURE 8 | U-NET was used to extract iris regions from slit-lamp images, and then random forest (RF) and convolutional neural network (CNN) were used to extract iris color chromatography as descriptors to distinguish UM patients from nontumor patients. Meanwhile, the extracted iris images were directly input into the CNN network to identify UM patients and nontumor groups.

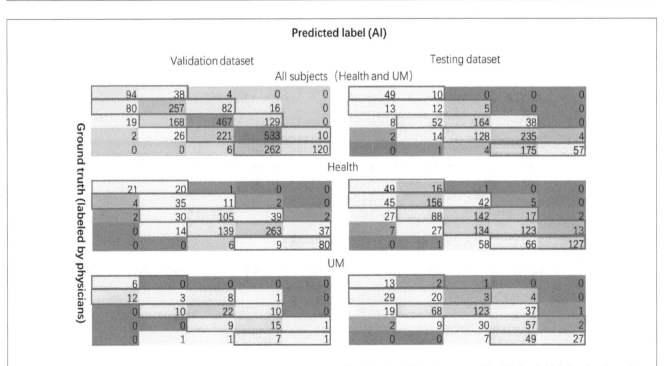

FIGURE 9 | The performance for evaluating the color of iris (RF). The left-hand side is listed as the validation dataset, and the right-hand side is listed as the testing dataset. The first line shows all subjects, the second one shows the nontumor control datasets, the third one shows the tumor patient datasets.

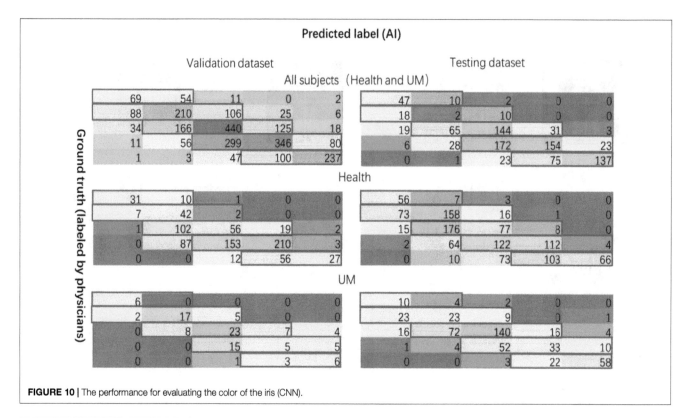

FIGURE 10 | The performance for evaluating the color of the iris (CNN).

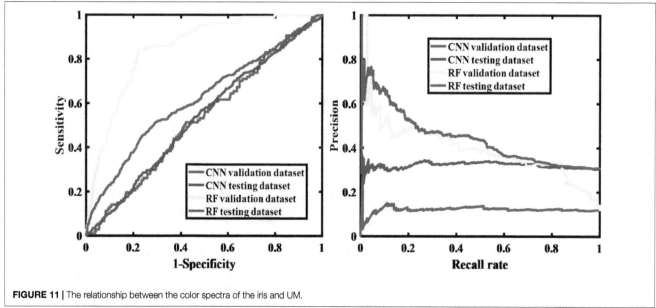

FIGURE 11 | The relationship between the color spectra of the iris and UM.

highest incidence in Northern Europe (Denmark and Norway) (Schmidt-Pokrzywniak et al., 2009). Regional differences may be attributed to ethnicity (lower risks among Asians and populations with higher levels of melanin production in the iris) or to environmental factors, including UV (Vajdic et al., 2002). In whites, a light iris color is an identified risk factor for UM. Our study is the first to verify the relationship between iris color and UM in East Asian ethnicity using deep learning methods. The results showed that there

was no significant correlation between the incidence of UM and iris color.

We compared our findings with other studies that have published cohorts of UM patients with known iris colors (Gallagher et al., 1985; Holly et al., 1990; Seddon et al., 1990; Pane and Hirst, 2000; Guénel et al., 2001; Stang et al., 2003; Schmidt-Pokrzywniak et al., 2009; Houtzagers et al., 2020), the size of our control group ($n = 2,239$) was much larger than in any of the other studies, and the number of UM patients in our study was also relatively large. Compared to the methods used in other studies, deep learning is a more novel and efficient method. In recent years, due to the unique advantages of artificial intelligence in intelligent identification, data mining, information classification, and other aspects, it has brought new scientific research technology to the medical industry, has accelerated the mining of medical information, and has been gradually widely used in the medical field. The accuracy of deep learning for image recognition depends on the number of cases, which often requires a long process of training and learning and optimization. The more image data available for learning, the more accurate the classification results will be. In our study, even though we eliminated many factors that may affect the judgment of iris color, we still included a considerable number of patients and control groups, which is conducive to improving the accuracy of machine learning algorithms.

At the same time, its limitations should be taken into account. First of all, the study population included only that of Chinese so that future studies may address patients of different races. Second, the method of iris color grading was susceptible to subjective factors; therefore, our three raters made their own judgments independently and did not know the classification results of others. Third, it is well known that the observation of color is heavily dependent on light sources; the color rendering index (Ra = color seen under a certain light source/color that can be seen under natural light irradiation) and color temperature are best in natural light, but it is difficult to capture all images in the same natural light. Therefore, we shot in a dark room and used the illumination head LI 900 combined with slit-lamp types BQ 900 BM 900 and BP 900. LI 900 is equipped with two individually adjustable LEDs. The first LED is used for slit illumination and the second for the background illumination. The diffuse light illumination is evenly balanced; the background light and the diffuse light illumination of the slit light gave a free shadow illumination, natural color, and two kinds of reflected light. Besides, since the color temperature and color rendering index of the illumination light sources of the two slit lamps we used were slightly different, and the years of image acquisition span a wide range (5 years), it might have affected the manual judgment of iris color to a certain extent. To solve this problem, we tried to balance the patients included and randomly selected nontumor patients who came to the hospital at the same time as the UM patients.

All in all, the reason why our results differ from previous studies is considered to be mainly the variability of ethnicity. Our study complements the relationship between UM and iris color, laying a foundation for further studies of host susceptibility factors and their molecular mechanisms. We intend to further explore the molecular verification of our research results, and the possible mechanism should be discussed by comparing with the Caucasian ancestry.

ETHICS STATEMENT

Written informed consent was obtained from the individual(s), and minor(s)' legal guardian/next of kin, for the publication of any potentially identifiable images or data included in this article.

AUTHOR CONTRIBUTIONS

HZ, YuL, KZ, YaL, and WW: design of the study. HZ and KZ: development of the algorithm. YuL, YaL, and WW: gathering of the data. HZ, YuL, KZ, SH, YF, and JL: performing of the data analysis. HZ, YuL, and KZ: drafting of the first version of the manuscript. All authors revision and approval of the manuscript.

REFERENCES

Boyle, P., Day, N. E., and Magnus, K. (1983). Mathematical modelling of malignant melanoma trends in Norway, 1953-1978. *Am. J. Epidemiol.* 118, 887–896. doi: 10.1093/oxfordjournals.aje.a113706

Cerbone, L., Van Ginderdeuren, R., Van den Oord, J., Fieuws, S., Spileers, W., Van Eenoo, L., et al. (2014). Clinical presentation, pathological features and natural course of metastatic UM, an orphan and commonly fatal disease. *Oncology* 86, 185–189. doi: 10.1159/000358729

Cumming, R. G., Mitchell, P., and Lim, R. (2000). Iris color and cataract: the blue mountains eye study. *Am. J. Ophthalmol.* 130, 237–238. doi: 10.1016/s0002-9394(00)00479-7

Damato, E. M., and Damato, B. E. (2012). Detection and time to treatment of UM in the United Kingdom: an evaluation of 2,384 patients. *Ophthalmology* 119, 1582–1589. doi: 10.1016/j.ophtha.2012.01.048

Dogrusöz, M., Jager, M. J., and Damato, B. (2017). UM treatment and prognostication. *Asia Pac. J. Ophthalmol.* 6, 186–196. doi: 10.22608/APO.201734

Egan, K. M., Seddon, J. M., Glynn, R. J., Gragoudas, E. S., and Albert, D. M. (1988). Epidemiologic aspects of UM. *Surv. Ophthalmol.* 32, 239–251.

Gallagher, R. P., Elwood, J. M., Rootman, J., Spinelli, J. J., Hill, G. B., Threlfall, W. J., et al. (1985). Risk factors for ocular melanoma: Western Canada melanoma study. *J. Natl. Cancer Inst.* 74, 775–778.

Guénel, P., Laforest, L., Cyr, D., Févotte, J., Sabroe, S., Dufour, C., et al. (2001). Occupational risk factors, ultraviolet radiation, and ocular melanoma: a case-control study in France. *Cancer Causes Control.* 12, 451–459.

Hamuda, E., Mc Ginley, B., Glavin, M., and Jones, E. (2017). Automatic crop detection under field conditions using the HSV colour space and morphological operations. *Comput. Electron. Agric.* 133, 97–107.

Holly, E. A., Aston, D. A., Char, D. H., Kristiansen, J. J., and Ahn, D. K. (1990). UM in relation to ultraviolet light exposure and host factors. *Cancer Res.* 50, 5773–5777.

Houtzagers, L. E., Wierenga, A. P. A., Ruys, A. A. M., Luyten, G. P. M., and Jager, M. J. (2020). Iris colour and the risk of developing UM. *Int. J. Mol. Sci.* 21:7172. doi: 10.3390/ijms21197172

Hu, D. N., Yu, G. P., McCormick, S. A., Schneider, S., and Finger, P. T. (2005). Population-based incidence of uveal melanoma in various races and ethnic groups. *Am. J. Ophthalmol.* 140, 612–617.

Li, W., Yang, Y., Zhang, K., Long, E., He, L., Zhang, L., et al. (2020). Dense anatomical annotation of slit-lamp images improves the performance of deep learning for the diagnosis of ophthalmic disorders. *Nat. Biomed. Eng.* 4, 767–777. doi: 10.1038/s41551-020-0577-y

Lin, D., Chen, J., Lin, Z., Li, X., Zhang, K., Wu, X., et al. (2020). A practical model for the identification of congenital cataracts using machine learning. *EBioMedicine* 51:102621. doi: 10.1016/j.ebiom.2019.102621

Noda, H., and Niimi, M. (2007). Colorization in YCbCr color space and its application to JPEG images. *Pattern Recognit.* 40, 3714–3720.

Pan, C.-W., Qiu, Q.-X., Qian, D.-J., Hu, D.-N., Li, J., Saw, S.-M., et al. (2018). Iris colour in relation to myopia among Chinese school-aged children. *Ophthalmic Physiol. Opt.* 38, 48–55.

Pane, A. R., and Hirst, L. W. (2000). Ultraviolet light exposure as a risk factor for ocular melanoma in Queensland, Australia. *Ophthalmic Epidemiol.* 7, 159–167.

Park, S. J., Oh, C. M., Kim, B. W., Woo, S. J., Cho, H., and Park, K. H. (2015). Nationwide incidence of ocular melanoma in South Korea by using the national cancer registry database (1999–2011). *Invest. Ophthalmol. Vis. Sci.* 56, 4719–4724.

Ronneberger, O., Fischer, P., and Brox, T. (2015). "U-net: convolutional networks for biomedical image segmentation," in *Medical Image Computing and Computer-Assisted Intervention–MICCAI 2015. MICCAI 2015. Lecture Notes in Computer Science*, Vol. 9351, eds N. Navab, J. Hornegger, W. Wells, and A. Frangi (Cham: Springer). doi: 10.1007/978-3-319-24574-4_28

Schmidt-Pokrzywniak, A., Jöckel, K. H., Bornfeld, N., Sauerwein, W., and Stang, A. (2009). Positive interaction between light iris color and ultraviolet radiation in relation to the risk of UM: a case-control study. *Ophthalmology* 116, 340–348.

Seddon, J. M., Gragoudas, E. S., Glynn, R. J., Egan, K. M., Albert, D. M., and Blitzer, P. H. (1990). Host factors, UV radiation,and risk of UM. A case-control study. *Arch. Ophthalmol.* 108, 1274–1280.

Shah, C. P., Weis, E., Lajous, M., Shields, J. A., and Shields, C. L. (2005). Intermittent and chronic ultraviolet light exposure and UM: a meta-analysis. *Ophthalmology* 112, 1599–1607. doi: 10.1016/j.ophtha.2005.04.020

Shields, C. L., Furuta, M., Thangappan, A., Nagori, S., Mashayekhi, A., Lally, D. R., et al. (2009). Metastasis of UM millimeter-by-millimeter in 8033 consecutive eyes. *Arch. Ophthalmol.* 127, 989–998. doi: 10.1001/archophthalmol.2009.208

Shih, H.-C., and Liu, E.-R. (2016). New quartile-based region merging algorithm for unsupervised image segmentation using color-alone feature. *Inform. Sci.* 342, 24–36.

Sidhartha, E., Gupta, P., Liao, J., Tham, Y. C., Cheung, C. Y., He, M., et al. (2014a). Assessment of iris surface features and their relationship with iris thickness in Asian eyes. *Ophthalmology* 121, 1007–1012.

Sidhartha, E., Nongpiur, M. E., Cheung, C. Y., He, M., Wong, T. Y., Aung, T., et al. (2014b). Relationship between iris surface features and angle width in Asian eyes. *Invest. Ophthalmol. Vis. Sci.* 55, 8144–8148.

Singh, A. D., Bergman, L., and Seregard, S. (2005). UM: epidemiologic aspects. *Ophthalmol. Clin. North Am.* 18, 75–84, viii. doi: 10.1016/j.ohc.2004.07.002

Singh, A. D., and Topham, A. (2003). Incidence of UM in the United States: 1973–1997. *Ophthalmology* 110, 956–961.

Stang, A., Ahrens, W., Anastassiou, G., and Jöckel, K. H. (2003). Phenotypical characteristics, lifestyle, social class and UM. *Ophthalmic Epidemiol.* 10, 293–302.

Stang, A., Parkin, D. M., Ferlay, J., and Jöckel, K. H. (2005). International uveal melanoma incidence trends in view of a decreasing proportion of morphological verification. *Int. J. Cancer* 114, 114–123.

Tomany, S. C., Klein, R., Klein, B. E., and Beaver Dam Eye Study (2003). The relationship between iris color, hair color, and skin sun sensitivity and the 10-year incidence of age-related maculopathy: the beaver dam eye study. *Ophthalmology* 110, 1526–1533. doi: 10.1016/s0161-6420(03)00539-6

Tomizuka, T., Namikawa, K., and Higashi, T. (2017). Characteristics of melanoma in Japan: a nationwide registry analysis 2011-2013. *Melanoma Res.* 27, 492–497.

Vajdic, C. M., Kricker, A., Giblin, M., McKenzie, J., Aitken, J., Giles, G. G., et al. (2002). Sun exposure predicts risk of ocular melanoma in Australia. *Int. J. Cancer* 101, 175–182. doi: 10.1002/ijc.10579

Wang, L., Zhang, K., Liu, X., Long, E., Jiang, J., An, Y., et al. (2017). Comparative analysis of image classification methods for automatic diagnosis of ophthalmic images. *Sci. Rep.* 7:41545. doi: 10.1038/srep41545

Weis, E., Shah, C. P., Lajous, M., Shields, J. A., and Shields, C. L. (2006). The association between host susceptibility factors and UM: a meta-analysis. *Arch. Ophthalmol.* 124, 54–60. doi: 10.1001/archopht.124.1.54

Yang, J., Zhang, K., Fan, H., Huang, Z., Xiang, Y., Yang, J., et al. (2019). Development and validation of deep learning algorithms for scoliosis screening using back images. *Commun. Biol.* 2:390. doi: 10.1038/s42003-019-0635-8

Zhang, K., Li, X., He, L., Guo, C., Yang, Y., Dong, Z., et al. (2020). A human-in-the-loop deep learning paradigm for synergic visual evaluation in children. *Neural Netw.* 122, 163–173. doi: 10.1016/j.neunet.2019.10.003

Zhang, K., Liu, X., Jiang, J., Li, W., Wang, S., Liu, L., et al. (2019). Prediction of postoperative complications of pediatric cataract patients using data mining. *J. Transl. Med.* 17:2. doi: 10.1186/s12967-018-1758-2

Zhang, K., Liu, X., Liu, F., He, L., Zhang, L., Yang, Y., et al. (2018). An interpretable and expandable deep learning diagnostic system for multiple ocular diseases: qualitative study. *J. Med. Internet Res.* 20:e11144. doi: 10.2196/11144

Zhang, Y., Li, F., Yuan, F., Zhang, K., Huo, L., Dong, Z., et al. (2020). Diagnosing chronic atrophic gastritis by gastroscopy using artificial intelligence. *Dig. Liver Dis.* 52, 566–572. doi: 10.1016/j.dld.2019.12.146

13

Metagenomic Analysis Reveals the Heterogeneity of Conjunctival Microbiota Dysbiosis in Dry Eye Disease

Qiaoxing Liang[1†], Jing Li[1†], Yanli Zou[1,2], Xiao Hu[1], Xiuli Deng[1], Bin Zou[1], Yu Liu[1], Lai Wei[1]*, Lingyi Liang[1]* and Xiaofeng Wen[1]*

[1]State Key Laboratory of Ophthalmology, Guangdong Provincial Key Laboratory of Ophthalmology and Visual Science, Zhongshan Ophthalmic Center, Sun Yat-sen University, Guangzhou, China, [2]Department of Ophthalmology, Foshan Hospital Affiliated to Southern Medical University, Foshan, China

*Correspondence:
Xiaofeng Wen
wenxiaofeng@gzzoc.com
Lingyi Liang
lianglingyi@gzzoc.com
Lai Wei
weil9@mail.sysu.edu.cn

[†]These authors have contributed equally to this work

Background: Dry eye disease (DED) is a multifactorial inflammatory disease of the ocular surface. It is hypothesized that dysbiosis of the conjunctival microbiota contributes to the development of DED. However, species-level compositions of the conjunctival microbiota in DED and the potential dysbiosis involving microorganisms other than bacteria remain largely uncharacterized.

Methods: We collected conjunctival impression samples from a cohort of 95 individuals, including 47 patients with DED and 48 healthy subjects. We examined the conjunctival microbiota of these samples using shotgun metagenomic sequencing and analyzed microbial dysbiosis in DED at the species level.

Results: The conjunctival microbiota in DED exhibited a decreased α-diversity and an increased inter-individual variation. The α-diversity of female patients with DED was higher than that of male patients. Despite a decreased prevalence in DED, 23 microbial species were identified to show abnormally high abundance in DED samples positive for the species. Among these species, a fungal species *Malassezia globosa* was enriched female patients. In addition, distinct patterns of associations with disease status were observed for different species of the same genus. For DED subtypes, *Staphylococcus aureus* and *S. capitis* were associated with meibomian gland dysfunction (MGD), whereas *S. hominis* was enriched in patients solely with aqueous tear deficiency (ATD). The microbiota of patients with a mixed type of diagnosis was more similar to MGD patients than ATD patients.

Conclusion: We demonstrated that the conjunctival microbiota dysbiosis in DED is characterized by significant heterogeneity. Microbial signatures may offer novel insights into the complicated etiology of DED and potentially promote the development of personalized treatment for DED in the future.

Keywords: dry eye disease, conjunctival microbiota, metagenomic shotgun sequencing, aqueous tear deficiency, meibomian gland dysfunction

INTRODUCTION

Dry eye disease (DED) is a multifactorial ocular surface disease with a prevalence ranging from 5 to 50% worldwide (Craig et al., 2017; Stapleton et al., 2017). There are two major types of dry eye, including aqueous deficient and evaporative dry eye (Craig et al., 2017). Aqueous deficient dry eye is featured by decreased tear secretion, whereas evaporative dry eye is featured by increased tear evaporation caused by meibomian gland dysfunction (MGD). The two types of dry eye are not exclusive. A significant number of patients are diagnosed with both aqueous tear deficiency (ATD) and MGD (Tsubota et al., 2020). Therefore, a hybrid form of dry eye (i.e., a mixed type diagnosis of ATD and MGD) has been proposed (Craig et al., 2017).

Emerging evidence suggests that alteration in the ocular surface microbiota is involved in DED (Gomes et al., 2020). However, the majority of prior studies have focused on specific types of DED, such as MGD and Sjögren's syndrome (de Paiva et al., 2016; Watters et al., 2017; Jiang et al., 2018; Dong et al., 2019; Zhao et al., 2020). In contrast, patients with other types of DED were less represented, especially those with a mixed type of diagnosis. Moreover, most studies have examined the ocular surface microbiota in DED by 16S rRNA sequencing (Jiang et al., 2018; Dong et al., 2019). As a result, microbial dysbiosis at the species level and involving microorganisms other than bacteria remain largely uncharacterized. Most importantly, the DED-associated microbial dysbiosis that was reported by different studies exhibits a high level of inconsistency (Watters et al., 2017; Andersson et al., 2021).

Given the complicated etiology of DED, we hypothesized that the ocular microbial dysbiosis in DED is characterized by significant heterogeneity. The heterogeneity potentially explains the inconsistency between conclusions from previous studies. To test this hypothesis and have a better understanding of the ocular microbial dysbiosis in DED, we surveyed the conjunctival microbiota of patients with DED and healthy individuals using shotgun metagenomic sequencing. We observed the polarization of the abundance of microbial species in DED. In addition, we detected DED-specific sex-related differences in the conjunctival microbiota. Finally, we identified the microbial species signatures of different types of dry eye, including ATD, MGD, and the mixed type of dry eye.

MATERIALS AND METHODS

Participant Recruitment

This study adhered to the tenets of the Declaration of Helsinki. All procedures were performed in compliance with the protocol (#2015MEKY011) approved by the Ethics Committee of Zhongshan Ophthalmic Center, Sun Yat-sen University (Guangzhou, China). Written informed consent was obtained from all participants. Participants were recruited at Zhongshan Ophthalmic Centre from January 2018 through December 2019. DED was diagnosed according to diagnostic criteria proposed by the International Dry Eye Workshop II (Craig et al., 2017). Objective tear film and ocular surface parameters of both eyes were examined, including an evaluation of tear break up time, Schirmer test, meibomian gland and an assessment of subjective symptoms. For DED subtype analysis, patients were classified into the three groups: 1) pure MGD (reduced expressibility and/or quality of the meibum, as well as morphological changes of the lid margins, such as telangiectasia, irregularity and a shifting of the openings of the meibomian glands); 2) pure ATD (Schirmer values $\leq$ 5 mm/5 min in at least one eye); 3) mixed type, MGD + ATD (both MGD and ATD criteria met).

The exclusion criteria included a history of: 1) topical and systemic anti-bacterial, anti-fungal, or anti-viral treatment within the past 90 days; 2) receiving immunosuppressants within the past 90 days; 3) receiving topical or systemic corticosteroids within one week; 4) any ocular surgery or trauma within the past 6 months; 5) any ocular surface diseases other than dry eye, such as infection, blepharitis, allergic conjunctivitis, Stevens-Johnson syndrome, pterygium, etc.; 6) concurrent systemic diseases; 7) contact lens wearing; 8) smoking; 9) receiving eye drops within the past 90 days.

Sample Collection

Both eyes of the patients diagnosed with DED were screened and the conjunctival impression sample was collected from the eye with severer symptoms than the other. Before sample collection, the eyes were topically anesthetized with 1–2 drops of alcaine Eye Drop (Alcon, Fort Worth, TX, United States). As previously described (de Paiva et al., 2016; Wen et al., 2017), a sterile semicircle MF membrane filter (REF: HAWP01300, 0.45 l m in diameter; Merck Millipore, Burlington, MA, United States) was placed on the inferior bulbar conjunctiva for 10 s. The membrane was then immediately placed in a sterile tube with 300 μL of Tissue and Cell Lysis Solution (Epicentre, Ambleside, United Kingdom) and stored at −80°C.

Metagenomic Shotgun Sequencing

DNA was extracted from conjunctival samples using the MasterPure Complete DNA and RNA Purification Kit (Epicentre) according to the manufacturer's instructions. A total of 100 ng DNA per sample was sonicated into 300–400 bp fragments using Bioruptor (Diagenode, Seraing, Belgium). Sequencing libraries were prepared using the VAHTS universal DNA library Prep Kit for Illumina (Vazyme, Nanjing, China) and quantified by qPCR using the KAPA SYBR FAST qPCR Kit (Kapa Biosystems, Wilmington, MA, United States). Paired-end 2 × 150-bp sequencing was performed on a NovaSeq 6,000 instrument (Illumina, San Diego, CA, United States). Negative blank controls, which had reagents from DNA extraction through sequencing, were processed along with the samples.

Taxonomic Profiling

Raw sequencing reads were first quality filtered using Trimmomatic (Bolger et al., 2014) v0.36 and PRINSEQ

(Schmieder and Edwards, 2011) v0.20.4. Human reads were removed using KneadData v0.6.1 (https://bitbucket.org/biobakery/kneaddata). Filtered reads were mapped using Kraken2 (Wood et al., 2019) v2.0.9 against a custom database composed of 29,943 complete microbial genomes downloaded on May 3, 2020. Complete bacterial, archaeal, and viral genomes were downloaded from the RefSeq database, whereas complete fungal genomes were downloaded from the GenBank database. Taxonomic classification results were filtered using a confidence score of 0.2. Species with more than 10 reads in at least one sample were included in analysis. Contaminant species were detected and removed using the decontam R package (Davis et al., 2018). The most stringent hyperparameter value ($p^* = 0.5$) was applied for frequency-based and prevalence-based contaminant identification of the *isContaminant* function. For the frequency-based method, DNA concentrations were measured by qPCR and obtained during library preparation. The scores from the frequency-based and prevalence-based methods were combined using the "minimum" approach. We further excluded the species whose relative abundance was greater than 0.05% in at least one negative blank control and the species whose relative abundance showed a significant inverse correlation with DNA concentrations ($\rho < -0.2$, $p < 0.05$, Spearman's correlation) (Jervis-Bardy et al., 2015).

Statistical Analysis

Statistical analysis was performed using R v4.0.2 software packages. The Shannon diversity index and Bray-Curtis dissimilarity index were computed using the vegan R package. Group differences of the Shannon diversity and Bray-Curtis dissimilarity were analyzed by two-sided Wilcoxon's rank sum test. Principal coordinates analysis (PCoA) was performed using the ade4 R package. For all boxplots, the box edges denoted the first and third quartiles and the horizontal line denoted the median, with the whiskers extending up to the 1.5-fold interquartile ranges. Associations between disease status and the abundance of microbial species were determined using multivariable regression models implemented in MaAsLin2 (https://huttenhower.sph.harvard.edu/maaslin). Microbial species present in at least 10% samples were included in the association analysis. Transformation and normalization were applied on the microbial species features using default options of MaAsLin2. Transformed abundances were fit with per-feature general linear model (GLM) in which the abundance of each species was modelled as a function of diagnosis (dry eye versus healthy, ATD versus non-ATD, and MGD versus non-MGD) as a categorical variable, age as a continuous covariate, and sex as a binary covariate. For assessment of sex-related differences, the abundance of each species was modelled as a function of sex with age as a covariate.

RESULTS

Dysbiosis of Conjunctival Microbiota in DED

The study cohort was composed of 47 patients with DED and 48 healthy individuals (**Supplementary Table S1**). The group of

DED comprised six patients with ATD, 14 with MGD, and 27 with mixed dry eye (**Supplementary Table S2**). We performed shotgun metagenomic sequencing on the conjunctival impression samples to characterize the taxonomic composition of the conjunctival microbiota. Overall, the phylum-level composition was similar between patients with DED and healthy individuals (**Figure 1A**). For healthy individuals and patients with different subtypes of DED, Actinobacteria, Firmicutes, Proteobacteria, and Bacteroidetes accounted for the majority of the conjunctival microbiota. Consistent with prior studies (Zilliox et al., 2020; Andersson et al., 2021), the α-diversity of patients with DED was significantly lower than that of healthy individuals (**Figure 1B**). The β-diversity within patients with DED was higher than that within healthy individuals, suggesting an increased inter-individual variation in the conjunctival microbiota of patients with DED (**Figure 1C**). We performed the principal coordinates analysis based on species-level composition and observed a clear delineation between DED and healthy samples (**Figure 1D**). These results demonstrate that DED is associated with microbial dysbiosis of the conjunctival microbiota.

To characterize the microbial species-level alterations related to the microbial dysbiosis, we compared the species profiles between samples from patients with DED and those from healthy individuals. We identified a total of 206 species that were more abundant in healthy individuals ($p < 0.05$). However, we did not detect any species that were significantly enriched in DED (**Supplementary Figure S1A**). In addition, we found that the majority of microbial species exhibited a decreased prevalence in the DED group in contrast to the healthy group (**Supplementary Figure S1B**). Specifically, only 50 species were present in at least 10% samples in both the dry eye and healthy groups (**Supplementary Figure S1C**) and the number decreased to 16 for species present in at least 20% samples (**Supplementary Figure S1D**). These observations suggest that the dysbiosis of the conjunctival microbiota in dry eye is primarily characterized by the depletion of commensal species.

Polarization of Microbial Species Abundance in DED

We hypothesized that the lack of general enrichment of microbial species in dry eye might be due to the high level of inter-individual variation in patients with dry eye. To search for the microbial species that contributed prominently to the individuality, we performed principal coordinates analysis on the species-level composition of samples from patients with dry eye. For each species present in at least 10% samples in the dry eye group, we analyzed differences of sample positions in principal coordinate 1 (PCo1) or 2 (PCo2) between the DED samples with the species (denoted as P-DED) and those without the species (denoted as N-DED). We identified 25 species that significantly contributed to either PCo1 or PCo2 ($p < 0.05$). The species list is available in **Supplementary Table S3**. We found that species of the genera *Streptococcus* and *Corynebacterium* were overrepresented in the list. Other genera that were represented by at least two species included *Cutibacterium*, *Rothia*, and *Staphylococcus*.

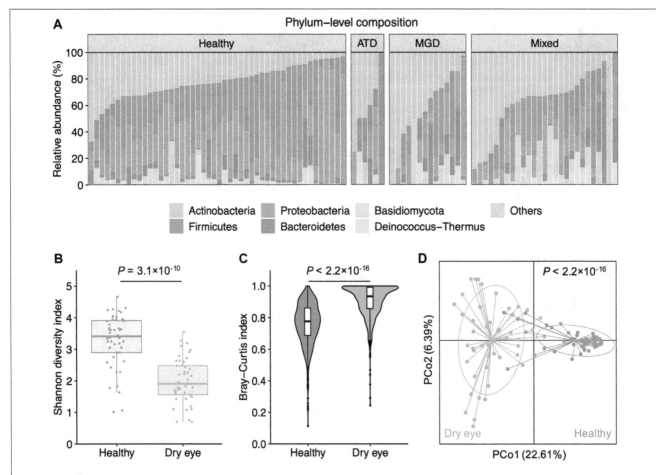

FIGURE 1 | Dry eye is associated with microbial dysbiosis of the conjunctival microbiota **(A)** Phylum-level composition of the conjunctival microbiota of healthy individuals ($n = 48$) and patients with dry eye ($n = 47$). Patients were diagnosed with aqueous tear deficiency (ATD, $n = 6$), meibomian gland dysfunction (MGD, $n = 14$), or a hybrid form of ATD and MGD (mixed, $n = 27$) **(B)** The α-diversity measured with the Shannon index was computed for healthy and dry eye samples **(C)** The β-diversity measured with Bray-Curtis dissimilarity within healthy and dry eye samples **(D)** Principal coordinates analysis of samples from all 95 participants based on the species-level Bray-Curtis distance. p values were computed for PCo1 using Wilcoxon's rank sum test.

Furthermore, given the dominant decrease in the prevalence of species in patients with DED in contrast to healthy individuals, we compared species relative abundance between P-DED and healthy samples. Intriguingly, we detected 23 species that were significantly enriched P-DED samples ($p < 0.05$). The species list is available in **Supplementary Table S4**. Notably, 46 out of 47 samples from patients with DED contained at least one of the 23 species. Among these species, 12 species significantly contributed to either PCo1 or PCo2 (**Figure 2A**). Examples of such species were shown in **Figure 2B**.

Of note, despite the absence in a part of patients with DED, the first quartiles of relative abundance of the microbial species enriched in P-DED samples were generally higher than the third quartiles of that in samples from healthy individuals (**Figure 2C**). This finding implies a polarized distribution of the abundance of microbial species in the conjunctival microbiota of patients with DED compared with healthy individuals. In other words, some microbial species might exhibit a relatively even distribution in healthy individuals, whereas they might be either depleted or with abnormally high abundance in patients with DED. Collectively, these results highlight the heterogeneous microbial dysbiosis in dry eye.

Distinct Sex-Related Differences in Conjunctival Microbiota

With a higher DED prevalence in women than men, female sex is considered as a risk factor for the development of DED (Sullivan et al., 2017). We therefore assessed whether sex factors are associated with the heterogeneity of the conjunctival microbiota in DED. Overall, sex was a minor factor accounting for inter-individual variation in DED (**Figure 3A**). We compared the α-diversity and the relative abundance of microbial species between female and male individuals in the healthy and dry eye groups, respectively, using multivariable regression models with age as a covariate. Consistent with previous observations (Ozkan et al., 2017), males harbor a more diverse conjunctival microbiota than

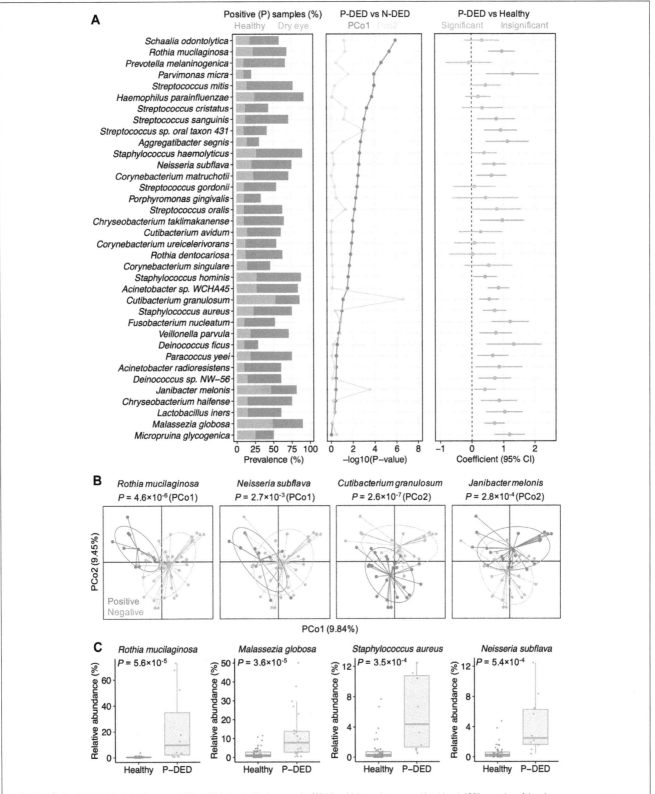

FIGURE 2 | Microbial dysbiosis in dry eye exhibits a high level of heterogeneity **(A)** Microbial species present in at least 10% samples of the dry eye group were shown if they significantly contributed to one of the top two principal coordinates of the dry eye samples or exhibited a polarized distribution in abundance. P-DED, DED samples in which a specific species was detected; N-DED, DED samples in which a specific species was not detected **(B)** Examples of species significantly contributing to PCo1 or PCo2. Samples are colored according to the detection of the species. p values were computed using Wilcoxon's rank sum test **(C)** Examples of species with a polarized distribution in abundance in DED samples compared to healthy samples.

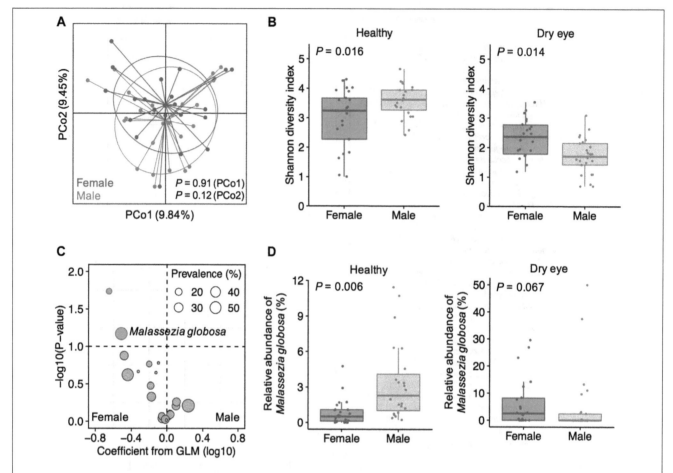

FIGURE 3 | Sex-related differences in the conjunctival microbiota of patients with dry eye **(A)** Principal coordinates analysis of samples from patients with dry eye. Samples are colored according to the sex of patients. *p* values were computed using Wilcoxon's rank sum test **(B)** Differences in the α-diversity between female and male individuals in the healthy and dry eye groups, respectively **(C)** The volcano plot demonstrating associations of the 23 species with polarized abundance with sex. Sizes of dots reflect their prevalence in the dry eye group. GLM, general linear model **(D)** Differences in the relative abundance of *Malassezia globosa* between female and male individuals in the healthy and dry eye groups, respectively.

females in healthy individuals (p = 0.016; **Figure 3B**). Unexpectedly, the α-diversity of female patients with DED was higher than male patients (p = 0.014).

Due to a major depletion of microbial species in DED, a few species were solely enriched in males for healthy individuals (**Supplementary Figure S1A, B**). For patients with DED, associations between sex and the relative abundance of species were different from or even in opposite ways of the trend in healthy individuals. For example, *Pseudomonas aeruginosa* and *Deinococcus* sp. NW-56 were exclusively detected in the samples from female patients with DED (**Supplementary Figure S2A, B**). However, in the healthy group, *Pseudomonas aeruginosa* was more abundant in males than females (p = 0.002), whereas *Deinococcus* sp. NW-56 showed no significant difference in abundance between females and males (p = 0.984). Among the 23 microbial species enriched in P-DED, we observed that *Malassezia globosa* was more abundant in female than male patients with DED (p = 0.067; **Figure 3C**). However, for healthy

individuals, *M. globosa* was positively associated with male sex (p = 0.006; **Figure 3D**). These results suggest that the sex-related differences in the conjunctival microbiota of patients with DED are distinct from that of healthy individuals.

Identification of Microbial Species Associated With Different Types of DED

We next examined the differences in the conjunctival microbiota among patients with different types of dry eye. To improve the representativeness of participants solely with ATD and MGD, 21 additional patients with DED recruited during the same period as the 47 patients were included in our analysis (**Supplementary Table S5**; **Supplementary Figure S3**). We first investigated the distribution of samples from patients with ATD, MGD, and mixed dry eye using principal coordinates analysis. We found a delineation between ATD and the other two types of dry eye (MGD and mixed dry eye). In contrast, the delineation between MGD and mixed dry eye were less clear (**Figure 4A**; **Supplementary Figure S4**). In

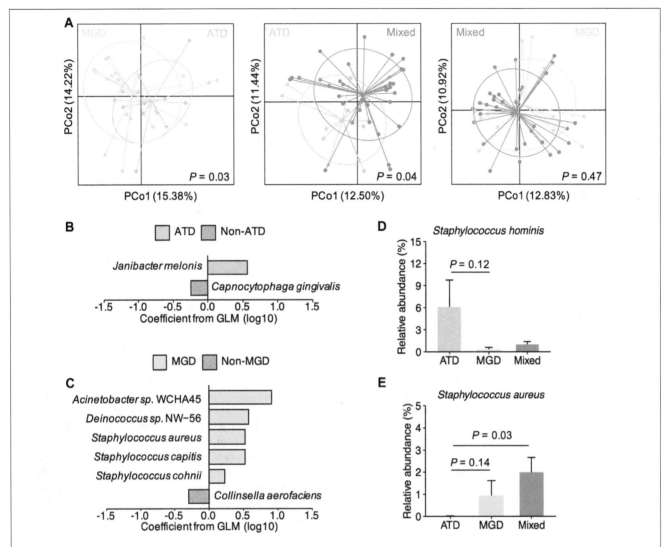

FIGURE 4 | Distinct microbial species signatures of different types of dry eye **(A)** Principal coordinates analysis of the microbial species composition of samples from patients with ATD (n = 14) and MGD (n = 19), ATD and mixed dry eye (n = 35), and MGD and mixed dry eye, respectively. p values were computed for PCo1 using Wilcoxon's rank sum test **(B)** Model coefficients of top-ranked species associated with either ATD or non-ATD dry eye (p < 0.1, coefficient >0.2) **(C)** Model coefficients of top-ranked species associated with either MGD or non-MGD dry eye (p < 0.1, coefficient >0.2) **(D)** Relative abundances of *Staphylococcus hominis* in the ATD, MGD, and mixed dry eye groups **(E)** Relative abundances of *Staphylococcus aureus* in the ATD, MGD, and mixed dry eye groups. Representative *Staphylococcus* species showing differences in abundance (p < 0.15) among the three groups are displayed. p values were computed using Wilcoxon's rank sum test. Relative abundances are represented as mean ± SEM. Error bars indicate standard error.

agreement with this finding, the microbial diversity in ATD was lower than mixed dry eye (p = 0.056). However, the difference in diversity was insignificant between MGD and mixed dry eye (p = 0.65; **Supplementary Figure S4**). These results indicate that the conjunctival microbiota of patients with mixed dry eye is more similar to MGD than ATD.

We hypothesized that different types of DED have distinct species-level signatures of the conjunctival microbiota. To test this hypothesis, we performed multivariable analysis to identify species that were associated with either ATD or MGD. Specifically, the relative abundance of each species was modelled as a function of ATD and MGD as variables and age and sex as covariates. We also examined the overlap between the 23 species with polarized abundance in DED and

the species associated with either ATD or MGD. Among the top-ranked associated species (p < 0.1, coefficient >0.2), *Janibacter melonis*, which is one of the DED-polarized species, was enriched in ATD (**Figure 4B**). Moreover, the top three species associated with MGD were all DED-polarized species, including *Acinetobacter* sp. WCHA45, *Deinococcus* sp. NW-56, and *Staphylococcus aureus* (**Figure 4C**).

We further compared the relative abundance of ATD or MGD associated species among ATD, MGD, and mixed dry eye groups. Notably, species of the genus *Staphylococcus* exhibited different patterns in the three types of DED (**Supplementary Figure S5**). For instance, *S. hominis* was more abundant in the ATD group than the MGD and mixed dry eye groups (**Figure 4D**), whereas *S. aureus* was more abundant in the MGD and mixed dry eye groups than the ATD group (**Figure 4E**). This finding potentially explains the inconsistent observations of associations between *Staphylococcus* and disease status in previous studies that either focused on dry eye or MGD (Gomes et al., 2020). Taken together, these results demonstrate that aqueous deficient, evaporative, and mixed dry eye are associated with distinct microbial species signatures in the conjunctival microbiota.

DISCUSSION

DED is a multifactorial ocular surface disease whose pathogenesis is not fully understood. Nonetheless, it is recognized that the breakdown of immune homeostasis at the ocular surface plays an important role in the development of DED (Stevenson et al., 2012). Prior studies have revealed the involvement of the ocular microbiota in DED (Gomes et al., 2020). However, conclusions in the alteration of the microbiota can be inconsistent between studies. In this study, we characterized the heterogeneity of conjunctival microbial dysbiosis in DED using data derived from shotgun metagenomic sequencing. We identified 23 species that showed abnormally high abundance in a portion of patients while absent in other patients. Sex is associated with different patterns of microbial dysbiosis in DED. ATD, MGD, and mixed dry eye have distinct signatures of the conjunctival microbiota. The microbial dysbiosis of mixed dry eye is more similar to MGD than ATD.

We observed that the majority of commensal microorganisms in the conjunctival microbiota exhibited a decreased prevalence in DED. Additionally, the α-diversity of patients with DED was lower than that of healthy individuals. These observations are consistent with previous studies (Zilliox et al., 2020; Andersson et al., 2021). Despite the depletion in a portion of DED samples, a group of species exhibited abnormally high abundance in patients with DED compared with healthy individuals. We defined this phenomenon in this study as the polarization in abundance. These findings highlight the heterogeneity of the microbial dysbiosis in DED.

Shotgun metagenomic sequencing enables us to assess the microbial dysbiosis at the species level and survey microorganisms other than bacteria. We detected different patterns of associations with disease status between species of the same genus. These results potentially explained a part of the inconsistent conclusions made at the genus level by previous studies using 16S rRNA sequencing. We believe that strain-level characterization in the future will provide further insight into the heterogeneity of microbial dysbiosis in DED. Furthermore, we identified the polarized abundance of a fungal species *M. globosa*. This species also showed different sex associations between patients with DED and healthy individuals. Therefore, the fungal dysbiosis in DED warrants further investigation.

We found that sex-related differences in the conjunctival microbiota of patients with DED were distinct from that of healthy individuals. Notably, the α-diversity and the abundance of a few microbial species were positively associated with female sex in patients with DED but were positively associated with male sex in healthy individuals. A possible explanation for this inverse trend is that males could tolerate a higher level of perturbations in the conjunctival microbiota than females before the development of DED. Whether the sex differences in the microbiota are associated with a high prevalence of DED in women remains unknown. Furthermore, future studies ideally with sex and age stratification are needed to clarify the associations among sex, DED, and the microbiota.

The conjunctival microbiota in mixed dry eye was more similar to MGD than ATD. An implication of this observation is that the microbial dysbiosis in DED patients with a mixed type of diagnosis is mainly associated with the occurrence of MGD. In agreement with previous studies (Dong et al., 2019), we found that *S. aureus* was positively associated with MGD. We further detected enrichment of *S. aureus* in samples from participants with MGD and mixed dry eye, when compared with ATD samples. This result highlights the involvement of *S. aureus* in MGD. However, the underlying mechanism remains unknown, warranting further investigation.

It has been recognized that DED is a multifactorial disease. According to the TFOS DEWS II definition, tear film instability and hyperosmolarity, ocular surface inflammation and damage, and neurosensory abnormalities can play etiological roles (Craig et al., 2017). The heterogeneity of microbial dysbiosis observed here potentially reflects the complicated etiology of DED. Further research is warranted to explore the link between patterns of microbial dysbiosis and specific etiology of DED. For instance, it may be fruitful to adopt multi-omics approaches integrating data from microbiome and metabolome. Additionally, differences in the microbiota before and after dry eye treatment is worth investigating.

A limitation of this study is that it remains unclear which aspects of the observed microbial dysbiosis are causes or consequences of the onset of DED. Both genetic and environmental factors can influence the conjunctival microbiota. The dysbiosis of microbiota can lead to loss of mucosal tolerance, thereby contributing to inflammation at the ocular surface. On the other hand, loss of homeostasis of the tear film can itself have an effect on the conjunctival microbiota. Furthermore, given the cyclical disease process of DED (Craig et al., 2017), the microbial dysbiosis may be both a cause and a result of DED.

A number of factors may contribute to the inter-individual variation in the microbiota, including host genetic and environmental variables. Importantly, these factors potentially influence both hosts and the microbiota. As a result, it can be difficult to determine whether the microbial dysbiosis mediates the effects of risks factors on the development and exacerbation of DED (Stapleton et al., 2017). To fully characterize the role of the ocular surface microbiota in DED, future studies may perform systemic analysis taking into consideration comprehensive factors like host genetic variants known to affect the composition of the microbiota, lifestyles, and other environmental exposures.

In summary, our study characterized the heterogeneity of conjunctival microbial dysbiosis in DED. It is worth investigating in the future whether microbiota signatures can refine our understanding of DED subtypes. Taken together, our findings offer novel insights into the ocular surface microbial dysbiosis in dry eye and potentially promote the development of microbiota-based personalized strategies for dry eye treatment.

ETHICS STATEMENT

The studies involving human participants were reviewed and approved by The Ethics Committee of Zhongshan Ophthalmic Center, Sun Yat-sen University (Guangzhou, China). The patients/participants provided their written informed consent to participate in this study.

AUTHOR CONTRIBUTIONS

LW and XW conceived the study. LL supervised the overall clinical sample collection and data analysis. JL, YZ, XH, and XD collected clinical samples. JL, YZ and XH carried out experiments. QL, BZ and YL performed data analysis. QL and XW drafted the manuscript. All authors read and approved the final version of the manuscript.

ACKNOWLEDGMENTS

We thank all members of the Wei and Liang Laboratories for their support and discussion.

REFERENCES

Andersson, J., Vogt, J. K., Dalgaard, M. D., Pedersen, O., Holmgaard, K., and Heegaard, S. (2021). Ocular Surface Microbiota in Patients with Aqueous Tear-Deficient Dry Eye. *Ocul. Surf.* 19, 210–217. doi:10.1016/j.jtos.2020.09.003

Bolger, A. M., Lohse, M., and Usadel, B. (2014). Trimmomatic: A Flexible Trimmer for Illumina Sequence Data. *Bioinformatics* 30, 2114–2120. doi:10.1093/bioinformatics/btu170

Craig, J. P., Nichols, K. K., Akpek, E. K., Caffery, B., Dua, H. S., Joo, C.-K., et al. (2017). TFOS DEWS II Definition and Classification Report. *Ocul. Surf.* 15, 276–283. doi:10.1016/j.jtos.2017.05.008

Davis, N. M., Proctor, D. M., Holmes, S. P., Relman, D. A., and Callahan, B. J. (2018). Simple Statistical Identification and Removal of Contaminant Sequences in Marker-Gene and Metagenomics Data. *Microbiome* 6, 226. doi:10.1186/s40168-018-0605-2

de Paiva, C. S., Jones, D. B., Stern, M. E., Bian, F., Moore, Q. L., Corbiere, S., et al. (2016). Altered Mucosal Microbiome Diversity and Disease Severity in Sjögren Syndrome. *Sci. Rep.* 6, 23561. doi:10.1038/srep23561

Dong, X., Wang, Y., Wang, W., Lin, P., and Huang, Y. (2019). Composition and Diversity of Bacterial Community on the Ocular Surface of Patients with Meibomian Gland Dysfunction. *Invest. Ophthalmol. Vis. Sci.* 60, 4774–4783. doi:10.1167/iovs.19-27719

Gomes, J. Á. P., Frizon, L., and Demeda, V. F. (2020). Ocular Surface Microbiome in Health and Disease. *Asia-pacific J. Ophthalmol.* 9, 505–511. doi:10.1097/APO.0000000000000330

Jervis-Bardy, J., Leong, L. E. X., Marri, S., Smith, R. J., Choo, J. M., Smith-Vaughan, H. C., et al. (2015). Deriving Accurate Microbiota Profiles from Human Samples with Low Bacterial Content through post-sequencing Processing of Illumina MiSeq Data. *Microbiome* 3, 19. doi:10.1186/s40168-015-0083-8

Jiang, X., Deng, A., Yang, J., Bai, H., Yang, Z., Wu, J., et al. (2018). Pathogens in the Meibomian Gland and Conjunctival Sac: Microbiome of normal Subjects and Patients with Meibomian Gland Dysfunction. *Infect. Drug Resist.* 11, 1729–1740. doi:10.2147/IDR.S162135

Ozkan, J., Nielsen, S., Diez-Vives, C., Coroneo, M., Thomas, T., and Willcox, M. (2017). Temporal Stability and Composition of the Ocular Surface Microbiome. *Sci. Rep.* 7, 9880. doi:10.1038/s41598-017-10494-9

Schmieder, R., and Edwards, R. (2011). Quality Control and Preprocessing of Metagenomic Datasets. *Bioinformatics* 27, 863–864. doi:10.1093/bioinformatics/btr026

Stapleton, F., Alves, M., Bunya, V. Y., Jalbert, I., Lekhanont, K., Malet, F., et al. (2017). TFOS DEWS II Epidemiology Report. *Ocul. Surf.* 15, 334–365. doi:10.1016/j.jtos.2017.05.003

Stevenson, W., Chauhan, S. K., and Dana, R. (2012). Dry Eye Disease. *Arch. Ophthalmol.* 130, 90–100. doi:10.1001/archophthalmol.2011.364

Sullivan, D. A., Rocha, E. M., Aragona, P., Clayton, J. A., Ding, J., Golebiowski, B.,

et al. (2017). TFOS DEWS II Sex, Gender, and Hormones Report. *Ocul. Surf.* 15, 284–333. doi:10.1016/j.jtos.2017.04.001

Tsubota, K., Yokoi, N., Watanabe, H., Dogru, M., Kojima, T., Yamada, M., et al. (2020). A New Perspective on Dry Eye Classification: Proposal by the Asia Dry Eye Society. *Eye Contact Lens Sci. Clin. Pract.* 46, S2–S13. doi:10.1097/ICL.0000000000000643

Watters, G. A., Turnbull, P. R., Swift, S., Petty, A., and Craig, J. P. (2017). Ocular Surface Microbiome in Meibomian Gland Dysfunction. *Clin. Exp. Ophthalmol.* 45, 105–111. doi:10.1111/ceo.12810

Wen, X., Miao, L., Deng, Y., Bible, P. W., Hu, X., Zou, Y., et al. (2017). The Influence of Age and Sex on Ocular Surface Microbiota in Healthy Adults. *Invest. Ophthalmol. Vis. Sci.* 58, 6030. doi:10.1167/iovs.17-22957

Wood, D. E., Lu, J., and Langmead, B. (2019). Improved Metagenomic Analysis with Kraken 2. *Genome Biol.* 20, 257. doi:10.1186/s13059-019-1891-0

Zhao, F., Zhang, D., Ge, C., Zhang, L., Reinach, P. S., Tian, X., et al. (2020). Metagenomic Profiling of Ocular Surface Microbiome Changes in Meibomian Gland Dysfunction. *Invest. Ophthalmol. Vis. Sci.* 61, 22. doi:10.1167/iovs.61.8.22

Zilliox, M. J., Gange, W. S., Kuffel, G., Mores, C. R., Joyce, C., de Bustros, P., et al. (2020). Assessing the Ocular Surface Microbiome in Severe Ocular Surface Diseases. *Ocul. Surf.* 18, 706–712. doi:10.1016/j.jtos.2020.07.007

14

Platelet-Derived Growth Factor-D Activates Complement System to Propagate Macrophage Polarization and Neovascularization

Zhen Xiong[†], Qianqian Wang[†], Wanhong Li, Lijuan Huang, Jianing Zhang, Juanhua Zhu, Bingbing Xie, Shasha Wang, Haiqing Kuang, Xianchai Lin, Chunsik Lee, Anil Kumar* and Xuri Li*

State Key Laboratory of Ophthalmology, Zhongshan Ophthalmic Center, Sun Yat-sen University, Guangzhou, China

*Correspondence:
Anil Kumar
kumar8@mail.sysu.edu.cn
Xuri Li
lixr6@mail.sysu.edu.cn

[†] These authors have contributed equally to this work

Platelet-derived growth factor-D (PDGF-D) is highly expressed in immune cells. However, the potential role of PDGF-D in immune system remains thus far unclear. Here, we reveal a novel function of PDGF-D in activating both classical and alternative complement pathways that markedly increase chemokine and cytokine responses to promote macrophage polarization. Pharmacological targeting of the complement C3a receptor using SB290157 alleviated PDGF-D-induced neuroinflammation by blocking macrophage polarization and inhibited pathological choroidal neovascularization. Our study thus suggests that therapeutic strategies targeting both PDGF-D and the complement system may open up new possibilities for the treatment of neovascular diseases.

Keywords: PDGF-D, C1qa, C3, macrophage polarization, inflammation

INTRODUCTION

Tissue inflammation is a cellular response initiated by various factors, such as invasion of foreign material and microbes and clearance of damaged cellular debris to maintain tissue homeostasis (Medzhitov, 2008). Low levels of inflammatory responses also help maintain normal homeostasis (Chen and Xu, 2015). Dysfunction or hyperactivation of inflammation results in various inflammatory neurodegenerative disorders, such as age-related macular degeneration (AMD), Alzheimer's disease, Parkinson's disease, and uveitis (Tan et al., 2020; Yang et al., 2020). AMD remains a significant cause for progressive loss of central vision, if uncontrolled, leading to legal blindness (DeAngelis et al., 2017). Microglia, resident immune cells in the retina, choroidal macrophages (Yu et al., 2020) and retinal pigment epithelial (RPE) cells play a central role during inflammation by secreting various chemokines, cytokines, growth factors and elements of the complement system (Holtkamp et al., 2001; Shi et al., 2008; de Oliveira Dias et al., 2011). Additionally, several studies have identified alterations of the complement pathway in AMD pathogenesis (Wu and Sun, 2019). Small menagerie of complement proteins can activate the complement system via classical, lectin and alternative pathways, converging on the critical complement component C3, to generate C3a, C5a and membrane-attacking complex (MAC) C5b-C9, acknowledged in the drusen of AMD patients (Crabb et al., 2002; Mullins et al., 2014; Kim et al., 2020). Increasing evidence suggests that persisting inflammatory milieu supports the classical macrophage activation (M1 polarization) to generate tissue-destructing proinflammatory signals, and alternative macrophage activation (M2 polarization) generates anti-inflammatory signals to promote pathological angiogenesis (Apte, 2010). However, currently, it is not well understood how the complement system in CNV is activated, although its components are found in neovascular lesions of wet AMD patients.

Platelet-derived growth factor-D (PDGF-D), a member of the PDGF family, has been shown to exert diverse functions under physiological and pathological conditions (Bergsten et al., 2001; Kazlauskas, 2017; Folestad et al., 2018; Kumar and Li, 2018). Several studies have implicated PDGF-D in the promotion of inflammation and in the increased migration of monocytes and macrophages under pathological conditions. During intracerebral hemorrhage, PDGF-D promotes neuroinflammation and enhances macrophage infiltration (Yang et al., 2016). Adipocyte-derived PDGF-D promotes adventitial fibrosis with inflammation, thereby contributing to the development of aortic aneurysm in obesity (Zhang et al., 2018). Ostendorf et al. (2006) and Boor et al. (2007) demonstrated that the administration of human mAb CR002, a PDGF-D antibody, reduced glomerular infiltration of monocytes/macrophages and prevented epithelial-mesenchymal transition. In our previous work, we have shown that *Pdgfd* knockdown by shRNA inhibited the macrophage infiltration and reduced choroidal neovascularization (Kumar et al., 2010). These studies highlight the effects of PDGF-D on inflammatory cell infiltration under pathological conditions. However, the mechanism by which PDGF-D induces inflammatory cell activation and migration is not well understood. Notably, a recent study has shown that PDGF-D inhibits tumor growth by binding to natural killer (NK) cell receptor NKp44, leading to the production of tumor-suppressive cytokines by NK cells (Barrow et al., 2018), in contrast to many previous reports showing angiogenic and oncogenic effects of PDGF-D (Li et al., 2003; Kumar et al., 2010; Kumar and Li, 2018). Thus, more in-depth studies are warranted to verify the functions of PDGF-D and the underlying mechanisms.

MATERIALS AND METHODS

Animals

All animal experiments were approved by the Animal Use and Care Committee of Zhongshan Ophthalmic Center at the Sun Yat-sen University, Guangzhou, People's Republic of China. C57BL/6J (6–8 weeks old) mice were purchased from Pengyue Company (Shandong, China). All mice were maintained on a 12-h light/dark cycle with water and chow provided *ad libitum* and were housed in an SPF facility in the Ophthalmic

Animal Laboratory of Zhongshan Ophthalmic Center at the Sun Yat-sen University. Five minutes after intraperitoneal injection of 4% chloral hydrate (10 ml/kg body weight), mice were anesthetized before treatment or euthanized directly by cervical dislocation.

Cell Culture

RAW264.7 cells (Zhong Qiao Xin Zhou Biotechnology Co., Ltd., China, cat: ZQ0098) were cultured in the Dulbecco's modified Eagle's medium (DMEM) (Corning, cat: 10–013–CV) supplemented with 10% heat inactivated FBS (ExCell Bio, China, cat: FSS050) and 1% penicillin/streptomycin (Corning, cat: 30-002-Cl). THP-1 cells (Zhong Qiao Xin Zhou Biotechnology Co., Ltd, China, cat: ZQ0086) were cultured in RPMI-1640 medium (Corning, cat: 10-040-CV) supplemented with 10% heat inactivated FBS and 1% penicillin/streptomycin as mentioned above. THP-1 cells were differentiated (dTHP1) by incubation with 150 nM phorbol-12-myristate-13-acetate (PMA) (Sigma, cat: P8139) in complete medium for 24 h followed by 24 h PMA-free and serum-free medium treatment to reduce cell detachment (Spano et al., 2013).

Preparation of Conditioned Medium

Primary human retinal pigment epithelial (HRPE) cells (Sciencell, cat: 6540) at passage 5 were used for collecting the conditioned medium (CM). Briefly, HRPE cells were cultured in epithelial cell medium (EpiCM, Sciencell, cat: 4101) containing 10% FBS (Sciencell, cat: 0010), 1% epithelial cell growth supplement (EpiCGS, Sciencell, cat: 4152) and 1% penicillin/streptomycin (P/S, Sciencell, cat: 0503). After reaching 80–90% confluence HRPE cells were starved in EpiCM without any supplements for 12 h, followed by 12 h treatment with/without 50 ng/ml recombinant human PDGF-D protein (R&D, cat: 1159-SB/CF). Cells were rinsed and cultured in the supplement-free Dulbecco's modified Eagle Medium / Ham's F-12 Mix (DMEM/F-12) (Corning, cat:10-092-CV) and after 24 h collected medium was filtered through 0.22 μm filter (Millex™ GP Filter Unit, Millipore, cat: SLGP033NB), and stored at –80°C until use.

Proliferation Assay

RAW264.7 and dTHP1 cell proliferation assays were performed using a Cell Counting Kit-8 assay (CCK8, Dojindo, Japan). Cells were seeded in 96-well culture plates (5,000 cells/well for RAW264.7 cells and 10,000 cells/well for dTHP1 cells, respectively) and 450 nm absorption values were recorded after treatment with the CCK-8 reagent.

Migration Assay

RAW264.7 cells were seeded in the cell culture inserts (Ibidi, Germany, cat: 80209) at 1×10^5 cells/chamber and the inserts were removed after 12 h to generate cell-free gaps. dTHP1 cells were seeded in 48-well plates (3×10^5 cells/well) and the cell-free area was produced by scratching the wells with a 200 μl pipette tip. Images were obtained at 0 and 24 h, respectively, after treatment and were analyzed using the ImageJ software.

Construction of Adeno-Associated Virus (AAV) for RPE-Specific PDGF-D Overexpression

The CMV promoter of the AAV vector pAV-CMV-C-FH (Vigenebio, China, cat: pAV100001–OE) was replaced with the human *VMD2* promoter (–598 bp upstream to 378 bp downstream of the transcription start site), known to drive efficient and specific transgene expression in RPE (Alexander and Hauswirth, 2008). The multi-cloning site of the vector was replaced by the coding sequence of human *PDGFD* gene (NM_025208). The AAV was packaged by Vigene Biosciences (Shandong, China) and stored at –80°C.

Subretinal AAV Injection in Mice

Mouse pupils were dilated by topical application of tropicamide. An intraperitoneal injection of 4% chloral hydrate (10 ml/kg body weight) was performed for anesthesia. Topical anesthesia was performed on the cornea using procainamide. Carboxymethyl cellulose sodium was used to avoid the development of cornea xerosis. Subretinal injection was performed using a sterilized 5 μl syringe (Hamilton, cat: 7633-01) with a 33-gauge blunt needle (Hamilton, cat: 7803-05, 33/15mm/3) through a puncture hole of 0.2 mm in diameter behind the cornea limbus, and AAV (1 μl/eye, 5 × 10^{13} vg/ml) was injected. A successful subretinal injection was indicated by the visualization of the semicircular retinal detachment around the injection site under a microscope or by fundus imaging.

Intraperitoneal Injection of C3a Antagonist

The 20 mg/ml stock solution of the C3a antagonist SB290157 (MCE, cat: HY-101502A) was prepared by dissolving the compound in a minimal volume of sterile dimethyl sulfoxide (DMSO, Sigma, cat: D4540). SB290157 was further diluted using corn oil to a final concentration of 2 mg/ml for injection at a dose of 30 mg/kg body weight. Three weeks after AAV injection, SB290157 or vehicle was injected intraperitoneally every 2 days for 3 times. In the laser-induced CNV model, the antagonist was intraperitoneally injected 3 times after laser photocoagulation.

Immunofluorescence Tissue Staining

Sections (10-μm thick) of eyeballs were incubated in 0.5% Triton™ X–100 (Sigma, X100) prepared in phosphate buffered saline for 15 min for permeabilization and then blocked using 5% normal goat serum for 1 h followed by overnight incubation with the primary antibody at 4°C. Primary antibodies used were: anti-IA/IE (BD, 562564), anti-C1q (Abcam, ab182451), anti-PDGFRα (CST, 3169), anti-PDGFRβ (CST, 3174), anti-CD16/32 (BD, 553141), anti-CD206 (Bio-Rad, MCA2235GA), anti-IBA1 (WAKO,

019-19741), anti-CD31 (Bio-Rad, MCA2388), anti-NG2 (Millipore, AB5320), and anti-α-SMA (Sigma, A2547). After three washes, slides were incubated for 1h at room temperature with secondary antibodies (Invitrogen) followed by a 10 min DAPI (Sigma, D9542) incubation. Immunostained sections were imaged using the Zeiss LSM710 laser scanning confocal microscope. Images were processed using ZEN 2012 (Zeiss) and quantified using ImageJ.

For analysis of flat-mounted retinas, 1 week after AAV-PDGF-D subretinal injection, SB290157 (MCE, cat: HY-101502A) was injected intraperitoneally (30 mg/kg body weight) every 2 days. After 1 week, the mice were sacrificed, and the eyes harvested and fixed in 4% PFA for the analysis of flat-mounted retinas. The anterior segment of the eye and lens were removed. The retinas were separated from the sclera and flattened on a glass slide and dissected by making four radial cuts. Flat-mounted retinas were stained with I isolectin B4 (IB4, Thermo Fisher, cat: 121411) and analyzed using a fluorescent microscope AX10 imager.Z2 (ZEISS). The vascular branch points were analyzed using Angio Tool (version 0.5).

RNA Sequencing and Transcriptomic Analysis

Four weeks after AAV injection, the mice were sacrificed. The eyeballs were removed and the fascial tissues and muscles around the eyeballs dissected on ice. Choroidal tissue was quickly dissected and put into the reagent for RNA isolation. RNA was sent to Shanghai Pharmaceutical Kangde Co., Ltd. (Shanghai, China) for RNA sequencing. Sequenced raw reads were mapped to mouse mm10 reference genome using STAR (v2.4.2a). After alignment, RSEM (V1.2.29) was used to generate FPKM values for known gene models. Differentially expressed genes were identified using DESeq2 (v1.22.2). Fold-changes were estimated according to each sample's FPKM. Differentially expressed genes were selected using the following filter criteria: P-value $\leq$ 0.1, FDR $\leq$ 0.1, fold-change $\geq$ 1.5, mean FPKM $\geq$ 1. Gene set functional enrichment analysis was performed using cluster Profiler (v3.17.0) with gene set size set to 5–500, P-value cutoff set to 0.05, and adjusted P-value set to 0.25. Volcano plots were generated using ggplot2 (v3.3.0). Heatmap plots were generated using pheatmap (v1.0.12). Gene-function networks for differentially expressed chemokine genes and related biological processes were visualized using Cytoscape (v3.6.1).

RNA Isolation and Real-Time Quantitative PCR

Total RNA was isolated using the TRNzol reagent (TIANGEN, cat: DP424) and converted to cDNA using the Fast King RT Kit (TIANGEN, cat: KR116) according to the manufacturer's instructions. Real-time quantitative PCR was carried out in a 10 μl reaction containing the SYBR Select Master Mix (Vazyme, cat: Q331) in technical quadruplicate using a Quantstudio 6K Flex system (Life Technologies). Results were analyzed using the Quantstudio 12 K Flex Software v1.2.2 (Thermo Fisher

Scientific). Relative mRNA levels were calculated based on the $2^{-\Delta\Delta CT}$ method, using the 18S rRNA as references.

Protein Extraction and Western Blots

Protein extraction was performed using RIPA lysis buffer with a cocktail of protease and phosphatase inhibitors (Thermo Fisher Scientific, cat: A32961). Lysates were separated using SDS-PAGE under reducing conditions and transferred onto a PVDF membrane (Bio-Rad, cat: 162-0177). Membranes were blocked using 5% defatted milk and immunoblotted with the primary antibodies overnight at 4°C, followed by incubation with the secondary antibodies conjugated with horseradish peroxidase (HRP). The following antibodies were used: anti-PDGFRα (CST, cat: 3169), anti-PDGFRβ (CST, cat: 3174), anti-NRP1 (Abcam, cat: ab81321), anti-PDGF-D (Santa Cruz, cat: sc137030), anti-PDGF-D (R&D, AF1159), anti-C1q (Abcam, cat: ab235454), and anti-C3 (Abcam, cat: 200999). Bands were detected using a Syngene GBOX/CHEMI-XT16 device.

Choroid Explant Assay

C57BL/6J mice at postnatal day eight were sacrificed, and eyes were enucleated and kept in ice-cold phosphate buffered saline before dissection. After removing the cornea and lens from the anterior of the eye, the peripheral choroid-scleral complex was separated from the retina and cut into pieces (approximately 1 mm × 1 mm). Choroid pieces were transferred into growth factor-reduced Matrigel (BD, Cat: 356231) and seeded in 24-well plates followed by Matrigel solidification for 10 min. A volume of 500 μl of medium was added to each well and incubated at 37°C with 5% CO_2 for 48 h. The medium was changed every 48 h. Individual explants were imaged daily using an inverted microscope. Areas of choroidal sprouts were quantified using ImageJ.

Laser Induced CNV

The laser-induced CNV mouse model was performed as described previously (Zhang et al., 2009). Briefly, 8 weeks old female mice were anesthetized by intraperitoneal injection of 4% chloral hydrate (10 ml/kg body weight), and eyes were dilated by topical application of tropicamide. Four laser spots were made by laser photocoagulation (90 mV power, 75 ms duration, 75 μm spot size, Oculight Infrared Laser System 810 nm, IRIDEX Corporation) at an equal distance from the optic nerve in each eye for CNV. The cornea of mice were treated with antibiotic tobramycin ointment locally after laser photocoagulation and mice were placed on a 37°C electric blanket until wake. After 7 days, the eyecups were flat-mounted and the immunohistochemical staining were performed as described (Zhang et al., 2009).

Statistical Analysis

Gene expression analysis by Q-PCR are expressed as means ± SD. While other results are expressed as means ± SEM. The statistical significance between the control and PDGF-D, or between AAV-GFP and AAV-PDGF-D groups were assessed with the unpaired student's two-tailed t test. Multiple group comparisons were performed with ordinary one-way ANOVA test. Differences between groups were tested with GraphPad Prism software (version 7.04) and considered statistically significant for $P < 0.05$.

RESULTS

PDGF-D-Induced Retinal Epithelial Cell Secretome Promotes Macrophage Migration

Under pathological conditions, PDGF-D has been shown to promote macrophage migration (Uutela et al., 2004). However, the mechanism by which PDGF-D promotes macrophage migration is not well understood. To address this, we stimulated murine macrophages (RAW264.7) and differentiated human macrophages (dTHP1) with PDGF-D. Murine macrophages expressed PDGFR-β and the PDGF-D co-receptor NRP1 but not PDGFR-α (**Figure 1A** and **Supplementary Figure 1A**). The human monocytic cell line (THP1) did not express PDGF receptors (**Figure 1A** and **Supplementary Figure 1B**). However, upon differentiation to macrophages by PMA, they expressed PDGFR-α, PDGFR-β and NRP1 (**Figure 1A** and **Supplementary Figure 1B**). PDGF-D stimulation did not promote proliferation (**Figure 1B** and **Supplementary Figures 1C,D**) or migration (**Figures 1C,D** and **Supplementary Figures 1E,F**) of mouse or human macrophages. Human retinal pigment epithelial (HRPE) cells play a crucial role in the pathophysiology of AMD, and PDGF-D has been shown to promote proliferation and migration of RPE cells (Li et al., 2007). PDGF-D activated the PDGFR-β on HRPE (**Supplementary Figure 2A**), and conditioned medium (CM) from cultured HRPE cells treated with PDGF-D (PDGF-D-CM) did not affect human or mouse macrophage proliferation (**Figure 1E** and **Supplementary Figures 1G,H**). However, and noteworthy, PDGF-D-CM significantly promoted migration of both types of macrophages (**Figures 1F,G** and **Supplementary Figures 2B,C**). Hence, PDGF-D-induced HRPE secretome promoted macrophage migration, while PDGF-D did not show a direct effect on them.

PDGF-D Overexpression in Mouse Retinal Epithelial Cells

Recombinant adeno-associated virus (AAV) has been shown to be effective for retinal gene therapy due to their efficient transduction of RPE cells with low toxicity (Vandenberghe and Auricchio, 2012). To over-express PDGF-D in mouse RPE cells, we constructed AAV type 8 (AAV8) vector expressing human PDGF-D (AAV-PDGF-D) driven by the retinal pigment epithelium specific *VMD2* promoter (**Figure 2A**). PDGF receptors are expressed in both mouse retinae and choroid (Hou et al., 2010; **Supplementary Figures 3A–D**). Four weeks after subretinal injection of AAV-PDGF-D or AAV-GFP (as a control), overexpression of *PDGF-D* mRNA and protein in the RPE-choroid complex were detected (**Figures 2B–D**). Moreover, immunofluorescence staining identified PDGF-D or GFP in the

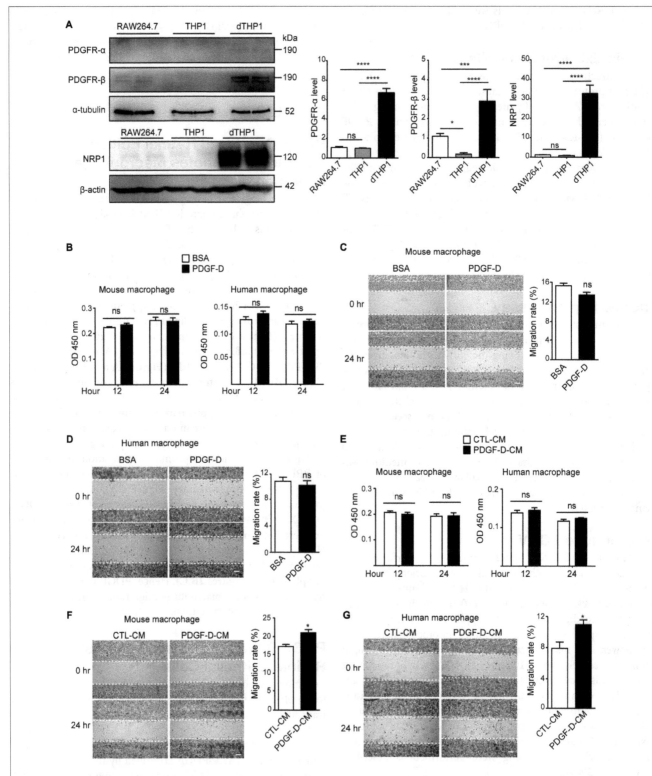

FIGURE 1 | Effect of PDGF-D on macrophage proliferation and migration. **(A)** Immunoblotting showing the expression of PDGFR-α, PDGFR-β and NRP1 in RAW264.7 mouse macrophages, THP1 human monocytes and dTHP1 human macrophages. **(B)** Proliferation of mouse and human macrophages treated with PDGF-D protein for 12 or 24 h. **(C,D)** Migration of mouse **(C)** and human **(D)** macrophages stimulated with PDGF-D protein for 24 h. **(E)** Proliferation of mouse and human macrophages treated with conditioned medium from PDGF-D-treated HRPE cells (PDGF-D-CM). Conditioned medium from HRPE cells without PDGF-D treatment (CTL-CM) was used as a control. **(F,G)** Migration of mouse **(F)** and human **(G)** macrophages treated with conditioned medium from PDGF-D-treated HRPE cells (PDGF-D-CM). Conditioned medium from HRPE cells without PDGF-D treatment (CTL-CM) was used as a control. Scale bars: 400 μm. All the experiments were performed in triplicates. Unpaired two-tailed Student's t-test was used for statistical analysis. $*p < 0.05$, $***p < 0.001$, $****p < 0.0001$, ns: not significant.

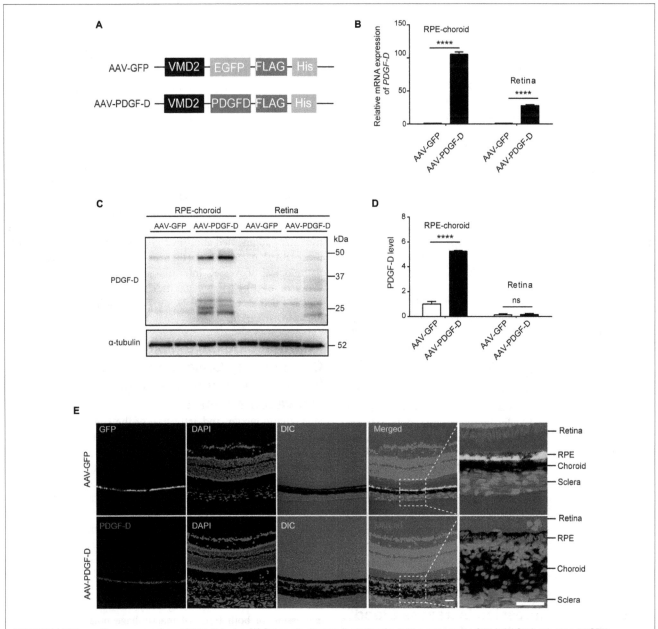

FIGURE 2 | RPE-specific overexpression of PDGF-D *in vivo*. **(A)** Schematic diagram illustrating the AAV vector carrying GFP (AAV-GFP) or human *PDGF-D* (AAV-PDGF-D) gene and RPE specific *VDM2* promoter. **(B)** Real-time PCR results of relative mRNA expression of *PDGF-D* in retinae or RPE-choroid complex from mice injected with AAV-GFP or AAV-PDGF- D for 4 weeks. **(C)** Representative immunoblotting showing PDGF-D expression in mouse retinae or RPE-choroid complex. **(D)** Quantifications of PDGF-D protein levels in **(C)**. **(E)** Immunofluorescence images highlighting RPE-specific expression of GFP or PDGF-D in mouse RPE-choroid complex with 4 weeks AAV-GFP or AAV-PDGF-D injection, respectively. Scale bar: 50 μm. $n = 5$, $****p < 0.0001$, ns: not significant.

RPE layer, respectively (**Figure 2E**), demonstrating successful RPE-specific PDGF-D overexpression *in vivo*.

Activation of the Complement Pathway Revealed by Transcriptomic Analysis of PDGF-D-Overexpressing RPE-Choroids

To identify PDGF-D-induced downstream pathways, we performed unbiased transcriptomic analysis using the PDGF-D-overexpressing RPE-choroid complex. A total of 2,486

differentially expressed genes (DEGs) were identified. Among them, 1697 were up-regulated and 789 were down-regulated (**Figure 3A**). Biological function enrichment gene ontology analysis showed that the most enriched biological processes were related to the regulation of immune system (**Figure 3B**), particularly, the complement pathway (**Figure 3C**). Other pathways included chemokine and its receptor (**Figure 3D** and **Supplementary Figure 4B**), cytokine signaling (**Supplementary Figures 4C,E**) and regulation of extracellular matrix and growth factors (**Supplementary Figures 4D,F**). Importantly, both gene

(**Supplementary Figure 4A**) and protein analysis confirmed the activation of both classical (**Figure 3E**) and alternative complement pathways (**Figure 3F**). Immunofluorescence staining further identified C1q expression in both RPE and choroids of PDGF-D-overexpressing samples (**Figure 3G**), where PDGF-D overexpression led to increased accumulation of IA/IE$^+$ macrophages in the choroids, which were also positive for C1q staining (**Figures 3G,H**). Further functional network analysis of DEGs demonstrated pathways related to activation of the complement system, immune cell migration and activation of immune responses in PDGF-D-overexpressing RPE-choroids (**Figure 3I**). These findings thus underscore PDGF-D overexpression-induced inflammation by activating the complement pathway and chemokine/cytokine signaling.

PDGF-D-Induced Complement Activation Promotes Macrophage Polarization

The complement component C1qa has been implicated in the promotion of the of M2 microphage polarization to mitigate tissue inflammation (Spivia et al., 2014), while complement anaphylatoxin C3a and C5a are acknowledged to promote tissue inflammation by activating monocytes and macrophages (Bohlson et al., 2014). Interestingly, PDGF-D overexpression upregulated both M1 polarization markers, such as *Tnfα*, *Il1β*, *Nos2* and *Cxcl10*, and M2 polarization markers, such as *Arg1*, *Il10*, and *Chi3i3* (**Figure 4A**). Furthermore, immunofluorescence staining revealed that PDGF-D promoted IBA1$^+$ macrophages in both retinae and choroids, which were also positive for CD16/32 staining, an M1 polarization marker (**Figure 4B**), with higher percentages in the PDGF-D overexpressing retinae and choroids (**Figure 4C**). In addition, IBA1$^+$ macrophages were positive for CD206 staining, an M2 polarization marker (**Figure 4D**), with higher proportions in PDGF-D overexpressing choroids and retinae (**Figure 4E**). Together, these findings underline the presence of both pro- and anti-inflammatory milieu triggered by PDGF-D overexpression.

PDGF-D Overexpression Increases Blood Vessel Density and Mural Cell Coverage

Neural retina is supported by the inner retinal blood vessels and outer retinal choriocapillaris beneath the RPE layer and Bruch membrane, which interacts with retinal microglia (McMenamin et al., 2019) and choroidal macrophages (Kumar et al., 2014). Since PDGF-D induced marked macrophage activation, we examined whether this affected retinal and choroidal blood vessel. In the PDGF-D overexpressing RPE-choroid complex, mRNA levels of genes encoding proangiogenic and extracellular matrix (ECM) regulators, such as *Tgfβ1*, *Fgf2*, *Mmp9*, *Mmp12* and *Mmp2*, were upregulated (**Figure 5A**). The PDGF family members are known to promote proliferation and recruitment of mural cells (Li et al., 2003; Uutela et al., 2004). PDGF-D overexpression increased CD31$^+$ endothelial cell density in both retinae and choroids, while αSMA$^+$ smooth muscle cell coverage increased only in choroids (**Figures 5B,C**). Thus, increased

PDGF-D expression levels promoted retinal and choroidal blood vessel growth and maturation.

Inflammatory Pathological Angiogenesis Triggered by PDGF-D

Choroidal blood vessels and RPE cells possess a unique symbiotic relationship by nourishing each other. The disruption of this association results in RPE degeneration or choroidal neovascularization (Lutty et al., 1999). Since PDGF-D overexpression increased choroidal endothelial cell density, we tested the effect of PDGF-D on choroids by stimulating choroidal explants with PDGF-D. PDGF-D promoted robust choroidal endothelial cell sprouting (**Figures 6A,B**) in a dose-dependent manner (**Supplementary Figures 5A,B**). Moreover, injury of the PDGF-D-overexpressing RPE cells by laser treatment augmented abnormal growth of IB4$^+$ neovessels with more IBA1$^+$ macrophages (**Figures 6C,D**). Furthermore, CD31$^+$ pathological neovessels intermingled with IBA1$^+$ macrophages (**Figures 6E,F**). These data indicated that the inflammatory milieu elicited by PDGF-D nurtured pathological choroidal neovascularization.

Pharmacological Inhibition of the Complement Cascade Alleviates Inflammation and Pathological Neovascularization

Since the induction and activation of the complement pathway by PDGF-D overexpression led to more macrophages and higher blood vessel density in the retinae and choroids, we tested whether blocking complement activation could inhibit pathological neovascularization and treated PDGF-D-stimulated macrophages and RPE with a C3a-receptor antagonist SB290157, which is known to block complement activation (Hutamekalin et al., 2010). SB290157 treatment inhibited migration of mouse and human macrophages (**Figure 7A** and **Supplementary Figure 6A**) *in vitro*. Furthermore, intraperitoneal injection of SB290157 to the RPE-specific PDGF-D overexpressing mice markedly reduced infiltration of IBA1$^+$ macrophages in the retinae and choroids (**Figures 7B,C**) and suppressed the expression of both types of macrophage polarization markers (**Supplementary Figure 6B**). Additionally, immunofluorescence staining of endothelial and mural cells showed a marked reduction in blood vessel density and smooth muscle cell coverage (**Figures 7D,E**) with concomitant reduction of angiogenic and chemokine gene signatures (**Figure 7F** and **Supplementary Figure 6C**). Moreover, analysis of flat-mounted retinas confirmed the above findings by showing that PDGF-D overexpression increased retinal vascular branch points, which was abolished by SB290157 treatment (**Supplementary Figures 7A,B**). Since complement components are found in CNV lesions of AMD patients, the complement pathway was inactivated by SB290157 treatment in a mouse CNV model. Importantly, intraperitoneal injection of SB290157 inhibited CNV by reducing immune cell density in neovascularization lesions (**Figures 7G,H**). Together, these observations suggested that PDGF-D-induced activation of the complement pathway

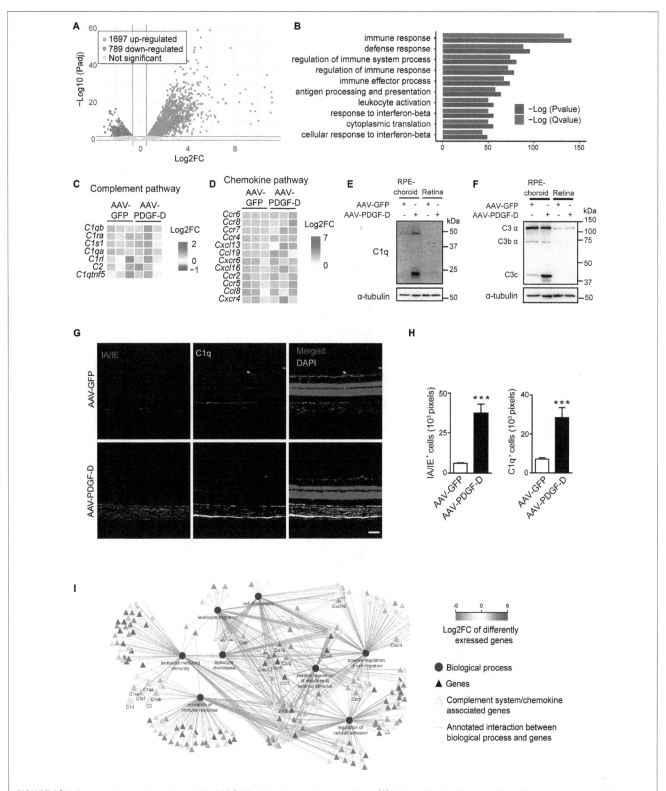

FIGURE 3 | RNA-seq and transcriptomic analysis of PDGF-D-induced complement pathway. **(A)** Volcano plot showing the differentially expressed genes (DEFs) from the RNA-seq data. **(B)** Biological function enrichment gene ontology (GO) analysis of DEGs showing the enriched biological processes in mouse PDGF-D-overexpressing RPE-choroids. **(C,D)** Heatmap of the DEGs associated to complement pathway **(C)** and chemokines and chemokine receptors **(D)** in mouse RPE-choroids injected with AAV-GFP or AAV-PDGF-D. **(E,F)** Immunoblot of C1q **(E)** and C3 **(F)** expression in RPE-choroid complex and retinae from mice with AAV-GFP or AAV-PDGF-D injection. **(G)** Immunofluorescence staining showing the IA/IE and C1q expression in mouse retinae and choroids with AAV-GFP or AAV-PDGF-D injection. **(H)** Quantification of IA/IE and C1q expression in **(G)**. **(I)** Functional network analysis of DEGs showing pathways related to activation of the complement system, immune cell migration and activation of immune responses in PDGF-D-overexpressing RPE-choroids. Scale bar: 50 μm. n = 5–6, ***p < 0.001.

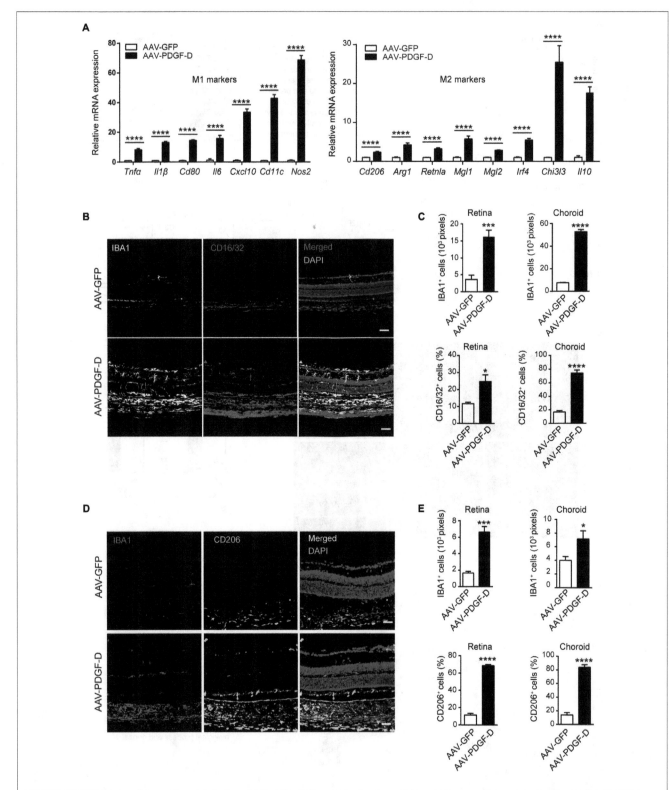

FIGURE 4 | PDGF-D induced macrophage polarizations. **(A)** Real-time PCR analysis of markers of M1 and M2 macrophage polarization regulated by PDGF-D in mouse retinal pigment epithelium. **(B)** Immunofluorescence staining for IBA1$^+$ and CD16/32$^+$ (M1 marker) cells in mouse retinae and choroids with AAV-GFP or AAV-PDGF-D injection. **(C)** Quantifications of IBA1$^+$ and CD16/32$^+$ macrophage densities in **(B)**. **(D)** Immunofluorescence staining of IBA1$^+$ and CD206$^+$ (M2 marker) cells in mouse retinae and choroids with AAV-GFP or AAV-PDGF-D injection. **(E)** Quantification of CD206$^+$ macrophage cell density in retinae and choroids in **(D)**. Scale bar: 50 μm. $n = 5$, *$p < 0.05$, ***$p < 0.001$, ****$p < 0.0001$.

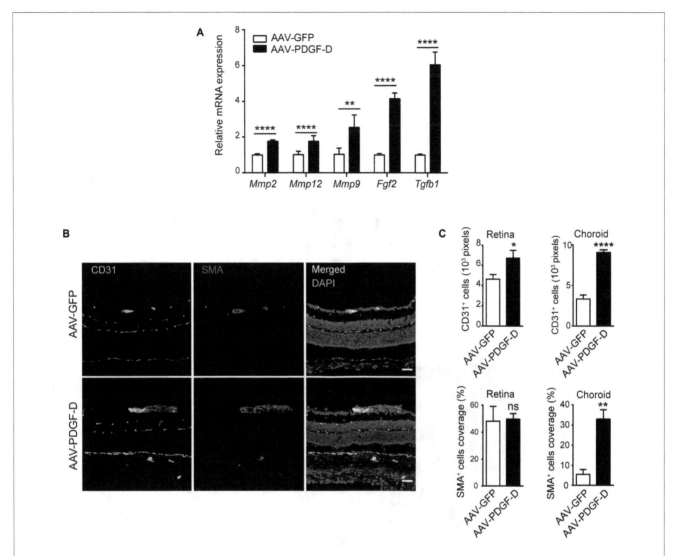

FIGURE 5 | PDGF-D overexpression increased vascular endothelial cell density and mural cell coverage in mouse retinae and choroids. **(A)** Real-time PCR results showing angiogenic genes upregulated by PDGF-D overexpression in RPE-choroid complex. **(B)** Immunofluorescence staining of CD31[+] endothelial cells (EC) and α-SMA [+] smooth muscle cells (SMC) in mouse retinae and choroids injected with AAV-GFP or AAV-PDGF-D. **(C)** Quantifications of CD31[+] cell density and SMC coverage in retinae and choroids in **(B)**. Scale bar: 50 μm. $n = 5$, $^*p < 0.05$, $^{**}p < 0.01$, $^{****}p < 0.0001$, ns: not significant.

is critical for the promotion of macrophage infiltration and CNV formation.

DISCUSSION

The pathogenesis of AMD is associated with degenerative conditions in the neural retina, and dysfunctional RPE cells or choroids. A growing body of evidence has demonstrated that many inflammatory signals, such as chemokines, cytokines, growth factors and alterations in the complement pathway, can modify the functions of neuronal, vascular, glial, and immune cells to promote macular degeneration and pathological neovascularization. Our current work, for the first time, provides evidence that increased PDGF-D expression activated complement pathway to orchestrate tissue milieu by altering

the expression of chemokines and cytokines responses to initiate macrophage activation and triggering neuroinflammatory conditions that exacerbate the pathogenesis of AMD.

The migration and activation of infiltrating inflammatory macrophages is detrimental to tissue function. Apart from exogenous stimuli, endogenously secreted molecules, such as cytokines, chemokines and growth factors, are essential to initiate macrophage migration (Lu et al., 1998; Apte, 2010; Qian et al., 2011; Jenkins et al., 2013; Gordon et al., 2014). PDGF-D expression in the synovial membranes of patients with rheumatoid arthritis and osteoarthritis is escorted with accumulation of synovial fibroblasts and macrophages (Pohlers et al., 2006). In chronic atherosclerotic lesions, PDGF-D was found to be colocalized with macrophages and promoted migration of THP1 monocytes in a dose-dependent manner (Wågsäter et al., 2009). Intriguingly, in our work, PDGF-D

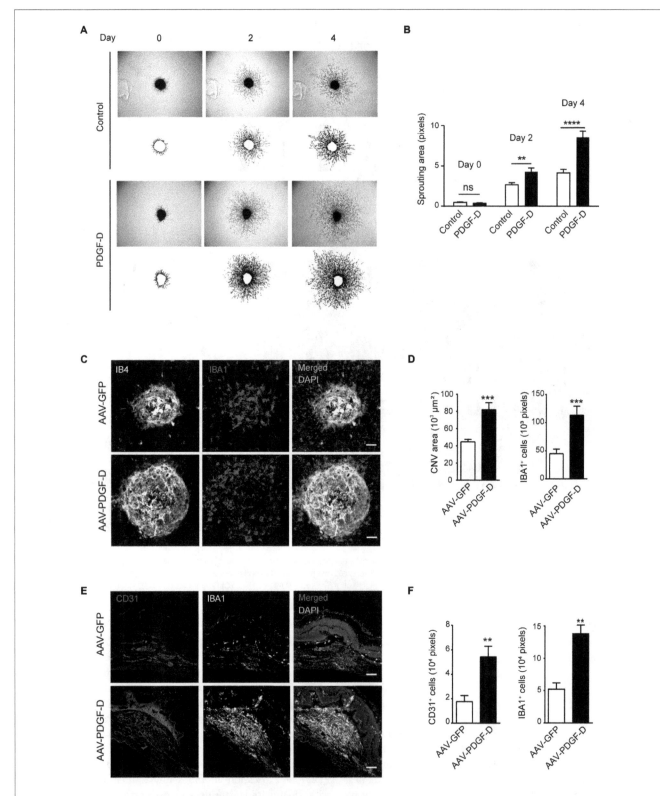

FIGURE 6 | PDGF-D promotes choroid sprouting and pathological choroidal neovascularization (CNV).**(A)** PDGF-D protein treatment increased mouse choroidal sprouting at different days. **(B)** Quantifications of choroidal sprouting areas in **(A)**. **(C)** RPE-choroid wholemount immunofluorescence staining of IB4+ neovessels and IBA1+ macrophages in laser-induced CNVs with AAV-GFP or AAV-PDGF-D overexpression. **(D)** Quantifications of neovascular areas and IBA1+ macrophages in **(C)**. **(E)** Immunofluorescence staining of CD31+ ECs and IBA1+ macrophages in laser-induced CNVs. **(F)** Quantifications of the CD31+ ECs and IBA1+ macrophages in e. Scale bar: 50 μm. $n = 5$, **$p < 0.01$, ***$p < 0.001$, ****$p < 0.0001$, ns: not significant.

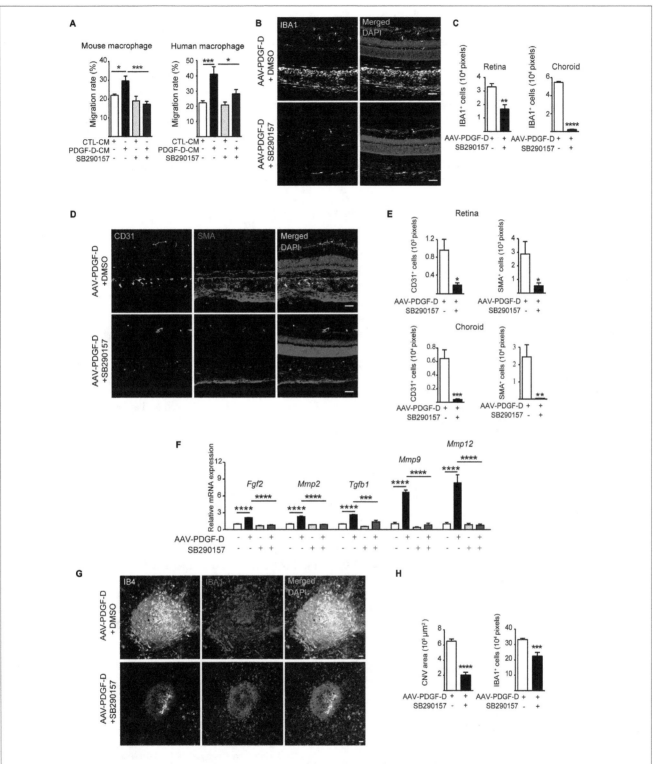

FIGURE 7 | Inhibiting complement C3 cascade by SB290157 alleviates PDGF-D-induced inflammation and pathological neovascularization. **(A)** SB290157 (20 μM) inhibited migration of mouse and human macrophages treated with conditioned medium from PDGF-D-treated HRPE cells (PDGF-D-CM) for 24 h. Conditioned medium from HRPE cells without PDGF-D treatment (CTL-CM) was used as a control. **(B)** Immunofluorescence staining of IBA1+ macrophages in PDGF-D-overexpressing RPE-choroids treated with or without SB290157. **(C)** Quantification of IBA1+ macrophages in retinae and choroids in **(B)**. **(D)** Immunofluorescence staining of CD31+ ECs, NG2+ pericytes and α-SMA+ SMCs in PDGF-D-overexpressing RPE-choroids treated with or without SB290157. **(E)** Quantification of the CD31+, SMA+, and NG2+ cells in retinae and choroids in **(D)**. **(F)** Real-time PCR results showing that SB290157 inhibited PDGF-D-induced upregulation of angiogenic genes. **(G)** RPE-choroid wholemount immunofluorescence staining showing SB290157 reduced IB4+ neovessels and IBA1+ macrophages in laser-induced CNVs with AAV-GFP or AAV-PDGF-D overexpression. **(H)** Quantification of IB4+ and IBA1+ cells in **(G)**. Scale bar: 50 μm. $n = 6$, $*p < 0.05$, $**p < 0.01$, $***p < 0.001$, $****p < 0.0001$.

failed to promote migration of mouse or human macrophages directly. While we do not know the exact reasons for this discrepancy, it could be attributed to different experimental conditions. However, intriguingly, while PDGF-D did not promote macrophage migration by itself, conditioned medium from PDGF-D-stimulated RPE cells did promote the migration of mouse and human macrophages. Since PDGF-D is a potent stimulant of RPE proliferation and migration (Li et al., 2007; Kumar and Li, 2018), and RPE can secrete a wide array of immunomodulatory cytokines (Holtkamp et al., 2001) and chemokines (Ma et al., 2009) that can regulate macrophage response, PDGF-D-induced RPE secretome hence can promote the migration and activation of macrophages.

Over the last decade, mounting evidence has shown that the complement system plays an important role in the pathogenesis of AMD (Sparrow et al., 2012). With the initial finding of complement factor H (CFH) as a high-risk factor for AMD, additional studies identified C3a, C5a and the membrane-attacking complex C5b-9 in the drusen of AMD patients (Nozaki et al., 2006; Mullins et al., 2014). Indeed, transcriptomic analysis of PDGF-D-overexpressing RPE-choroid samples indicated that the presence of classical complement component C1qa and its activated product C3a. C1q expression was strongly associated with RPE cells and IA/IE^{+} macrophages, and C3a protein expression was seen in both the retinae and choroids. Interestingly, it has been shown that inhibition of PDGF-D using the monoclonal antibody CR002 decreased C5b-9 deposition in an experimental glomerulonephritis model (Ostendorf et al., 2006), supporting a role of PDGF-D in the regulation of the complement system. Several reports have also shown that activation of the complement pathway and C5b-9 can regulate the expression of numerous chemokines and cytokines (Kilgore et al., 1996; Selvan et al., 1998; Risnes et al., 2003). Additionally, under inflammatory conditions, RPE cells can generate a myriad of cytokines that can activate macrophages (Holtkamp et al., 2001). Indeed, engagement of both the classical (C1qa) and alternative (C3) complement pathways by PDGF-D overexpression markedly increased the levels of numerous chemokines and cytokines, and triggered polarization of both M1 and M2 macrophages. In fact, C1qa can downregulate inflammasome activation and promote the polarization of inflammation-resolving M2-like macrophages to engulf atherogenic lipoproteins (Bohlson et al., 2014; Spivia et al., 2014). While enhanced C3a signaling facilitates M1 polarization to exacerbate renal interstitial fibrosis, C3 gene deletion increased neovascularization in a mouse retinopathy model (Langer et al., 2010; Cui et al., 2019). PDGF-D has been demonstrated to have pleiotropic effects on vascular and non-vascular cells to stimulate pathological angiogenesis (Li et al., 2003; Kumar et al., 2010). Here, our data highlight yet another VEGF-A-independent function of PDGF-D by regulating the complement system and immune cells to promote CNV formation. Thus, PDGF-D imparted its effects by modulating the complement pathway to polarize macrophages, thereby promoting pathological neovascularization.

Targeting the complement system has been shown to protect mice from accumulating inflammatory mononuclear phagocytes in the subretinal space to maintain tissue homeostasis (Calippe et al., 2017). Complement fragments C3a, C5a, and C5b-9 are generated from C3 during complement activation. Treatment with SB290157, a potent and selective C3a-receptor antagonist, suppressed inflammation by blocking macrophage activation in animal models (Ames et al., 2001; Lim et al., 2013; Rowley et al., 2020). Indeed, we also observed that SB290157 treatment constrained macrophage polarization and blocked infiltration of macrophages by suppressing the expression of various chemokines, cytokines and growth factors, thus decreasing inflammatory neovascularization in the eye.

Collectively, our data reveal that increased PDGF-D levels activate the complement pathway, subsequently leading to marked macrophage activation and inflammation, the key pathologies of neovascular AMD. Therapeutic strategies targeting PDGF-D signaling and complement-mediated inflammation may provide new possibilities for the treatment of neovascular diseases.

ETHICS STATEMENT

The animal study was reviewed and approved by the Zhongshan Ophthalmic Center at the Sun Yat-sen University, Guangzhou, People's Republic of China.

AUTHOR CONTRIBUTIONS

ZX and QW designed and performed the experiments, analyzed the data, and wrote a part of the manuscript. WL, LH, JiZ, and JuZ performed the experiments and analyzed the data. BX, SW, HK, XCL, and CL provided critical experimental tools and suggestions. XRL and AK designed the experiments, provided resources and supervision, analyzed the data, and wrote the manuscript. All authors contributed to the article and approved the submitted version.

SUPPLEMENTARY MATERIAL

Supplementary Figure 1 | PDGF-D does not affect macrophage proliferation. **(A)** Real-time PCR results showing expression of *Pdgfrα*, *Pdgfrβ*, and *Nrp1* in RAW264.7 mouse macrophages. **(B)** Real-time PCR results showing expression of *PDGFRα*, *PDGFRβ*,and *NRP1* in THP1 human monocytes and differentiated dTHP1 human macrophages. **(C,D)** PDGF-D protein treatment at different concentrations did not affect proliferation of mouse **(C)** or human **(D)** macrophages at 12 or 24 h. **(E,F)** PDGF-D protein treatment at different concentrations did not affect migration of mouse **(E)** or human **(F)** macrophages at 24 h. **(G,H)** Proliferation of mouse **(G)** and human **(H)** macrophages treated with conditioned medium from PDGF-D-treated HRPE cells (PDGF-D-CM). Scale bar: 400 μm. All the experiments were performed in triplicates, ****$p < 0.0001$, ns: not significant.

Supplementary Figure 2 | PDGF-D-induced RPE secretome promotes macrophage migration. (A) Immunoblot showing the activation of PDGFR-β by PDGF-D in HRPE. (B,C) Migration of mouse (B) and human (C) macrophages treated with conditioned medium from PDGF-D-treated HRPE cells (PDGF-D-CM). Scale bar: 400 μm. All the experiments were performed in triplicates. *$p < 0.05$, **$p < 0.01$, ***$p < 0.001$.

Supplementary Figure 3 | Expression of PDGF-D receptors in mouse retina and choroid. (A) Real-time PCR results showing expression of PDGF receptors in retinae and RPE-choroid complex of normal C57BL6 mice. (B) Immunoblot analysis showing PDGF receptor expression in normal mouse retinae and RPE-choroid. (C) Immunofluorescence staining reveling PDGF receptor expression in normal mouse retina and choroids. Scale bar: 50 μm. $n = 5$, *$p < 0.05$, **$p < 0.01$, ns, not significant.

Supplementary Figure 4 | RNA-seq and transcriptomic analysis showing PDGF-D induced. complement pathway, chemokine and cytokine signaling, extracellular matrix and growth factors. (A,B) Real-time PCR results showing PDGF-D-induced upregulation of complement pathway genes (A) and chemokine and their receptors (B) in mouse RPE-choroids. (C,D) Heatmaps of PDGF-D-induced DEGs associated to cytokine family (C) and extracellular matrix (ECM) and growth factors (D) n mouse RPE-choroids. (E,F) Real-time PCR results

showing PDGF-D-induced upregulation of Il7r (E) and extracellular matrix genes (F). $n = 5$, *$p < 0.05$, ***$p < 0.001$, ****$p < 0.0001$.

Supplementary Figure 5 | PDGF-D promotes mouse choroid sprouting in a dose-dependent manner. (A) PDGF-D protein treatment induced mouse choroidal sprouting. (B) Quantifications of the choroidal sprouting in (A). $n = 5$, **$p < 0.01$, ***$p < 0.001$, ****$p < 0.0001$, ns: not significant.

Supplementary Figure 6 | SB290157 inhibits PDGF-D-induced macrophage migration and gene expression. (A) SB290157 inhibited mouse (upper penal) and human (lower panel) macrophage migration induced by conditioned medium from PDGF-D-treated HRPE cells (PDGF-D-CM). (B,C) Real-time PCR results showing that SB290157 inhibited AAV-PDGF-D-induced upregulation of M1 and M2 macrophage polarization genes (B) and cytokine and chemokine genes (C). Scale bar: 500 μm. All the experiments were performed in triplicates, **$p < 0.01$, ***$p < 0.001$, ****$p < 0.0001$.

Supplementary Figure 7 | Vascular changes in the flat-mounted retinas with PDGF-D overexpression with or without SB290157 treatment. (A) Analysis of flat-mounted retinas after IB4 staining (green) showing that PDGF-D overexpression increased retinal vascular branch points, which was abolished by SB290157 treatment. (B) Quantifications of vascular branch points in the mouse retinas with PDGF-D overexpression with or without SB290157 treatment. Scale bars in (A): upper panel 500 μm, lower panel 50 μm, $n = 8$, ***$p < 0.001$.

REFERENCES

Alexander, J. J., and Hauswirth, W. W. (2008). Adeno-associated viral vectors and the retina. Adv. Exp. Med. Biol. 613, 121–128. doi: 10.1007/978-0-387-74904-4_13

Ames, R. S., Lee, D., Foley, J. J., Jurewicz, A. J., Tornetta, M. A., Bautsch, W., et al. (2001). Identification of a selective nonpeptide antagonist of the anaphylatoxin C3a receptor that demonstrates antiinflammatory activity in animal models. J. Immunol. 166, 6341–6348. doi: 10.4049/jimmunol.166.10.6341

Apte, R. S. (2010). Regulation of angiogenesis by macrophages. Adv. Exp. Med. Biol. 664, 15–19. doi: 10.1007/978-1-4419-1399-9_2

Barrow, A. D., Edeling, M. A., Trifonov, V., Luo, J., Goyal, P., Bohl, B., et al. (2018). Natural killer cells control tumor growth by sensing a growth factor. Cell 172, 534–548.e519. doi: 10.1016/j.cell.2017.11.037

Bergsten, E., Uutela, M., Li, X., Pietras, K., Ostman, A., Heldin, C. H., et al. (2001). PDGF-D is a specific, protease-activated ligand for the PDGF beta-receptor. Nat. Cell. Biol. 3, 512–516. doi: 10.1038/35074588

Bohlson, S. S., O'Conner, S. D., Hulsebus, H. J., Ho, M. M., and Fraser, D. A. (2014). Complement, c1q, and c1q-related molecules regulate macrophage polarization. Front. Immunol. 5:402. doi: 10.3389/fimmu.2014.00402

Boor, P., Konieczny, A., Villa, L., Kunter, U., van Roeyen, C. R., LaRochelle, W. J., et al. (2007). PDGF-D inhibition by CR002 ameliorates tubulointerstitial fibrosis following experimental glomerulonephritis. Nephrol. Dial. Trans. 22, 1323–1331. doi: 10.1093/ndt/gfl691

Calippe, B., Augustin, S., Beguier, F., Charles-Messance, H., Poupel, L., Conart, J. B., et al. (2017). Complement factor H inhibits CD47-mediated resolution of inflammation. Immunity 46, 261–272. doi: 10.1016/j.immuni.2017.01.006

Chen, M., and Xu, H. (2015). Parainflammation, chronic inflammation, and age-related macular degeneration. J. Leukoc. Biol. 98, 713–725. doi: 10.1189/jlb.3RI0615-239R

Crabb, J. W., Miyagi, M., Gu, X., Shadrach, K., West, K. A., Sakaguchi, H., et al. (2002). Drusen proteome analysis: an approach to the etiology of age-related macular degeneration. Proc. Natl. Acad. Sci. U.S.A. 99, 14682–14687. doi: 10.1073/pnas.222551899

Cui, J., Wu, X., Song, Y., Chen, Y., and Wan, J. (2019). Complement C3 exacerbates renal interstitial fibrosis by facilitating the M1 macrophage phenotype in a mouse model of unilateral ureteral obstruction. Am. J. Physiol. Renal. Physiol. 317, F1171–F1182. doi: 10.1152/ajprenal.00165.2019

de Oliveira Dias, J. R., Rodrigues, E. B., Maia, M., Magalhães, O. Jr.,

Penha, F. M., and Farah, M. E. (2011). Cytokines in neovascular age-related macular degeneration: fundamentals of targeted combination therapy. Br. J. Ophthalmol. 95, 1631–1637. doi: 10.1136/bjo.2010.186361

DeAngelis, M. M., Owen, L. A., Morrison, M. A., Morgan, D. J., Li, M., Shakoor, A., et al. (2017). Genetics of age-related macular degeneration (AMD). Hum. Mol. Genet. 26:R246. doi: 10.1093/hmg/ddx343

Folestad, E., Kunath, A., and Wågsäter, D. (2018). PDGF-C and PDGF-D signaling in vascular diseases and animal models. Mol. Aspects Med. 62, 1–11. doi: 10.1016/j.mam.2018.01.005

Gordon, S., Plüddemann, A., and Martinez Estrada, F. (2014). Macrophage heterogeneity in tissues: phenotypic diversity and functions. Immunol. Rev. 262, 36–55. doi: 10.1111/imr.12223

Holtkamp, G. M., Kijlstra, A., Peek, R., and de Vos, A. F. (2001). Retinal pigment epithelium-immune system interactions: cytokine production and cytokine-induced changes. Prog. Retin. Eye. Res. 20, 29–48. doi: 10.1016/s1350-9462(00)00017-3

Hou, X., Kumar, A., Lee, C., Wang, B., Arjunan, P., Dong, L., et al. (2010). PDGF-CC blockade inhibits pathological angiogenesis by acting on multiple cellular and molecular targets. Proc. Natl. Acad. Sci. U.S.A. 107, 12216–12221. doi: 10.1073/pnas.1004143107

Hutamekalin, P., Takeda, K., Tani, M., Tsuga, Y., Ogawa, N., Mizutani, N., et al. (2010). Effect of the C3a-receptor antagonist SB 290157 on anti-OVA polyclonal antibody-induced arthritis. J. Pharmacol. Sci. 112, 56–63. doi: 10.1254/jphs.09180fp

Jenkins, S. J., Ruckerl, D., Thomas, G. D., Hewitson, J. P., Duncan, S., Brombacher, F., et al. (2013). IL-4 directly signals tissue-resident macrophages to proliferate beyond homeostatic levels controlled by CSF-1. J. Exp. Med. 210, 2477–2491. doi: 10.1084/jem.20121999

Kazlauskas, A. (2017). PDGFs and their receptors. Gene 614, 1–7. doi: 10.1016/j.gene.2017.03.003

Kilgore, K. S., Flory, C. M., Miller, B. F., Evans, V. M., and Warren, J. S. (1996). The membrane attack complex of complement induces interleukin-8 and monocyte chemoattractant protein-1 secretion from human umbilical vein endothelial cells. Am. J. Pathol. 149, 953–961.

Kim, B. J., Mastellos, D. C., Li, Y., Dunaief, J. L., and Lambris, J. D. (2020). Targeting complement components C3 and C5 for the retina: key concepts and lingering questions. Prog. Retin. Eye. Res. 100936. doi: 10.1016/j.preteyeres.2020.100936 [Epub ahead of print].

Kumar, A., Hou, X., Lee, C., Li, Y., Maminishkis, A., Tang, Z., et al. (2010). Platelet-derived growth factor-DD targeting arrests pathological angiogenesis by modulating glycogen synthase kinase-3beta phosphorylation. J. Biol. Chem.

285, 15500–15510. doi: 10.1074/jbc.M110.113787

Kumar, A., and Li, X. (2018). PDGF-C and PDGF-D in ocular diseases. *Mol. Aspects Med.* 62, 33–43. doi: 10.1016/j.mam.2017.10.002

Kumar, A., Zhao, L., Fariss, R. N., McMenamin, P. G., and Wong, W. T. (2014). Vascular associations and dynamic process motility in perivascular myeloid cells of the mouse choroid: implications for function and senescent change. *Invest. Ophthalmol. Vis. Sci.* 55, 1787–1796. doi: 10.1167/iovs.13-13522

Langer, H. F., Chung, K. J., Orlova, V. V., Choi, E. Y., Kaul, S., Kruhlak, M. J., et al. (2010). Complement-mediated inhibition of neovascularization reveals a point of convergence between innate immunity and angiogenesis. *Blood* 116, 4395–4403. doi: 10.1182/blood-2010-01-261503

Li, H., Fredriksson, L., Li, X., and Eriksson, U. (2003). PDGF-D is a potent transforming and angiogenic growth factor. *Oncogene* 22, 1501–1510. doi: 10.1038/sj.onc.1206223

Li, R., Maminishkis, A., Wang, F. E., and Miller, S. S. (2007). PDGF-C and -D induced proliferation/migration of human RPE is abolished by inflammatory cytokines. *Invest. Ophthalmol. Vis. Sci.* 48, 5722–5732. doi: 10.1167/iovs.07-0327

Lim, J., Iyer, A., Suen, J. Y., Seow, V., Reid, R. C., Brown, L., et al. (2013). C5aR and C3aR antagonists each inhibit diet-induced obesity, metabolic dysfunction, and adipocyte and macrophage signaling. *Faseb J.* 27, 822–831. doi: 10.1096/fj.12-220582

Lu, B., Rutledge, B. J., Gu, L., Fiorillo, J., Lukacs, N. W., Kunkel, S. L., et al. (1998). Abnormalities in monocyte recruitment and cytokine expression in monocyte chemoattractant protein 1-deficient mice. *J. Exp. Med.* 187, 601–608. doi: 10.1084/jem.187.4.601

Lutty, G., Grunwald, J., Majji, A. B., Uyama, M., and Yoneya, S. (1999). Changes in choriocapillaris and retinal pigment epithelium in age-related macular degeneration. *Mol. Vis.* 5:35.

Ma, W., Zhao, L., Fontainhas, A. M., Fariss, R. N., and Wong, W. T. (2009). Microglia in the mouse retina alter the structure and function of retinal pigmented epithelial cells: a potential cellular interaction relevant to AMD. *PLoS One* 4:e7945. doi: 10.1371/journal.pone.0007945

McMenamin, P. G., Saban, D. R., and Dando, S. J. (2019). Immune cells in the retina and choroid: two different tissue environments that require different defenses and surveillance. *Prog. Retin. Eye. Res.* 70, 85–98. doi: 10.1016/j.preteyeres.2018.12.002

Medzhitov, R. (2008). Origin and physiological roles of inflammation. *Nature* 454, 428–435. doi: 10.1038/nature07201

Mullins, R. F., Schoo, D. P., Sohn, E. H., Flamme-Wiese, M. J., Workamelahu, G., Johnston, R. M., et al. (2014). The membrane attack complex in aging human choriocapillaris: relationship to macular degeneration and choroidal thinning. *Am. J. Pathol.* 184, 3142–3153. doi: 10.1016/j.ajpath.2014.07.017

Nozaki, M., Raisler, B. J., Sakurai, E., Sarma, J. V., Barnum, S. R., Lambris, J. D., et al. (2006). Drusen complement components C3a and C5a promote choroidal neovascularization. *Proc. Natl. Acad. Sci. U.S.A.* 103, 2328–2333. doi: 10.1073/pnas.0408835103

Ostendorf, T., Rong, S., Boor, P., Wiedemann, S., Kunter, U., Haubold, U., et al. (2006). Antagonism of PDGF-D by human antibody CR002 prevents renal scarring in experimental glomerulonephritis. *J. Am. Soc. Nephrol.* 17, 1054–1062. doi: 10.1681/asn.2005070683

Pohlers, D., Huber, R., Ukena, B., and Kinne, R. W. (2006). Expression of platelet-derived growth factors C and D in the synovial membrane of patients with rheumatoid arthritis and osteoarthritis. *Arthr. Rheum.* 54, 788–794. doi: 10.1002/art.21670

Qian, B. Z., Li, J., Zhang, H., Kitamura, T., Zhang, J., Campion, L. R., et al. (2011). CCL2 recruits inflammatory monocytes to facilitate breast-tumour metastasis. *Nature* 475, 222–225. doi: 10.1038/nature10138

Risnes, I., Ueland, T., Aukrust, P., Lundblad, R., Baksaas, S. T., Mollnes, T. E., et al. (2003). Complement activation and cytokine and chemokines release during mediastinitis. *Ann. Thorac. Surg.* 75, 981–985. doi: 10.1016/s0003-4975(02)04556-3

Rowley, J. A., Reid, R. C., Poon, E. K. Y., Wu, K. C., Lim, J., Lohman, R. J., et al. (2020). Potent thiophene antagonists of human complement C3a receptor with anti-inflammatory activity. *J. Med. Chem.* 63, 529–541. doi: 10.1021/acs.jmedchem.9b00927

Selvan, R. S., Kapadia, H. B., and Platt, J. L. (1998). Complement-induced expression of chemokine genes in endothelium: regulation by IL-1-dependent and -independent mechanisms. *J. Immunol.* 161, 4388–4395.

Shi, G., Maminishkis, A., Banzon, T., Jalickee, S., Li, R., Hammer, J., et al. (2008). Control of chemokine gradients by the retinal pigment epithelium. *Invest. Ophthalmol. Vis. Sci.* 49, 4620–4630. doi: 10.1167/iovs.08-1816

Spano, A., Barni, S., and Sciola, L. (2013). PMA withdrawal in PMA-treated monocytic THP-1 cells and subsequent retinoic acid stimulation, modulate induction of apoptosis and appearance of dendritic cells. *Cell Prolif.* 46, 328–347. doi: 10.1111/cpr.12030

Sparrow, J. R., Ueda, K., and Zhou, J. (2012). Complement dysregulation in AMD: RPE-Bruch's membrane-choroid. *Mol. Aspects Med.* 33, 436–445. doi: 10.1016/j.mam.2012.03.007

Spivia, W., Magno, P. S., Le, P., and Fraser, D. A. (2014). Complement protein C1q promotes macrophage anti-inflammatory M2-like polarization during the clearance of atherogenic lipoproteins. *Inflamm. Res.* 63, 885–893. doi: 10.1007/s00011-014-0762-0

Tan, W., Zou, J., Yoshida, S., Jiang, B., and Zhou, Y. (2020). The role of inflammation in age-related macular degeneration. *Int. J. Biol. Sci.* 16, 2989–3001. doi: 10.7150/ijbs.49890

Uutela, M., Wirzenius, M., Paavonen, K., Rajantie, I., He, Y., Karpanen, T., et al. (2004). PDGF-D induces macrophage recruitment, increased interstitial pressure, and blood vessel maturation during angiogenesis. *Blood* 104, 3198–3204. doi: 10.1182/blood-2004-04-1485

Vandenberghe, L. H., and Auricchio, A. (2012). Novel adeno-associated viral vectors for retinal gene therapy. *Gene. Ther.* 19, 162–168. doi: 10.1038/gt.2011.151

Wågsäter, D., Zhu, C., Björck, H. M., and Eriksson, P. (2009). Effects of PDGF-C and PDGF-D on monocyte migration and MMP-2 and MMP-9 expression. *Atherosclerosis* 202, 415–423. doi: 10.1016/j.atherosclerosis.2008.04.050

Wu, J., and Sun, X. (2019). Complement system and age-related macular degeneration: drugs and challenges. *Drug. Des. Devel. Ther.* 13, 2413–2425. doi: 10.2147/dddt.s206355

Yang, P., Manaenko, A., Xu, F., Miao, L., Wang, G., Hu, X., et al. (2016). Role of PDGF-D and PDGFR-β in neuroinflammation in experimental ICH mice model. *Exp. Neurol.* 283(Pt. A), 157–164. doi: 10.1016/j.expneurol.2016.06.010

Yang, Q., Wang, G., and Zhang, F. (2020). Role of peripheral immune cells-mediated inflammation on the process of neurodegenerative diseases. *Front. Immunol.* 11:582825. doi: 10.3389/fimmu.2020.582825

Yu, C., Roubeix, C., Sennlaub, F., and Saban, D. R. (2020). Microglia versus Monocytes: distinct roles in degenerative diseases of the retina. *Trends Neurosci.* 43, 433–449. doi: 10.1016/j.tins.2020.03.012

Zhang, F., Tang, Z., Hou, X., Lennartsson, J., Li, Y., Koch, A. W., et al. (2009). VEGF-B is dispensable for blood vessel growth but critical for their survival, and VEGF-B targeting inhibits pathological angiogenesis. *Proc. Natl. Acad. Sci. U.S.A.* 106, 6152–6157. doi: 10.1073/pnas.0813061106

Zhang, Z. B., Ruan, C. C., Lin, J. R., Xu, L., Chen, X. H., Du, Y. N., et al. (2018). Perivascular adipose tissue-derived PDGF-D contributes to aortic aneurysm formation during obesity. *Diabetes* 67, 1549–1560. doi: 10.2337/db18-0098

15

An Optical Coherence Tomography-Based Deep Learning Algorithm for Visual Acuity Prediction of Highly Myopic Eyes after Cataract Surgery

Ling Wei[1,2,3†], Wenwen He[1,2,3†], Jinrui Wang[4], Keke Zhang[1,2,3], Yu Du[1,2,3], Jiao Qi[1,2,3], Jiaqi Meng[1,2,3], Xiaodi Qiu[1,2,3], Lei Cai[1,2,3], Qi Fan[1,2,3], Zhennan Zhao[1,2,3], Yating Tang[1,2,3], Shuang Ni[5], Haike Guo[5], Yunxiao Song[6], Xixi He[4], Dayong Ding[4], Yi Lu[1,2,3*] and Xiangjia Zhu[1,2,3*]

[1] Department of Ophthalmology, Eye and ENT Hospital, Eye Institute, Fudan University, Shanghai, China, [2] Key Laboratory of Myopia, NHC Key Laboratory of Myopia, Fudan University, Chinese Academy of Medical Sciences, Shanghai, China, [3] Shanghai Key Laboratory of Visual Impairment and Restoration, Shanghai, China, [4] Visionary Intelligence Ltd, Beijing, China, [5] Department of Ophthalmology, Heping Eye Hospital, Shanghai, China, [6] Illinois Computer Science, University of Illinois, Champaign, IL, United States

*Correspondence:
Xiangjia Zhu
zhuxiangjia1982@126.com
Yi Lu
luyieent@163.com
[†] These authors have contributed equally to this work

Background: Due to complicated and variable fundus status of highly myopic eyes, their visual benefit from cataract surgery remains hard to be determined preoperatively. We therefore aimed to develop an optical coherence tomography (OCT)-based deep learning algorithms to predict the postoperative visual acuity of highly myopic eyes after cataract surgery.

Materials and Methods: The internal dataset consisted of 1,415 highly myopic eyes having cataract surgeries in our hospital. Another external dataset consisted of 161 highly myopic eyes from Heping Eye Hospital. Preoperative macular OCT images were set as the only feature. The best corrected visual acuity (BCVA) at 4 weeks after surgery was set as the ground truth. Five different deep learning algorithms, namely ResNet-18, ResNet-34, ResNet-50, ResNet-101, and Inception-v3, were used to develop the model aiming at predicting the postoperative BCVA, and an ensemble learning was further developed. The model was further evaluated in the internal and external test datasets.

Results: The ensemble learning showed the lowest mean absolute error (MAE) of 0.1566 logMAR and the lowest root mean square error (RMSE) of 0.2433 logMAR in the validation dataset. Promising outcomes in the internal and external test datasets were revealed with MAEs of 0.1524 and 0.1602 logMAR and RMSEs of 0.2612 and 0.2020 logMAR, respectively. Considerable sensitivity and precision were achieved in the BCVA < 0.30 logMAR group, with 90.32 and 75.34% in the internal test dataset and 81.75 and 89.60% in the external test dataset, respectively. The percentages of the prediction errors within ± 0.30 logMAR were 89.01% in the internal and 88.82% in the external test dataset.

Conclusion: Promising prediction outcomes of postoperative BCVA were achieved by the novel OCT-trained deep learning model, which will be helpful for the surgical planning of highly myopic cataract patients.

Keywords: machine learning, visual acuity, high myopia, cataract, optical coherence tomography

INTRODUCTION

A predicted number of 938 million people of the world's population may suffer from high myopia by the year 2050 (Holden et al., 2016), leading to a major worldwide concern. Eyes with high myopia were prone to early-onset and nuclear-type cataracts (Hoffer, 1980; Zhu et al., 2018). Yet, nowadays, surgery is the only effective therapeutic method for cataracts (Thompson and Lakhani, 2015). With the advancement of techniques, cataract surgery can now provide a promising visual outcome in nonmyopes (Liu et al., 2017). However, for highly myopic cataract patients, due to the more complicated fundus conditions such as foveoschisis, chorioretinal atrophy, or cicatrices from previous choroidal neovascularization (Chang et al., 2013; Todorich et al., 2013; Gohil et al., 2015; Lichtwitz et al., 2016; Li et al., 2018), their visual benefit from cataract surgery remains hard to be determined preoperatively.

With the wide application of optical coherence tomography (OCT), surgeons could assess the fundus status of highly myopic eyes on an anatomical scale (Huang et al., 2018; Li et al., 2018), but the morphological diagnoses were hard to be directly associated with the actual manifested visual acuity (VA). Therefore, difficulties might occur when surgeons want to predict the postoperative VA and explain the prognosis to the highly myopic patients during preoperative conversations, which might thereby affect the overall surgical planning and patients' satisfaction with the surgery later.

Recently, deep learning was found promising in automated classification. Particularly, the ResNet and Inception algorithms have their advantages on medical image analysis (Gulshan et al., 2016; Fu et al., 2018; Grassmann et al., 2018). Such techniques have the potential to revolutionize the diagnosis and clinical prediction by rapidly reviewing large amounts of morphological features and by performing integrations difficult for human experts (Kermany et al., 2018). Hence, prediction of the clinical manifestation based on deep learning analysis of relevant morphological features is becoming possible and important (Chen et al., 2018; Rohm et al., 2018). However, due to the more complicated and variable morphological changes of the fundus, no appropriate deep learning model has been developed for highly myopic eyes currently.

In this study, on the basis of the OCT scans of highly myopic eyes, we aim to predict their postoperative VA of cataract surgery by developing and comparing five machine learning algorithms and consequently evaluating the model on real-world datasets.

MATERIALS AND METHODS

Ethics

The Institutional Review Board of the Eye and Ear, Nose, and Throat (ENT) Hospital of Fudan University (Shanghai, China) approved this study. The study adhered to the tenets of the Declaration of Helsinki and was registered at www.clinicaltrials.gov (accession number NCT03062085). Written consent was obtained from the patients and all private information was removed in advance.

Patients

An internal dataset including 1,415 highly myopic eyes from 1,415 patients was drawn from the database of the Shanghai High Myopia Study between 2015 and 2020 at the Eye and ENT Hospital of Fudan University (Shanghai, China). Eligible criteria were as follows: (1) cataract patients with axial length (AL) over 26.0 mm, (2) had reliable macular OCT measurements before cataract surgery, (3) underwent uneventful cataract surgeries, and (4) had credible postoperative best corrected visual acuity (BCVA) measured at 4 weeks after surgery. Exclusion criteria were eyes with (1) corneal opacity or other corneal diseases that may significantly influence the visual pathway, (2) congenital ocular abnormalities, (3) neuropathies that may influence the visual acuity, (4) ocular trauma, and (5) other severe oculopathies that may affect the surgical outcomes. The OCT images in the internal dataset were taken from Spectralis OCT (Heidelberg Engineering, Heidelberg, Germany) or Cirrus OCT (Carl Zeiss Meditec, Dublin, CA, United States).

Another external dataset consisted of 161 highly myopic eyes of 161 patients drawn from the database of the Heping Eye Hospital (Shanghai, China) with the same inclusion and exclusion criteria. The OCT images in this external dataset were taken from Spectralis OCT (Heidelberg Engineering, Heidelberg, Germany).

Datasets

The eligible internal database was randomly divided into a training dataset, a validation dataset, and an internal test dataset with a fixed ratio of 6:2:2. The eligible external database was all used as an external test dataset. The actual BCVAs at 4 weeks after cataract surgery were set as the ground truth. The Snellen VA was converted to its logarithm of minimal angle of resolution (logMAR) equivalent as previously described, with counting fingers being assigned a value of 1.9, hand motion 2.3, light perception 2.7, and no light perception 3.0 (Lange et al., 2009). Eyes with actual BCVAs < 0.30 logMAR (Snellen 6/12 or higher) were defined as the good VA group, while eyes with actual BCVAs ≥ 0.30 logMAR (Snellen 6/12 and lower) were defined as the poor VA group (Quek et al., 2011).

Data Normalization

The e2e files from Spectrialis OCT or scan figures from Cirrus OCT were extracted and preprocessed. All OCT images were down-sized to 224 × 224 pixels, the default choice for deep learning-based image classification. In order to simulate more real-world situations and to improve model generalization ability, it was performed on the image by changing the brightness, saturation, and contrast with a factor uniformly sampled from [0, 2], respectively. After the color space normalization, the macular OCT images were set as model input.

Deep Learning Models

In our study, to predict the BCVA after cataract surgery for highly myopic patients, we constructed an ensemble learning using five different deep convolutional neural networks (CNN) algorithms, including Deep Residual Learning for Image Recognition (ResNet, Microsoft Research) with 18, 34, 50, and 101 layers (ResNet-18, ResNet-34, ResNet-50, and ResNet-101) (He et al., 2016) and Inception-v3 (Szegedy et al., 2016). The postfix number of ResNet referred to diverse depths of ResNet networks that lead to different parameter scales. All five models were pretrained on the ImageNet dataset. For each model, the last fully connected layer which originally output 1,000 class was replaced to output a single value to suit our task. The parameters of this layer were randomly initialized.

Based on the training dataset, the model was optimized with a target of minimizing the mean square error (MSE) loss function using the Adam optimizer (Fu et al., 2018). The final output score was calculated as the mean value of the ensemble model. MSE loss was defined as:

$$MSE = \frac{1}{N} \sum_{i=1}^{N} (\widetilde{y}_i - y_i)^2, \tag{1}$$

where N indicates the number of input OCT images, $\widetilde{y}_i$ indicates the actual BCVA, and y_i indicates the predicted BCVA.

The maximal number of training epochs was set to be 80. We adopted an early stop strategy, which is the training procedure stops when there is no performance improvement on the validation dataset in 15 consecutive epochs. The initial learning rate was set to 0.001 and would be decayed by 0.1 every 30 epochs. Each CNN algorithm was trained five times repeatedly, and only the model with the best performance on the validation dataset was reserved for the ensemble learning.

Evaluation

The metrics used to show the differences in logMAR postoperative BCVA between the prediction and the ground truth were mean absolute error (MAE, calculated for the predictions of the algorithms compared to the ground truth) and the root mean square error (RMSE), which were defined as:

$$MAE = \frac{1}{N} \sum_{i=1}^{N} |\widetilde{y}_i - y_i|, \tag{2}$$

$$RMSE = \sqrt{\frac{1}{N} \sum_{i=1}^{N} (\widetilde{y}_i - y_i)^2}, \tag{3}$$

where N, $\widetilde{y}_i$, and y_i were defined as above.

Furthermore, sensitivity is defined as the proportion of correctly predicted eyes with VA < 0.30 logMAR (or ≥0.30 logMAR) in the overall eyes having actual VA < 0.30 logMAR (or ≥0.30 logMAR). Precision is defined as the proportion of correctly predicted eyes with VA < 0.30 logMAR (or ≥0.30 logMAR) in the overall eyes having predicted VA < 0.30 logMAR (or ≥0.30 logMAR).

The ensemble learning of the five CNN models was adopted to develop the prediction model and then further evaluated using the internal and external test datasets, which contain data the model has not seen. The OCT reports in pdf format from both test datasets were adopted and evaluated. The prediction error was calculated by subtracting the predicted BCVA from the actual BCVA. The percentage of BCVA prediction errors within ± 0.30 logMAR (Snellen 6/12, $R_{e0.30logMAR}$) was then calculated (Gao et al., 2015), which was defined as:

$$R_{e0.3logMAR} = \frac{1}{N} \sum_{i=1}^{N} I\left(|\widetilde{y}_i - y_i| \leq 0.3\, logMAR\right), \tag{4}$$

where N, $\widetilde{y}_i$, and y_i were defined as above. $I(\cdot)$ is the function which returns 1 if the · is true, else return 0.

In order to make the performance more comparable, fixed randomly generated seeds were used to shuffle the data and initialize the models' parameter. To better visualize the prediction, gradient-weighted class activation mapping (Grad-CAM) was used to highlight the model's interests in the OCT images in prediction VA (Selvaraju et al., 2020).

The illustration of the pipeline of our work is demonstrated in **Figure 1**.

Statistics

Continuous variables were described as the mean ± standard deviation. The Student's t test or one-way ANOVA test followed by Tukey's test was used to compare the continuous variables and the χ^2 test was used to compare categorical variables. The alignment of the predicted BCVA and ground truth was demonstrated by scatter plots. Pearson correlation analysis was used to evaluate the relationship between the predicted outcome and the ground truth, and the Bland–Altman plot was used to assess the agreement between the predicted outcome and the ground truth. The information of the computer used in this study was as follows: Intel Xeon 4144 (2.20 GHz), 128 gigabytes of RAM, and three pieces of GeForce RTX 2080 Ti Ubuntu 18.04 LTS. Model development was performed by Python (version 3.7.5) with libraries of torch (version 1.4.0) and torchvision

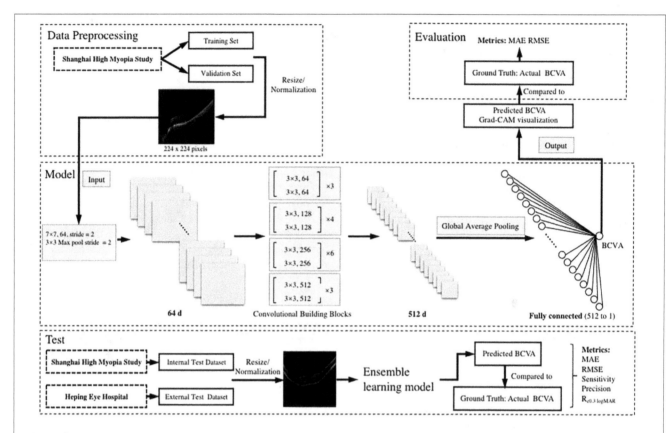

FIGURE 1 | An illustration of the pipeline of the tasks. The preoperative b-scan OCT image is fed into the model. It eventually outputs the prediction of postoperative BCVA. BCVA, best corrected visual acuity; logMAR, logarithm of the minimum angle of resolution; MAE, mean absolute error; RMSE, root mean square error; $R_{e0.30logMAR}$, the percentage of BCVA prediction errors within ± 0.30 logMAR.

(version 0.4.0), and statistical analyses were performed with a commercially available statistical software package (SPSS Statistics 20.0; IBM, Armonk, NY).

RESULTS

The clinical characteristics of the patients are demonstrated in **Table 1**. No difference was found in age, sex, and mean actual postoperative BCVA among the training, validation, internal test, and external test datasets ($p > 0.05$).

The performances of all five CNN algorithms were compared after training and validating for five times. The average values of the five-time performances of the five models separately and the ensemble learning outcomes combining all models' decisions using the validation dataset are presented in **Table 2**. Notably, the ensemble learning showed the lowest MAE (0.1566 logMAR) and the lowest RMSE (0.2433 logMAR). Therefore, the ensemble learning model with the most promising performance was then chosen for further development and evaluations.

The internal and external test datasets were used to determine the performance of our prediction model using the ensemble learning and to confirm the generalizability. As shown in **Table 3**, the prediction model demonstrated stably promising outcomes with MAEs of 0.1524 and 0.1602 logMAR and RMSEs of 0.2612

and 0.2020 logMAR in the internal and external test datasets, respectively. In the internal test dataset, the sensitivity of our model was 90.32% in the good VA group and 42.71% in the poor VA group; the precision was 75.34% in the good VA group and 69.49% in the poor VA group. In the external test dataset, the sensitivity of our model was 81.75% in the good VA group and 45.83% in the poor VA group; the precision was 89.60% in the good VA group and 30.55% in the poor VA group. The scatter plot of the predicted BCVA and the ground truth (actual BCVA) was demonstrated in the internal (**Figure 2A**) and external test datasets (**Figure 2B**). Pearson correlation analysis revealed the significant relationships between the predicted BCVA and the ground truth in the internal test dataset ($r = 0.55$; $p < 0.001$) and external test dataset (Pearson coefficients $r = 0.50$; $p < 0.001$). The Grad-CAM visualization was used for the CNN models. Representative cases in the good VA group (**Figure 2C**) and in the poor VA group (**Figure 2D**) were demonstrated, showing the highly discriminative region of OCT scans when predicting the VA.

The Bland–Altman plots assessing the agreement between predictions and the ground truth are shown in **Figure 3**. The 95% confidence limits of agreement ranged from −0.52 to 0.50 logMAR in the internal test dataset and −0.22 to 0.44 logMAR in the external test dataset, while no statistically significant evidence of proportional bias was found (both $p > 0.05$).

TABLE 1 | Demographic and clinical characteristics.

	Internal datasets			External test dataset
	Training	Validation	Test	
Number of eyes	851	282	282	161
Female gender (%)	391 (45.9%)	158 (56.0%)	150 (53.2%)	86 (53.4%)
Age (mean ± SD, years)	61.37 ± 10.45	61.93 ± 11.15	61.19 ± 9.47	62.45 ± 9.32
Actual postoperative BCVA (LogMAR, mean ± SD)	0.26 ± 0.33	0.25 ± 0.30	0.25 ± 0.31	0.14 ± 0.19
Number of OCT images in each BCVA range				
<0.30 logMAR (Snellen 6/12 or higher)	559	186	186	137
≥0.30 logMAR (Snellen 6/12 or lower)	292	96	96	24

LogMAR, logarithm of the minimum angle of resolution; BCVA, best corrected distance visual acuity.

TABLE 2 | The performances of five algorithms and the ensemble learning using the validation dataset (n = 282).

Algorithms	ResNet-18	ResNet-34	ResNet-50	ResNet-101	Inception-v3	Ensemble
MAE	0.1648	0.1737	0.1729	0.1723	0.1842	0.1566*
RMSE	0.2540	0.2677	0.2682	0.2600	0.2857	0.2433*

MAE, mean absolute error; RMSE, root mean square error.
*The best performances in MAE and RMSE.

TABLE 3 | The performances of the prediction model in the internal (n = 282) and external test datasets (n = 161).

Algorithms	Internal test dataset	External test dataset
MAE	0.1524	0.1602
RMSE	0.2612	0.2020
Sensitivity in each VA group*		
<0.30 logMAR (Snellen 6/12 or higher)	90.32% (168/186)	81.75% (112/137)
≥0.30 logMAR (Snellen 6/12 and lower)	42.71% (41/96)	45.83% (11/24)
Precision in each VA group†		
<0.30 logMAR (Snellen 6/12 or higher)	75.34% (168/223)	89.60% (112/125)
≥0.30 logMAR (Snellen 6/12 and lower)	69.49% (41/59)	30.55% (11/36)

MAE, mean absolute error; RMSE, root mean square error.
*Sensitivity = number of correctly predicted eyes with VA < 0.30 logMAR (or ≥0.30 logMAR) / overall number of eyes having actual VA < 0.30 logMAR (or ≥0.30 logMAR).
†Precision = number of correctly predicted eyes with VA < 0.30 logMAR (or ≥0.30 logMAR) / overall number of eyes having predicted VA < 0.30 logMAR (or ≥0.30 logMAR).

Figure 4 shows the distributions of the difference between the ground truth and the predicted BCVA in both test datasets. The percentages of the prediction errors within ± 0.30 logMAR were 89.01% in the internal test dataset and 88.82% in the external test dataset.

Further analysis was conducted on the falsely predicted cases in the test datasets. They can be divided into two groups: (1) underestimated cases: the ground truth < 0.30 logMAR (good VA) but the predicted VA ≥ 0.30 logMAR (poor VA), and (2) overestimated cases: the ground truth ≥ 0.30 logMAR (poor VA) but the predicted VA < 0.30 logMAR (good VA). **Supplementary Table 1** shows the distribution of all falsely predicted cases.

These cases can be attributed to the following four categories: (A) vague OCT images induced by extraordinarily cloudy cataract (under- or overestimated, 39.6%); (B) morphological changes on OCT scan exist but might have poor effect on VA (underestimated, 8.1%), e.g., changes located away from the macular, which were irregularly focused by the model; (C) morphological changes on OCT scan exist but might have unclear effect on VA (under- or overestimated VA, 46.8%), e.g., rough retinal pigment epithelium layer or irregular inner segment/outer segment layer; and (D) morphological changes on OCT scan exist which might have some effect on VA, but were presented as signal-deficient lesions and were accidentally ignored by the model (overestimated VA, 5.4%). Representative cases in the four categories with their Grad-CAM visualizations are presented in **Supplementary Figure 1**.

DISCUSSION

Highly myopic cataract patients usually inevitably have macular complications such as foveoschisis, chorioretinal atrophy, and cicatrices from previous choroidal neovascularization (Chang et al., 2013; Todorich et al., 2013; Gohil et al., 2015; Lichtwitz et al., 2016; Li et al., 2018), which could render the preoperative prediction of visual acuity after cataract surgery very difficult, even though an OCT scan can be used for morphological diagnosis (Jeon and Kim, 2011). In the present study, by using the preoperative OCT scans of macular as input, we developed and validated a deep learning algorithm to predict the postoperative BCVA of highly myopic eyes after cataract surgery and revealed that the ensemble model showed stably promising performance in both internal and external test datasets with MAEs of 0.1524 and 0.1602 logMAR and RMSEs of 0.2612 and 0.2020 logMAR, respectively.

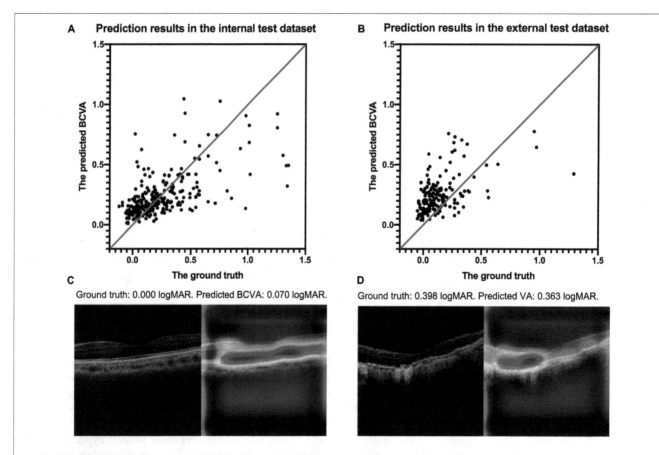

FIGURE 2 | The scatter plots of the predicted BCVA and the actual BCVA (ground truth) in the internal **(A)** and external **(B)** test datasets. Representative cases of Grad-CAM visualization in the good VA group **(C)** and in the poor VA group **(D)**. Red regions corresponds to highly discriminative areas of OCT scans when predicting the VA. All values were provided in logMAR units. BCVA, best corrected distance visual acuity; logMAR, logarithm of the minimum angle of resolution; Grad-CAM, gradient-weighted class activation mapping.

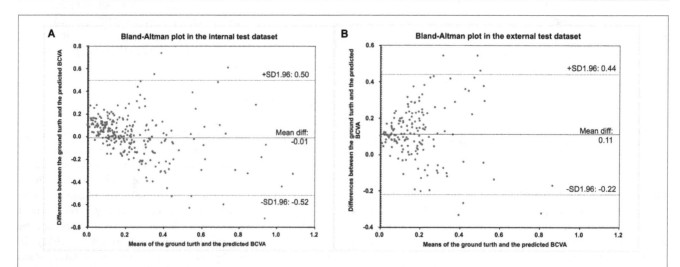

FIGURE 3 | The Bland–Altman plots of the predicted BCVA and the actual BCVA (ground truth) in the internal **(A)** and external **(B)** test datasets. All values were provided in logMAR units. BCVA, best corrected distance visual acuity; logMAR, logarithm of the minimum angle of resolution.

Cataract patients usually expect a significant improvement of VA after removal of the cloudy lens (Zhu et al., 2017). However, those with high myopia are more concerned about their VA improvement during the surgical planning stage. Myopic maculopathies are the main source of the gap between the expected outcomes and the actual potentials

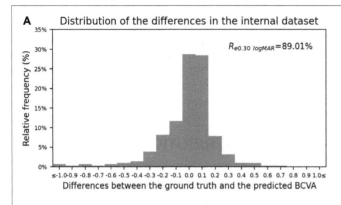
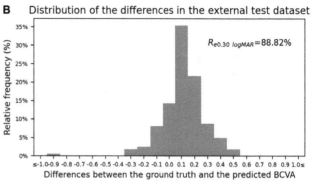

FIGURE 4 | The distribution of the difference between the predicted BCVA and the actual BCVA (ground truth) in the internal **(A)** and external **(B)** test datasets. All values were provided in logMAR units. The vertical axis indicates the relative frequency of each BCVA delta value. BCVA, best corrected visual acuity; logMAR, logarithm of the minimum angle of resolution; $R_{e0.30logMAR}$, the percentage of BCVA prediction errors within $\pm$ 0.30 logMAR.

their fundus have. Hence, a forecast model which could tell the patients their potential postoperative visual acuities might be helpful with their surgical decisions (Rönbeck et al., 2011). Nevertheless, the prediction of VA for highly myopic eyes has always been very difficult. Although high-resolution OCT may reveal morphological changes and thereby identify eyes at high risk of developing clinically significant macular complications affecting the postoperative visual outcomes (Hayashi et al., 2010), it is still hard for cataract surgeons to specifically determine the exact postoperative VA preoperatively.

In recent years, deep learning has been widely applied for its ability to process highly complex tasks through a neural network, which can be seen as a mathematical function composed of a large number of parameters provided by medical images. An OCT scan of macular could provide millions of morphological parameters affecting the VA (Abdolrahimzadeh et al., 2017; Chung et al., 2019). The neural network was able to identify the corresponding features and thereby automatically generate the target VA predictions. Therefore, using deep learning algorithms to predict the postoperative BCVA was practicable and meaningful. Compared with other types of neural networks, CNN can initially identify a few adjacent pixels as local lower-level features and then merge them into global higher-level features, and thus, it has been proven effective widely in the field of medical image analysis (Anwar et al., 2018). In the current study, when taking a preoperative OCT image as input, the ensemble learning showed the most promising performance, and the model automatically predicted the postoperative BCVA for highly myopic eyes having cataract surgeries with promising accuracies. With this model, surgeons only need to input an OCT image of macular, and a predicted postoperative BCVA together with a Grad-CAM visualization could be generated. The expectant surgical outcomes could be discussed between the surgeons and highly myopic patients before surgery. Patients might more thoroughly understand their macular status and how it might affect the visual outcome of cataract surgery. It might also help

with surgical decisions such as whether to choose premium IOL implantations.

Previous reports about applying deep learning approaches to predict VA outcomes were mainly in the field of retinal or macular diseases, such as age-related macular degeneration, diabetic retinopathy, or retinopathy of prematurity (Chen et al., 2018; Rohm et al., 2018; Huang et al., 2020). The morphologies of featured lesions for these diseases were relatively simple or identifiable. Yet, there are rare studies about implementing the deep learning approach on high myopia due to its more complicated and variable fundus status (Zhu et al., 2020). It might be more valuable to predict the VA outcomes based on the diverse fundus morphologies for highly myopic eyes. Moreover, dozens of features from the patients' medical history were adopted or annotated one by one to train their models (Chen et al., 2018; Rohm et al., 2018; Huang et al., 2020). It might be highly difficult to ensure that during applications, such many features from real-world patients were available simultaneously and completely. The data missing problem might be serious and may result in uncertain accuracies, thus restricting the generalizability of their models. Our study, mainly targeting VA prediction of highly myopic eyes, adopted the OCT scan as the only input feature, which examines almost every highly myopic patient before their cataract surgery. Hence, the data missing problem could be rare when clinically applying our model.

Notably, our model has shown considerable sensitivity and precision in the good VA group in both test datasets (all >75%), thus solving nearly 60% of the problems after cataract surgery according to a previous report (Barañano et al., 2008). As for the poor VA group, the model demonstrated relatively lower sensitivity and precision, which might due to the very complicated and changeable characteristic of the fundus status among these highly myopic patients. As for the falsely predicted cases in categories A and C, manually predicting the VA can still be tricky for experienced cataract surgeons. In the future, the accuracy could be further improved by the model training with larger sample sizes. As for the falsely predicted cases in categories B and D, they revealed less focus on the signal-deficient signs by the model intrinsically, but only made up very minimal proportions. This can be further improved by manual annotations of the signal-deficient lesions when more cases are included in model training in the future. Currently, as there are no perfect ways to accurately predict the surgical benefit of highly myopic patients with very poor fundus condition, our predictions by the deep learning model might still provide valuable references for preoperative communications and clinical decisions for this special population.

In conclusion, based on macular OCT images taken before cataract surgery, we are taking the lead to originally develop the deep learning prediction model for highly myopic eyes, which can provide promising predictions of postoperative BCVA for cataract patients with high myopia. Our model will be helpful for surgical planning and preoperative conversations with highly myopic cataract patients.

ETHICS STATEMENT

The studies involving human participants were reviewed and approved by The Institutional Review Board of the Eye and Ear, Nose, and Throat Hospital of Fudan University (Shanghai, China). The patients/participants provided their written informed consent to participate in this study.

AUTHOR CONTRIBUTIONS

LW and WH collected the data, performed the analyses, and wrote the manuscript. JW, XH, and DD programmed the model and performed the analyses. KZ, YD, JQ, and JM collected the data and performed the analyses. XQ, LC, QF, ZZ, YT, SN, and HG collected the data. YS performed the analyses. YL and XZ gained the fund and supervised the process. XZ revised the manuscript, gained the fund, and supervised the process. All authors contributed to the article and approved the submitted version.

REFERENCES

Abdolrahimzadeh, S., Parisi, F., Plateroti, A. M., Evangelista, F., Fenicia, V., Scuderi, G., et al. (2017). Visual acuity, and macular and peripapillary thickness in high myopia. *Curr. Eye Res.* 42, 1468–1473. doi: 10.1080/02713683.2017.1347692

Anwar, S. M., Majid, M., Qayyum, A., Awais, M., Alnowami, M., and Khan, M. K. (2018). Medical image analysis using convolutional neural networks: a review. *J. Med. Syst.* 42:226.

Barañano, A. E., Wu, J., Mazhar, K., Azen, S. P., and Varma, R. (2008). Visual acuity outcomes after cataract extraction in adult latinos. The Los Angeles latino eye study. *Ophthalmology* 115, 815–821. doi: 10.1016/j.ophtha.2007.05.052

Chang, L., Pan, C. W., Ohno-Matsui, K., Lin, X., Cheung, G. C., Gazzard, G., et al. (2013). Myopia-related fundus changes in Singapore adults with high myopia. *Am. J. Ophthalmol.* 155, 991–999.e1.

Chen, S. C., Chiu, H. W., Chen, C. C., Woung, L. C., and Lo, C. M. (2018). A novel machine learning algorithm to automatically predict visual outcomes in intravitreal ranibizumab-treated patients with diabetic macular edema. *J. Clin. Med.* 7:475. doi: 10.3390/jcm7120475

Chung, Y. W., Choi, M. Y., Kim, J. S., and Kwon, J. W. (2019). The association between macular thickness and axial length in myopic eyes. *Biomed. Res. Int.* 2019:8913582.

Fu, H., Cheng, J., Xu, Y., Zhang, C., Wong, D. W. K., Liu, J., et al. (2018). Disc-aware ensemble network for glaucoma screening from fundus image. *IEEE Trans. Med. Imaging* 37, 2493–2501. doi: 10.1109/tmi.2018.2837012

Gao, X., Lin, S., and Wong, T. Y. (2015). Automatic feature learning to grade nuclear cataracts based on deep learning. *IEEE Trans. Biomed. Eng.* 62, 2693–2701. doi: 10.1109/tbme.2015.2444389

Gohil, R., Sivaprasad, S., Han, L. T., Mathew, R., Kiousis, G., and Yang, Y. (2015). Myopic foveoschisis: a clinical review. *Eye (Lond.)* 29, 593–601. doi: 10.1038/eye.2014.311

Grassmann, F., Mengelkamp, J., Brandl, C., Harsch, S., Zimmermann, M. E., Linkohr, B., et al. (2018). Deep learning algorithm for prediction of age-related eye disease study severity scale for age-related macular degeneration from color fundus photography. *Ophthalmology* 125, 1410–1420. doi: 10.1016/j.ophtha.2018.02.037

Gulshan, V., Peng, L., Coram, M., Stumpe, M. C., Wu, D., Narayanaswamy, A., et al. (2016). Development and validation of a deep learning algorithm for detection of diabetic retinopathy in retinal fundus photographs. *JAMA* 316, 2402–2410. doi: 10.1001/jama.2016.17216

Hayashi, K., Ohno-Matsui, K., Shimada, N., Moriyama, M., Kojima, A., Hayashi, W., et al. (2010). Long-term pattern of progression of myopic maculopathy: a natural history study. *Ophthalmology* 117, 1595–1611, 1611.e1591–e1594..

He, K., Zhang, X., Ren, S., and Sun, J. (2016). "Identity mappings in deep residual networks," in *Computer Vision – Eccv 2016, Part IV*, Vol. 9908, eds B. Leibe, J. Matas, N. Sebe, and M. Welling (Cham: Springer), 630–645. doi: 10.1007/978-3-319-46493-0_38

Hoffer, K. J. (1980). Biometry of 7,500 cataractous eyes. *Am. J. Ophthalmol.* 90, 360–368. doi: 10.1016/s0002-9394(14)74917-7

Holden, B. A., Fricke, T. R., Wilson, D. A., Jong, M., Naidoo, K. S., Sankaridurg, P., et al. (2016). Global prevalence of myopia and high myopia and temporal trends from 2000 through 2050. *Ophthalmology* 123, 1036–1042. doi: 10.1016/j.ophtha.2016.01.006

Huang, C. Y., Kuo, R. J., Li, C. H., Ting, D. S., Kang, E. Y., Lai, C. C., et al. (2020). Prediction of visual outcomes by an artificial neural network following intravitreal injection and laser therapy for retinopathy of prematurity. *Br. J. Ophthalmol.* 104, 1277–1282.

Huang, X., Zhang, Z., Wang, J., Meng, X., Chen, T., and Wu, Z. (2018). Macular assessment of preoperative optical coherence tomography in ageing Chinese undergoing routine cataract surgery. *Sci. Rep.* 8:5103.

Jeon, S., and Kim, H. S. (2011). Clinical characteristics and outcomes of cataract surgery in highly myopic Koreans. *Korean J. Ophthalmol.* 25, 84–89. doi: 10.3341/kjo.2011.25.2.84

Kermany, D. S., Goldbaum, M., Cai, W., Valentim, C. C. S., Liang, H., Baxter, S. L., et al. (2018). Identifying medical diagnoses and treatable diseases by image-based deep learning. *Cell* 172, 1122–1131.e9.

Lange, C., Feltgen, N., Junker, B., Schulze-Bonsel, K., and Bach, M. (2009). Resolving the clinical acuity categories "hand motion" and "counting fingers" using the Freiburg Visual Acuity Test (FrACT). *Graefes Arch. Clin. Exp. Ophthalmol.* 247, 137–142. doi: 10.1007/s00417-008-0926-0

Li, T., Wang, X., Zhou, Y., Feng, T., Xiao, M., Wang, F., et al. (2018). Paravascular abnormalities observed by spectral domain optical coherence tomography are risk factors for retinoschisis in eyes with high myopia. *Acta Ophthalmol.* 96, e515–e523.

Lichtwitz, O., Boissonnot, M., Mercié, M., Ingrand, P., and Leveziel, N. (2016). Prevalence of macular complications associated with high myopia by multimodal imaging. *J. Fr. Ophtalmol.* 39, 355–363. doi: 10.1016/j.jfo.2015.11.005

Liu, Y. C., Wilkins, M., Kim, T., Malyugin, B., and Mehta, J. S. (2017). Cataracts. *Lancet* 390, 600–612.

Quek, D. T., Jap, A., and Chee, S. P. (2011). Risk factors for poor visual outcome following cataract surgery in Vogt-Koyanagi-Harada disease. *Br. J. Ophthalmol.* 95, 1542–1546. doi: 10.1136/bjo.2010.184796

Rohm, M., Tresp, V., Müller, M., Kern, C., Manakov, I., Weiss, M., et al. (2018). Predicting visual acuity by using machine learning in patients treated for neovascular age-related macular degeneration. *Ophthalmology* 125, 1028–1036. doi: 10.1016/j.ophtha.2017.12.034

Rönbeck, M., Lundström, M., and Kugelberg, M. (2011). Study of possible predictors associated with self-assessed visual function after cataract surgery. *Ophthalmology* 118, 1732–1738. doi: 10.1016/j.ophtha.2011.04.013

Selvaraju, R. R., Cogswell, M., Das, A., Vedantam, R., Parikh, D., and Batra, D. (2020). Grad-CAM: visual explanations from deep networks via gradient-based localization. *Int. J. Comput. Vis.* 128, 336–359. doi: 10.1007/s11263-019-01228-7

Szegedy, C., Vanhoucke, V., Ioffe, S., Shlens, J., and Wojna, Z. (2016). "Rethinking the inception architecture for computer vision," in *Proceedings of the 2016 IEEE Conference on Computer Vision and Pattern Recognition*, (Las Vegas, NV: IEEE), 2818–2826.

Thompson, J., and Lakhani, N. (2015). Cataracts. *Prim. Care* 42, 409–423.

Todorich, B., Scott, I. U., Flynn, H. W. Jr., and Chang, S. (2013). Macular retinoschisis associated with pathologic myopia. *Retina* 33, 678–683. doi: 10.1097/iae.0b013e318285d0a3

Zhu, X., Li, D., Du, Y., He, W., and Lu, Y. (2018). DNA hypermethylation-mediated downregulation of antioxidant genes contributes to the early onset of cataracts in highly myopic eyes. *Redox Biol.* 19, 179–189. doi: 10.1016/j.redox.2018.08.012

Zhu, X., Meng, J., Wei, L., Zhang, K., He, W., and Lu, Y. (2020). Cilioretinal arteries and macular vasculature in highly myopic eyes. *Ophthalmol. Retina* 4, 965–972. doi: 10.1016/j.oret.2020.05.014

Zhu, X., Ye, H., He, W., Yang, J., Dai, J., and Lu, Y. (2017). Objective functional visual outcomes of cataract surgery in patients with good preoperative visual acuity. *Eye (Lond.)* 31, 452–459. doi: 10.1038/eye.2016.239

16

Generation and Staging of Human Retinal Organoids Based on Self-Formed Ectodermal Autonomous Multi-Zone System

Jinyan Li†, Yijia Chen†, Shuai Ouyang, Jingyu Ma, Hui Sun, Lixia Luo*, Shuyi Chen* and Yizhi Liu*

State Key Laboratory of Ophthalmology, Zhongshan Ophthalmic Center, Sun Yat-sen University, Guangzhou, China

Correspondence:
Lixia Luo
luolixia@mail.sysu.edu.cn
Shuyi Chen
chenshy23@mail.sysu.edu.cn
Yizhi Liu
liuyizh@mail.sysu.edu.cn

†These authors have contributed equally to this work

Methods for stem cell-derived, three-dimensional retinal organoids induction have been established and shown great potential for retinal development modeling and drug screening. Herein, we reported an exogenous-factors-free and robust method to generate retinal organoids based on "self-formed ectodermal autonomous multi-zone" (SEAM) system, a two-dimensional induction scheme that can synchronously generate multiple ocular cell lineages. Characterized by distinct morphological changes, the differentiation of the obtained retinal organoids could be staged into the early and late differentiation phases. During the early differentiation stage, retinal ganglion cells, cone photoreceptor cells (PRs), amacrine cells, and horizontal cells developed; whereas rod PRs, bipolar cells, and Müller glial cells were generated in the late differentiation phase, resembling early-phase and late-phase retinogenesis *in vivo*. Additionally, we modified the maintenance strategy for the retinal organoids and successfully promoted their long-term survival. Using 3D immunofluorescence image reconstruction and transmission electron microscopy, the substantial mature PRs with outer segment, inner segment and ribbon synapse were demonstrated. Besides, the retinal pigment epithelium (RPE) was induced with distinct boundary and the formation of ciliary margin was observed by co-suspending retina organoids with the zone containing RPE. The obtained RPE could be expanded and displayed similar marker expression, ultrastructural feature and functional phagocytosis to native RPE. Thus, this research described a simple and robust system which enabled generation of retina organoids with substantial mature PRs, RPE and the ciliary margin without the need of exogenous factors, providing a new platform for research of retinogenesis and retinal translational application.

Keywords: human retinal organoid, RPE, ciliary margin, photoreceptor cell, SEAM system, retinogenesis

INTRODUCTION

The human eye is composed of the refractive system (lens and cornea) and the visual neural system (retina). Being the sensory structure in the eye, the retina is highly stratified and retinogenesis is orchestrated by a series of networks of extrinsic and intrinsic signaling. During retinogenesis, the eye field first appears as an optic vesicle and eventually invaginates into a double-layered optic cup. The outer layer gives rise to the retinal pigment epithelium (RPE) and the inner layer becomes the neural retina (NR), which further form the lamellae that comprise the six retinal cell types (Chow and Lang, 2001).

Substantial progress has been made in the modeling of three-dimensional retinal organoids "in a dish." Up to now, existed retinal organoid induction strategies could be briefly divided into four categories, including direct 3D induction-based, embryoid body-based, lumen cyst-based and confluent adherent culture-based induction system (Meyer et al., 2009, 2011; Nakano et al., 2012; Reichman et al., 2014; Zhong et al., 2014; Mellough et al., 2015; Lowe et al., 2016; Sridhar et al., 2016; Gonzalez-Cordero et al., 2017; Wahlin et al., 2017; Hallam et al., 2018; Ovando-Roche et al., 2018; Phillips et al., 2018; Capowski et al., 2019; Shrestha et al., 2019; Pan et al., 2020; Regent et al., 2020; Zhang and Jin, 2021); these can mimic retinogenesis *in vitro* and have malignant application value (see the systematic reviews (Artero Castro et al., 2019; Jin et al., 2019; Kruczek and Swaroop, 2020; Nguyen et al., 2020; O'Hara-Wright and Gonzalez-Cordero, 2020; Sharma et al., 2020). To be noted that most of these existed protocols required various exogenous factors treatment, including growth factors and small-molecule inhibitors, which might render undesired complexity when applied for candidate signaling molecule research or drug screening (Hyun, 2010; Daley, 2012; Wan et al., 2015). Thus, we aimed to set up an exogenous-factors-free retina organoids construction system.

Nishida's research group reported an interesting two-dimensional induction system, termed "self-formed ectodermal autonomous multi-zones" (SEAMs) (Hayashi et al., 2016, 2017), which was capable of generating substantial colonies comprising multiple ocular lineages without the need of exogenous factors. The generated corneal components have the capacity to recover corneal function, indicating its potential for clinical translation of the SEAM system. Hence, we wondered whether substantial and mature retinal organoids could be also achieved by modifying the SEAM system.

In this study, we established a robust method for retinal organoids induction based on the SEAM system. After our modifications, three-dimensional retinal organoids were substantially induced without the need of exogenous factors. Moreover, we showed that the morphogenesis of the obtained organoids could be staged into two phases, resembling to early-phase and late-phase retinogenesis *in vivo*, and developed substantial mature PRs, spontaneous differentiated RPE as well as the ciliary margin like structure. Taken together, we herein reported an exogenous-factors-free and robust method for the induction of retinal organoids, which were additional to the field of retina organoid induction system and might be a powerful tool for retinogenesis modeling and drug screening.

MATERIALS AND METHODS

Human Embryonic Stem Cell Culture

The hESC H9 cell line was a generous gift from Xiaoyan Ding at the Institute of Biochemistry and Cell Biology, obtained from the National Stem Cell Bank (c/o WiCell Research Institute). The cells were cultured on Matrigel (BD Biosciences)-coated plates in mTeSR medium (STEMCELL Technologies). Cells were regularly passaged and approximately 4.5–6.0×10^4 cells per well were cultured in 6-well plates to promote colony formation.

Retinal Organoid Differentiation

The starting cell density was crucial, as a cell density either below 70% or above 90% affected the differentiation efficiency. hESCs were transferred to SEAM medium containing G-MEM (Gibco), 10% knockout serum replacement (KSR; Life Technologies), 0.1 mM non-essential amino acids (NEAA; Life Technologies), 1 mM sodium pyruvate (Life Technologies), 1% penicillin-streptomycin solution (PS; Life Technologies), and 55 μM 2-mercaptoethanol (Life Technologies) for the first Week 2–3 to form cell clusters. After colony formation, the induction medium was switched to retinal induction medium (RDM) containing DMEM: F12 3:1, 2% B-27 supplement (Thermo Fisher Scientific), 0.1 mM NEAA, and 1% PS. Around Week 4–6, the cup-like retina aggregates became visible and were isolated using fine forceps (Dumont) under a dissecting microscope. We modified the long-term suspension culture strategy by using low-attachment 96-well plates in RDM supplemented with 10% fetal bovine serum (FBS, HyClone), 100 mM taurine (Sigma) and 0.1 mM GlutaMAX (Life Technologies) (retinal maturation medium (RMM). All-*trans* retinoic acid (RA, 1 μM, Sigma) was additionally added after 2 weeks of suspension culture. An Axio Observer D1 microscope (Carl Zeiss) was used to acquire phase-contrast and bright-field images.

Retinal Pigment Epithelium Expansion

The RPE spheres were manually collected from the retinal organoids at Week 5–7. 10–20 spheres were digested with Accutase (Innovative Cell Technologies) at 37°C for 8 min into individualized cells and seeded into a Matrigel pre-coated well of a six-well plate. During the first week, RDM supplemented with 10% FBS and 100 mM taurine was used. When the cells reached to 100% confluence, FBS was removed from the medium, which was beneficial for RPE maturation. The medium was exchanged every 2–3 days.

Immunofluorescence Staining

Immunofluorescence staining of cells cultured on plates was performed as previously described (Han et al., 2018). In brief, cells were fixed in 4% paraformaldehyde (PFA; Sigma) at room temperature for 10 min and permeabilized with 0.5% Triton X-100 (Sigma) for 10 min. Cells were then blocked by 5% normal donkey serum (NDS; Jackson ImmunoResearch) for 30 min. Subsequently, the cells were incubated with primary antibodies overnight at 4°C, followed by incubation with the corresponding Alexa Fluor-conjugated secondary antibodies at room temperature for 1 h. The nuclei were counterstained with DAPI (Invitrogen). Fluorescence images were acquired using a ZEISS Axio Observer Z1 (Carl Zeiss).

The obtained retinal organoids were fixed in 4% PFA at 4°C overnight, and immersed in 15% sucrose followed by 30% sucrose in PBS before cryopreservation. The frozen sections were incubated in citrate buffer (pH 6.0) at 95°C for 30 min and cooled to room temperature for antigen retrieval. The sections were then incubated with primary antibody diluted in 5% NDS at 4°C overnight. After washing with PBS-Tween, the sections then were incubated with Alexa Fluor-conjugated secondary antibodies for 1 h. The nuclei were counterstained with DAPI. Fluorescence images were acquired with ZEISS LSM880 confocal microscope (Carl Zeiss).

For whole-mount immunocytochemistry, the organoids were fixed in 4% PFA at room temperature for 10 min. After washing with PBS containing 1% Triton X-100 (PBSTr), the organoids were rinsed with H_2O and treated with acetone at –20°C for 7 min. The organoids were incubated with the primary antibody diluted in PBSTr containing 10% NDS overnight at 4°C. On the following day, the organoids were washed with PBSTr (three times for 30 min). Incubation with the secondary antibody was performed at room temperature for 3 h. The nuclei were counterstained with DAPI. A ZEISS LSM880 confocal microscope were used to acquired fluorescence images using the Z-stack scan modes, and 3D reconstruction was performed by Zen software (Carl Zeiss). Alexa Fluor 488 or 568-conjugated donkey anti-rabbit, mouse, sheep or goat secondary antibodies (1:500; Invitrogen) were used. The primary antibodies, suppliers, and dilutions used are presented in **Supplementary Table 1**.

Transmission Electron Microscopy

Samples were fixed in EM fixative (2.5% glutaraldehyde/2% PFA) at 4°C and immediately sent for dehydration, embedding, sectioning and staining at Electron Microscopy Core Facility of Sun Yat-sen College of Medical Science, Sun Yat-sen University (Guangzhou, China). Ultrastructural analysis were performed by transmission electron microscope (Tecnai G2 Spirit; FEI, Inc., Carlsbad, CA, United States).

Phagocytosis Assay

Phagocytosis Assay was performed using 1 μm polystyrene FluoSpheres (Invitrogen) (Shrestha et al., 2020). In brief, confluent monolayers of RPE cells were incubated with FluoSpheres (cell counts/particles, around 1:100) at 37°C for 4 h. Then, the cultures were washed, fixed with 4% PFA and performed immunofluorescence staining as described above. Fluorescence images were acquired with ZEISS LSM880 confocal microscope.

Statistical Analysis

Statistical comparisons were conducted using GraphPad Prism (GraphPad software). All experiments were conducted at least in triplicate. The values are expressed as mean ± SEM (standard error of mean) or mean ± SD (standard deviation). $P < 0.05$ was considered statistically significant.

RESULTS

Robust Retinal Organoid Induction After Self-Formed Ectodermal Autonomous Multi-Zone System Modification

First, to examine how well the retinal fate was established in the SEAM system, we examined the expression of retina

development-related transcription factors in the SEAM system. As shown in **Figure 1A**, after approximately 2 weeks into the SEAM induction, cell aggregates had acquired eye field fate, expressing PAX6 and centrally located SIX3 (Bailey et al., 2004; Miesfeld and Brown, 2019). A few Chx10+ cells (a specific markers of retinal progenitor cells) were observed at this time (**Figure 1A'**), indicating the low efficiency of retinal fate induction. Hence, we wondered whether we could enhance the retinal fate induction by replacing the original SEAM medium with retinal differentiation medium (RDM), which is known to induce retinal progenitor cells (Zhong et al., 2014). As shown in **Figure 1B**, after RDM replacement, aggregates expressing neural progenitor marker SOX2 and OTX2 robustly emerged and gradually developed a horseshoe/dome-shaped structure. Compared with the original SEAM protocol, the use of RDM improved the number of clusters expressing OTX2, SOX2, and CHX10, which are crucial for retinal progenitor cell differentiation (**Figure 1C**; Livne-Bar et al., 2006; Danno et al., 2008).

After 3–4 weeks of differentiation, distinct colonies with multiple-zones had started to form. Cup-like structures were observed in the center of these colonies. The paracentrally distributed pigmentation were seen as well, surrounded by an identifiable border (**Figure 1D**). Immunofluorescence showed that the three-dimensional structure was CHX10-positive and the adjacent pigmented zone was MITF-positive, indicating the cell fate specification of NR and RPE, respectively (**Figure 1D'**; Bharti et al., 2008; Zou and Levine, 2012). Under RDM treatment, new retina organoids of various sizes emerged continuously from around week 4–6. After 40 days of differentiation, approximately 74 colonies with multiple-zones (±19, $n = 4$ technical replicates per well, in six-well plates) were harvested (**Figure 1E**). Thus, as illustrated in **Figure 1F**, without the need of exogenous factors, we achieved a substantial number of retinal organoids with RPE by modification of the SEAM protocol.

Staging of Retinal Organoid Morphogenesis

The cornea precursors cells in the SEAM system have been demonstrated their full potential to generate a mature corneal epithelium (Hayashi et al., 2016), but the retinal components have not. Thus, we next sought to investigate the differentiation capacity of the retinal organoids derived from the modified SEAM protocol. To normalize for the inconsistency of the retinal organoid formation, we defined the day of isolation of the suspension culture as Day 0.

The morphogenesis of retinal organoids was then documented. All organoids possessed a cup-like or horseshoe-like structure right after pinching (**Figure 2A**). As shown in **Figure 2B**, the organoids increased in size in the first 7–11 weeks, but with different growth rates. The growth rate was quantified by sphere size and neuroepithelium thickness. During the first 5–6 weeks, the organoids grew rapidly, with relatively slower growth afterward (**Figure 2C**). A similar increase was found for the thickness over the first 5 weeks; subsequently, it started to thin (**Figure 2D**). Moreover, the lamination of the neuroepithelium

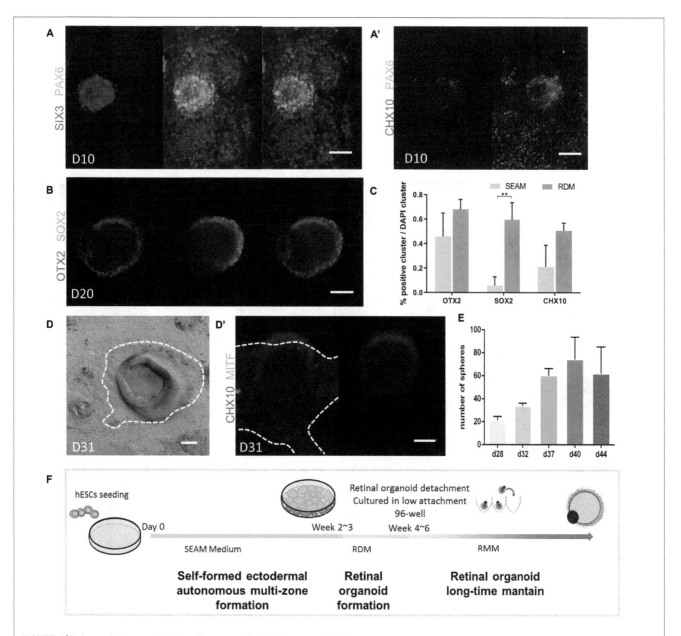

FIGURE 1 | Robust retinal organoids induced by the modified SEAM method. **(A,B)** Expression pattern of key transcription factors during the induction of retinal organoids. Immunofluorescent staining of eye field marker SIX3 (red) and PAX6 (green) on Day 10 **(A)**; the retinal progenitor cell marker CHX10 (red) on Day 10 **(A')**; the neural progenitor cell markers OTX2 (red) and SOX2 (green) on Day 20 **(B)**. Scale bar = 100 μm. **(C)** The ratio of OTX2-, SOX2-, and CHX10-labeled clusters to total clusters (marked by DAPI) on Day 28 in the SEAM- and RDM-treated groups, respectively. The bars represent the mean ± SEM. **P < 0.01 (n = 3).
(D) Bright-field imaging showing the derivation of cup-like neural structure and the surrounding pigment cell on Day 31. The identification of the retinal progenitor cell marker CHX10 (red, in the 3D cup-like neural structure) and retinal pigment epithelial cell marker MITF (green, at the bottom of the 3D cup-like neural structure) **(D')**. Scale bar = 100 μm. **(E)** Average number of retinal organoids obtained per well in 6-well plates on Day 28, Day 32, Day 37, Day 40, and Day 44 (n = 3).
(F) Schematic diagram of the induction of human retinal using the modified SEAM method.

was well-defined during the rapid growth period (before Week 6), and generally became blurred (**Figure 2E**). Along with the morphologic changes, immunostaining for Ki67 showed the extensive proliferative activity throughout the neuroepithelium in Week 3–7. As the maintenance time was prolonged, Ki67$^+$-cells could only be detected in the inner layer (Week 19) and were finally barely visible (**Figure 2F**), indicating the decreased proliferation of retinal cells. Hence, we defined two patterns of retinal organoids differentiation as early (Week 0–6/7) and late stage (after Week 6/7), respectively.

Early-Stage Differentiation Resembled Early-Phase Retinogenesis *in vivo*

Retinal cell differentiation follows an established pattern *in vivo*. Retinal ganglion cells (RGCs), cone photoreceptor cells (PRs),

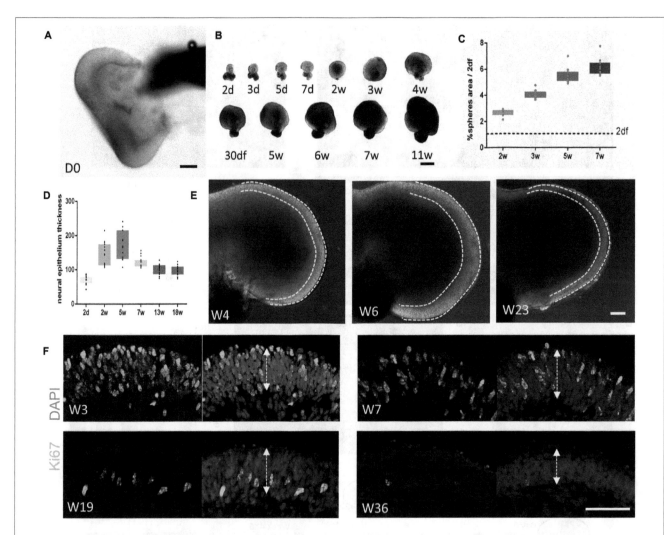

FIGURE 2 | Morphogenesis of retinal organoids. **(A)** Bright-field imaging showing the cup-like structure of the retinal organoid immediately after isolation. Scale bar = 100 µm. **(B)** Variation in the growth rate of retinal organoids at different time points. Scale bar = 500 µm. **(C,D)** The growth rate was quantified by sphere size [**(C)**, n = 10 retinal organoids from three independent experiments] and neural retina thickness [**(D)**, n = 15 retinal organoids from three independent experiments]. **(E)** Representative images at Week 4, Week 6, and Week 23 showing the changes in the thickness of the neural retina (dashed line). Scale bar = 100 µm. **(F)** Ki67 immunostaining of the neural retina at Week 3, Week 7, Week 19, and Week 36, indicating the downregulation of proliferation as differentiation proceeded. The neural retina thickness was measured as illustrated by the arrows. Scale bar = 50 µm.

horizontal cells, and amacrine cells originate from early retina progenitors in sequence (Jin and Xiang, 2017; O'Hara-Wright and Gonzalez-Cordero, 2020). In our system, BRN3$^+$/TUJ1$^+$ RGCs occurred first and were observed at 2 weeks after isolation. Subsequently, the number of BRN3$^+$ RGCs increased sharply, lining the innermost layer of neuroepithelium. However, we noticed that the number of RGCs decreased (**Figure 3A**). As shown in **Figure 3B**, compared to that of Week 5, the average ratio of BRN3 + cells versus total cells (marked by DAPI) of Week 8 was significantly decrease (36.32% ± 13.22% at Week 5 and 11.72% ± 5.7% at Week 8, respectively, n = 7 independent replicates).

CRX$^+$ cone PRs emerged after robust RGCs generation, starting from the basal side of the neuroepithelium and gradually migrating to the corresponding apical layers (**Figure 3C**). Furthermore, a small proportion of AP2α$^+$ amacrine cells and

AP2α$^+$/PROX1$^+$ horizontal cells (Zhong et al., 2014) were detected at Week 5, as further confirmed by CALBINDIN labeling (**Figures 3D,D'**). Therefore, these findings suggested that in early differentiation stage, RGCs, cone PRs, amacrine cells, and horizontal cells had developed, thus mimicking the early-born retinal lineage differentiation pattern during vertebrate retinogenesis.

Late-Stage Differentiation Recapitulated Late-Phase Retinogenesis *in vivo*

We continued to study the cellular dynamics of retinogenesis in the late-stage differentiation of our system. In addition to CRX$^+$ cells, a wave of Recoverin$^+$ cells were observed at the apical side at Week 13 (**Figure 4A**), implying the generation of rod PRs. CHX10 and SOX9 are markers of retinal progenitor cells

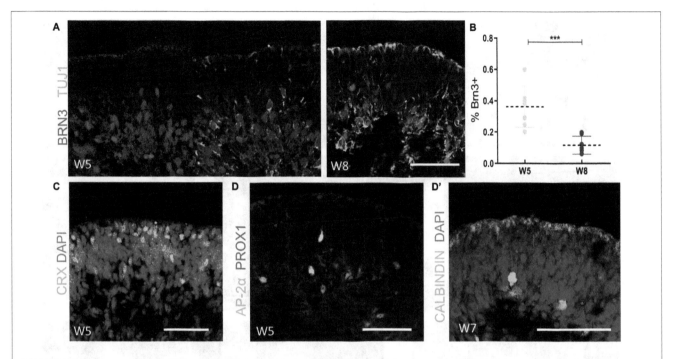

FIGURE 3 | The cellular composition of retinal organoids during the early-stage differentiation. **(A)** The cellular dynamics of retinal ganglion cells were marked at Week 5 (BRN3, red; TUJ1, green), and Week 8 (BRN3, red; TUJ1, green). **(B)** Statistics analysis of the ratio of BRN3 + cells versus total cells (marked by DAPI) at Week 5 and Week 8, respectively. Mean ± SD, ***P < 0.0005. **(C)** Localization of CRX$^+$ cone photoreceptor cells at Week 5. **(D)** The onset of AP2α + amacrine cells and AP2α$^+$/PROX1$^+$ horizontal cells were detected (AP-2α, green; PROX1-red) at Week 5 and confirmed by CALBINDIN (green, **D'**) staining at Week 7. Scale bar = 50 μm.

during development, and their expression are restricted to bipolar cells and Müller glial cells in the mature retina, respectively (Liu et al., 1994; Poche et al., 2008). In our system, CHX10- or SOX9-labeled retinal progenitor cells were found throughout the neuroepithelium until Week 5 (**Supplementary Figure 1A**). Their expression were gradually restricted in the deep, relative to the outermost layer during the late differentiation stage (**Supplementary Figure 1B**). CHX10$^+$/α-PKC$^+$ bipolar cells were generated at Week 18 and migrated to a progressively distinguishable layer, which was indicative of the developing presumptive inner nuclear layer (INL) (**Figure 4B**). In addition, a thin, nuclei-free layer was gradually established, in a position indicative of the outer plexiform layer (**Figure 4C**; Capowski et al., 2019). A few SOX9$^+$/GS$^+$ Müller glia cells could be detected at Week 23 (**Figure 4D**). Subsequently, more Müller glia cells were generated, confined to a near single layer of cells within the presumptive INL, with their projection extending to the outermost layer in a radial orientation (**Figure 4D'**). Collectively, these results suggested that during the late-stage differentiation, rod PRs, bipolar cells, and Müller glia cells were generated, with the development of the INL and the outer plexiform layer, which corresponded to late-born retina differentiation phase *in vivo*.

Efficient Long-Term Survival and Maturation of Photoreceptor Cells

To make retinal organoids capable of long-term survival, the maintenance protocol was further modified. As spheres in a

mixed suspension culture tend to adhere to each other, resulting in disruption of the laminar morphology, we transferred them into low-attachment 96-well plates after isolation to provide an undisturbed environment. It turned out this small change efficiently promoted survival, as well as reducing reagent costs.

At Week 21 (or earlier in some cases), the organoids began to grow hair-like microvilli on the surface, which has been shown to represent the developing PR outer segments (**Figures 5A,A'**; Gonzalez-Cordero et al., 2017; Phillips et al., 2018; Capowski et al., 2019). Most of the organoids were able to develop these hair-like surface appendages in the separated culture (**Figure 5B**). Indeed, expression of the cone PR marker Green/Red Opsin and the rod PR marker Rhodopsin clearly showed the typical morphogenesis of both types of PRs (**Figures 5C,D**). CRX$^+$/Arrestin 3$^+$ PRs were arranged in a continuous, uniform, 4/5-nuclei–thick layer when the outer segments formed (**Figure 5E,E'**). The vesicular transporter marker VGLUT1 was shown to be lining underneath Arrestin 3$^+$ cells, indicating that the PR synapse had been generated (**Figure 5F**). Transmission electron microscopy analysis showed that the hair-like microvilli, which extended through the outer limiting membrane, was found to contain mitochondria-rich inner segments-like and disk-containing rudimentary outer segments-like structures, indicating the maturation of photoreceptors (**Figures 5G, H**). Besides, ribbon synapse, a specialized form of synapse connecting photoreceptor cells, bipolar and the interneurons, was found at the basal side of photoreceptors (**Figures 5H, I**; Capowski et al., 2019). Taken

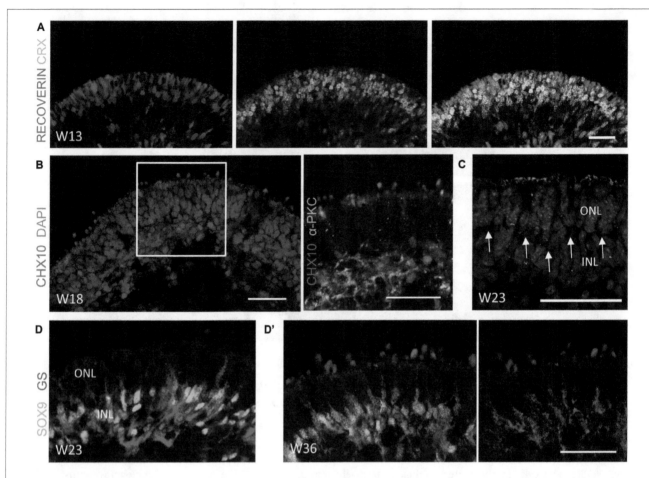

FIGURE 4 | The cellular composition of retinal organoids during the late-stage differentiation. **(A)** Robust derived cone and rod photoreceptor cells at Week 13 as indicated by CRX (green) and RECOVERIN (red), respectively. Scale bar = 100 μm. **(B)** The co-localization of CHX10 (red) and α-PKC (green) in the presumptive inner nuclear layer (INL), suggesting the generation of bipolar cells at Week 18. **(C)** The nuclei-free layer between the outer nuclear layer (ONL) and the INL was illustrated by DAPI immunostaining, indicating the outer plexiform layer (OPL, arrowhead). **(D)** Müller glial cells were detected at Week 23 and were rapidly generated at Week 36 **(D')**, as shown by immunostaining of the Müller glial cell markers SOX9 (green) and GS (red). Scale bar = 50 μm.

together, these results have demonstrated that the obtained retinal organoids were capable to develop photoreceptor cells with a high degree of maturation containing outer segment, inner segment and the synaptic connectivity between PR axon terminals and cells of the INL.

To have a comprehensive analysis of the distribution of rod and cone PRs in our retinal organoids, we performed whole-mount immunostaining using mature markers of both types of PRs. The 3D reconstruction showed the high performance of our retinal organoid induction protocol, as the external surface of our organoids was densely filled with needle-like mature rod and cone PRs. Furthermore, rod and cone PRs were unevenly distributed in our system (**Figures 6A,B** and **Supplementary Figure 2**). The fluorescence intensity assay showed that the rod PRs were mainly located in the RPE proximal part, whereas the cone PRs were in the distal part (**Figure 6B'**). The average ratio of the numbers of cone PRs versus rod PRs were 1.12 ($\pm$0.60, ranging 0.44–1.80, $n = 8$) in the proximal part and 4.56 ($\pm$2.29, ranging 1.34–8.54, $n = 8$) in the distal part, respectively (**Figure 6C**). Taken together, these results indicated

the potential of long-term survival and the maturation of the PRs obtained in our system.

Autonomous Generation of Retinal Pigment Epithelium and the Ciliary Margin

As the original SEAM system was able to generate multiple ocular cell lineages, we wondered whether we could produce other ocular cell lineages after modification. As shown in **Figure 7A**, when the centrally located retinal spheres were developing, the peripheral domain progressively formed three other identifiable concentric zones within 4–6 weeks. Unlike the original SEAM methods, cells in zone 1 were Chx10[+] NR progenitor cells and MITF[+] RPE-commitment cells were in zone 2, with a distinct boundary to other zones. Apart from that, the distribution of PAX6[+]/p63[+] corneal precursors in zone 3 and αA-crystallin[+]/PAX6[+] lens primordial cells at the margin of zones 2 and 3 was similar to that of the original SEAM system (**Supplementary Figure 3A**; Shibata et al., 2018).

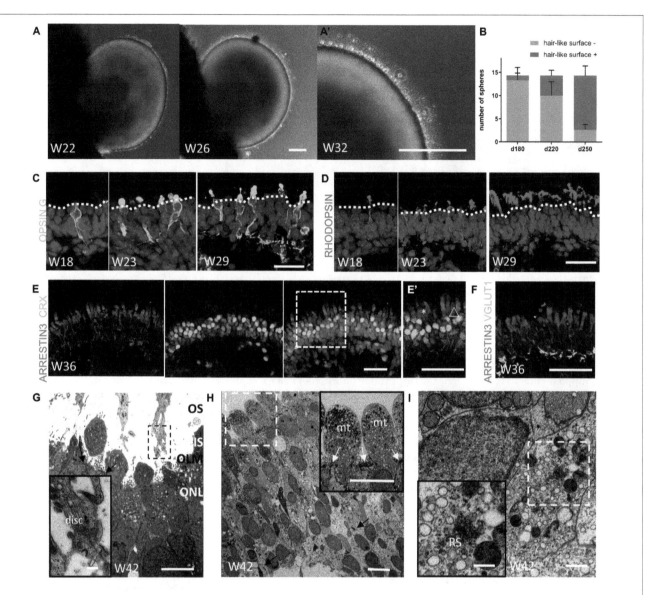

FIGURE 5 | Maturation of photoreceptor cells in retinal organoids. **(A)** Representative images showing the onset of hair-like microvilli on the surface of the retinal organoid at Week 22, Week 26, and **(A')** Week 32. Scale bar = 100 μm. **(B)** Progressive increase in the number of retinal organoids with hair-like microvilli (n = 3 independent experiments per group; each group contained 18, 12, and 13 retinal organoids, respectively). **(C,D)** Representative images showing the maturation of cone and rod PRs, as indicated by the mature PRs markers Opsin Green/Red **(C**, Opsin G/R, green) and RHODOPSIN **(D**, red) at Week 18, Week 23, and Week 29. Scale bar = 50 μm. **(E)** Immunofluorescent staining of the PR marker ARRESTIN 3 (red) and CRX (green) showed that a 4/5-nuclei–thick layer was formed. **(E')** Higher magnification of **(E)** showing the distinct morphology of the cone outer segment (asterisks) and the rod outer segment (triangle). Scale bar = 50 μm. **(F)** The co-staining of ARRESTIN 3 (red) and vesicular transporter marker VGLUT1 (green) indicated the formation of the PR synapse. Scale bar = 50 μm. **(G)** Electron microscopy showed the formation of outer segments-like (OS) and inner segments-like structure (IS), outer limiting membrane (OLM, indicated by black arrow) and outer nuclear layer (ONL). Scale bar = 5 μm. The insert image showed the infolding disk-like structure in OS. Scale bar = 0.5 μm. **(H)** The 4/5-nuclei–thick ONL was shown. The black arrow indicated that the ribbon synapses-like structure were present at basal side of photoreceptors. Scale bar = 10 μm. The insert image showed the mitochondria-rich inner segment-like structure. The white arrow indicated the OLM. Scale bar = 2 μm. **(I)** The clearer image of ribbon synapse-like structure (RS) was shown, surrounded by various vesicles. Scale bar = 500 nm (The insert image scale bar = 50 nm).

Therefore, by simply scratching the border around the underlying RPE domain (zone 2), it was simple to obtain retinal organoids suspended with the RPE-commitment cells. As illustrated in **Figure 7B**, isolation of zone 1–3 yielded retinal organoids with a 64% frequency (±14%, n = 3) of RPE spheres on Day 78, which was significantly higher than that without isolation of zone 2. Moreover, 21% (±6%, n = 3)

of lens/corneal spheres could be harvested (**Figure 7B** and **Supplementary Figure 3B**). Hence, these results demonstrated that the simultaneous differentiation of retinal organoids and RPE was achieved in our system.

Given that the interaction of NR and RPE during retinogenesis is crucial for the development of the ciliary margin (CM) *in vivo* (Cicero et al., 2009; Fischer et al., 2013), we examined

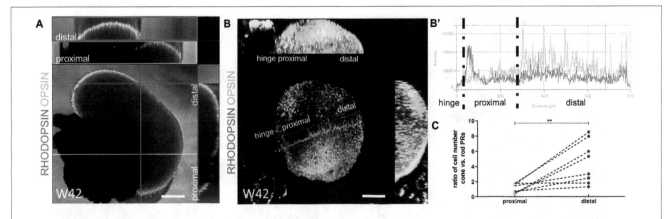

FIGURE 6 | The uneven distribution of rod and cone photoreceptor cells. **(A)** The ortho X-Z display of a random section of the organoid at Week 42 showed that the hinge distal part was mainly composed of cone PRs (Opsin B/G/R, green, purple frame) and rod PRs (Rhodopsin, red, green frame) mainly located at the hinge proximal part. **(B)** Ortho display of maximum intensity projection of the whole organoid at Week 42. The fluorescence intensity from the hinge proximal to distal part (marker by the red box) was calculated in **(B')**. Scale bar = 200 μm. **(C)** The ratio of the numbers of cone PRs versus rod PRs were paired calculated in the proximal and distal part, respectively. **P < 0.005.

the morphological dynamics of retinal organoids coupled with RPE spheres. During the first few days after zone 1–3 suspension, these semi-spherical aggregates gradually became spherical (**Supplementary Figure 3C**). As the suspension culture proceeded, part of the NR that was adjacent to the presumptive RPE region, extended, grew increasingly thinner, and finally obtained peripheral-NR-like morphology (**Figure 7C**), consistent with the researches of CM induction (Kuwahara et al., 2015; Kinoshita et al., 2016). Finally, a distinct extended domain expressing PAX6[+]/CX43[+] (markers of the CM) were clearly observed at the junction between the NR and the RPE, indicating the formation of the CM-like structure in the retinal organoids (**Figure 7D**). Collectively, these results indicated that our retina organoid induction system enabled the simultaneous generation of RPE and the CM.

Expansion and Validation of Retinal Pigment Epithelium Differentiation Capacity

Given the translational value of RPE induction, the differentiation and expansion capacity of the RPE component were further examined. We isolated the RPE spheres from retinal organoids at Week 5–7, when the RPE spheres could be clearly distinguished. The collected RPE spheres were then digested into small clusters and seeded. Consistent with previous reports (Hu et al., 2010; Liu et al., 2018), these cells proliferated vigorously and reached 100% confluence within 1 week, accompanied by pigment loss (**Figure 8A**). An increasing number of cells exhibited typical polygonal appearance in the following 2–4 weeks and the re-pigmentation gradually occurred in these cells with phase-bright borders, forming a honeycomb monolayer (**Figure 8B**). After that, spontaneously formed elevated domes were observed, suggesting the formation of apical-basal polarization and the underlying barrier function of RPE (**Figure 8B'**; Hu et al., 2010). Immunofluorescence analysis showed that the cells expressed naive RPE markers OTX2 and PAX6 in the first week during

RPE expansion, but were negative for RPE65 (a mature RPE marker) (**Figure 8C**). The expression of RPE65 was detected when pigmentation re-appeared in cells, coupled with MITF and ZO-1 expression, indicating the maturation of RPE at this time (**Figure 8D**). Transmission electron microscopy showed that the RPE has developed microvilli and the abundant apical tight junctions (**Figures 8E,F**; Liu et al., 2018). Additionally, as shown in **Figure 8G**, through phagocytosis assay, we found that the RPE sheet was able to phagocytose polystyrene FluoSpheres, suggesting the functional ability of phagocytosis. In conclusion, mature and functional RPE could be yielded through the expansion of RPE spheres obtain from retinal organoids.

DISCUSSION

The SEAM system was reported as a two-dimensional eye-like colonies induction system without exogenous factors treatment. In the present study, our attempts showed that by improving the retinal components in the SEAM system, substantial 3D retinal organoids could be induced without the need of exogenous factors.

The differentiation of obtained retina oganoids mimics the early and late-phase of retinogenesis *in vivo*. From the morphologic changes observed under the microscope, two development stages with different growth rates could be defined. The early differentiation stage was characterized by a well-defined laminar neural epithelium and rapid growth rate, with ongoing thickness compression and relatively slower proliferation in the late differentiation stage. During retinogenesis *in vivo*, the differentiation capacity of neuroepithelial progenitors gradually changed; they tend to be restricted to the production of two or three types of cells at different stages, termed early- and late-phase retinogenesis (Livesey and Cepko, 2001; Bassett and Wallace, 2012). In our system, we found the development of RGCs, cone PRs, horizontal cells, and amacrine cells in the early differentiation stage; whereas in late stage, the

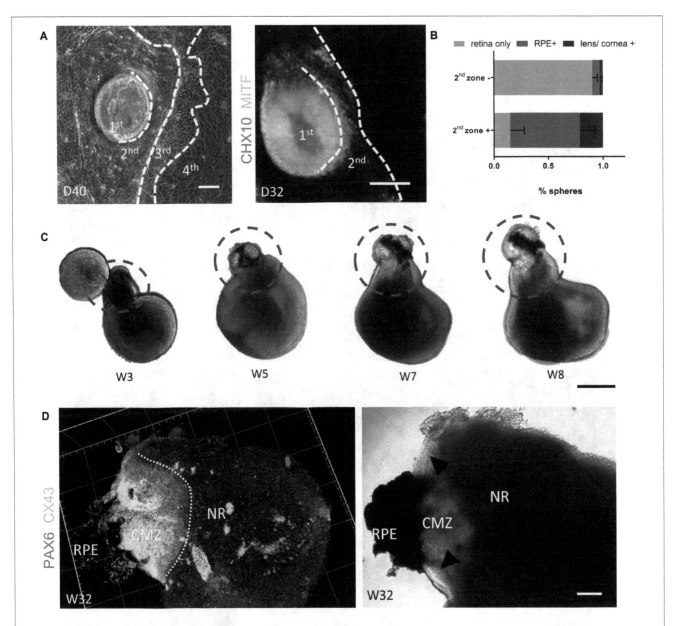

FIGURE 7 | Autonomous generation of the retinal pigment epithelium and the ciliary margin. **(A)** Representative images showed the autonomous formation of a four concentric-zone cluster. Immunofluorescent staining showed that zone 1 and zone 2 were CHX10- (green) and MITF- (red) positive, respectively. Scale bar = 100 μm. **(B)** Compared with isolation without zone 2 [zone 2 (–)], isolation of retinal organoids with zone 2 [zone 2 (+)] generated more RPE spheres (n = 3 independent experiments per group; each group contained 20 or more retinal organoids). **(C)** Representative images showing the gradual formation of the peripheral neural retina between the neural retina and the RPE (dashed circle). Scale bar = 500 μm. **(D)** Co-staining of the ciliary margin marker PAX6 (green) and CX43 (red) confirmed the generation of ciliary margin zone at Week 32 (triangle). Scale bar = 200 μm.

occurrence of rod PRs, bipolar cells, and Müller glial cells were observed, resembling the early-born and late-born retinal lineages differentiation *in vivo*. Considering the great potential of retinal organoids in retinal replacement therapies, our study suggested that the underlying limited differentiation capacity should be taken into consideration when performing translational research using retinal organoids-derived retinal progenitor cells. To be noted that the efficiency of our protocol was based on hESC H9 cell line, the induction of other source of ESCs/iPSCs needs further test.

Along with retina organoid, our system enabled the spontaneous induction of RPE and ciliary margin-like domain. The interaction between the NR and the RPE is crucial for the ciliary margin formation, a potential retinal stem cells region in adult retina (Bhatia et al., 2010; Fischer et al., 2013). The Sasai group has previously developed an *in vitro* method for the co-induction of retinal organoids and the RPE that generates the CM. However, precise control of treatment time and drug dose are required, making it hard to replicate the results. We herein showed that the RPE could be co-induced

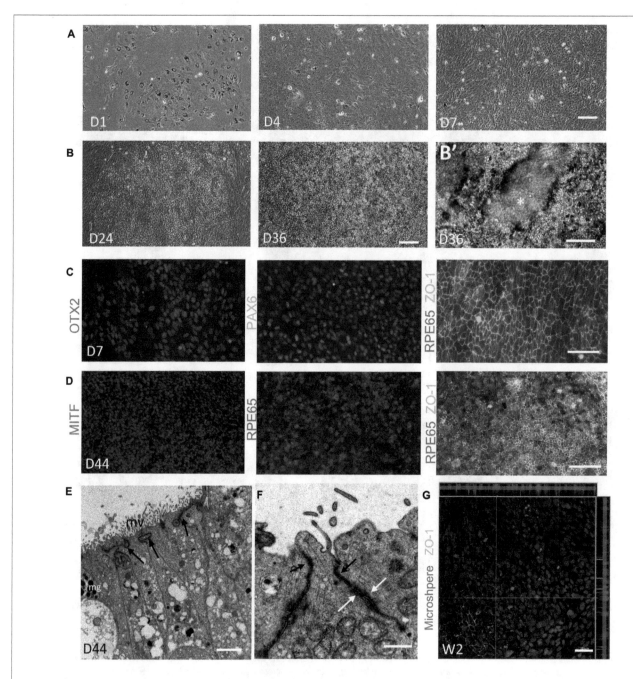

FIGURE 8 | Expansion and validation of the retina pigment epithelium (RPE). **(A,B)** Representative images showing the expansion and pigmentation loss of the RPE on Day 1, Day 4, and Day 7 **(A)**; and the re-pigmentation on Day 24 and Day 36 **(B)**. **(B')** Higher magnification images showing the formation of elevated domes (asterisks). **(C)** Expression of the naïve RPE marker OTX2 (red, left), PAX6 (green, middle) and the RPE marker ZO-1 (green, right) was shown on Day 7, while the mature RPE marker RPE65 (red, right) was not found. **(D)** On Day 44, RPE65 (red, left) coupled with the RPE marker MITF (red, middle) and ZO-1 (green, right) indicated the maturation of the RPE. Scale bar = 100 μm. **(E)** Electron microscopy showed that on Day 44, RPE sheet has developed melanin granules (mg), microvilli (mv) and the abundant tight junctions at the apical side (indicated by black arrow). Scale bar = 2 μm. **(F)** Different cell junctions of RPE were clearly shown (apical tight junctions, indicated by black arrow; desmosomes, indicated by white arrow). Scale bar = 500 nm. **(G)** Phagocytosis assay showed that the 2-week-old RPE sheets, labeled by ZO-1 (green), were able to phagocytose FluoroSpheres (red). Scale bar = 20 μm.

in a recognizable domain, termed as zone 2, adjacent to the retinal organoid zone (zone 1) after modification based on SEAM method. By simply isolating zone 1 and zone 2, we could simultaneously induce retina organoids along with the RPE. Later, the interaction between the NR and the RPE domains resulted in the gradual formation of a CM-like domain at the NR-RPE boundary. Moreover, the obtained RPE spheres could be expanded and displayed similar marker expression, ultrastructural feature as native RPE, and exhibited the functional ability of phagocytosis. The presence of abundant apical tight junction and the elevated domes suggested that to some extent, our RPE sheets might be able to function as biological barrier. More biological characterization such as transepithelial resistance measurement is needed to verify the function of our RPE sheets. Taken together, we have established an exogenous-factors-free retinal organoid induction system, which also enabled the spontaneous generation of RPE and ciliary margin.

With the use of low-attachment microwell plates, we have improved the long-term survival rate, so as to improve the efficiency of obtaining retinal organoids with hair-like surface appendages, which indicated the developing PR outer segment. The gain of opsin expression, the patterned outer-segment formation, and the onset of phototransduction are considered to be hallmarks of the terminal differentiation of PRs (Swaroop et al., 2010). We herein have presented the morphological changes from precursors to the terminal differentiation of both PR types in our system, starting from the time when the outer-segment began to form. Moreover, unlike previous rod-cone analysis performed on slide sections, which may induce bias, we developed whole-mount staining and 3D reconstruction imaging to analyze the long-term maintained retina organoids. Combining the result of whole-mount staining and electron microscopy, it turned out that substantial mature PRs has developed, which contained mitochondria-rich inner segments-like, disk-containing rudimentary outer segments-like, and ribbon synapse structures. Additionally, the rod and cone PRs were unevenly distributed. To some extent, this may be related to the distance from NR-RPE hinge. We showed that rod PRs were mainly located in the hinge proximal region, while cone PRs occurred more frequently in the distal region; these were correlated with PR distribution *in vivo* (Szel et al., 2000).

Owing to the limitations of *in vitro* culture system, generating retinal organoid with microglia remains an unsolved problem (Cora et al., 2019; Zerti et al., 2020). In our induction system, we have found the expression of mesodermal marker Brachyury and classical microglia marker IBA1 in some cases (**Supplementary Figure 3D**), suggesting the presence of mesodermal progenitors and the transition status from mesodermal progenitors to microglia-like cells. However, they were located at the bottom of the NR spheres and no sign of migration into the inner retina

was observed (Li et al., 2019). More attempts to verify the identity of these IBA1-expressing microglia is needed. In this regard, our integration of retinal generation with other ocular component may be a new solution for retinal organoid optimization.

Retinal organoid is a powerful system for the modeling of developmental mechanisms, for the testing and screening of drugs, and for the investigation of retinal replacement. Our exogenous-factors-free system features several advantages such as the fine reproducibility and repeatability, as well as the lower cost. Besides, when it comes to the application of our system, unpredictable cross reactivity with candidate signaling pathway, small molecule or drug could be minimum due to the absence of exogenous factor during retinal organoid induction.

In summary, we have established a simple and robust retinal organoid induction system based on the SEAM method. The overview of the cellular dynamics of the obtained retinal organoids presented above has demonstrated the potential to mimic early-phase and late-phase retinogenesis *in vivo*. In addition, our further modifications has enabled the generation of substantial mature PRs, the simultaneously induced RPE and the CM. Thus, we believe our exogenous-factors-free system may be a valuable new platform for studying retinogenesis and retinal translational application.

AUTHOR CONTRIBUTIONS

LL, SC, and YL contributed to conceptualization. JL and YC performed the induction experiments and writing. SO analyzed the data. JM performed the immunofluorescence staining imaging. HS maintained the induction system. All authors contributed to the article and approved the submitted version.

ACKNOWLEDGMENTS

We thank Xiaoyan Ding (Chinese Academy of Sciences, China) and Hong Ouyang (Sun Yat-sen University, China) for the generous gift of the hESC H9 cell line and p63 antibody, respectively. We also thank Guilan Li (Sun Yat-sen University, China) for retinal organoids induction assistance.

REFERENCES

Artero Castro, A., Rodriguez Jimenez, F. J., Jendelova, P., and Erceg, S. (2019). Deciphering retinal diseases through the generation of three dimensional stem cell-derived organoids: concise Review. *Stem Cells* 37, 1496–1504.

Bailey, T. J., El-Hodiri, H., Zhang, L., Shah, R., Mathers, P. H., and Jamrich, M. (2004). Regulation of vertebrate eye development by Rx genes. *Int. J. Dev. Biol.* 48, 761–770. doi: 10.1387/ijdb.041878tb

Bassett, E. A., and Wallace, V. A. (2012). Cell fate determination in the vertebrate retina. *Trends Neurosci.* 35, 565–573. doi: 10.1016/j.tins.2012.05.004

Bharti, K., Liu, W., Csermely, T., Bertuzzi, S., and Arnheiter, H. (2008). Alternative promoter use in eye development: the complex role and regulation of the transcription factor MITF. *Development* 135, 1169–1178. doi: 10.1242/dev.014142

Bhatia, B., Singhal, S., Jayaram, H., Khaw, P. T., and Limb, G. A. (2010). Adult retinal stem cells revisited. *Open Ophthalmol. J.* 4, 30–38. doi: 10.2174/1874364101004010030

Capowski, E. E., Samimi, K., Mayerl, S. J., Phillips, M. J., Pinilla, I., Howden, S. E., et al. (2019). Reproducibility and staging of 3D human retinal organoids across multiple pluripotent stem cell lines. *Development* 146:dev171686. doi: 10.1242/dev.171686

Chow, R. L., and Lang, R. A. (2001). Early eye development in vertebrates. *Annu. Rev. Cell Dev. Biol.* 17, 255–296. doi: 10.1146/annurev.cellbio.17.1.255

Cicero, S. A., Johnson, D., Reyntjens, S., Frase, S., Connell, S., Chow, L. M., et al. (2009). Cells previously identified as retinal stem cells are pigmented ciliary epithelial cells. *Proc. Natl. Acad. Sci. U. S. A.* 106, 6685–6690. doi: 10.1073/pnas.0901596106

Cora, V., Haderspeck, J., Antkowiak, L., Mattheus, U., Neckel, P. H., Mack, A. F., et al. (2019). A Cleared View on Retinal Organoids. *Cells* 8:391. doi: 10.3390/cells8050391

Daley, G. Q. (2012). The promise and perils of stem cell therapeutics. *Cell Stem Cell* 10, 740–749. doi: 10.1016/j.stem.2012.05.010

Danno, H., Michiue, T., Hitachi, K., Yukita, A., Ishiura, S., and Asashima, M.

(2008). Molecular links among the causative genes for ocular malformation: Otx2 and Sox2 coregulate Rax expression. *Proc. Natl. Acad. Sci. U. S. A.* 105, 5408–5413. doi: 10.1073/pnas.0710954105

Fischer, A. J., Bosse, J. L., and El-Hodiri, H. M. (2013). The ciliary marginal zone (CMZ) in development and regeneration of the vertebrate eye. *Exp. Eye Res.* 116, 199–204. doi: 10.1016/j.exer.2013.08.018

Gonzalez-Cordero, A., Kruczek, K., Naeem, A., Fernando, M., Kloc, M., Ribeiro, J., et al. (2017). Recapitulation of Human Retinal Development from Human Pluripotent Stem Cells Generates Transplantable Populations of Cone Photoreceptors. *Stem Cell Rep.* 9, 820–837. doi: 10.1016/j.stemcr.2017.07.022

Hallam, D., Hilgen, G., Dorgau, B., Zhu, L., Yu, M., Bojic, S., et al. (2018). Human-Induced Pluripotent Stem Cells Generate Light Responsive Retinal Organoids with Variable and Nutrient-Dependent Efficiency. *Stem Cells* 36, 1535–1551. doi: 10.1002/stem.2883

Han, C., Li, J., Wang, C., Ouyang, H., Ding, X., Liu, Y., et al. (2018). Wnt5a Contributes to the Differentiation of Human Embryonic Stem Cells into Lentoid Bodies Through the Noncanonical Wnt/JNK Signaling Pathway. *Invest. Ophthalmol. Vis. Sci.* 59, 3449–3460. doi: 10.1167/iovs.18-23902

Hayashi, R., Ishikawa, Y., Katori, R., Sasamoto, Y., Taniwaki, Y., Takayanagi, H., et al. (2017). Coordinated generation of multiple ocular-like cell lineages and fabrication of functional corneal epithelial cell sheets from human iPS cells. *Nat. Protoc.* 12, 683–696. doi: 10.1038/nprot.2017.007

Hayashi, R., Ishikawa, Y., Sasamoto, Y., Katori, R., Nomura, N., Ichikawa, T., et al. (2016). Co-ordinated ocular development from human iPS cells and recovery of corneal function. *Nature.* 531, 376–380. doi: 10.1038/nature17000

Hu, Q., Friedrich, A. M., Johnson, L. V., and Clegg, D. O. (2010). Memory in induced pluripotent stem cells: reprogrammed human retinal-pigmented epithelial cells show tendency for spontaneous redifferentiation. *Stem Cells* 28, 1981–1991. doi: 10.1002/stem.531

Hyun, I. (2010). The bioethics of stem cell research and therapy. *J. Clin. Invest.* 120, 71–75. doi: 10.1172/JCI40435

Jin, K., and Xiang, M. (2017). Transitional Progenitors during Vertebrate Retinogenesis. *Mol. Neurobiol.* 54, 3565–3576. doi: 10.1007/s12035-016-9899-x

Jin, Z. B., Gao, M. L., Deng, W. L., Wu, K. C., Sugita, S., Mandai, M., et al. (2019). Stemming retinal regeneration with pluripotent stem cells. *Prog. Retin. Eye Res.* 69, 38–56. doi: 10.1016/j.preteyeres.2018.11.003

Kinoshita, H., Suzuma, K., Kaneko, J., Mandai, M., Kitaoka, T., and Takahashi, M. (2016). Induction of Functional 3D Ciliary Epithelium-Like Structure From Mouse Induced Pluripotent Stem Cells. *Invest. Ophthalmol. Vis. Sci.* 57, 153–161. doi: 10.1167/iovs.15-17610

Kruczek, K., and Swaroop, A. (2020). Pluripotent stem cell-derived retinal organoids for disease modeling and development of therapies. *Stem Cells* 38, 1206–1215. doi: 10.1002/stem.3239

Kuwahara, A., Ozone, C., Nakano, T., Saito, K., Eiraku, M., and Sasai, Y. (2015). Generation of a ciliary margin-like stem cell niche from self-organizing human retinal tissue. *Nat. Commun.* 6:6286. doi: 10.1038/ncomms7286

Li, F., Jiang, D., and Samuel, M. A. (2019). Microglia in the developing retina. *Neural Dev.* 14:12. doi: 10.1186/s13064-019-0137-x

Liu, I. S., Chen, J. D., Ploder, L., Vidgen, D., van der Kooy, D., Kalnins, V. I., et al. (1994). Developmental expression of a novel murine homeobox gene (Chx10): evidence for roles in determination of the neuroretina and inner nuclear layer. *Neuron* 13, 377–393. doi: 10.1016/0896-6273(94)90354-9

Liu, S., Xie, B., Song, X., Zheng, D., He, L., Li, G., et al. (2018). Self-Formation of RPE Spheroids Facilitates Enrichment and Expansion of hiPSC-Derived RPE Generated on Retinal Organoid Induction Platform. *Invest. Ophthalmol. Vis. Sci.* 59, 5659–5669. doi: 10.1167/iovs.17-23613

Livesey, F. J., and Cepko, C. L. (2001). Vertebrate neural cell-fate determination: lessons from the retina. *Nat. Rev. Neurosci.* 2, 109–118. doi: 10.1038/35053522

Livne-Bar, I., Pacal, M., Cheung, M. C., Hankin, M., Trogadis, J., Chen, D., et al. (2006). Chx10 is required to block photoreceptor differentiation but is dispensable for progenitor proliferation in the postnatal retina. *Proc. Natl. Acad. Sci. U. S. A.* 103, 4988–4993. doi: 10.1073/pnas.0600083103

Lowe, A., Harris, R., Bhansali, P., Cvekl, A., and Liu, W. (2016). Intercellular Adhesion-Dependent Cell Survival and ROCK-Regulated Actomyosin-Driven Forces Mediate Self-Formation of a Retinal Organoid. *Stem Cell Rep.* 6, 743–756. doi: 10.1016/j.stemcr.2016.03.011

Mellough, C. B., Collin, J., Khazim, M., White, K., Sernagor, E., Steel, D. H., et al. (2015). IGF-1 Signaling Plays an Important Role in the Formation of Three-

Dimensional Laminated Neural Retina and Other Ocular Structures From Human Embryonic Stem Cells. *Stem Cells* 33, 2416–2430. doi: 10.1002/stem.2023

Meyer, J. S., Howden, S. E., Wallace, K. A., Verhoeven, A. D., Wright, L. S., Capowski, E. E., et al. (2011). Optic vesicle-like structures derived from human pluripotent stem cells facilitate a customized approach to retinal disease treatment. *Stem Cells* 29, 1206–1218. doi: 10.1002/stem.674

Meyer, J. S., Shearer, R. L., Capowski, E. E., Wright, L. S., Wallace, K. A., McMillan, E. L., et al. (2009). Modeling early retinal development with human embryonic and induced pluripotent stem cells. *Proc. Natl. Acad. Sci U. S. A.* 106, 16698–16703. doi: 10.1073/pnas.0905245106

Miesfeld, J. B., and Brown, N. L. (2019). Eye organogenesis: a hierarchical view of ocular development. *Curr. Top. Dev. Biol.* 132, 351–393. doi: 10.1016/bs.ctdb.2018.12.008

Nakano, T., Ando, S., Takata, N., Kawada, M., Muguruma, K., Sekiguchi, K., et al. (2012). Self-formation of optic cups and storable stratified neural retina from human ESCs. *Cell Stem Cell* 10, 771–785. doi: 10.1016/j.stem.2012.05.009

Nguyen, T., Urrutia-Cabrera, D., Liou, R. H., Luu, C. D., Guymer, R., and Wong, R. C. (2020). New Technologies to Study Functional Genomics of Age-Related Macular Degeneration. *Front. Cell Dev. Biol.* 8:604220. doi: 10.3389/fcell.2020.604220

O'Hara-Wright, M., and Gonzalez-Cordero, A. (2020). Retinal organoids: a window into human retinal development. *Development* 147:dev189746. doi: 10.1242/dev.189746

Ovando-Roche, P., West, E. L., Branch, M. J., Sampson, R. D., Fernando, M., Munro, P., et al. (2018). Use of bioreactors for culturing human retinal organoids improves photoreceptor yields. *Stem Cell Res. Ther.* 9:156. doi: 10.1186/s13287-018-0907-0

Pan, D., Xia, X. X., Zhou, H., Jin, S. Q., Lu, Y. Y., Liu, H., et al. (2020). COCO enhances the efficiency of photoreceptor precursor differentiation in early human embryonic stem cell-derived retinal organoids. *Stem Cell Res. Ther.* 11:366. doi: 10.1186/s13287-020-01883-5

Phillips, M. J., Capowski, E. E., Petersen, A., Jansen, A. D., Barlow, K., Edwards, K. L., et al. (2018). Generation of a rod-specific NRL reporter line in human pluripotent stem cells. *Sci. Rep.* 8:2370. doi: 10.1038/s41598-018-20813-3

Poche, R. A., Furuta, Y., Chaboissier, M. C., Schedl, A., and Behringer, R. R. (2008). Sox9 is expressed in mouse multipotent retinal progenitor cells and functions in Muller glial cell development. *J. Comp. Neurol.* 510, 237–250. doi: 10.1002/cne.21746

Regent, F., Chen, H. Y., Kelley, R. A., Qu, Z., Swaroop, A., and Li, T. (2020). A simple and efficient method for generating human retinal organoids. *Mol. Vis.* 26, 97–105.

Reichman, S., Terray, A., Slembrouck, A., Nanteau, C., Orieux, G., Habeler, W., et al. (2014). From confluent human iPS cells to self-forming neural retina and retinal pigmented epithelium. *Proc. Natl. Acad. Sci. U. S. A.* 111, 8518–8523. doi: 10.1073/pnas.1324212111

Sharma, K., Krohne, T. U., and Busskamp, V. (2020). The Rise of Retinal Organoids for Vision Research. *Int. J. Mol. Sci.* 21:8484. doi: 10.3390/ijms21228484

Shibata, S., Hayashi, R., Okubo, T., Kudo, Y., Katayama, T., Ishikawa, Y., et al. (2018). Selective Laminin-Directed Differentiation of Human Induced Pluripotent Stem Cells into Distinct Ocular Lineages. *Cell Rep.* 25, 1668–1679.e5. doi: 10.1016/j.celrep.2018.10.032

Shrestha, R., Wen, Y. T., Ding, D. C., and Tsai, R. K. (2019). Aberrant hiPSCs-Derived from Human Keratinocytes Differentiates into 3D Retinal Organoids that Acquire Mature Photoreceptors. *Cells* 8:36. doi: 10.3390/cells8010036

Shrestha, R., Wen, Y. T., and Tsai, R. K. (2020). Effective Differentiation and Biological Characterization of Retinal Pigment Epithelium Derived from Human Induced Pluripotent Stem Cells. *Curr. Eye Res.* 45, 1155–1167. doi: 10.1080/02713683.2020.1722180

Sridhar, A., Ohlemacher, S. K., Langer, K. B., and Meyer, J. S. (2016). Robust Differentiation of mRNA-Reprogrammed Human Induced Pluripotent Stem Cells Toward a Retinal Lineage. *Stem Cells Transl. Med.* 5, 417–426. doi: 10.5966/sctm.2015-0093

Swaroop, A., Kim, D., and Forrest, D. (2010). Transcriptional regulation of photoreceptor development and homeostasis in the mammalian retina. *Nat. Rev. Neurosci.* 11, 563–576. doi: 10.1038/nrn2880

Szel, A., Lukats, A., Fekete, T., Szepessy, Z., and Rohlich, P. (2000). Photoreceptor distribution in the retinas of subprimate mammals. *J. Opt. Soc. Am. A Opt. Image Sci. Vis.* 17, 568–579. doi: 10.1364/josaa.17.000568

Wahlin, K. J., Maruotti, J. A., Sripathi, S. R., Ball, J., Angueyra, J. M., Kim, C., et al. (2017). Photoreceptor Outer Segment-like Structures in Long-Term 3D Retinas from Human Pluripotent Stem Cells. *Sci. Rep.* 7:766. doi: 10.1038/s41598-017-00774-9

Wan, P. X., Wang, B. W., and Wang, Z. C. (2015). Importance of the stem cell microenvironment for ophthalmological cell-based therapy. *World J. Stem Cells* 7, 448–460. doi: 10.4252/wjsc.v7.i2.448

Zerti, D., Collin, J., Queen, R., Cockell, S. J., and Lako, M. (2020). Understanding the complexity of retina and pluripotent stem cell derived retinal organoids with single cell RNA sequencing: current progress, remaining challenges and future prospective. *Curr. Eye Res.* 45, 385–396. doi: 10.1080/02713683.2019.1697453

Zhang, X., and Jin, Z. B. (2021). Directed Induction of Retinal Organoids from Human Pluripotent Stem Cells. *J. Vis. Exp.* 2021:e62298. doi: 10.3791/62298

Zhong, X., Gutierrez, C., Xue, T., Hampton, C., Vergara, M. N., Cao, L. H., et al. (2014). Generation of three-dimensional retinal tissue with functional photoreceptors from human iPSCs. *Nat. Commun.* 5:4047. doi: 10.1038/ncomms5047

Zou, C., and Levine, E. M. (2012). Vsx2 controls eye organogenesis and retinal progenitor identity via homeodomain and non-homeodomain residues required for high affinity DNA binding. *PLoS Genet.* 8:e1002924. doi: 10.1371/journal.pgen.1002924

17

The Regulatory NOD-Like Receptor NLRC5 Promotes Ganglion Cell Death in Ischemic Retinopathy by Inducing Microglial Pyroptosis

Yang Deng[†], Yunzhao Fu[†], Longxiang Sheng[†], Yixin Hu, Lishi Su, Jiawen Luo, Chun Yan and Wei Chi*

State Key Laboratory of Ophthalmology, Zhongshan Ophthalmic Center, Sun Yat-sen University, Guangzhou, China

*Correspondence:
Wei Chi
chiwei@mail.sysu.edu.cn
[†] These authors have contributed equally to this work

Retinal ischemia is a common pathological event that can result in retinal ganglion cell (RGC) death and irreversible vision loss. The pathogenic mechanisms linking retinal ischemia to RGC loss and visual deficits are uncertain, which has greatly hampered the development of effective treatments. It is increasingly recognized that pyroptosis of microglia contributes to the indirect inflammatory death of RGCs. In this study, we report a regulatory NOD-like receptor, NOD-, LRR- and CARD-containing 5 (NLRC5), as a key regulator on microglial pyroptosis and the retinal ischemia process. Through an in-depth analysis of our recently published transcriptome data, we found that NLRC5 was significantly up-regulated in retina during ischemia–reperfusion injury, which were further confirmed by subsequent detection of mRNA and protein level. We further found that NLRC5 was upregulated in retinal microglia during ischemia, while NLRC5 knockdown significantly ameliorated retinal ischemic damage and RGC death. Mechanistically, we revealed that knockdown of NLRC5 markedly suppressed gasdermin D (GSDMD) cleavage and activation of interleukin-1β (IL-1β) and caspase-3, indicating that NLRC5 promotes both microglial pyroptosis and apoptosis. Notably, we found that NLRC5 directly bound to NLRP3 and NLRC4 in inflammasomes to cooperatively drive microglial pyroptosis and apoptosis mediating retinal ischemic damage. Overall, these findings reveal a previously unidentified key contribution of NLRC5 signaling to microglial pyroptosis under ischemia or hypoxia conditions. This NLRC5-dependent pathway may be a novel therapeutic target for treatment of ischemic retinopathy.

Keywords: NLRC5, retinal ischemia–reperfusion injury, pyroptosis, apoptosis, microglia

INTRODUCTION

Ischemic retinopathy is one of the leading causes of visual impairment and irreversible blindness worldwide. It is a common clinical entity associated with various ocular disorders in which retinal blood flow is insufficient to meet the metabolic demands of the retina (the highest of any tissue), including acute glaucoma, retinal vein occlusion, retinopathy of prematurity, and diabetic retinopathy (Hardy et al., 2005; Jo et al., 2015). While it is well known that interruption of retinal blood flow causes retinal ischemia–reperfusion (RIR) injury and eventually leads to retinal ganglion cell (RGC) death (Fouda et al., 2018), molecular pathomechanisms of RGC death and associated treatment targets are still obscure. Microglia are the main immunological sentinels in the central nervous system (CNS), including retinal tissues. Under inflammatory conditions, microglia are activated and secret pro-inflammatory cytokines and cytotoxic mediators that can induce the death of neurons (Brown and Vilalta, 2015). Our previous studies demonstrated that this microglia-driven neuroinflammation mediates retinal tissue damage and RGC death during RIR injury (Chi et al., 2014).

In recent years, an increasing attention has been paid to the NOD-like receptors (NLRs) family which are the largest and most diverse cytoplasmic pattern recognition receptors in terms of the structure and function, as well as the signals they recognize (Meunier and Broz, 2017). Innate immune responses can be induced by the recognition of NLRs for endogenous danger signals, termed damage-associated molecular patters (DAMPs), or conservative microbial components, termed pathogen-associated molecular patterns (PAMPs) (Brubaker et al., 2015). According to their primary or best-characterized functions, NLRs can be categorized into three subgroups: inflammasome-forming NLRs, reproductive NLRs (functioning during reproduction and embryogenesis), and regulatory NLRs (Coutermarsh-Ott et al., 2016). While inflammasome-forming NLRs are well described, regulatory NLRs such as NOD1, NOD2, NLRX1, NLRC3, and NLRC5 are less studied and mainly refer to function as either positive or negative regulators of inflammatory signaling cascades (Coutermarsh-Ott et al., 2016; Fekete et al., 2018). In the past several years, accumulated evidence from *in vitro* and *in vivo* studies has clearly shown that inflammasome-forming NLRs, such as NLRP3, NLRP1, NLRP6, and NLRC4, play an important role in RIR injury (Chi et al., 2014; Wan et al., 2019; Chen et al., 2020). However, the contributions of regulatory NLRs to RIR injury are still unknown.

NLRC5 (NLR family, CARD domain containing 5) is a newly discovered NLRs family protein, belonging to the regulatory NLRs, which plays an important regulatory role in both adaptive and innate immune signaling (Meng et al., 2015; Benko et al., 2017). The role of NLRC5 in the regulation of major histocompatibility complex (MHC) class I genes is well established. However, the exact functions of NLRC5 in innate immune responses are unclear due to discrepancies and inconsistencies in reported data. Ma and Xie (2017) reported that NLRC5 deficiency aggravated fibrosis and inflammatory responses following heart injury, whereas Zhou et al. (2017) reported that NLRC5 silencing significantly ameliorated cardiac fibrosis. Others have reported that NLRC5 can act as a negative regulator of stress-associated nuclear factor kappa B (NF-κB) signaling, while other studies have found no influence of NLRC5 deficiency on the expression of NF-κB-dependent genes (Cui et al., 2010; Kumar et al., 2011; Yao et al., 2012). Moreover, the function of NLRC5 in the regulation of inflammasomes is even less well studied.

Programmed cell death (PCD), such as apoptosis, pyroptosis and necroptosis, is a fundamental cellular process essential for the homeostasis and development of multicellular organisms (Man et al., 2017). Our recent studies revealed that

a NLRP12/NLRP3/NLRC4 inflammasome-initiated pyroptosis pathway contributes to RGCs death in elevated intraocular pressure (IOP)-induced retinal ischemia (Chen et al., 2020). Recent breakthroughs reveal that the different types of PCD are highly interconnected and could be regarded as a single, coordinated cell death system that allows for flexible mutual compensation, just like in some conditions inflammatory caspases can trigger apoptosis while apoptotic triggers can induce pyroptosis (Bedoui et al., 2020). However, the exact molecular mechanisms inducing RGC death by the microglial PCD, especially apoptosis and pyroptosis, are still not fully understood under ischemia or hypoxia conditions. Furthermore, whether and how NLRC5 regulates microglial PCD to mediate RIR injury is currently unknown.

In the present study, we elucidate novel regulatory functions of NLRC5 in promoting microglial pyroptosis and ensuing RGCs death under retinal ischemia. We further reveal the relationship between the canonical inflammasomes NLRP3/NLRC4 and NLRC5 in mediating microglial pyroptosis and apoptosis.

MATERIALS AND METHODS

Ethics Statement

The adult female wild type C57BL/6 mice used in this study were purchased from GemPharmatech Co. Ltd., and raised in the Experimental Animal Center of Zhongshan Ophthalmic Center, Sun Yat-sen University, under specific pathogen-free conditions. All procedures involving animals were conducted strictly in accordance with the Association for Research in Vision and Ophthalmology (ARVO) Statement for the use of Animals in Ophthalmic and Vision Research. All animal experiments were formally reviewed and approved by the Animal Care and Ethics Committee of the Zhongshan Ophthalmic Center (Approval number: 2018-073). All efforts were made to ensure the welfare and alleviate the suffering of animals.

Retinal Ischemic Injury Model

All animals were 6–8 weeks of age, 18–20 g, and in good health at the time of experiments. The RIR ischemic retinopathy model was established as described in our previous article (Chen et al., 2020). In brief, mice were injected intraperitoneally with 50 mg/kg pentobarbital sodium for general anesthesia and locally dropped with 0.5% tetracaine hydrochloride for corneal anesthesia. Pupils were dilated with 1% tropicamide, and then a 30-gauge needle (BD, Franklin Lakes, NJ, United States) linked to an elevated saline reservoir was inserted into the anterior chamber of the right eye to maintain IOP at 110 mmHg for 90 min. The contralateral eye served as a sham control. Retinal ischemia was confirmed by the disappearance of the fundus red-light reflex, conjunctival edema, and corneal haze, while subsequent reperfusion was confirmed by recovery of the red-light reflex. At different times during reperfusion, mice were sacrificed and eyeballs or retina tissues isolated for subsequent experiments.

A small interfering (si) RNA targeting NLRC5 (siNLRC5) was used to silence NLRC5 expression in mouse retina. To avoid degradation *in vivo*, the siRNA was specifically designed and modified by methylation and cholesterol. A 1-nM solution of either siNLRC5 or a negative control siRNA (siNC) was injected into the vitreous cavity before the onset of reperfusion. The negative control siRNA was used to illustrate the specificity of siNLRC5 action and serve as a reference to analyze the siNLRC5 action. Both siRNAs were purchased from Ribobio Co., Ltd. The target sequence for the NLRC5-siRNA was TGACCAGCAGACTCTTTGA. The mice were sacrificed 3 days after intravitreal siRNA injection.

Histology and Immunohistochemistry

At designated times post-reperfusion, mice were sacrificed and their eyeballs isolated for histology and immunohistochemistry assays. The enucleated eyes were fixed with 4% paraformaldehyde overnight and then embedded in paraffin. Three, 4-μm thick slices through the optic disk of each eye were selected for hematoxylin and eosin (HE) staining. To quantitatively assess retinal tissue damage, total retinal thickness between the inner and outer limiting membranes was measured at a distance of 1 mm from the optic disk using CaseViewer software (3DHISTECH). Measurements were averaged to yield a representative retinal thickness for each eye. Slices selected for immunohistochemical analysis were deparaffinized and treated with antigen retrieval. According to the manufacturer's instructions, TUNEL assay was performed to detect and quantify the PCD at single cell level by using *In Situ* Cell Death Detection Kit (Roche). TUNEL-positive cells were manually counted in inner retina and the number of TUNEL-positive cells was expressed as the average per 1-mm length area using Image Pro Plus 7.0 as previously described (Sun et al., 2010; Sato et al., 2020). For TUNEL assay on cultured cells, the average TUNEL positive cell number in the percentage of total DAPI-stained nuclei was calculated. For immunofluorescence staining of the retina, the sections after antigen retrieval were first permeabilized with 0.3% Triton X-100 at room temperature for 30 min, blocked with 10% goat serum at room temperature for 1 h, and then incubated at 4°C overnight with primary antibodies targeting Rabbit polyclonal anti-RBPMS (1:200, Abclonal, Cat#ab152101), Rabbit polyclonal anti-Iba-1 (1:200, Wako, Cat#019-19741), Goat polyclonal anti-Iba-1 (1:100, abcam, Cat#ab48004), Mouse monoclonal anti-GSDMD (1:200, Santa Cruz, Cat#sc-393581), and Mouse monoclonal anti-NLRC5 (1:100, Santa Cruz, Cat#sc-515668). Sections were incubated with appropriate secondary antibodies at room temperature under darkness for 1 h and then cell nuclei were counterstained with DAPI. Fluorescence images were acquired using an Olympus fluorescence microscope or a Nikon A1 spectral confocal microscope. RBPMS is a specific and reliable marker for RGCs (Kwong et al., 2010). To perform RGC survival counts, each RBPMS-positive cell was merged with DAPI and counted individually to represent number of RGCs. RGC survival counts of each group were determined by counting average RBPMS-positive cells from four retina of four different animals (per retina including three 4-μm thick slices from ora serrata to ora serrata through the optic disk). The average of the RBPMS-positive cells counts in the NC siRNA normal control group as the denominator to

calculate the percentages in the remaining groups. To detect the expression of NLRC5 protein, immunohistochemical staining was performed using a DAB kit (Servicebio) following the standard protocol. Briefly, sections were deparaffinized, subjected to antigen retrieval, incubated in 3% hydrogen peroxide to eliminate endogenous peroxidase activity, blocked in solution containing 3% bovine serum albumin (BSA) and 0.3% Triton X-100, and incubated with primary antibody targeting NLRC5 (1:100, abcam, Cat#ab105411). Images were acquired using an Olympus light microscope.

Cell Culture and Treatment

The BV2 microglial cell line was purchased from Procell Co. Ltd. (#CL-0493, Wuhan, China) and cultured in a humidified atmosphere of 5% CO_2 at 37°C. The growth medium consisted of Dulbecco's Modified Eagle's Medium (DMEM) supplemented with 10% fetal bovine serum (FBS) and 1% penicillin-streptomycin. For gene silencing, BV2 cells were transfected with NLRC5-targeted or control siRNA when the cell density reached 60%–80% confluence using Lipofectamine RNAiMAX (Invitrogen) according to the manufacturer's instructions. Briefly, the Lipofectamine RNAiMAX reagent and siRNA were both diluted in Opti-MEM(Gibco) medium, then the diluted siRNA and the diluted Lipofectamine RNAiMAX solution were mixed in a 1:1 ratio and incubated for 5 min and finally the siRNA-lipid complex was added to the cells. After incubation for 24 h, the cells were treated with oxygen–glucose deprivation and reperfusion.

In vitro Oxygen–Glucose Deprivation and Reperfusion (OGDR) Model

The OGDR model was used to simulate the effects of retinal ischemia on microglia in isolation. Cultures of BV2 cells were first starved with a serum-free and glucose-free DMEM for 1 h under normoxic conditions, and then exposed to hypoxia (95% N_2, 5% CO_2) for 3 h in an incubator chamber. Alternatively, control cultures were incubated in serum-free DMEM under normoxic conditions for the same duration. Reperfusion was started by replacing medium with DMEM containing 10% FBS and 4.5 g/L glucose, and culturing them at 37°C for 24 h under normoxic conditions.

Western Blotting

Total protein was extracted using M-PER mammalian protein lysis buffer (Thermo Fisher Scientific, Rockford, IL, United States) supplemented with protease inhibitor cocktail (Thermo Fisher Scientific, Rockford, IL, United States) (1:100) according to the manufacturer's instructions. The protein concentration was determined using a quantitative BCA protein kit (Generay, Shanghai, China). Proteins were then separated using 8% or 10% polyacrylamide gels and transferred onto polyvinylidene difluoride (PVDF) membranes following standard protocols. Membrane were blocked with 5% non-fat milk diluted in Tris-buffered saline plus Triton-X (TBST) for 1 h at room temperature, and then incubated at 4°C overnight with the following primary antibodies: Rabbit polyclonal anti-NLRP3 (1:500, ABclonal, Cat#A14223), Rabbit polyclonal anti-NLRC5

(1:250, abcam, Cat#ab105411), Rabbit monoclonal anti-caspase-3 (1:200, Cell Signaling Technology, Cat#9665), Rabbit polyclonal anti-cleaved caspase-3 (1:200, Cell Signaling Technology, Cat#9661), Rabbit polyclonal anti-caspase-8 (1:200, ABclonal, Cat#A11324), Rabbit monoclonal anti-cleaved caspase-8 (1:200, Cell Signaling Technology, Cat#8592), Rabbit polyclonal anti-caspase-1 (1:200, ABclonal, Cat#A0964), Mouse monoclonal anti-caspase-1 p20 (1:200, AdipoGen, Cat#AG-20B-0042), Rabbit monoclonal anti-GSDMD (1:200, abcam, Cat#ab209845), Rabbit polyclonal anti-IL-1β (1:200, Immunoway, Cat#YT5201), Rabbit polyclonal anti-NLRC4 (1:500, ABclonal, Cat#A7382), and Rabbit monoclonal anti-β-actin (1:80000, ABclonal, Cat#AC026) as the gel loading control. Finally, after incubation in corresponding secondary antibodies, the immunoblots were detected by an enhanced chemiluminescence kit (ECL, eBioscience), captured using an Image Lab system (Bio-Rad, United States), and quantified using ImageJ software.

Immunoprecipitation

After the protein supernatant was extracted, immunoprecipitation antibody targeting Mouse monoclonal anti-NLRC5 (1:100, Santa Cruz, Cat#sc-515668) or negative control mouse IgG (1:100, ABclonal, Cat#AC011) was added and incubated overnight at 4°C. Next, 30 mL Protein A/G-agarose beads (Abmart, A10001) were added and incubated for 3 h. After incubation, the agarose beads were separated by instantaneous centrifugation and washed three times with cell lysis buffer. Then, beads were added with 60 mL 2 × loading buffer and boiled for 5 min, and removed after centrifugation. The eluted immune complexes in the supernatant were analyzed by western blotting. Cell lysates directly used for western blot analysis without immunoprecipitation processing were used as positive controls.

Quantitative Real-Time PCR (RT-qPCR)

Total RNA was extracted from cells or retinal tissue samples using TRIzol reagent (Thermo Fisher Scientific) according to the instruction manual and reverse-transcribed into cDNA using HiScript® III RT SuperMix (Vazyme). Real-time quantitative PCR (RT-qPCR) was conducted using ChamQ™ SYBR® Color qPCR Master Mix (Vazyme) according to the manufacturer's standard procedure and recorded by a Light Cycler 480 Real-Time PCR system. The sequences of primers were listed in **Table 1**.

Statistical Analysis

All statistical analyses were conducted using GraphPad Prism 6.0 software (GraphPad Software, Inc., San Diego, CA, United States). After checking the data for the normal distribution by Shapiro-Wilk test using SPSS 25.0 (IBM SPSS, Inc., Chicago, IL, United States), data are expressed as mean ± SD. Two group means were compared using the two-tailed independent samples Student's t-test while three or more group means were compared using one-way or two-way ANOVA with *post hoc* Bonferroni tests. A $P < 0.05$ was considered statistically significant for all tests.

RESULTS

NLRC5 Expression Is Markedly Elevated During RIR Injury

First, we established a high IOP-induced RIR injury model simulating the pathological process of ischemic retinopathy. Model mice demonstrated the typical morphological changes of retinal tissue damage during reperfusion as well as a significant reduction in retinal thickness, especially of the inner retina, from the third day of reperfusion and continuing thereafter (**Figure 1A**). Additionally, immunofluorescence staining revealed a gradual decrease in the number of RGCs and a concomitant increase in the number of activated microglia as evidenced by the transition from a ramified to amoeboid morphology (**Figures 1B,C**).

Mounting evidence implicates inflammasome-forming NLRs such as NLRP3, NLRP1, and NLRP6 in RIR injury (Chi et al., 2014; Wan et al., 2019), but the potential roles of regulatory NLRs have not been explored. By analyzing transcriptome sequencing data obtained from our recently published study (Chen et al., 2020), we discovered that the mRNA expression level of regulatory NLRC5 was significantly upregulated in the retina of RIR injury model mice, and this upregulation was further confirmed by RT-qPCR (**Figures 1D,E**). Both western blot and immunohistochemical staining also demonstrated significantly upregulated expression of NLRC5 in the retina at different times during reperfusion (**Figures 1F–H**). Moreover, dual immunofluorescence staining further revealed upregulated NLRC5 expression in retinal microglia (**Figure 1I**).

NLRC5 Deficiency Ameliorates Retinal Damage and RGC Death During RIR Injury

To examine the functions of NLRC5 in RIR injury, we compared retinal responses to high IOP between mice receiving intravitreal injection of a siRNA targeting the NLRC5 gene and mice receiving control siRNA. First, NLRC5 gene silencing was

TABLE 1 | Primer sequences used for this study.

Targeted genes	Forward primer sequence (5′–3′)	Reverse primer sequence (5′–3′)
mNLRC4	ACCTGGAAAAGGATGGGAATGAA	AAGTTTGGCAAGTCCTGGGG
mGSDMD	GCGATCTCATTCCGGTGGACAG	TTCCCATCGACGACATCAGAGAC
mNLRP3	ATTACCCGCCCGAGAAAGG	TCGCAGCAAAGATCCACACAG
mNLRC5	TCAGCCCAGAACAAGTATCC	TGGGCACAGACTTCCATTAG
mIL-1β	CTCCATGAGCTTTGTACAAGG	TGCTGATGTACCAGTTGGGG
mCaspase-1	CAGGCAAGCCAAATCTTTATCACT	GTGCCATCTTCTTTGTTCTGTTCTT
mCaspase-8	GTCACCGTGGGATAGGATACA	AGACATAACCCAACTCCGAAAA
mCaspase-3	TGGTGATGAAGGGGTCATTTATG	TTCGGCTTTCCAGTCAGACTC
mβ-Actin	TCCAGCCTTCCTTCTTGGGT	GCACTGTGTTGGCATAGAGGTC

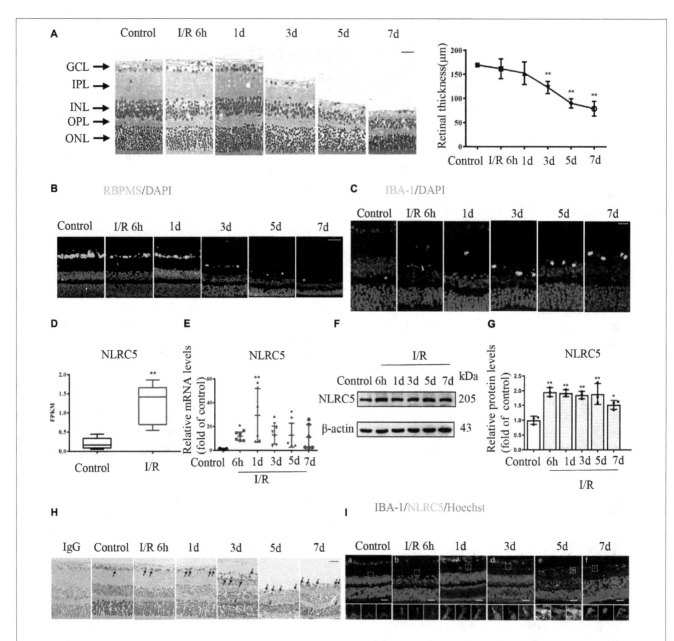

FIGURE 1 | The regulatory NOD-like receptor NLRC5 is upregulated during elevated intraocular pressure (IOP)-induced retinal ischemia–reperfusion (RIR) injury. **(A)** Hematoxylin and eosin (HE) staining of retinal sections showing the evolution of tissue and cellular damage during reperfusion and corresponding quantitative analysis demonstrating progressively reduced retinal thickness between the inner and outer limiting membranes (Scale bar: 30 μm, Magnification: ×400, n = 5). **(B,C)** Immunofluorescence images showing reduced numbers of anti-RBPMS-labeled retinal ganglion cells (RGCs) (Scale bar: 50 μm, Magnification: ×200) and elevated numbers of anti-Iba-1-labeled microglia (Scale bar: 15 μm, Magnification: ×400) during RIR. **(D)** Box plot illustrating significantly increased NLRC5 mRNA expression in the retina of RIR injury based on RNA sequencing data from our recently published article (n = 5). **(E–G)** RT-qPCR and western blot analysis showing elevated NLRC5 expression following RIR at mRNA (n = 6) and protein levels (n = 3), respectively. **(H)** Immunohistochemical analysis showing elevated NLRC5 expression during RIR (Scale bar: 30 μm, Magnification: ×400, n = 3). **(I)** Dual immunofluorescence image indicating anti-Iba-1-labeled microglia (red) and NLRC5 (green) (Scale bar: 25 μm, Magnification: ×400). I/R, retinal ischemia–reperfusion; ONL, outer nuclear layer; OPL, outer plexiform layer; INL, inner nuclear layer; IPL, inner plexiform layer; GCL, ganglion cell layer. Results **(A,D,E,G)** are presented as mean ± SD. *P < 0.05, **P < 0.01. Two-tailed unpaired Student's t-test and one-way ANOVA with *post hoc* Bonferroni tests was applied.

confirmed by RT-qPCR analysis, which showed that the siRNA targeting NLRC5 significantly down-regulated the expression of NLRC5 in RIR injury compared to the control siRNA (**Figure 2A**). HE staining revealed that NLRC5 knockdown notably reduced the severity of retinal tissue damage and the decrease in total retinal thickness observed during reperfusion, compared with the control siRNA (**Figure 2B**). Further, immunofluorescence staining also showed greater numbers of surviving RGCs (**Figure 2C**) and reduced numbers of TUNEL-positive cells (**Figure 2D**) in the retinal ganglion cell layer (GCL)

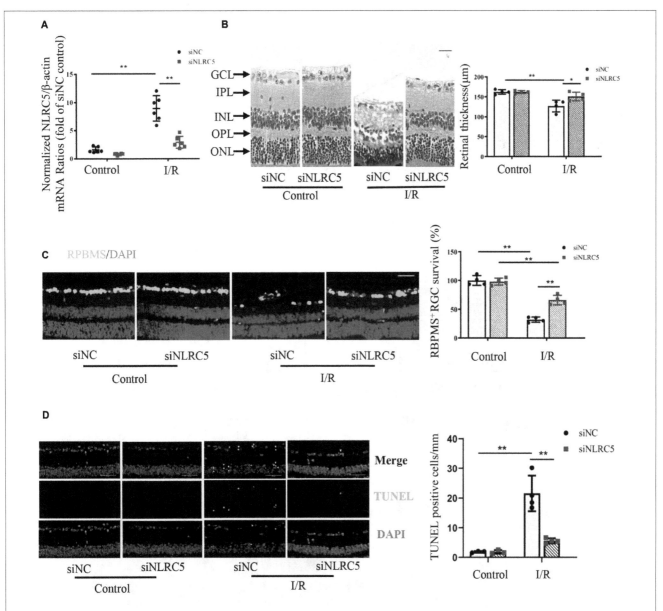

FIGURE 2 | NLRC5 knockdown effectively ameliorates retinal damage following ischemia–reperfusion. **(A)** RT-qPCR analysis of retinal NLRC5 gene knockdown efficiency using a targeted siRNA (*n* = 6). **(B)** HE staining of mouse retina showing that intravitreal injection of NLRC5 siRNA ameliorates tissue damage and reverses the reduction in retinal thickness following ischemia–reperfusion compared to retinas transfected with control siRNA (Scale bar: 30 μm, Magnification: ×400, *n* = 4). **(C)** Retinal immunofluorescence images and corresponding quantitative analysis of anti-RBPMS-labeled RGCs showing that the reduction in RGC number following RIR is reversed by NLRC5 knockdown (Scale bar: 50 μm, Magnification: ×200, *n* = 4). **(D)** TUNEL staining of retina following RIR (Scale bar: 50 μm, Magnification: ×400, *n* = 4). The white arrow indicates TUNEL-positive cells. All samples were obtained on the third day of reperfusion. I/R, retinal ischemia–reperfusion; ONL, outer nuclear layer; OPL, outer plexiform layer; INL, inner nuclear layer; IPL, inner plexiform layer; GCL, ganglion cell layer. Results are presented as mean ± SD. *$P < 0.05$, **$P < 0.01$. Two-way ANOVA with *post hoc* Bonferroni tests was applied.

and inner nuclear layer (INL) of the NLRC5 knockdown group compared to the control siRNA group.

Pyroptosis and Apoptosis Are Essential to the Development of Retinal Ischemic Injury

Multiple processes, including neuroinflammation, oxygen free radical generation, intracellular calcium overload, and activation

of apoptosis signaling pathways contribute to the development of RIR injury (Takahashi et al., 1992; Kuriyama et al., 2001; Oz et al., 2005; Madeira et al., 2016). Our recent study also indicated a key role for pyroptosis in elevated IOP-induced retinal ischemic injury (Chen et al., 2020). Consistent with these findings, protein levels of the apoptosis markers cleaved caspase-8 and cleaved caspase-3 were significantly upregulated starting on day 3 after reperfusion *in vivo*, while the protein levels of pyroptosis markers cleaved caspase-1 and N-terminal GSDMD

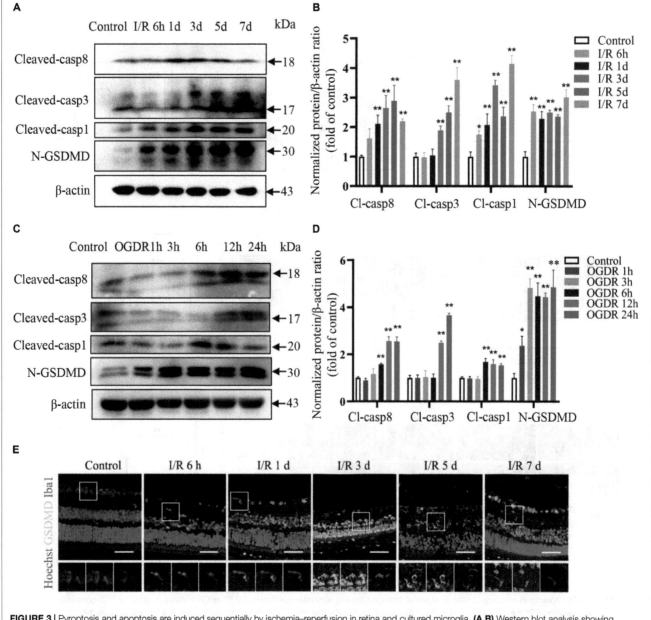

FIGURE 3 | Pyroptosis and apoptosis are induced sequentially by ischemia–reperfusion in retina and cultured microglia. **(A,B)** Western blot analysis showing induction of pyroptosis and apoptosis markers in retinal tissue following RIR (*n* = 3). **(C,D)** Western blot analysis showing upregulation of pyroptosis and apoptosis markers in BV2 microglia following OGDR (*n* = 3). **(E)** Dual immunofluorescence staining of retina showing induction of the pyroptosis markers GSDMD in retinal microglia following RIR (Scale bar: 50 μm, Magnification: ×400). I/R, retinal ischemia–reperfusion; OGDR, oxygen-glucose deprivation and reperfusion. *P < 0.05, **P < 0.01. One-way ANOVA with *post hoc* Bonferroni tests was applied.

increased significantly as early as 6 h following reperfusion (**Figures 3A,B**).

To examine pyroptotic and apoptotic signaling specifically in microglia, we established an *in vitro* OGDR model using BV2 microglia and found that the protein expression levels of pyroptosis markers increased more rapidly than apoptosis markers during reperfusion (**Figures 3C,D**), consistent with *in vivo* results. Dual immunofluorescence staining further confirmed increased expression level of pyroptosis marker GSDMD in retinal microglia during reperfusion (**Figure 3E**).

NLRC5 Is an Essential Mediator of Microglial Pyroptosis

Microglia, the primary resident immune cell in the retina, make pathologic contributions to augmenting RGC degeneration by producing neurotoxic proinflammatory cytokines and by clearing stressed but still living neurons (Silverman and Wong, 2018). However, the contributions of NLRC5 signaling to the proinflammatory activity of microglia as well as to the observed microglial pyroptosis and apoptosis during RIR injury have not been examined.

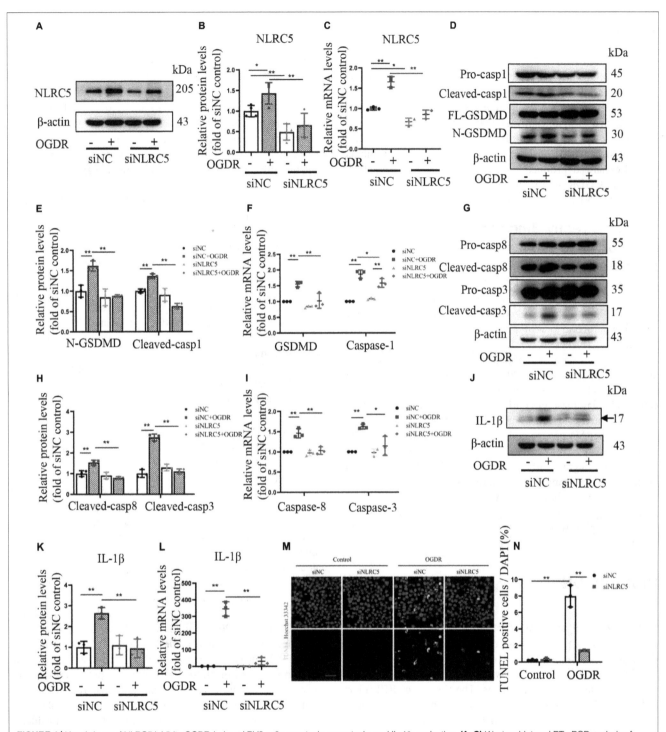

FIGURE 4 | Knockdown of NLRC5 inhibits OGDR-induced BV2 cells apoptosis, pyroptosis, and IL-1β production. **(A–C)** Western blot and RT-qPCR analysis of NLRC5 expression to verify gene knockdown efficiency. **(D–L)** Western blot and RT-qPCR analysis showing that NLRC5 knockdown reverses the OGDR-induced upregulation of pyroptosis markers **(D–F)**, apoptosis markers **(G–I)** and mature IL-1β **(J–L)**. **(M,N)** TUNEL staining of BV2 cells following OGDR (Scale bar: 50 μm, Magnification: ×400). All samples were obtained after 24 h of reperfusion. All data shown are representative of at least three independent experiments and presented as mean ± SD. *$P < 0.05$, **$P < 0.01$. Two-way ANOVA with *post hoc* Bonferroni tests was applied. I/R, retinal ischemia–reperfusion; OGDR, oxygen-glucose deprivation and reperfusion.

Therefore, we explored the influence of NLRC5 knockdown on pyroptosis and apoptosis of BV2 microglia subjected to *in vitro* OGDR. Transfection with a siRNA targeting NLRC5 significantly inhibited its expression at both protein and mRNA levels regardless of OGDR exposure, compared with the control siRNA (**Figures 4A–C**). In the control siRNA groups, OGDR induced pyroptosis and apoptosis of BV2 microglia, as demonstrated by the increased expression of cleaved caspase-1, N-terminal GSDMD, cleaved caspase-3 and cleaved caspase-8, as well as increased numbers of TUNEL-positive cells (**Figure 4**). Silencing NLRC5 significantly reduced the elevation in cleaved caspase-1 and N-terminal GSDMD induced by OGDR at both the protein level and mRNA level (**Figures 4D–F**). Moreover, NLRC5 knockdown also significantly reduced OGDR-induced elevations in cleaved caspase-3 and -8 at both the protein level and mRNA level (**Figures 4G–I**). Furthermore, NLRC5 knockdown inhibited OGDR-enhanced production of mature IL-1β (**Figures 4J–L**) as well as OGDR-increased numbers of TUNEL-positive cells (**Figures 4M,N**) compared with the control siRNA.

NLRC5 Directly Binds and Promotes NLRP3/NLRC4 Inflammasomes to Mediate Pyroptosis

In response to PAMPs or DAMPs, canonical inflammasomes containing NLRP3 or NLRC4 recruit and activate pro-caspase-1, which then can cleave GSDMD to initiate pyroptosis, as well the precursors of proinflammatory IL-18 and IL-1β (Aglietti and Dueber, 2017). Recent work has also revealed that inflammasomes can recruit pro-caspase-8, thereby triggering apoptosis (Aachoui et al., 2013). However, it is unknown if NLRC5 can also induce pyroptosis and apoptosis by regulating canonical inflammasomes during RIR injury. Protein and mRNA expression levels of NLRP3 and NLRC4 increased significantly in the control siRNA groups under RIR *in vivo* and OGDR *in vitro* (**Figures 5A–F**). While these elevations induced by OGDR or RIR were significantly suppressed by NLRC5 knockdown (**Figures 5A–F**). Immunoprecipitation analysis further showed that NLRC5 can bind directly to NLRP3 and NLRC4 in BV2 microglia (**Figures 5G,H**), suggesting that NLRC5 may form a complex with NLRP3/NLRC4 and positively regulate NLRP3/NLRC4 inflammasome pathways.

DISCUSSION

Ischemia–reperfusion injury is the major pathogenic process underlying multiple forms of ischemic retinopathy, and often causes irreversible visual impairment or even blindness, severely damaging the patient's quality of life (Osborne et al., 2004). The retina is particularly sensitive to ischemia and hypoxia due to its high metabolic requirements. The process of RIR injury induces oxidative stress and a series of inflammatory cascades, which in turn can destroy retinal neurons, especially RGCs. Unfortunately, once dead, RGCs can hardly regenerate, just like other neurons in the CNS, and eventually causes irreversible loss of vision (Liu et al., 2019). Therefore, a better understanding of the molecular mechanisms leading to ischemia-induced RGC dysfunction and death is essential for the development of therapeutic strategies to delay or halt vision loss. In the current study, we provide the first evidence that the regulatory NOD-like receptor NLRC5 is critically involved in elevated IOP-induced retinal ischemic injury and RGC death. We also uncovered a crucial function for NLRC5 in mediating neuroinflammatory

responses and regulating both apoptosis and pyroptosis pathways in microglia. Furthermore, our findings for the first time reveal the connection between NLRC5 and NLRC4, and indicate that NLRC5 contributes to RIR injury mainly by directly binding to NLRP3/NLRC4 inflammasomes and promoting their activation.

High IOP-induced RIR injury model is a widely used and well-established model to simulate the pathological process of ischemic retinopathy (Hartsock et al., 2016). Successful modeling is commonly evaluated by whether neuron loss in the GCL and retinal tissue thinning are significant compared to normal controls, although the degree of ischemic damage varies due to differences in modeling methods in different studies, such as the difference in the degree of elevated IOP (Wang et al., 2016; Huang et al., 2018; Wan et al., 2019). In this study, IOP was elevated to 110 mmHg for 90 min and elevated IOP-induced ischemic damage was also confirmed by significant retinal tissue thinning and RGCs loss from the third day of reperfusion. The diverse functions of inflammasome-forming NLRs family members are well characterized, while the potential roles of regulatory NLRs are less extensively explored. We first discovered that regulatory NLRC5 expression was markedly upregulated in the murine retina under RIR injury, implying its potential association with ischemic damage. Evidence shows that microglial responses are associated with the severity of RGCs degeneration by producing pro-inflammatory and neurotoxic factors (Almasieh et al., 2012; Silverman and Wong, 2018). We found that NLRC5 was also upregulated in retinal microglia during ischemia, suggesting that NLRC5 may exert its function though retinal microglia. Indeed, knockdown of NLRC5 expression in cultured microglia reduced cytotoxic IL-1b production in response to *in vitro* ischemia, further supporting this notion.

NLRC5 is the largest and most recently discovered member of the NLRs family, and has recently been implicated in the development of inflammatory diseases (Wang et al., 2019); however, precise functions in innate immune responses remain controversial. Ma and Xie (2017) reported that NLRC5 deficiency aggravated fibrosis and inflammatory responses triggered by high fat-induced heart injury). Conversely, Zhou et al. (2017) reported that NLRC5 silencing significantly inhibited cardiac fibroblast proliferation and migration, and ameliorated TGF-β1-induced fibrosis. Li et al. (2020) reported that NLRC5 partially aggravated inflammatory lung injury, while Wang et al. (2020) concluded that NLRC5 negatively regulated this inflammatory response. The contributions of NLRC5 to ophthalmopathy are similarly unclear. We therefore explored the potential role of NLRC5 *in vivo* and *in vitro* models that simulate the pathological process of ischemic retinopathy. Our findings provide the first evidence that NLRC5 deficiency can ameliorate retinal damage and RGCs death in mice subjected to high IOP-induced retinal ischemic injury, suggesting that NLRC5 is an important contributor to the pathophysiology of ischemic retinopathy and a promising therapeutic target.

An electron microscopy study of degenerating retinal cells in the GCL and INL at several time points after RIR injury by Büchi et al. revealed three morphologically distinct types of cell death, one consistent with necrosis, one resembling apoptosis, and one sharing several features with necrosis (Büchi, 1992). Also,

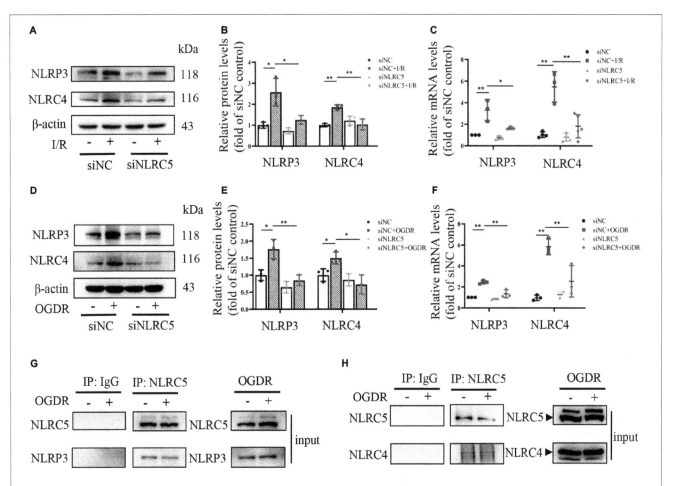

FIGURE 5 | NLRC5 binds to and activates NLRP3/NLRC4 inflammasomes during RIR or OGDR. **(A–F)** Western blot and RT-qPCR analysis of NLRP3 and NLRC4 expression in BV2 microglial cultures and mouse retina following OGDR and RIR, respectively. Expression levels of both proteins and mRNAs were elevated *in vivo* and *in vitro* by RIR or OGDR. Elevated expression levels following OGDR were markedly suppressed by NLRC5 knockdown. **(G,H)** Co-immunoprecipitation assay showing that NLRC5 interacts with NLRP3/NLRC4 in BV2 cells subjected to OGDR. All data shown are representative of at least three independent experiments and presented as mean ± SD. *P < 0.05, **P < 0.01. Two-way ANOVA with *post hoc* Bonferroni tests was applied. I/R, retinal ischemia–reperfusion; OGDR, oxygen-glucose deprivation and reperfusion.

accumulating evidence suggests that inhibition of the apoptosis pathway attenuates retinal ischemic injury (Ishikawa et al., 2012; Gencer et al., 2014; Han et al., 2020). In the current study as well, we confirmed activation of the apoptosis pathway in high IOP-induced retinal ischemic injury. Recently, a newly identified form of pro-inflammatory PCD called pyroptosis has also been implicated in various neurodegenerative diseases. Pyroptosis involves activation of caspase-1 or caspase-11/4/5, which then cleaves GSDMD to form N-terminal GSDMD. These cleaved N-terminal GSDMD proteins accumulate in the plasma membrane and form pores, eventually leading to plasma membrane rupture and release of cytosolic contents (Kovacs and Miao, 2017). This study, together with our recently published study, provide compelling evidence that pyroptosis of activated microglia contributes to retinal ischemic injury, including the death of RGCs (Chen et al., 2020). We also found that both apoptosis and pyroptosis pathways were activated in OGDR-stimulated microglia, and that the expression of pyroptotic marker proteins increased more rapidly than apoptotic marker

proteins. Poh et al. (2018) also found apoptotic and pyroptotic cell death of microglia under cerebral ischemia. These distinct PCD pathways are interconnected functionally and at the molecular levels, and thus may not operate in isolation but rather act cooperatively or synergistically for mutual compensation (Bedoui et al., 2020). Bedoui et al. (2020) also provide an explanation for the phenomenon that the onset of apoptosis is delayed than that of pyroptosis, that is, they believe that it is because the onset of apoptosis involves more steps to ensure coordinated operation. Clearly, more work will be needed to understand the precise molecular and physiological interrelationships between pyroptosis and apoptosis pathways and how they work together to induce RGCs death.

Previous studies have shown that NLRC5 can mediate apoptosis in acute kidney injury, cerebral ischemia/reperfusion injury, and acute myocardial infarction (Han et al., 2018; Liu et al., 2020; Yang et al., 2020). However, little is known about the function of NLRC5 in the apoptosis pathway during RIR injury. We found that NLRC5 knockdown reduced production of the key apoptotic effector cleaved caspase-3, suggesting that NLRC5 can promote microglial apoptosis. Moreover, to our knowledge, no reports have shown whether NLRC5 plays a role in the pyroptosis pathway. We show for the first time that NLRC5 knockdown can also reduce production of both the key pyroptosis effector protein N-terminal GSDMD and bioactive IL-1β, suggesting that NLRC5 can promote microglial pyroptosis and the production and release of neurotoxic inflammatory mediators.

Inflammasomes are intracellular multiprotein signaling complexes that are classically composed of three parts: a cytosolic sensor such as nucleotide-binding domain and leucine-rich repeat receptor (NLR) or absent in melanoma 2-like receptor (ALR), an adaptor protein such as apoptosis-associated speck-like protein containing a CARD (ASC), and an effector caspase precursor such as pro-caspase-1 (Rathinam and Fitzgerald, 2016). Recent work indicates that inflammasomes can trigger pyroptotic and apoptotic cell death in response to DAMPs or PAMPs by recruiting and activating effector caspases including caspase-1 and/or caspase-8 (Aachoui et al., 2013; Sagulenko et al., 2013). In view of the novel function of NLRC5 in microglial pyroptosis and apoptosis, we therefore hypothesize that a regulatory link between NLRC5 and inflammasomes is essential for the development of RIR injury. Triantafilou et al. (2013) used fluorescence resonance energy transfer to reveal that NLRC5 synergistically promotes the assembly of NLRP3 inflammasome in response to rhinovirus infection, and Davis et al. (2011) used co-immunoprecipitation to demonstrate that NLRC5 directly binds with NLRP3 and ASC in a nucleotide-binding domain-dependent manner. However, the association between NLRC5 and other inflammasomes such as NLRC4 inflammasome is less studied. Our findings not only confirm that NLRC5 can bind with NLRP3 to mediate NLRP3 inflammasome activation but also reveal that NLRC5 directly acts with NLRC4 to synergistically promote NLRC4 inflammasome activation, suggesting that the regulation of pyroptosis and apoptosis

by NLRC5 depends primarily on its direct combination with NLRP3/NLRC4 to promote the activation of inflammasomes, co-inducing RGCs death.

In conclusion, this study demonstrates for the first time that the regulatory NLR NLRC5 can mediate retinal tissue injury and RGCs death during RIR injury. We also demonstrate that NLRC5 knockdown can reduce neuroinflammation and inhibit pyroptosis and apoptosis pathways in activated microglia under ischemia or hypoxia conditions by binding to NLRP3/NLRC4 and preventing the activation of inflammasomes and ensuing pro-inflammatory cytokine production. Our findings suggest that NLRC5 has an essential role in the regulation of high IOP-induced retinal ischemic injury and microglial pyroptosis, highlighting NLRC5 as a promising therapeutic target to treat ischemic retinopathy.

ETHICS STATEMENT

The animal study was reviewed and approved by the Animal Care and Ethics Committee of the Zhongshan Ophthalmic Center (Approval number: 2018-073).

AUTHOR CONTRIBUTIONS

WC and YD contributed to the study concept and design. WC, YD, LS, LoS, JL, and YF contributed to the experimental and technical support. WC, YD, LiS, CY, and YF contributed to the acquisition, analysis, or interpretation of data. WC, YD, and LiS contributed to the RNA sequence analysis. WC and YD contributed to the drafting of the manuscript. WC, YD, and LoS contributed to the critical revision of the manuscript for important intellectual content. WC, YD, and YF contributed to the statistical analysis. All authors contributed to the article and approved the submitted version.

REFERENCES

Aachoui, Y., Sagulenko, V., Miao, E. A., and Stacey, K. J. (2013). Inflammasome-mediated pyroptotic and apoptotic cell death, and defense against infection. *Curr. Opin. Microbiol.* 16, 319–326. doi: 10.1016/j.mib.2013.04.004

Aglietti, R. A., and Dueber, E. C. (2017). Recent insights into the molecular mechanisms underlying pyroptosis and gasdermin family functions. *Trends Immunol.* 38, 261–271. doi: 10.1016/j.it.2017.01.003

Almasieh, M., Wilson, A. M., Morquette, B., Cueva Vargas, J. L., and Di Polo, A. (2012). The molecular basis of retinal ganglion cell death in glaucoma. *Prog. Retin. Eye Res.* 31, 152–181. doi: 10.1016/j.preteyeres.2011.11.002

Bedoui, S., Herold, M. J., and Strasser, A. (2020). Emerging connectivity of programmed cell death pathways and its physiological implications. *Nat. Rev. Mol. Cell Biol.* 21, 678–695. doi: 10.1038/s41580-020-0270-8

Benko, S., Kovacs, E. G., Hezel, F., and Kufer, T. A. (2017). NLRC5 functions beyond MHC I regulation-what do we know so far? *Front. Immunol.* 8:150. doi: 10.3389/fimmu.2017.00150

Brown, G. C., and Vilalta, A. (2015). How microglia kill neurons. *Brain Res.* 1628(Pt B), 288–297. doi: 10.1016/j.brainres.2015.08.031

Brubaker, S. W., Bonham, K. S., Zanoni, I., and Kagan, J. C. (2015). Innate immune pattern recognition: a cell biological perspective. *Annu. Rev. Immunol.* 33, 257–290. doi: 10.1146/annurev-immunol-032414-112240

Büchi, E. R. (1992). Cell death in the rat retina after a pressure-induced ischaemia-reperfusion insult: an electron microscopic study. I. Ganglion cell layer and inner nuclear layer. *Exp. Eye Res.* 55, 605–613. doi: 10.1016/s0014-4835(05)80173-3

Chen, H., Deng, Y., Gan, X., Li, Y., Huang, W., Lu, L., et al. (2020). NLRP12 collaborates with NLRP3 and NLRC4 to promote pyroptosis inducing ganglion cell death of acute glaucoma. *Mol. Neurodegener.* 15:26. doi: 10.1186/s13024-020-00372-w

Chi, W., Li, F., Chen, H., Wang, Y., Zhu, Y., Yang, X., et al. (2014). Caspase-8 promotes NLRP1/NLRP3 inflammasome activation and IL-1beta production in acute glaucoma. *Proc. Natl. Acad. Sci. U.S.A.* 111, 11181–11186. doi: 10.1073/pnas.1402819111

Coutermarsh-Ott, S., Eden, K., and Allen, I. C. (2016). Beyond the inflammasome: regulatory NOD-like receptor modulation of the host immune response following virus exposure. *J. Gen. Virol.* 97, 825–838. doi: 10.1099/jgv.0.000401

Cui, J., Zhu, L., Xia, X., Wang, H. Y., Legras, X., Hong, J., et al. (2010). NLRC5 negatively regulates the NF-kappaB and type I interferon signaling pathways. *Cell* 141, 483–496. doi: 10.1016/j.cell.2010.03.040

Davis, B. K., Roberts, R. A., Huang, M. T., Willingham, S. B., Conti, B. J., Brickey, W. J., et al. (2011). Cutting edge: NLRC5-dependent activation of the inflammasome. *J. Immunol.* 186, 1333–1337. doi: 10.4049/jimmunol.1003111

Fekete, T., Bencze, D., Szabo, A., Csoma, E., Biro, T., Bacsi, A., et al. (2018). Regulatory NLRs control the RLR-mediated Type I interferon and inflammatory responses in human dendritic cells. *Front. Immunol.* 9:2314. doi: 10.3389/fimmu.2018.02314

Fouda, A. Y., Xu, Z., Shosha, E., Lemtalsi, T., Chen, J., Toque, H. A., et al. (2018). Arginase 1 promotes retinal neurovascular protection from ischemia through suppression of macrophage inflammatory responses. *Cell Death Dis.* 9:1001. doi: 10.1038/s41419-018-1051-6

Gencer, B., Karaca, T., Tufan, H. A., Kara, S., Arikan, S., Toman, H., et al. (2014). The protective effects of dexmedetomidine against apoptosis in retinal ischemia/reperfusion injury in rats. *Cutan Ocul. Toxicol.* 33, 283–288. doi: 10.3109/15569527.2013.857677

Han, F., Gao, Y., Ding, C. G., Xia, X. X., Wang, Y. X., Xue, W. J., et al. (2018). Knockdown of NLRC5 attenuates renal I/R injury in vitro through the activation of PI3K/Akt signaling pathway. *Biomed. Pharmacother.* 103, 222–227. doi: 10.1016/j.biopha.2018.04.040

Han, Y., Bing Zhu, X., Ye, Y., Yu Deng, K., Yang Zhang, X., and Ping Song, Y. (2020). Ribonuclease attenuates retinal ischemia reperfusion injury through inhibition of inflammatory response and apoptosis in mice. *Int. Immunopharmacol.* 85:106608. doi: 10.1016/j.intimp.2020.106608

Hardy, P., Beauchamp, M., Sennlaub, F., Gobeil, F. Jr., Tremblay, L., Mwaikambo, B., et al. (2005). New insights into the retinal circulation: inflammatory lipid mediators in ischemic retinopathy. *Prostaglandins Leukot Essent Fatty Acids* 72, 301–325. doi: 10.1016/j.plefa.2005.02.004

Hartsock, M. J., Cho, H., Wu, L., Chen, W. J., Gong, J., and Duh, E. J. (2016). A mouse model of retinal ischemia-reperfusion injury through elevation of intraocular pressure. *J. Vis. Exp.* 54065. doi: 10.3791/54065

Huang, R., Liang, S., Fang, L., Wu, M., Cheng, H., Mi, X., et al. (2018). Low-dose minocycline mediated neuroprotection on retinal ischemia-reperfusion injury of mice. *Mol. Vis.* 24, 367–378.

Ishikawa, S., Hirata, A., Nakabayashi, J., Iwakiri, R., and Okinami, S. (2012). Neuroprotective effect of small interfering RNA targeted to caspase-3 on rat retinal ganglion cell loss induced by ischemia and reperfusion injury. *Curr. Eye Res.* 37, 907–913. doi: 10.3109/02713683.2012.688161

Jo, D. H., Kim, J. H., and Kim, J. H. (2015). A platform of integrative studies from in vitro to in vivo experiments: towards drug development for ischemic retinopathy. *Biomed. Pharmacother.* 69, 367–373. doi: 10.1016/j.biopha.2014.12.027

Kovacs, S. B., and Miao, E. A. (2017). Gasdermins: effectors of pyroptosis. *Trends Cell Biol.* 27, 673–684. doi: 10.1016/j.tcb.2017.05.005

Kumar, H., Pandey, S., Zou, J., Kumagai, Y., Takahashi, K., Akira, S., et al. (2011). NLRC5 deficiency does not influence cytokine induction by virus and bacteria infections. *J. Immunol.* 186, 994–1000. doi: 10.4049/jimmunol.1002094

Kuriyama, H., Waki, M., Nakagawa, M., and Tsuda, M. (2001). Involvement of oxygen free radicals in experimental retinal ischemia and the selective vulnerability of retinal damage. *Ophthalmic Res.* 33, 196–202. doi: 10.1159/000055670

Kwong, J. M., Caprioli, J., and Piri, N. (2010). RNA binding protein with multiple splicing: a new marker for retinal ganglion cells. *Invest. Ophthalmol. Vis. Sci.* 51, 1052–1058. doi: 10.1167/iovs.09-4098

Li, N. N., Cao, T., Yu, F., Luo, L., and Liu, P. (2020). MiR-520c-3p alleviates LPS-induced A549 cell and mice lung injury via targeting NLRC5. *Pharmazie* 75, 275–278. doi: 10.1692/ph.2020.0355

Liu, W., Xia, F., Ha, Y., Zhu, S., Li, Y., Folorunso, O., et al. (2019). Neuroprotective effects of HSF1 in retinal ischemia-reperfusion injury. *Invest. Ophthalmol. Vis. Sci.* 60, 965–977. doi: 10.1167/iovs.18-26216

Liu, Z., Liu, J., Wei, Y., Xu, J., Wang, Z., Wang, P., et al. (2020). LncRNA MALAT1 prevents the protective effects of miR-125b-5p against acute myocardial infarction through positive regulation of NLRC5. *Exp. Ther. Med.* 19, 990–998. doi: 10.3892/etm.2019.8309

Ma, S. R., and Xie, X. W. (2017). NLRC5 deficiency promotes myocardial damage induced by high fat diet in mice through activating TLR4/NF-κB. *Biomed. Pharmacother.* 91, 755–766. doi: 10.1016/j.biopha.2017.03.062

Madeira, M. H., Boia, R., Elvas, F., Martins, T., Cunha, R. A., Ambrosio, A. F., et al. (2016). Selective A2A receptor antagonist prevents microglia-mediated neuroinflammation and protects retinal ganglion cells from high intraocular pressure-induced transient ischemic injury. *Transl. Res.* 169, 112–128. doi: 10.1016/j.trsl.2015.11.005

Man, S. M., Karki, R., and Kanneganti, T. D. (2017). Molecular mechanisms and functions of pyroptosis, inflammatory caspases and inflammasomes in infectious diseases. *Immunol. Rev.* 277, 61–75. doi: 10.1111/imr.12534

Meng, Q., Cai, C., Sun, T., Wang, Q., Xie, W., Wang, R., et al. (2015). Reversible ubiquitination shapes NLRC5 function and modulates NF-kappaB activation switch. *J. Cell Biol.* 211, 1025–1040. doi: 10.1083/jcb.201505091

Meunier, E., and Broz, P. (2017). Evolutionary convergence and divergence in NLR function and structure. *Trends Immunol.* 38, 744–757. doi: 10.1016/j.it.2017.04.005

Osborne, N. N., Casson, R. J., Wood, J. P., Chidlow, G., Graham, M., and Melena, J. (2004). Retinal ischemia: mechanisms of damage and potential therapeutic strategies. *Prog. Retin. Eye Res.* 23, 91–147. doi: 10.1016/j.preteyeres.2003.12.001

Oz, O., Gurelik, G., Akyurek, N., Cinel, L., and Hondur, A. (2005). A short duration transient ischemia induces apoptosis in retinal layers: an experimental study in rabbits. *Eur. J. Ophthalmol.* 15, 233–238. doi: 10.1177/112067210501500210

Poh, L., Kang, S. W., Baik, S. H., Yong Quan Ng, G., She, D. T., Balaganapathy, P., et al. (2018). Evidence that NLRC4 inflammasome mediates apoptotic and pyroptotic microglial death following ischemic stroke. *Brain Behav. Immun.* 75, 34–47. doi: 10.1016/j.bbi.2018.09.001

Rathinam, V. A., and Fitzgerald, K. A. (2016). Inflammasome complexes: emerging mechanisms and effector functions. *Cell* 165, 792–800. doi: 10.1016/j.cell.2016.03.046

Sagulenko, V., Thygesen, S. J., Sester, D. P., Idris, A., Cridland, J. A., Vajjhala, P. R., et al. (2013). AIM2 and NLRP3 inflammasomes activate both apoptotic and pyroptotic death pathways via ASC. *Cell Death Differ.* 20, 1149–1160. doi: 10.1038/cdd.2013.37

Sato, K., Mochida, S., Tomimoto, D., Konuma, T., Kiyota, N., Tsuda, S., et al. (2020). A pyruvate dehydrogenase kinase inhibitor prevents retinal cell death and improves energy metabolism in rat retinas after ischemia/reperfusion injury. *Exp. Eye Res.* 193:107997. doi: 10.1016/j.exer.2020.107997

Silverman, S. M., and Wong, W. T. (2018). Microglia in the retina: roles in development, maturity, and disease. *Annu. Rev. Vis. Sci.* 4, 45–77. doi: 10.1146/annurev-vision-091517-034425

Sun, M. H., Pang, J. H., Chen, S. L., Han, W. H., Ho, T. C., Chen, K. J., et al. (2010). Retinal protection from acute glaucoma-induced ischemia-reperfusion injury through pharmacologic induction of heme oxygenase-1. *Invest. Ophthalmol. Vis. Sci.* 51, 4798–4808. doi: 10.1167/iovs.09-4086

Takahashi, K., Lam, T. T., Edward, D. P., Buchi, E. R., and Tso, M. O. (1992). Protective effects of flunarizine on ischemic injury in the rat retina. *Arch. Ophthalmol.* 110, 862–870. doi: 10.1001/archopht.1992.01080180134041

Triantafilou, K., Kar, S., van Kuppeveld, F. J., and Triantafilou, M. (2013). Rhinovirus-induced calcium flux triggers NLRP3 and NLRC5 activation in bronchial cells. *Am. J. Respir. Cell Mol. Biol.* 49, 923–934. doi: 10.1165/rcmb.2013-0032OC

Wan, P., Su, W., Zhang, Y., Li, Z., Deng, C., Li, J., et al. (2019). LncRNA H19 initiates microglial pyroptosis and neuronal death in retinal ischemia/reperfusion injury. *Cell Death Differ.* 27, 176–191. doi: 10.1038/s41418-019-0351-4

Wang, J. Q., Liu, Y. R., Xia, Q., Chen, R. N., Liang, J., Xia, Q. R., et al. (2019). Emerging roles for NLRC5 in immune diseases. *Front. Pharmacol.* 10:1352. doi: 10.3389/fphar.2019.01352

Wang, Y., Huang, C., Bian, E., Lei, T., Lv, X., and Li, J. (2020). NLRC5 negatively regulates inflammatory responses in LPS-induced acute lung injury through NF-κB and p38 MAPK signal pathways. *Toxicol. Appl. Pharmacol.* 403:115150. doi: 10.1016/j.taap.2020.115150

Wang, Y., Lopez, D., Davey, P. G., Cameron, D. J., Nguyen, K., Tran, J., et al. (2016). Calpain-1 and calpain-2 play opposite roles in retinal ganglion cell degeneration induced by retinal ischemia/reperfusion injury. *Neurobiol. Dis.* 93, 121–128. doi: 10.1016/j.nbd.2016.05.007

Yang, J., Yang, N., Luo, J., Cheng, G., Zhang, X., He, T., et al. (2020). Overexpression of S100A4 protects retinal ganglion cells against retinal ischemia-reperfusion injury in mice. *Exp. Eye Res.* 201:108281. doi: 10.1016/j.exer.2020.108281

Yao, Y., Wang, Y., Chen, F., Huang, Y., Zhu, S., Leng, Q., et al. (2012). NLRC5 regulates MHC class I antigen presentation in host defense against intracellular pathogens. *Cell Res.* 22, 836–847. doi: 10.1038/cr.2012.56

Zhou, H., Yu, X., and Zhou, G. (2017). NLRC5 silencing ameliorates cardiac fibrosis by inhibiting the TGF-β1/Smad3 signaling pathway. *Mol. Med. Rep.* 16, 3551–3556. doi: 10.3892/mmr.2017.6990

18

The Metabolic Reprogramming of *Frem2* Mutant Mice Embryos in Cryptophthalmos Development

Xiayin Zhang[1†], Ruixin Wang[1†], Ting Wang[1†], Xulin Zhang[1†], Meimei Dongye[1],
Dongni Wang[1], Jinghui Wang[1], Wangting Li[1], Xiaohang Wu[1], Duoru Lin[1] and
Haotian Lin[1,2]*

[1] State Key Laboratory of Ophthalmology, Zhongshan Ophthalmic Center, Sun Yat-sen University, Guangzhou, China,
[2] Center for Precision Medicine, Sun Yat-sen University, Guangzhou, China

Correspondence:
Haotian Lin
linht5@mail.sysu.edu.cn
orcid.org/0000-0003-4672-9721

[†] *These authors have contributed*
equally to this work

Background: Cryptophthalmos is characterized by congenital ocular dysplasia with eyelid malformation. The pathogenicity of mutations in genes encoding components of the FRAS1/FREM protein complex is well established, but the underlying pathomechanisms of this disease are still unclear. In the previous study, we generated mice carrying *Frem2[R725X/R2156W]* compound heterozygous mutations using CRISPR/Cas9 and showed that these mice recapitulated the human cryptophthalmos phenotype.

Methods: In this study, we tracked changes in the metabolic profile of embryos and expression of metabolism-related genes in *Frem2* mutant mice on E13.5 compared with wild-type mice. RNA sequencing (RNA-seq) was utilized to decipher the differentiated expression of genes associated with metabolism. Untargeted metabolomics and targeted metabolomics analyses were performed to detect and verify the shifts in the composition of the embryonic metabolome.

Results: Differentially expressed genes participating in amino acid metabolism and energy metabolism were observed by RNA-seq. Transcriptomic analysis suggests that 821 (39.89%) up-regulated genes and 320 (32.99%) down-regulated genes were involved in the metabolic process in the enriched GO terms. A total of 92 significantly different metabolites were identified including creatine, guanosine 5′-monophosphate, cytosine, cytidine 5′-monophosphate, adenine, and L-serine. Interestingly, major shifts related to ATP binding cassette transporters (ABC transporters) and the biosynthesis of amino acids in the composition of the embryonic metabolome were observed by KEGG metabolic analysis, indicating that these pathways could also be involved in the pathogenesis of cryptophthalmos.

Conclusion: We demonstrate that *Frem2* mutant fetal mice have increased susceptibility to the disruption of eye morphogenesis in association with distinct transcriptomic and metabolomic signatures. Our findings suggest that the metabolomic signature established before birth may play a role in mediating cryptophthalmos in *Frem2* mutant mice, which may have important implications for the pathogenesis of cryptophthalmos.

Keywords: metabonomics, *Frem2* mutation, cryptophthalmos, development of eyelids, transcriptomics

INTRODUCTION

Cryptophthalmos (MIM: 123570) is a rare congenital ocular dysplasia accompanied by fusion of the eyelids (François, 1969). Mutations in the *FREM2* gene result in reduced epithelial-mesenchymal coupling and transient embryonic epidermal blistering, leading to the development of cryptophthalmos (Jadeja et al., 2005; Haelst et al., 2010). However, the underlying pathomechanisms of this disease are still not known.

Metabolomics is considered as a sensitive approach for the development of novel targeted therapeutics because of its direct elucidation of pathophysiological mechanisms and its mediation as signals that directly or indirectly trigger adaptive responses (Piazza et al., 2018). Nutritional states, stress, and ecological conditions can all influence the intracellular levels of metabolites, and the development of the eye has been proven to be associated with intermediates of multiple metabolites by accumulating evidence (Robciuc et al., 2013; Cherif et al., 2018; Paramita et al., 2018). It is unclear whether the absence of metabolites drives epithelial–mesenchymal coupling in either mice or humans and whether the metabolic disorder is a consequence of cryptophthalmos.

Our objective, therefore, was to define the contribution of the metabolic disorder in driving cryptophthalmos as a predisposing factor. In our previous study, we established a mouse model that recapitulates the human complete cryptophthalmos phenotype characterized by abnormal eyelids, microphthalmia, and severe ocular anterior segment developmental defects (Zhang et al., 2019). Here, we used untargeted metabolomics analysis in conjunction with RNA-seq, to examine the contribution of metabolites and metabolism-related genes in modulating cryptophthalmos susceptibility in *Frem2* mutant fetal mice. Real-time quantitative PCR and targeted metabolomics analysis were performed to verify the shifts in the composition of the embryonic metabolome. We suggest that the metabolites established before birth may have an impact on cryptophthalmos susceptibility in *Frem2* mutant mice.

MATERIALS AND METHODS

Animals

All animals used in this study were *Mus musculus*, C57BL/6J mice. All mouse procedures were approved by the Institutional Animal Care and Use Committee of Zhongshan Ophthalmic Center, Sun Yat-sen University. All experiments were carried out in accordance with the ARVO Statement for the Use and Care of Animals in Ophthalmic and Vision Research. The mice were maintained on a 12-h: 12-h light-dark cycle with unlimited access to food and water. All animals used for experiments were killed humanely and quickly by cervical dislocation (adult mice) or decapitation (embryos).

The generation of mice carrying the c.2173C > T (R725X) or c.6466A > T (R2156W) point mutation in the murine *Frem2* gene was designed as previously reported using CRISPR/Cas9 technology (Zhang et al., 2019). According to our previous study, the phenotypes exhibited by the $Frem2^{R725X/R2156W}$ adult mice were bilateral or unilateral cryptophthalmos. Furthermore, 8/11 mice exhibited a single kidney and 4/11 mice exhibited syndactyly (Zhang et al., 2019).

Histological Analysis

The embryos from *Frem2* mutant and wild-type mice were fixed with 4% paraformaldehyde and subsequently embedded in paraffin for at least 24 h. Tissues were sectioned in a vertical pupillary optic nerve plane and stained with H&E.

RNA-Seq Analysis and Real-Time Quantitative PCR Analysis

We compared embryonic transcriptome changes between three *Frem2* mutant mice and one wild-type littermates. Total RNA was extracted with TRIzol reagent (Invitrogen). The RNA-seq libraries were generated using Illumina TruSeq RNA Sample Preparation Kits. RNA-seq was performed using an Illumina HiSeq 2000 platform as previously reported (Robciuc et al., 2013). Genes with q ≤ 0.05 and | log2_ratio| ≥ 1 were identified as differentially expressed genes. GO enrichment analyses of the differentially expressed genes were performed using DAVID.[1] GO terms with a Bonferroni corrected *P* value of < 0.05 were considered significantly enriched functional annotations.

Real-time quantitative PCR was performed in three *Frem2* mutant mice embryos and three wild-type embryos on a 7900HT Real-time PCR system (Applied Biosystems) using real-time primers and TaqMan probes from Applied Biosystems. The first strand was reverse-transcribed using the Omniscript Reverse Transcription Kit (Qiagen) and random primers. The fold changes in gene expression were calculated using the $\Delta\Delta Ct$ (cycle threshold) values. Expression was normalized to *Actin*. All primers used are listed in **Supplementary Table S1**.

Untargeted Metabolomics Analysis

Untargeted high-throughput metabolomic profiling was conducted in six embryos of *Frem2* mutant mice and compared with that in six wild-type embryos. Frozen embryos of $Frem2^{R725X/R2156W}$ and wild-type mice were thawed and analyzed using an UHPLC (1290 Infinity LC, Agilent Technologies) coupled with an AB SCIEX Triple TOF 6600 System (AB SCIEX, Framingham, MA, United States). In parallel to the preparation of the test samples (in a group of six), pooled quality control samples were prepared by mixing equal amounts (30 μL) of each sample. The quality control samples were utilized to monitor the LC-MS response in real time.

Abbreviations: ABC transporters, ATP binding cassette transporters; ESI, electrospray ionization; H&E, hematoxylin-eosin; KEGG; Kyoto Encyclopedia of Genes and Genomes; LC-MS, liquid chromatography-mass spectrometry; MRM, multiple reaction monitoring; MS, mass spectrometry; PCR, polymerase chain reaction; RNA-seq, RNA sequencing; TOF, time-of-flight; UHPLC, ultra high-performance liquid chromatography; VIP, variable influence on projection.

---

[1]http://david.abcc.ncifcrf.gov/

All samples were analyzed using a 2.1 mm × 100 mm ACQUIY UPLC BEH 1.7 μm column (Waters, Ireland). In both ESI positive and negative modes, the mobile phase contained the following: A, 25 mM ammonium acetate, and 25 mM ammonium hydroxide in water; B, acetonitrile (Merck, 1,499,230–935). The gradient elution program was 95% B for 1 min, linearly reduced to 65% in 13 min, reduced to 40% in 2 min, kept for 2 min, and then increased to 85% in 0.1 min, with a 5 min re-equilibration.

The ESI source conditions were set as follows: ion source gas1, 60; ion source gas2, 60; curtain gas, 30; source temperature, 600°C, ion spray voltage floating ± 5500 V, TOF MS scan m/z range, 60–1000 Da; and accumulation time, 0.20 s/spectra; production scan m/z range, 25–1000 Da; and accumulation time, 0.05 s/spectra for MS/MS acquisition. The production scan is acquired using information-dependent acquisition by high sensitivity mode with collision energy as 35 V with ±15 eV and declustering potential as ±60 V.

The raw MS data (wiff. scan files) were converted to mzXML files through ProteoWizard and processed by XCMS. The metabolites were identified by accuracy mass (<25 ppm) and MS/MS data that were matched with the lab database (Shanghai Applied Protein Technology Co., Ltd.). The variables having more than 50% of the valid values in at least one group were kept and handled for the multivariate statistical analysis by MetaboAnalyst[2], as well as unidimensional statistical analysis by R software. The significantly different metabolites were determined based on the combination of a statistically significant threshold of VIP values obtained from supervised partial least squares-discriminate analysis and a two-tailed Student's t-test. The VIP can measure the impact strength and interpretation capability of each metabolite pattern to distinguish samples in each group. Metabolites with VIP > 1.0 and P < 0.1 were considered significant. For metabolite annotation and pathway analysis, metabolites that showed differences between groups were analyzed by the KEGG[3] database.

Targeted Metabolomics Analysis

Targeted high-throughput metabolomic profiling was conducted in five embryos of *Frem2* mutant mice and compared with that in six wild-type mice. To precipitate proteins, the samples were incubated for 1 h at −20°C, followed by 15 min centrifugation at 13,000 r/min and 4°C. The resulting supernatant was removed and evaporated to dryness in a vacuum concentrator. The dry extracts were then reconstituted in 100 mL ACN: H2O (1:1, v/v), sonicated for 10 min, and centrifuged for 15 min at 13,000 r/min and 4°C to remove insoluble debris. The supernatants were transferred to HPLC vials for LC-MS analysis. The LC-MS analysis was performed using a UHPLC system (Agilent Technologies) coupled to a triple quadrupole mass spectrometer in the MRM mode. For the argininosuccinate and arginine tests alone, metabolites were monitored in positive

mode only. For high-throughput metabolic profiling, metabolites were monitored in both ESI positive and ESI negative modes. A WATERS ACQUITY UPLC BEH Amino column (particle size, 1.7 mm, 100 mm length × 2.1 mm ID) was used for argininosuccinate and arginine tests. Phenomenex Luna amino column (particle size, 3 mm; 100 mm length 3 2.1 mm ID) was used for metabolic profiling. The column temperature was kept at 25°C. The flow rate was 300 mL/min and the sample injection volume was 2 mL. Mobile phase A was 25 mM ammonium acetate and 25 mM ammonium hydroxide in 100% water, and B was 100% acetonitrile. The linear gradient for argininosuccinate and arginine tests was set as follows: 0–1 min: 85% B, 1–6 min: 85% B to 70% B, 6–10 min: 70% B to 0% B, 10–15 min: 0% B, 15–15.1 min: 0% B to 85% B, 15.1–20 min: 85% B. The linear gradient for metabolic profiling was set as follows: 0–1 min: 85% B, 1–14 min: 95% B to 65% B, 14–16 min: 65% B to 40% B, 16–18 min: 40% B, 18–18.1 min: 40% B to 95% B, 18.1–23 min: 95% B. ESI source conditions were set as follows: sheath gas temperature, 350°C; dry gas temperature, 350°C; sheath gas flow, 12 L/min for argininosuccinate and arginine tests, 11 L/min for metabolic profiling; dry gas flow, 16 L/min for argininosuccinate and arginine tests, 10 L/min for metabolic profiling; capillary voltage, 3000 V in positive mode for argininosuccinate and arginine tests, 4000 or −3500 V in positive or negative modes for metabolic profiling; nozzle voltage, 1000 V for argininosuccinate and arginine tests, 500 V for metabolic profiling; nebulizer pressure, 40 psi for argininosuccinate and arginine tests, 30 psi for metabolic profiling. For argininosuccinate and arginine tests, four MRM transitions representing the two metabolites were simultaneously monitored. The dwell time for each MRM transition is 50 ms, and the total cycle time is 535 ms. For metabolic profiling, the dwell time for each MRM transition is 3 ms, and the total cycle time is 1.263 s. Original MRM raw data were processed by MRMAnalyzer based on detection and area integration of peaks from individual target metabolites. Protein concentration was used for sample normalization.

To construct the metabolite MRM library, each metabolite standard (100 mg/mL) was first analyzed in ESI positive/negative mode via flow injection using the software MassHunter Optimizer (Agilent Technologies) to obtain the optimal MRM transition parameters. Then the retention time of each metabolite was determined by measuring the corresponding MRM transition individually on the column. The significantly different metabolites were determined based on the combination of a statistically significant threshold from fold change analysis (fold change > 1.5) and a two-tailed Student's t-test (P < 0.05).

Statistical Analysis

The principal component analysis was performed to examine intrinsic clusters of metabolomics data. Heatmaps were generated using a hierarchical clustering algorithm to visualize metabolite differences. All statistical analyses were performed using SPSS (version 19.0) and R (version 3.3.1). Significance levels of P values are graphically represented with: * for P values between 0.05 and 0.01.

---

[2] www.metaboanalyst.ca

[3] http://www.genome.jp/kegg/

RESULTS

Ocular Abnormalities in *Frem2* Mutant Embryos

As formation of the eyelids in the mouse begins at approximately 13–14 days of gestation (Pei and Rhodin, 1970), we studied E13.5 mice. H&E staining confirmed microphthalmia and showed dysplastic eye structures in the *Frem2* mutant embryo (**Figure 1**). At the beginning of eyelid formation, the lower eyelid fold cannot be defined in the *Frem2* mutant embryo, whereas small grooves developing from the surface ectoderm to form the eyelid folds above and below the developing eye have been well formed in wild-type mice. The corneal epithelium of the *Frem2* mutant embryo stratifies unclearly with the reduction in corneal epithelial thickness. In addition, the dysplastic eyes exhibited a reduced axial length and reduced lens thickness compared to the wild-type mice.

Identification of Differentially Expressed Genes Enriched in the Metabolic Process

To identify other genes that potentially contribute to the ocular phenotype, RNA-seq was performed with RNA from the whole embryos of E13.5 mice. RNA-seq results confirmed decreased expression of *Frem2* and genes contributing to extracellular matrix organization and cell-matrix adhesion, including *Ecm2*, *Col6a1*, *Col5a3*, *Colla1*, and *Lama5* in *Frem2* mutant mice (Zhang et al., 2019). In addition, we observed differentially expressed genes including *Stat5a*, *Cbs*, *Dpys*, *Adssl1*, and *Pm20d1* participating in amino acid metabolism, and *Ldhb*, *Hk1*, *Chchd10* participating in energy metabolism in fetal *Frem2*$^{R725X/R2156W}$ mice.

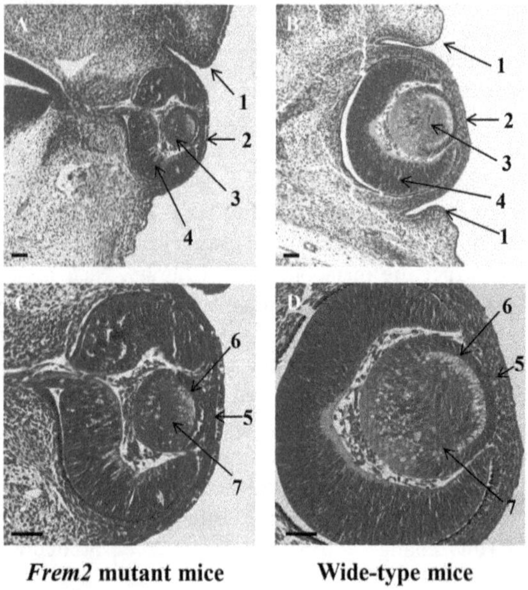

FIGURE 1 | Abnormal ocular development in fetal *Frem2* mutant mice. Histology of eyes from E13.5 *Frem2*$^{R725X/R2156W}$ mice **(A,C)** and wild-type mice **(B,D)**. **(A)** The lower eyelid fold cannot be defined in *Frem2* mutant mice, and the axial length and size of the lens are significantly reduced. **(C)** The corneal epithelium stratifies unclearly with the reduction in corneal epithelial thickness. The primary lens fibers are significantly shortened. Numbered arrows refer to the following: 1. eyelid; 2.cornea; 3. lens vesicle; 4. retina; 5. cornea epithelium; 6. lens epithelium; 7. primary lens fiber. Scale bars in all panels = 200 μm.

Moreover, there were 821 (39.89%) up-regulated genes and 320 (32.99%) down-regulated genes involved in the metabolic process in the enriched GO terms of biological processes (**Figure 2A**). The decreased expressions of *Ldhb* and increased expression levels of *Stat5a*, *Pm20d1*, *Chchd10*, and *Hk1* were verified by performing real-time quantitative PCR in the embryos of *Frem2*$^{R725X/R2156W}$ mice (**Figure 2B**).

Frem2 Mutant Fetal Mice Have a Distinct Metabolomic Profile

To determine whether the metabolomic signatures were consistent with the transcriptomic signatures, a total of 92 metabolites that differed significantly between the mutant and wild-type embryos of E13.5 mice were identified by untargeted metabolomics analysis (**Supplementary Table S2**). Principal component analysis plots were performed for both positive and negative modes, showing that metabolite profiles in embryos from *Frem2* mutant mice with ocular hypoplasia were very different from those in embryos from wild-type mice (**Figures 3A,B**). We identified the top 50 most different biologically significant metabolites, displayed by volcano plots in **Figures 3C,D**. Heatmaps of differentially expressed metabolites within fetal *Frem2* mutant mice were visualized in **Figure 4**. Metabolites including creatine, guanosine 5′-monophosphate, cytosine, cytidine 5′-monophosphate, adenine, and L-serine were identified to be altered in the whole embryos of *Frem2* mutant mice by targeted LC-MS analyses (**Figure 3E**).

Metabolites determined in untargeted metabolomics analysis were screened and placed into the KEGG database to determine chemical and metabolic pathways that could be involved in the development of cryptophthalmos. A total of 153 possible pathways were found to be involved, covering 74 specific metabolites. KEGG metabolic pathway analysis of different metabolites annotated significant features related to ABC transporters and biosynthesis of amino acids, indicating that these substances could also be involved in the pathogenesis of cryptophthalmos (**Table 1** and **Figure 3F**). Consistent with the KEGG analysis, real-time quantitative PCR confirmed the higher expression of ABC genes including *Abcc3*, *Abcc6*, and *Abcc9*, as well as genes contributing to the biosynthesis of amino acids in the embryos of *Frem2*$^{R725X/R2156W}$ mice (**Figure 2B**).

DISCUSSION

Ocular and eyelid development occurs in a step-wise fashion, and any misstep will be followed by the failure of subsequent steps (Tawfik et al., 2016). Our results confirmed that the phenotype of *Frem2* mutant embryonic mice shows consistent results with that of the adult mice characterized by abnormal eyelids,

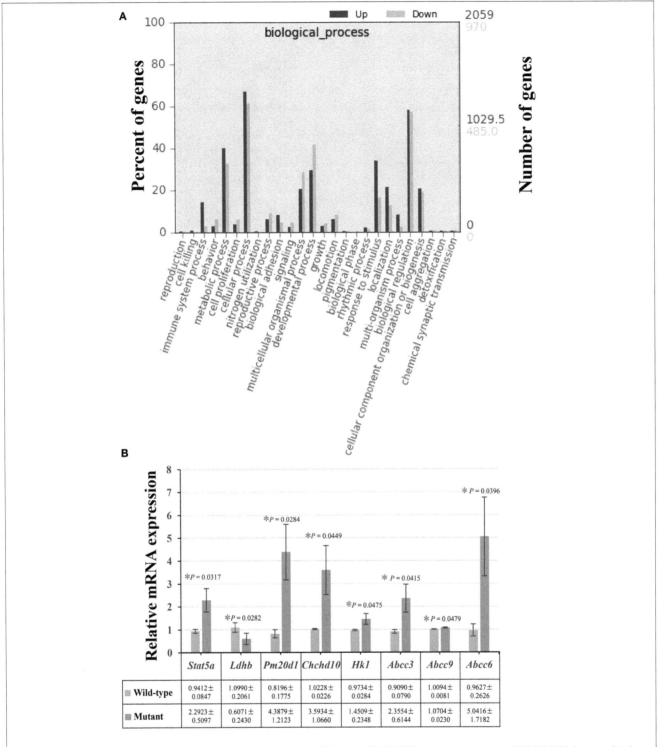

FIGURE 2 | Differentially expressed genes enriched in the metabolic process. **(A)** A total of 821 (39.89%) up-regulated genes and 320 (32.99%) down-regulated genes involved in the metabolic process were identified in the enriched GO terms of biological processes. **(B)** The decreased expressions of *Ldhb*, and increased expression levels of *Stat5a*, *Pm20d1*, *Chchd10*, *Hk1*, *Abcc3*, *Abcc9*, and *Abcc6* were verified by performing real-time quantitative PCR in the whole embryos of *Frem2*[R725X/R2156W] mice (*$P < 0.05$). Data are presented as the mean ± standard deviation ($n = 3$).

microphthalmia, and developmental defects in the anterior segment. In addition, these congenital ocular dysplasias begin to appear at E13.5.

This study has highlighted the impact of loss-of-function mutations of *Frem2* on the mouse embryonic metabolome. In particular, the data show connections between transcriptomic

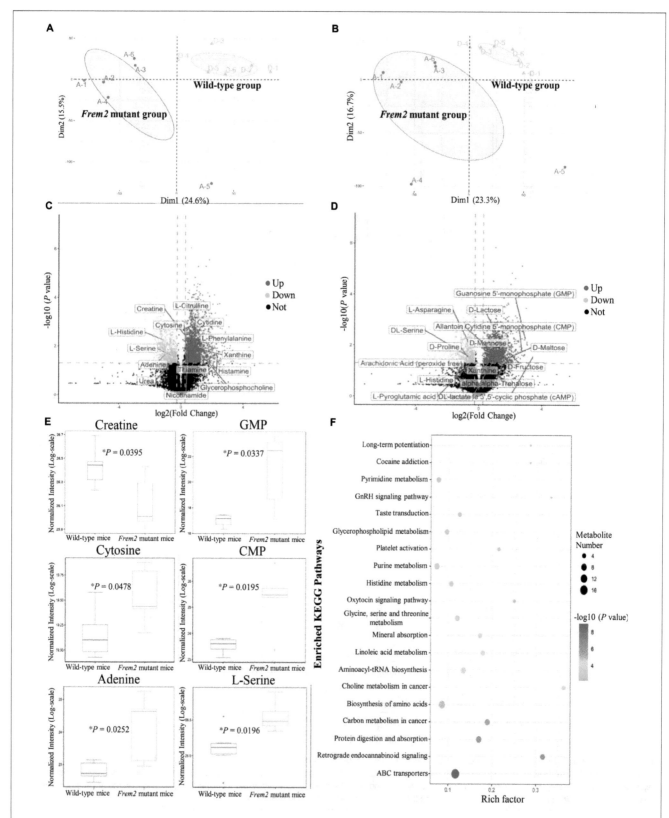

FIGURE 3 | Metabolites profiles in fetal $Frem2^{\Delta R725X/R2156W}$ mice. **(A,B)** Principal component analysis plots were performed under positive and negative modes. **(C,D)** Volcano plot showing the top 50 most different biologically significant metabolites under positive and negative modes. **(E)** Metabolites including creatine, guanosine 5′-monophosphate, cytosine, cytidine 5′-monophosphate, adenine, and L-serine were quantified in the embryos of Frem2 mutant mice compared with wild-type mice by targeted LC-MS analyses (*P < 0.05). **(F)** KEGG metabolic pathway analysis of different metabolites.

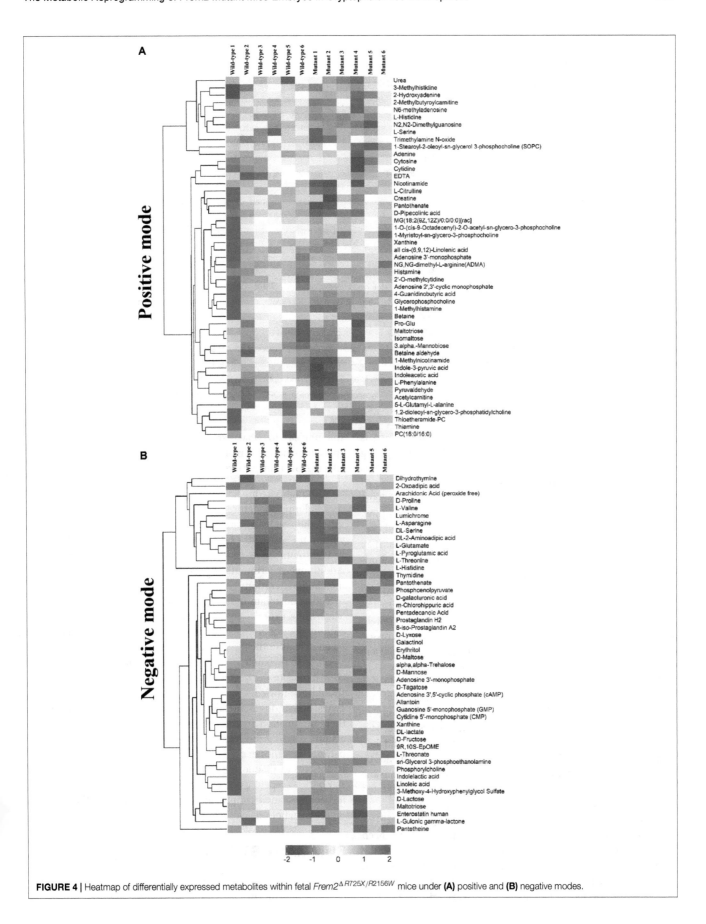

FIGURE 4 | Heatmap of differentially expressed metabolites within fetal $Frem2^{\Delta R725X/R2156W}$ mice under **(A)** positive and **(B)** negative modes.

TABLE 1 | The significantly altered pathways including more than ≥5 different metabolites.

Map ID	Map name	Metabolites name
map02010	ABC transporters	L-Histidine, Cytidine, Maltotriose, L-Phenylalanine, L-Serine, Thiamine, Urea, Betaine, D-galacturonic acid, D-Lactose, D-Mannose, Erythritol, D-Maltose, L-Threonine, L-Valine, L-Glutamate
map01230	Biosynthesis of amino acids	L-Citrulline, L-Histidine, L-Phenylalanine, L-Serine, L-Asparagine, Phosphoenolpyruvate, DL-2-Aminoadipic acid, L-Threonine, L-Valine, L-Glutamate, 2-Oxoadipic acid
map04974	Protein digestion and absorption	L-Histidine, L-Phenylalanine, Histamine, L-Serine, L-Asparagine, L-Threonine, L-Valine, L-Glutamate
map00970	Aminoacyl-tRNA biosynthesis	L-Histidine, L-Phenylalanine, L-Serine, L-Asparagine, L-Threonine, L-Valine, L-Glutamate
map05230	Central carbon metabolism in cancer	L-Histidine, L-Phenylalanine, L-Serine, L-Asparagine, Phosphoenolpyruvate, L-Valine, L-Glutamate
map00230	Purine metabolism	Xanthine, Adenine, Adenosine 3′-monophosphate, Urea, Adenosine 2′,3′-cyclic monophosphate, Guanosine 5′-monophosphate (GMP), Adenosine 3′,5′-cyclic phosphate (cAMP)
map00260	Glycine, serine, and threonine metabolism	Creatine, Pyruvaldehyde, L-Serine, Betaine aldehyde, Betaine, L-Threonine
map04723	Retrograde endocannabinoid signaling	PC(16:0/16:0), 1-Stearoyl-2-oleoyl-sn-glycerol 3-phosphocholine (SOPC), cAMP, Arachidonic Acid, Prostaglandin H2, L-Glutamate
map04978	Mineral absorption	L-Phenylalanine, L-Serine, L-Asparagine, L-Threonine, L-Valine
map00591	Linoleic acid metabolism	PC(16:0/16:0), SOPC, all cis-(6,9,12)-Linolenic acid, Arachidonic Acid, Linoleic acid
map00330	Arginine and proline metabolism	Creatine, 4-Guanidinobutyric acid, Urea, D-Proline, L-Glutamate
map00590	Arachidonic acid metabolism	PC(16:0/16:0), SOPC, Arachidonic Acid, 8-iso-Prostaglandin A2, Prostaglandin H2
map00340	Histidine metabolism	L-Histidine, 1-Methylhistamine, 3-Methylhistidine, Histamine, L-Glutamate
map01210	2-Oxocarboxylic acid metabolism	L-Phenylalanine, DL-2-Aminoadipic acid, L-Valine, L-Glutamate, 2-Oxoadipic acid
map00240	Pyrimidine metabolism	Cytidine, Cytosine, Urea, Cytidine 5′-monophosphate (CMP), Thymidine
map00564	Glycerophospholipid metabolism	PC(16:0/16:0), Glycerophosphocholine, SOPC, sn-Glycerol 3-phosphoethanolamine, Phosphorylcholine

and metabolomic signatures in *Frem2* mutant mice, which is intriguing coincides with reductions in metabolites participating in amino acid metabolism and energy metabolism. Metabolites identified to be altered in the *Frem2* mutant mice by targeted LC-MS analyses, including guanosine 5′-monophosphate, cytosine, cytidine 5′-monophosphate, adenine, and L-serine, were all essential in the ocular development. Overall, we demonstrate that changes in metabolome composition may have contributed to the development of the cryptophthalmos phenotype in *Frem2* mutant mice.

As shown in the KEGG metabolic pathway analysis, 16 different metabolites have been revealed to be related to the map of ABC transporters, which constitute a ubiquitous protein superfamily forming the largest transporter gene family expressed in various body tissues (Lee et al., 2016). ABC transporters translocate a wide variety of substrates, hydrophobic compounds, and metabolites across extra and intracellular membranes and play critical roles in maintaining intracellular balance (Gottesman et al., 2002; Szakacs et al., 2006). Mutations in these genes contribute to disorders including cystic fibrosis, neurological disease, retinal degeneration, cholesterol and bile transport defects, anemia, and drug response (Dean et al., 2001). Mutations in the ABCC6 gene were proved to be responsible for connective tissue disorder (Saux et al., 2000) and suggested to play a role in the transportation of toxic metabolites to which connective tissue cells are sensitive (Fung et al., 2019). In addition to these activities, ABC transporters have been shown to mediate epithelial to mesenchymal transition, and the cystic fibrosis transmembrane conductance regulator has been proven to function as a chloride/anion channel in epithelial cells around the body (Meng et al., 2016). However, it is

still unclear to what extent this transport effect is related to epithelial–mesenchymal coupling and how *FREM2* mutation affects ABC transporters.

Although connections between transcriptomic and metabolomic signatures have been shown in *Frem2* mutant mice, the results of our study should be cautiously interpreted within the context of C57BL/6J mice embryos, as postnatal validation in mice and humans should be further confirmed. Additional experiments are also required to study whether the metabolic alterations were paralleled to the genetic changes or served as upstream indicators in cryptophthalmos development. Meanwhile, experiments designed to clarify the chronology of the pathogenesis of cryptophthalmos are also essential for identifying when defects in the formation of the eye and other tissues occur.

Shifts in metabolome composition and functionality may have contributed to the cryptophthalmos phenotype. As a result, we should acknowledge the influence of both direct mutations in genes and indirect metabolic programming effects caused by their modulation in utero. This is suggestive of a cooperative action utilizing both metabolic detection and screening of pathogenic genes in prenatal diagnostic testing, as cryptothalmos is difficult to diagnose by prenatal B-ultrasound. Furthermore, as novel therapeutics of genome editing tools enter the market, it becomes increasingly important to consider their effects on the metabolome.

SUMMARY STATEMENT

Metabolomic and transcriptomic signatures provide a map of metabolism in the *Frem2* mutant mouse model of cryptophthalmos. These data provide insights into further mechanistic studies of the pathogenesis of cryptophthalmos.

ETHICS STATEMENT

All mouse procedures were approved by the Institutional Animal Care and Use Committee of Zhongshan Ophthalmic Center, Sun Yat-sen University.

AUTHOR CONTRIBUTIONS

HL and XYZ designed the study. XYZ, RW, XLZ, DW, and MD performed the experiments. XYZ analyzed the data and wrote the manuscript. TW, XW, DL, JW, and WL critically revised the manuscript. All authors discussed the results and commented on the manuscript.

REFERENCES

Cherif, H., François, D., Bruno, C., Bouchard, A., and Jean-François, B. (2018). Receptors of intermediates of carbohydrate metabolism, gpr91 and gpr99, mediate axon growth. *PLoS Biol.* 16:e2003619. doi: 10.1371/journal.pbio.2003619

Dean, M., Rzhetsky, A., and Allikmets, R. (2001). The human ATP-binding cassette (ABC) transporter superfamily. *Genom. Res.* 11:1156. doi: 10.1101/gr.gr-1649r

François, J. (1969). Malformative syndrome with cryptophthalmos. *Acta Genet. Med. Gemellol.* 18, 18–50. doi: 10.1017/s1120962300012294

Fung, S. W., Cheung, F. Y., Yip, C. W., Ng, W. C., and Cheung, S. T. (2019). The ATP-binding cassette transporter ABCF1 is a hepatic oncofetal protein that promotes chemoresistance, EMT and cancer stemness in hepatocellular carcinoma. *Cancer Lett.* 457, 98–109. doi: 10.1016/j.canlet.2019.05.010

Gottesman, M. M., Fojo, T., and Bates, S. E. (2002). Multidrug resistance in cancer: role of ATP-dependent transporters. *Nat. Rev. Cancer* 2, 48–58. doi: 10.1038/nrc706

Haelst, M. M. V., Maiburg, M., Baujat, G., Jadeja, S., and Scambler, P. J. (2010). Molecular study of 33 families with fraser syndrome new data and mutation review. *Am. J. Med. Genet. Part A* 146A, 2252–2257. doi: 10.1002/ajmg.a.32440

Jadeja, S., Smyth, I., Pitera, J. E., Taylor, M. S., van Haelst, M., Bentley, E., et al. (2005). Identification of a new gene mutated in Fraser syndrome and mouse myelencephalic blebs. *Nat. Genet.* 37, 520–525. doi: 10.1038/ng1549

Lee, J. Y., Kinch, L. N., Borek, D. M., Wang, J., and Rosenbaum, D. M. (2016). Crystal structure of the human sterol transporter abcg5/abcg8. *Nature* 533, 561–564. doi: 10.1038/nature17666

Meng, X., Clews, J., Kargas, V., Wang, X., and Ford, R. C. (2016). The cystic fibrosis transmembrane conductance regulator (CFTR) and its stability. *Cell. Mole. Life Sci.* 74, 23–38.

Paramita, P., Naik, A., Birbrair, K., and Bhutia, S. (2018). Mitophagy-driven metabolic switch reprograms stem cell fate. *Cell. Mole. Life Sci.* 76, 27–43. doi: 10.1007/s00018-018-2922-9

Pei, Y. F., and Rhodin, J. A. G. (1970). The prenatal development of the mouse eye. *Anatom. Record* 168, 105–125. doi: 10.1002/ar.1091680109

Piazza, I., Kochanowski, K., Cappelletti, V., Fuhrer, T., Noor, E., Sauer, U., et al. (2018). A map of protein-metabolite interactions reveals principles of chemical communication. *Cell* 172, 358–372.e.

Robciuc, A., Hyötyläinen, T., Jauhiainen, M., and Holopainen, J. M. (2013). Ceramides in the pathophysiology of the anterior segment of the eye. *Curr. Eye Res.* 38, 1006–1016. doi: 10.3109/02713683.2013.810273

Saux, O. L., Urban, Z., Tschuch, C., Csiszar, K., and Boyd, C. D. (2000). Mutations in a gene encoding an abc transporter cause pseudoxanthoma elasticum. *Nat. Genet.* 25, 223–227. doi: 10.1038/76102

Szakacs, G., Paterson, J. K., Ludwig, J. A., Booth-Genthe, C., and Gottesman, M. M. (2006). Targeting multidrug resistance in cancer. *Nat. Rev. Drug Discov.* 5, 219–234.

Tawfik, H. A., Abdulhafez, M. H., Fouad, Y. A., and Dutton, J. J. (2016). Embryologic and fetal development of the human eyelid. *Ophthal. Plastic Reconstru. Sur.* 32:407. doi: 10.1097/iop.0000000000000702

Zhang, X., Wang, D., Dongye, M., Zhu, Y., and Lin, H. (2019). Loss-of-function mutations in frem2 disrupt eye morphogenesis. *Exp. Eye Res.* 181, 302–312. doi: 10.1016/j.exer.2019.02.013

19

AI-Model for Identifying Pathologic Myopia Based on Deep Learning Algorithms of Myopic Maculopathy Classification and "Plus" Lesion Detection in Fundus Images

Li Lu[1†], Peifang Ren[2†], Xuyuan Tang[2†], Ming Yang[1], Minjie Yuan[1], Wangshu Yu[1], Jiani Huang[1], Enliang Zhou[3], Lixian Lu[4], Qin He[2], Miaomiao Zhu[2], Genjie Ke[3] and Wei Han[1]*

[1] Department of Ophthalmology, Eye Center of the Second Affiliated Hospital, School of Medicine, Zhejiang University, Hangzhou, China, [2] Department of Ophthalmology, The First Affiliated Hospital, School of Medicine, Zhejiang University, Hangzhou, China, [3] Department of Ophthalmology, The First Affiliated Hospital of University of Science and Technology of China, Hefei, China, [4] College of Computer Science and Technology, Zhejiang University, Hangzhou, China

*Correspondence:
Wei Han
hanweidr@zju.edu.cn

[†] These authors have contributed equally to this work and share the first authorship

Background: Pathologic myopia (PM) associated with myopic maculopathy (MM) and "Plus" lesions is a major cause of irreversible visual impairment worldwide. Therefore, we aimed to develop a series of deep learning algorithms and artificial intelligence (AI)–models for automatic PM identification, MM classification, and "Plus" lesion detection based on retinal fundus images.

Materials and Methods: Consecutive 37,659 retinal fundus images from 32,419 patients were collected. After excluding 5,649 ungradable images, a total dataset of 32,010 color retinal fundus images was manually graded for training and cross-validation according to the META-PM classification. We also retrospectively recruited 1,000 images from 732 patients from the three other hospitals in Zhejiang Province, serving as the external validation dataset. The area under the receiver operating characteristic curve (AUC), sensitivity, specificity, accuracy, and quadratic-weighted kappa score were calculated to evaluate the classification algorithms. The precision, recall, and F1-score were calculated to evaluate the object detection algorithms. The performance of all the algorithms was compared with the experts' performance. To better understand the algorithms and clarify the direction of optimization, misclassification and visualization heatmap analyses were performed.

Results: In five-fold cross-validation, algorithm I achieved robust performance, with accuracy = 97.36% (95% CI: 0.9697, 0.9775), AUC = 0.995 (95% CI: 0.9933, 0.9967), sensitivity = 93.92% (95% CI: 0.9333, 0.9451), and specificity = 98.19% (95% CI: 0.9787, 0.9852). The macro-AUC, accuracy, and quadratic-weighted kappa were 0.979, 96.74% (95% CI: 0.963, 0.9718), and 0.988 (95% CI: 0.986, 0.990) for algorithm II. Algorithm III achieved an accuracy of 0.9703 to 0.9941 for classifying the "Plus" lesions and an F1-score of 0.6855 to 0.8890 for detecting and localizing lesions. The performance metrics in external validation dataset were comparable to those of the experts and were slightly inferior to those of cross-validation.

Conclusion: Our algorithms and AI-models were confirmed to achieve robust performance in real-world conditions. The application of our algorithms and AI-models has promise for facilitating clinical diagnosis and healthcare screening for PM on a large scale.

Keywords: artificial intelligence, deep learning, pathologic myopia, myopic maculopathy, "Plus" lesion, fundus image

INTRODUCTION

It is now widely believed that myopia is epidemic across the world, especially in developed countries of East and Southeast Asia (Dolgin, 2015). Myopia also has a significant impact on public health and socioeconomic wellbeing (Smith, 2009; Zheng et al., 2013; Holden et al., 2016). Pathologic myopia (PM), a severe form of myopia defined as high myopia combined with a series of characteristic maculopathy lesions, involves a greater risk of adverse ocular tissue changes leading to associated sight-threatening complications (Wong et al., 2014; Cho et al., 2016). For this reason, PM is a major cause of severe irreversible vision loss and blindness in East Asian countries (Morgan et al., 2017; Ohno-Matsui et al., 2019).

Due to the irreversible pathologic alterations in the shape and structure of the myopic globe, effective therapies for PM are still lacking, and the prognosis of PM complications is often poor. Moreover, as the disease process progresses slowly (Hayashi et al., 2010), PM patients often ignore their ocular symptoms and attribute these changes to their unsuitable glasses. Therefore, a better strategy for PM may be regular screening in myopic populations to identify and stop the aggravation of PM at an early stage. The precise diagnosis and evaluation of PM requires ophthalmic work-up and is aided by a series of imaging examinations, including fundus imaging, optical coherence tomography (OCT), and three-dimensional magnetic resonance imaging (3D-MRI) (Faghihi et al., 2010; Moriyama et al., 2011) which can hardly be included in screening programs. A recent meta-analysis of a pathologic myopia system (META-PM) provided a new simplified systematic classification for myopic maculopathy (MM) and defined PM based on fundus photography, which offers us a practical screening criterion (Ohno-Matsui et al., 2015). According to this classification standard, eyes with MM, which is equal to or more serious than diffuse choroidal atrophy, or with at least one "Plus" lesion, can be defined as having PM (Ohno-Matsui, 2017). However, even with this criterion, PM screening still depends on careful examination of the whole retina by retinal specialists through a magnified slit lamp noncontact lens or fundus images (Baird et al., 2020), challenging the ophthalmic medical resources in terms of clinical data analysis, especially retinal fundus image reading. It is difficult to imagine that such a large-scale screening task could be carried out by humans alone.

Fortunately, with the rapid development of artificial intelligence (AI) technologies, a sophisticated subclass of machine learning known as deep learning plays important roles in automated clinical data processing and hence makes labor-intensive work feasible (Hamet and Tremblay, 2017). The AI-model, with a deep artificial neural network as its core, has shown great efficiency and excellent performance comparable to those of board-certified specialists with respect to massive medical analysis (Esteva et al., 2017; Zhao et al., 2018; Liao et al., 2020). AI-model related diagnosis software has been successfully applied to screening tasks of diabetic retinopathy and glaucoma (Bhaskaranand et al., 2019; Li et al., 2020).

This study aimed to design and train a series of deep learning algorithms and AI-models based on the META-PM classification system using a large dataset of color retinal fundus images obtained from the ophthalmic clinics of hospitals and annotated by expert teams. We hope our models could (1) identify PM, (2) classify the category of MM, and (3) detect and localize the "Plus" lesions automatically. These works would facilitate the PM identification for either clinical management in hospital or healthcare service in community.

MATERIALS AND METHODS

Data Collection

In this study, the use of images was approved by the Ethics Committee of First Affiliated Hospital, School of Medicine, Zhejiang University. As the study was a retrospective review and analysis of fully anonymized retinal fundus images, the medical ethics committee declared it exempt from informed consent.

Altogether, 37,659 original color retinal fundus images of 32,419 myopia patients were obtained from the eye centers of the First Affiliated Hospital of School of Medicine, Zhejiang University; the First Affiliated Hospital of University of Science and Technology of China; and the First Affiliated Hospital of Soochow University between July 2016 and January 2020, and analysis began February 2020. Three different desktop nonmydriatic retinal cameras (Canon, NIDEK, and Topcon) were used. Similar imaging protocols were applied for all three systems. All retinal fundus images were maculalutea-centered 45° color fundus photographs. Pupil dilation was decided by the examiners depending on the patient's ocular condition. All patient data displayed with the images were pseudonymized before study inclusion.

Subsequently, the ungradable images were excluded. The criteria applied to determine a gradable image are listed as follows:

(a) Image field definition: primary field must include the entire optic nerve head and macula.
(b) Images should have perfect exposure because dark and washed-out areas interfere with detailed grading.
(c) The focus should be good for grading of small retinal lesions.
(d) Fewer artifacts: Avoid dust spots, arc defects, and eyelash images.
(e) There should be no other errors in the fundus photograph, such as the absence of objects in the picture.

According to this criteria, 5,649 ungradable images were excluded. A total dataset of 32,010 color retinal fundus images was established and further annotated by ophthalmologists.

Definitions, Annotation, and the Reference Standard

According to the META-PM study classification, MM was classified into five categories: no myopic retinal degenerative lesion (Category 0), tessellated fundus (Category 1), diffuse chorioretinal atrophy (Category 2), patchy chorioretinal atrophy (Category 3), and macular atrophy (Category 4). Additionally, lacquer cracks (LCs), myopic choroidal neovascularization (CNV), and Fuchs' spot were defined as "Plus" lesions (Ohno-Matsui et al., 2015). Thus, in the present study, fundus image with MM $\geq$ Category 2 or with at least one of the "Plus" lesions were considered as a PM image, while the remaining images were defined as non-PM images including the MM of Category 0 or Category 1 without "Plus" lesions. All the images of PM or C1-C4 MM were from high myopia patients whose spherical equivalence is worse than -6.0 D. The relevant demographic data were shown in **Table 1**. It is worth mentioning that Category 0 in this study included normal fundus and other fundus diseases.

After learning the definition and testing the intra- and inter-rater reliability, a total of 20 ophthalmologists from three ophthalmic centers, who achieved a kappa value ≥ 0.81 (almost perfect), participated in manual grading and annotation and served as graders (Landis and Koch, 1977). Fifteen of them were general ophthalmologists with more than 5 years of experience, and five of them were senior retinal specialists with over 10 years of experience. They were randomly grouped into five teams, with each team having one senior specialist. The reference standard was determined based on the following protocol. Graders on the same team evaluated the same set of images. Each grader was blinded to the grades given by the others, and they made independent decisions on the fundus images. The results recognized unanimously by the three graders of the same team were taken as the reference standard. The results that differed among the general ophthalmologists in the same team were arbitrated by the retinal specialist for the final annotation decision. For the detailed workflow of data

processing, all available fundus images were involved ($n = 37,659$) at the beginning stage, and the ungradable images were then identified and excluded by the grader teams. Next, in the gradable images group ($n = 32,010$), image-level binary classification label was given by grader teams to describe whether the eye had PM, which was used to develop algorithm I. Simultaneously, all the gradable images would obtain a category label according to its MM category, which was used to develop algorithm II. These two kinds of labels were based on the criteria of META-PM classification, with PM or C1–C4 MM images confirmed by the refractive error data (spherical equivalence worse than -6.0 D). Lastly, in the PM image group, graders localized the "Plus" lesions within the image if they existed by drawing rectangular bounding boxes, which was used to develop algorithm III. Meanwhile, the image was labeled as having the corresponding "Plus" lesions.

Image Preprocessing and Augmentation

All the raw fundus images were preprocessed by cropping and resizing to a resolution of 512×512 pixels to meet the requirement of the input image format. Grayscale transformations, geometric variation, and image enhancement were applied to eliminate irrelevant information and recover useful or true information in the images.

Development of the Deep Learning Algorithms and AI-Models

Our training platform was implemented with the PyTorch framework, and all of the deep learning algorithms were trained in parallel on four NVIDIA 2080 Ti graphics processing units (Paszke et al., 2019). In this study, three deep learning algorithms were trained after annotation: (I) for the binary classification of non-pathologic myopia/pathologic myopia (NPM/PM), (II) for the five-class classification of MM categories, and (III) for "Plus" lesion detection and localization.

Based on the three algorithms, two AI-models, namely Model I and II, were developed. Model-1 was a one-step model, only containing algorithm I, to directly identify the NPM and PM. Model-2 was a two-step model, consisting of algorithm II, algorithm III, and a logical analysis module. The core of the logical analysis module was the META-PM classification. Step 1 was to obtain the output of the image by algorithm II and algorithm III, while step 2 was to use the logical analysis module to analyze the result of step 1 and then determine whether the image was of PM. The performance of two models was then compared in order to obtain the optimized model for PM identification. The detailed workflow is shown in **Figure 1**.

A five-fold cross-validation approach was employed to train and test the algorithms (Yang et al., 2019). The total dataset was randomly subgrouped into five equally sized folds at the image level, and each image was allowed to exist in one-fold. Effort was made to ensure that the rate of classification outcome was basically consistent from fold to fold (Herzig et al., 2020). The development process included two steps: first, we randomly selected four-folds for algorithm training and hyperparameter optimization and the remaining fold for testing. Then, this

TABLE 1 | Summary of the total dataset and external validation dataset.

	Number of images with labels	Number of participants	Number of ROI with labels	Mean age (years)	Sex (% female)	Spherical Equivalent (diopters)
Total dataset						
None PM	26,131	24,708	NA	50.39 ± 14.27(24 to 81)	56.3	−2.07 ± 3.79(−13 to −0.5)
Pathologic myopia	5,879	4,205	NA	52.39 ± 15.15(23 to 82)	66.0	−13.72 ± 4.54(−23.0 to −6)
Category 0	20,919	20,884	NA	50.52 ± 14.47(26 to 75)	54.5	−0.53 ± 0.33(−6.5 to −0.5)
Category 1	5,345	3,902	NA	49.59 ± 12.99(24 to 81)	65.8	−10.52 ± 2.98(−17.5 to −6)
Category 2	4,044	2,943	NA	50.10 ± 14.90(23 to 75)	64.5	−12.88 ± 4.02(−19.25 to −7.25)
Category 3	1,154	871	NA	56.90 ± 14.63(29 to 80)	71.1	−15.77 ± 4.89(−22.5 to −7.75)
Category 4	548	313	NA	63.22 ± 12.49(33 to 82)	68.7	−16.21 ± 5.38(−23.0 to −8.25)
CNV	734	442	857	55.28 ± 15.42(26 to 82)	60.6	−15.02 ± 3.98(−22 to -7)
Fuchs	746	411	3,020	58.24 ± 13.40(24 to 80)	58.2	−16.21 ± 4.23(−23 to −7.75)
LC	99	79	207	43.11 ± 12.76(25 to 73)	56.3	−15.47 ± 3.09(−21.75 to −6.75)
External validation dataset						
None PM	434	381	NA	51.28 ± 9.61(16 to 69)	55.1	−4.92 ± 5.16(−16 to −0.5)
Pathologic myopia	566	351	NA	54.71 ± 13.60(17 to 83)	61.3	−15.41 ± 6.05(−23.5 to −6)
Category 0	229	217	NA	50.85 ± 10.82(16 to 69)	49.3	−0.67 ± 0.72(−6.75 to −0.5)
Category 1	222	178	NA	50.21 ± 9.41(18 to 67)	59.6	−10.81 ± 2.68(−17.75 to −6)
Category 2	220	149	NA	51.60 ± 10.48(17 to 75)	61.7	−14.02 ± 5.54(−21 to −7.25)
Category 3	196	115	NA	55.93 ± 13.06(26 to 80)	66.1	−16.35 ± 6.14(−23.5 to −6.75)
Category 4	133	73	NA	63.71 ± 13.59(35 to 83)	60.3	−17.04 ± 6.58(−23.5 to −6.5)
CNV	67	41	97	51.27 ± 13.88(27 to 80)	54.5	−16.15 ± 5.57(−23 to −6.5)
Fuchs	205	130	878	59.24 ± 13.42(27 to 81)	58.6	−16.89 ± 5.81(−23.25 to −7)
LC	9	6	24	39.50 ± 11.26(26 to 53)	50.0	−15.96 ± 3.78(−22.25 to −7.5)

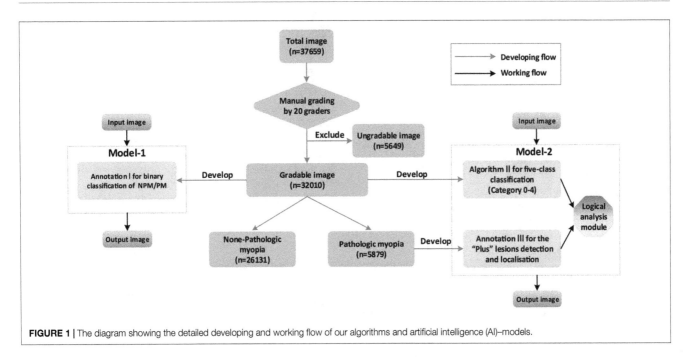

FIGURE 1 | The diagram showing the detailed developing and working flow of our algorithms and artificial intelligence (AI)–models.

process was repeated five times to confirm that each fold was set as the testing set (Keenan et al., 2019).

Architecture of Deep Learning Algorithms

Algorithm I and algorithm II in this study were based on a state-of-the-art convolutional neural network (CNN) architecture, namely, ResNet18, while algorithm III for "Plus" lesion localization was constructed using a feature pyramid network (FPN)–based faster region-based convolutional neural network (Faster R-CNN). These architectures were all pretrained on the ImageNet dataset. The details of the relevant CNN architectures are shown in **Supplementary Figure 1**.

Retrospective External Validation and Expert-Machine Comparison

To further evaluate our algorithms, we also retrospectively recruited 1,000 images from 732 patients from the three other hospitals in Zhejiang Province, serving as the external validation dataset (**Table 1**). Two different types of desktop nonmydriatic retinal cameras (Canon and ZEISS) were used to capture fundus images, and these were different from the cameras used to acquire training data. The annotation protocol for this dataset was the same as that for the total dataset. The images in the external validation dataset were simultaneously evaluated by the algorithms and two experts (one general ophthalmologist and one retinal specialist) who were not the participants in the aforementioned grading teams. The comparison results between the algorithms and experts were used to further quantify the performance of the algorithms.

Misclassification and Visualization Heatmap Analysis of Classification Algorithms

In the external validation dataset, the images misclassified by algorithms I and II were further analyzed by a senior retinal specialist. To provide detailed guidance for clinical analysis, a convolutional visualization layer was implanted at the end of algorithm II. Then, this layer generated a visualization heatmap highlighting the strongly predictive regions on retinal fundus images (Gargeya and Leng, 2017). The consistency analysis between the hot regions and the actual lesions was evaluated by a senior retinal specialist.

Statistics

According to the reference standard, all five-fold cross-validation results of the algorithms were recorded, and the average metrics were calculated. The performance of algorithm I was evaluated using the indices of sensitivity, specificity, accuracy, and area under the receiver operating characteristic curve (AUC). For the five-class classification of MM categories, the area under the macroaverage of ROC curve (macro-AUC) for each class in a one-vs.-all manner, the kappa score and the accuracy were calculated to evaluate algorithm II. Algorithm III was evaluated in two dimensions: (1) image classification and (2) region of interest (ROI) detection and lesion localization. Two groups of performance metrics were calculated. The former consisted of the accuracy, sensitivity, and specificity of binary classifications of the image with "Plus" lesions, while the latter included precision, recall, and F1-score. Model-1 and model-2 were compared with respect to the indices of sensitivity, specificity, precision, and accuracy. In the external validation dataset, the same indices were also calculated and compared with the experts of different expertise levels. All of the statistical tests in our study were two-sided, and a P-value less than 0.05 was considered significant. Additionally, the Clopper–Pearson method was used to calculate the 95% CIs. Statistical data analysis was implemented using IBM SPSS statistics for Windows version 26.0 (SPSS Inc., Chicago, IL, United States) and Python 3.7.3.

RESULTS

A total dataset of 32,010 color retinal fundus images from 28,913 patients was built and used for algorithm training and validation. Among the total dataset, approximately 13% of the graded images

with inconsistent diagnoses were submitted to retinal specialists for final grading. The characteristics of the total dataset are summarized in **Table 1**.

Performance of the Five-Fold Cross-Validation

The five-fold cross-validation was used to evaluate the three algorithms. Specifically, algorithm I achieved an AUC of 0.995 (95% CI: 0.993–0.996), accuracy of 0.973 (95% CI: 0.969–0.977), specificity of 0.981 (95% CI: 0.978–0.985) and sensitivity of 0.939 (95% CI: 0.933–0.945) (**Table 2** and **Figure 2A**). Algorithm II achieved a macro-AUC value of 0.979 (95% CI: 0.972–0.985), accuracy of 0.967 (95% CI: 0.963–0.971), and quadratic-weighted kappa of 0.988 (95% CI: 0.986–0.990) for differentiating the five MM categories (**Table 2** and **Figure 2B**). From C0 to C4 MM, the specific accuracy of algorithm II is 97.7, 97.8, 91.3, 96.1, and 90.0% respectively. The confusion matrices of algorithm I and algorithm II are shown in **Supplementary Figures 2A,B**. Algorithm III achieved an accuracy of 0.970 to 0.994 for identifying the "Plus" lesions and an F1-score of 0.685 to 0.889 for detecting and localizing lesions. The typical output images of algorithm III are shown in **Supplementary Figure 3**. The more detailed results are listed in **Table 2**. The accuracy of model-1 and model-2 was 0.973 (95% CI: 0.969–0.977) and 0.984 (95% CI: 0.981–0.987), respectively. The two-step model-2 showed better performance in identifying PM.

External Validation and Expert-Machine Comparison

Based on the results of better performance in identifying PM, model-2 and algorithms were further evaluated in the external validation dataset (**Supplementary Table 1** and **Supplementary Figures 2C,D**). The performance of model-2 and the three algorithms in the external validation dataset was slightly worse than that in the total dataset. Although there was significant difference in accuracy between the AI-models/deep learning algorithms and experts in terms of identifying PM ($P = 0.013$), distinguishing different MM lesions ($P < 0.001$), and detecting CNV ($P < 0.001$) and Fuchs' spot ($P < 0.001$), the AI-models/deep learning algorithms achieved an overall comparable performance to that of the experts (**Figure 3**). For PM identifying, model-2 exhibited even higher accuracy than the general ophthalmologist (96.9 vs. 96.1%). In each task of algorithm II and algorithm III, the difference in accuracy compared to the general ophthalmologist was within 3%. The detailed outcomes of the external validation are shown in **Supplementary Table 1**.

Misclassified Image Analysis in the External Validation Dataset

There were 49 images misclassified by algorithm I, including 21 false negatives and 28 false positives. All false negatives were produced in eyes with the other PM complications, such as retinal detachment and retinal vein obstruction. The false positives included 24 tessellated fundus images, 3 proliferative retinopathy images, and 1 exudative retinopathy image. The major error of algorithm II was that 38 Category 0 images were erroneously

AI-Model for Identifying Pathologic Myopia Based on Deep Learning Algorithms of Myopic Maculopathy Classification...

215

TABLE 2 | Five-fold cross-validation of the performance of the algorithms in the total dataset.

		AUC (95% CI)	Accuracy (95% CI)	Specificity (95% CI)	Sensitivity (95% CI)		
Algorithm I		0.995 (0.993, 0.996)	0.973 (0.969, 0.977)	0.981 (0.978, 0.985)	0.939 (0.933, 0.945)		

		Macro-AUC	Accuracy (95% CI)	Quadratic-weighted kappa (95% CI)			
Algorithm II		0.979 (0.972, 0.985)	0.967 (0.963, 0.971)	0.988 (0.986, 0.990)			

		Image classification			ROI detection and lesion localization		
	Classification	Accuracy (95% CI)	Specificity (95% CI)	Sensitivity (95% CI)	Recall	Precision	F1-score
Algorithm III	CNV	0.970 (0.966, 0.974)	0.970 (0.966, 0.974)	0.973 (0.969, 0.977)	0.916	0.789	0.848
	Fuchs	0.971 (0.967, 0.975)	0.971 (0.967, 0.975)	0.978 (0.975, 0.982)	0.915	0.864	0.889
	LC	0.994 (0.992, 0.995)	0.995 (0.993, 0.996)	0.684 (0.672, 0.695)	0.724	0.656	0.688

	Accuracy (95% CI)		Sensitivity (95% CI)	Specificity (95% CI)	Precision (95% CI)		
Model-1	0.973 (0.969, 0.977)		0.939 (0.933, 0.945)	0.981 (0.978, 0.985)	0.926 (0.920, 0.933)		
Model-2	0.984 (0.981, 0.987)		0.946 (0.941, 0.952)	0.992 (0.990, 0.995)	0.967 (0.963, 0.972)		

classified as Category 1 images. Additionally, 23 Category 3 images were identified as Category 4 images. Typical misclassified images are shown in **Supplementary Figures 4A–E**, and the confusion matrices are given in **Supplementary Figures 2C,D**.

Visualization Heatmap Analysis

The original images of different MM categories were input into algorithm II as exampled in **Figure 4A**. After generating a fundus heatmap by the visualization layer, the regions where the algorithm thought most critical for its choice were highlighted in a color scale as shown in **Figure 4B**. Subsequently, the senior retinal specialist checked the consistency of hot regions highlighted by the algorithm and actual typical MM lesions, including tessellated fundus, diffuse chorioretinal atrophy, patchy chorioretinal atrophy, and macular atrophy. The results by algorithm showed good alignment with the diagnosis by the specialists. Of note, in ophthalmic practice, these lesions are used to diagnose PM.

DISCUSSION

Based on retinal fundus images, the present work developed a series of deep learning algorithms implementing three tasks: (1) identify PM, (2) classify the category of MM, and (3) localize the "Plus" lesions. After comparing two AI-models comprising the three algorithms, we confirmed that the two-step AI-model (model-2) showed better performance. Although there were

still gaps between the AI-models/algorithms and the retinal specialists, metrics of our AI-models/algorithms at this stage were comparable to the general ophthalmologists. Our work was an exploratory and innovative effort to apply deep learning technologies to the diagnosis and management of PM.

Recently, several automatic detection systems for PM have been reported. Tan et al. (2009) introduced the PAMELA system, which could automatically identify PM based on the peripapillary atrophy features. Freire et al. (2020) reported their work of PM diagnosis and detection of retinal structures and some lesions which achieved satisfactory performance both in classification and segmentation tasks. Devda and Eswari (2019) developed a deep learning method with CNN for tasks of Pathologic Myopia Challenge (PALM) based on the dataset provided by International Symposium on Biomedical Imaging (ISBI). Their works showed a better performance when compared to the PAMELA system. However, both of these systems were developed from public databases, such as the Singapore Cohort Study of the Risk factors for Myopia and ISBI. The volumes of the training and test datasets involved in the development process of these systems have been relatively small. Moreover, authoritative criteria for identifying PM were lacking in these studies.

In this work, a large dataset of 37,659 retinal fundus images was used to develop the algorithms. The dataset from real world was able to provide more original disease information and data complexity than public databases. Nevertheless, one major challenge for algorithms is the general applicability to the data and hardware settings outside the development

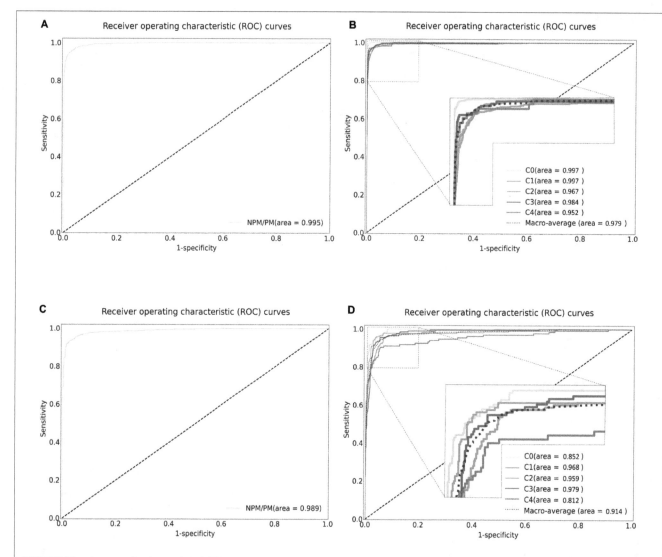

FIGURE 2 | Receiver operating characteristic (ROC) curves of Algorithm I and Algorithm II in five-fold cross-validation and external validation. **(A)** The ROC curve of the algorithm I for identifying pathologic myopia in five-fold cross-validation. **(B)** The ROC curve of the algorithm II for classifying the category of MM in five-fold cross-validation. **(C)** The ROC curve of the algorithm I for identifying pathologic myopia in external validation. **(D)** The ROC curve of the algorithm II for classifying the category of MM in external validation. NPM: non-pathologic myopia. PM: pathologic myopia. area: area under the receiver operating characteristic curve. C: Category.

site (Liu et al., 2019). One resolution is to maximize the diversity of data sources so as to prevent parameter overfitting and improve generalizability. For the present work, all the training images were obtained from three hospitals in three different provinces and captured by cameras from three different manufacturers, respectively. Meanwhile, we also constructed an external validation dataset including 1,000 fundus images from the other three additional hospitals to further test our algorithms and AI-models. As expected, the high diversity of the data source lowered the performance of our algorithms somewhat, but the results were still acceptable, with the accuracy of 96.9%, sensitivity of 98.8%, and specificity of 94.6% for model-2 especially, justifying the validity of our algorithms.

This study applied a systemic classification standard of META-PM, which was widely applied in clinical trials and epidemiologic

studies. Unlike the criteria used in other studies, META-PM classification is not only simpler but also has more clinical implications. The category of MM can reflect the severity of PM to a large extent, as the morphological and functional characteristics of highly myopic eyes were found to be positively correlated with MM category (from Category 0 to 3) (Zhao et al., 2020). The "Plus" lesions can be concurrent with any MM category and have a significant impact on vision (Wong et al., 2015). Therefore, our algorithms and AI-models can assist the clinicians with valuable and practical fundus information of PM.

There was a similar study that applied the META-PM classification. Du et al. (2021) reported a META-PM categorizing system (META-PM CS) integrating four DL algorithms and a special processing layer. This system could recognize the fundus images of Category 2 to 4 MM and CNV and detect PM

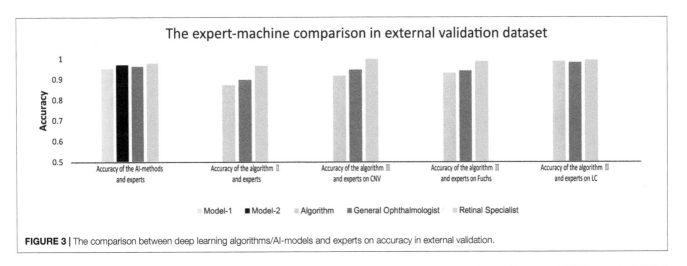

FIGURE 3 | The comparison between deep learning algorithms/AI-models and experts on accuracy in external validation.

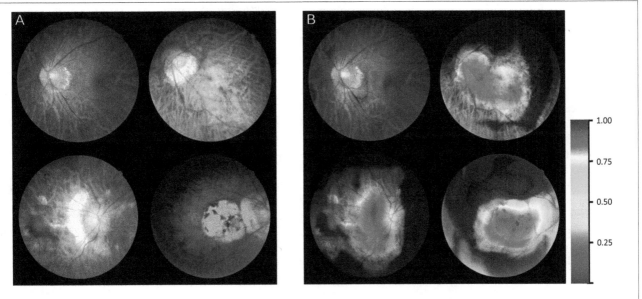

FIGURE 4 | Visualization of algorithm II for classifying the category of myopic maculopathy (MM). **(A)** The original images of different MM (Category 1–Category 4). **(B)** Heatmap generated from deep features overlaid on the original images. The typical MM lesions were observed in the hot regions.

defined as having MM equal to or more serious than diffuse atrophy (category 2). Compared with their system, our deep learning algorithms are more powerful and can automatically classify the category of MM and localize the "Plus" lesions based on retinal fundus images. Our AI-model could obtain the output of the algorithms mentioned above and use the logical analysis module to analyze the results of algorithms to determine whether the image was of PM. The core of the logical analysis module was the more precise PM definition (equal to or more serious than diffuse atrophy (category 2) or with at least one of the "plus" lesions) based on the META-PM classification.

In addition to the large training dataset and systemic META-PM standard, the other advantage of our work is the CNN architecture selected for development of algorithms and AI-models. The ResNet18 was used as the basic architecture for all the classification algorithms, and the Faster R-CNN+FPN was

used for the localization algorithm in our work. ResNet was proposed in 2015 after three classical CNN networks, namely, AlexNet, GoogLeNet, and VGG were established and had won the top prize in the ImageNet competition classification task. ResNet is arguably the most pioneering work in computer vision and deep learning in the past few years, as it can effectively solve the problem of accuracy saturation and decline while the network depth increases by introducing a shortcut mechanism (He et al., 2016; Zhu et al., 2019). Faster R-CNN is one of the most advanced object detection networks, which can integrate the feature and proposal extractions as well as the classification and bounding box regression (Ren et al., 2017; Ding et al., 2020). FPN, a densely connected feature pyramid network, can build high-level semantic feature maps at all scales for object detection (Tayara and Chong, 2018; Pan et al., 2019). With the same backbone network, the FPN-based Faster R-CNN system is thought to be superior to all existing single-model entries (Pan et al., 2019).

Therefore, our algorithms and AI-models were based on the advanced architectures and should be precise and efficient for the PM detection.

The distribution of misclassifications by our algorithms was also analyzed in the external validation dataset. The misclassified images generated by algorithm I were mainly due to the misjudgment of certain diseases that appeared less frequently in training. Meanwhile, algorithm II made some errors in distinguishing Category 3 and Category 4 MM. To minimize the errors, increasing the images of specific diseases into the training dataset and applying visual attention mechanisms to the CNN architecture will always be an effective approach (Pesce et al., 2019). Moreover, the visualization results demonstrated that the typical MM lesions of each category appeared in the regions where the algorithm made a positive contribution to the classification results, so that our algorithm is justified to be convincing from the clinical point of view. These results also indicated the directions of optimization and updating for the algorithms in our future's work.

This study still has limitations. First, our algorithm had the ability to automatically detect and localize "Plus" lesions, but the performance metrics were slightly lower if compared with that in the mission of MM classification, especially for the LC detection. LCs vary greatly in shape, size, color, and location. Combining with infrared reflectance or indocyanine green angiography image is certainly the more effective method to detect LCs than using the fundus images alone. However, the fundus images are relatively easy and economical for clinical practice in most medical institutes. At this stage, the "plus" lesions appeared in less than 15% of images containing MM of all severity in the total dataset. With the continuously accumulated data by our work, the performance of the algorithm will be further improved. Second, the presence of posterior staphyloma is also defined as PM according to the META-PM classification (Ohno-Matsui et al., 2016), but it is difficult to diagnose posterior staphyloma accurately from fundus images; MRI or OCT images are needed. Our algorithm does not yet have the capability to detect or localize posterior staphyloma. A multimodal imaging AI diagnostic platform involving fundus images, OCT, optical coherence tomography angiography (OCTA), fluorescein angiography, and MRI data is our ongoing effort to establish a more powerful automatic system to identify PM lesions (Ruiz-Medrano et al., 2019).

In conclusion, this study developed a series of deep learning algorithms and AI-models that have the ability to automatically identify PM, classify the category of MM, and localize the "Plus" lesions based on retinal fundus images. They have achieved performance comparable to that of experts. Due to such promising performance at this stage, we initiated the task of engineering relevant algorithms and hope that our research can make more contributions to clinical and healthcare screening work for myopia patients.

ETHICS STATEMENT

Written informed consent was not obtained from the individual(s) for the publication of any potentially identifiable images or data included in this article. As the study was a retrospective review and analysis of fully anonymized retinal fundus images, the medical ethics committee declared it exempt from informed consent.

AUTHOR CONTRIBUTIONS

LL and WH: design of the study. MYu, WY, JH, EZ, QL, XT, PR, QH, MZ, and GK: acquisition, analysis, or interpretation of the data. LL, PR, and XT: drafting of the manuscript. LL and LXL: development of the algorithms and models. LL, MY, WY, and QH: statistical analysis. LL and WH: obtaining the fund. WH: supervising the process. All authors: revision and approval of the manuscript.

REFERENCES

Baird, P. N., Saw, S. M., Lanca, C., Guggenheim, J. A., Smith, I. E., Zhou, X., et al. (2020). Myopia. *Nat. Rev. Dis. Primers.* 6:99. doi: 10.1038/s41572-020-00231-4

Bhaskaranand, M., Ramachandra, C., Bhat, S., Cuadros, J., Nittala, M. G., Sadda, S. R., et al. (2019). The value of automated diabetic retinopathy screening with the eyeart system: a study of more than 100,000 consecutive encounters from people with diabetes. *Diabetes Technol. Ther.* 21, 635–643. doi: 10.1089/dia.2019.0164

Cho, B. J., Shin, J. Y., and Yu, H. G. (2016). Complications of pathologic myopia. *Eye Contact Lens.* 42, 9–15. doi: 10.1097/ICL.0000000000000223

Devda, J., and Eswari, R. (2019). Pathological myopia image analysis using deep learning. *Proc. Computer Sci.* 165, 239–244. doi: 10.1016/j.procs.2020.01.084

Ding, L., Liu, G., Zhang, X., Liu, S., Li, S., Zhang, Z., et al. (2020). A deep learning nomogram kit for predicting metastatic lymph nodes in rectal cancer. *Cancer Med.* 9, 8809–8820. doi: 10.1002/cam4.3490

Dolgin, E. (2015). The myopia boom. *Nature* 519, 276–278. doi: 10.1038/519276a

Du, R., Xie, S., Fang, Y., Igarashi-Yokoi, T., Moriyama, M., Ogata, S., et al. (2021). Deep learning approach for automated detection of myopic maculopathy and pathologic myopia in fundus images. *Ophthalmol. Retina.* doi: 10.1016/j.oret.2021.02.006 [Epub ahead of print],

Esteva, A., Kuprel, B., Novoa, R. A., Ko, J., Swetter, S. M., Blau, H. M., et al. (2017). Dermatologist-level classification of skin cancer with deep neural networks. *Nature* 542, 115–118. doi: 10.1038/nature21056

Faghihi, H., Hajizadeh, F., and Riazi-Esfahani, M. (2010). Optical coherence tomographic findings in highly myopic eyes. *J. Ophthalmic. Vis. Res.* 5, 110–121.

Freire, C. R., Moura, J. C. D. C., Barros, D. M. D. S., and Valentim, R. A. D. M. (2020). *Automatic Lesion Segmentation and Pathological Myopia Classification in Fundus Images* [preprint]. arXiv:2002.06382.

Gargeya, R., and Leng, T. (2017). Automated identification of diabetic retinopathy using deep learning. *Ophthalmology* 124, 962–969. doi: 10.1016/j.ophtha.2017.02.008

Hamet, P., and Tremblay, J. (2017). Artificial intelligence in medicine. *Metabolism* 69, S36–S40. doi: 10.1016/j.metabol.2017.01.011

Hayashi, K., Ohno-Matsui, K., Shimada, N., Moriyama, M., Kojima, A., Hayashi, W., et al. (2010). Long-term pattern of progression of myopic maculopathy: a natural history study. *Ophthalmology* 117, 1595–1611. doi: 10.1016/j.ophtha.2009.11.003

He, K., Zhang, X., Ren, S., and Sun, J. (2016). "Deep residual learning for image recognition," in *Proceeding of the 2016 IEEE Conference on Computer Vision and Pattern Recognition (CVPR)*, 770–778. doi: 10.1109/CVPR.2016.90

Herzig, S. J., Stefan, M. S., Pekow, P. S., Shieh, M. S., Soares, W., Raghunathan, K., et al. (2020). Risk factors for severe opioid-related adverse events in a national cohort of medical hospitalizations. *J. Gen. Intern. Med.* 35, 538–545. doi: 10.1007/s11606-019-05490-w

Holden, B. A., Fricke, T. R., Wilson, D. A., Jong, M., Naidoo, K. S., Sankaridurg, P., et al. (2016). Global prevalence of myopia and high myopia and temporal trends from 2000 through 2050. *Ophthalmology* 123, 1036–1042. doi: 10.1016/j.ophtha.2016.01.006

Keenan, T. D., Dharssi, S., Peng, Y., Chen, Q., Agrón, E., Wong, W. T., et al. (2019). A deep learning approach for automated detection of geographic atrophy from color fundus photographs. *Ophthalmology* 126, 1533–1540. doi: 10.1016/j.ophtha.2019.06.005

Landis, J. R., and Koch, G. G. (1977). The measurement of observer agreement for categorical data. *Biometrics* 33, 159–174.

Li, F., Song, D., Chen, H., Xiong, J., Li, X., Zhong, H., et al. (2020). Development and clinical deployment of a smartphone-based visual field deep learning system for glaucoma detection. *NPJ Digit. Med.* 3:123. doi: 10.1038/s41746-020-00329-9

Liao, H., Long, Y., Han, R., Wang, W., Xu, L., Liao, M., et al. (2020). Deep learning-based classification and mutation prediction from histopathological images of hepatocellular carcinoma. *Clin. Trans. Med.* 10:102. doi: 10.1002/ctm2.102

Liu, H., Li, L., Wormstone, I. M., Qiao, C., Zhang, C., Liu, P., et al. (2019). Development and validation of a deep learning system to detect glaucomatous optic neuropathy using fundus photographs. *JAMA Ophthalmol.* 137, 1353–1360. doi: 10.1001/jamaophthalmol.2019.3501

Morgan, I. G., He, M., and Rose, K. A. (2017). Epidemic of pathologic myopia: what can laboratory studies and epidemiology tell us? *Retina* 37, 989–997. doi: 10.1097/IAE.0000000000001272

Moriyama, M., Ohno-Matsui, K., Hayashi, K., Shimada, N., Yoshida, T., Tokoro, T., et al. (2011). Topographic analyses of shape of eyes with pathologic myopia by high-resolution three-dimensional magnetic resonance imaging. *Ophthalmology* 118, 1626–1637. doi: 10.1016/j.ophtha.2011.01.018

Ohno-Matsui, K. (2017). What is the fundamental nature of pathologic myopia? *Retina* 37, 1043–1048.

Ohno-Matsui, K., Fang, Y., Shinohara, K., Takahashi, H., Uramoto, K., and Yokoi, T. (2019). Imaging of pathologic myopia. *Asia. Pac. J. Ophthalmol. (Phila)* doi: 10.22608/APO.2018494 [Epub ahead of print],

Ohno-Matsui, K., Kawasaki, R., Jonas, J. B., Cheung, C. M. G., Saw, S., Verhoeven, V. J. M., et al. (2015). International photographic classification and grading system for myopic maculopathy. *Am. J. Ophthalmol.* 159, 877–883. doi: 10.1016/j.ajo.2015.01.022

Ohno-Matsui, K., Lai, T. Y., Lai, C. C., and Cheung, C. M. (2016). Updates of pathologic myopia. *Prog. Retin. Eye Res.* 52, 156–187. doi: 10.1016/j.preteyeres.2015.12.001

Pan, H., Chen, G., and Jiang, J. (2019). Adaptively dense feature pyramid network for object detection. *IEEE Access.* 7, 81132–81144. doi: 10.1109/access.2019.2922511

Paszke, A., Gross, S., Massa, F., Lerer, A., Bradbury, J., Chanan, G., et al. (2019). Pytorch: an imperative style, high-performance deep learning library. *arXiv* [preprint]. arXiv:1912.01703,

Pesce, E., Joseph, W. S., Ypsilantis, P. P., Bakewell, R., Goh, V., and Montana, G. (2019). Learning to detect chest radiographs containing pulmonary lesions using visual attention networks. *Med. Image Anal.* 53, 26–38. doi: 10.1016/j.media.2018.12.007

Ren, S., He, K., Girshick, R., and Sun, J. (2017). Faster r-cnn: towards real-time object detection with region proposal networks. *IEEE Trans. Pattern Anal. Mach. Intell.* 39, 1137–1149. doi: 10.1109/TPAMI.2016.2577031

Ruiz-Medrano, J., Montero, J. A., Flores-Moreno, I., Arias, L., García-Layana, A., and Ruiz-Moreno, J. M. (2019). Myopic maculopathy: current status and proposal for a new classification and grading system (atn). *Prog. Retin. Eye Res.* 69, 80–115. doi: 10.1016/j.preteyeres.2018.10.005

Smith, T. (2009). Potential lost productivity resulting from the global burden of uncorrected refractive error. *B. World Health Organ.* 87, 431–437. doi: 10.2471/BLT.08.055673

Tan, N. M., Liu, J., Wong, D. K., Lim, J. H., Zhang, Z., Lu, S., et al. (2009). Automatic detection of pathological myopia using variational level set. *Conf. Proc. IEEE Eng. Med. Biol. Soc.* 2009, 3609–3612. doi: 10.1109/IEMBS.2009.5333517

Tayara, H., and Chong, K. (2018). Object detection in very high-resolution aerial images using one-stage densely connected feature pyramid network. *Sensors* *Basel.* 18:3341. doi: 10.3390/s18103341

Wong, T. Y., Ferreira, A., Hughes, R., Carter, G., and Mitchell, P. (2014). Epidemiology and disease burden of pathologic myopia and myopic choroidal neovascularization: an evidence-based systematic review. *Am. J. Ophthalmol.* 157, 9–25. doi: 10.1016/j.ajo.2013.08.010

Wong, T. Y., Ohno-Matsui, K., Leveziel, N., Holz, F. G., Lai, T. Y., Yu, H. G., et al. (2015). Myopic choroidal neovascularisation: current concepts and update on clinical management. *Br. J. Ophthalmol.* 99, 289–296. doi: 10.1136/bjophthalmol-2014-305131

Yang, J., Zhang, K., Fan, H., Huang, Z., Xiang, Y., Yang, J., et al. (2019). Development and validation of deep learning algorithms for scoliosis screening using back images. *Commun. Biol.* 2:390. doi: 10.1038/s42003-019-0635-8

Zhao, X., Ding, X., Lyu, C., Li, S., Liu, B., Li, T., et al. (2020). Morphological characteristics and visual acuity of highly myopic eyes with different severities of myopic maculopathy. *Retina* 40, 461–467. doi: 10.1097/IAE.0000000000002418

Zhao, X., Wu, Y., Song, G., Li, Z., Zhang, Y., and Fan, Y. (2018). A deep learning model integrating fcnns and crfs for brain tumor segmentation. *Med. Image Anal.* 43, 98–111. doi: 10.1016/j.media.2017.10.002

Zheng, Y. F., Pan, C. W., Chay, J., Wong, T. Y., Finkelstein, E., and Saw, S. M. (2013). The economic cost of myopia in adults aged over 40 years in singapore. *Invest. Ophthalmol. Vis. Sci.* 54, 7532–7537. doi: 10.1167/iovs.13-12795

Zhu, Y., Wang, Q., Xu, M., Zhang, Z., Cheng, J., Zhang, Y., et al. (2019). Application of convolutional neural network in the diagnosis of the invasion depth of gastric cancer based on conventional endoscopy. *Gastrointest. Endosc.* 89, 806–815. doi: 10.1016/j.gie.2018.11.011

20

Novel Corneal Protein Biomarker Candidates Reveal Iron Metabolic Disturbance in High Myopia Eyes

Jingyi Chen[1,2], Wenjing Wu[2], Zhiqian Wang[3], Chuannan Zhai[4], Baocheng Deng[5], Mohammad Alzogool[1] and Yan Wang[1,2]*

[1] School of Medicine, NanKai University, Tianjin, China, [2] Tianjin Key Lab of Ophthalmology and Visual Science, Tianjin Eye Hospital, Tianjin Eye Institute, Nankai University Eye Hospital, Tianjin, China, [3] Department of Optometry, Shenyang Eye Institute, The 4th People's Hospital of Shenyang, Shenyang, China, [4] Department of Cardiology, Tianjin Chest Hospital, Tianjin, China, [5] Department of Infectious Disease, The 1st Affiliated Hospital of China Medical University, Shenyang, China

*Correspondence:
Yan Wang
wangyan7143@vip.sina.com

Myopia is a major public health concern with increasing global prevalence and is the leading cause of vision loss and complications. The potential role of the cornea, a substantial component of refractive power and the protective fortress of the eye, has been underestimated in the development of myopia. Our study acquired corneal stroma tissues from myopic patients undergoing femtosecond laser-assisted small incision lenticule extraction (SMILE) surgery and investigated the differential expression of circulating proteins between subjects with low and high myopia by means of high-throughput proteomic approaches—the quantitative tandem mass tag (TMT) labeling method and parallel reaction monitoring (PRM) validation. Across all corneal stroma tissue samples, a total of 2,455 proteins were identified qualitatively and quantitatively, 103 of which were differentially expressed between those with low and high myopia. The differentially abundant proteins (DAPs) between the groups of stroma samples mostly demonstrated catalytic activity and molecular function regulator and transporter activity and participated in metabolic processes, biological regulation, response to stimulus, and so forth. Pathway enrichment showed that mineral absorption, ferroptosis, and HIF-1 signaling pathways were activated in the human myopic cornea. Furthermore, TMT analysis and PRM validation revealed that the expression of ferritin light chain (FTL, P02792) and ferritin heavy chain (FTH1, P02794) was negatively associated with myopia development, while the expression of serotransferrin (TF, P02787) was positively related to myopia status. Overall, our results indicated that subjects with low and high myopia could have different proteomic profiles or signatures in the cornea. These findings revealed disturbances in iron metabolism and corneal oxidative stress in the more myopic eyes. Iron metabolic proteins could serve as an essential modulator in the pathogenesis of myopia.

Keywords: myopia, cornea, protein biomarkers, signal, iron metabolism, protein–protein interaction, oxidative stress

INTRODUCTION

Myopia, as a complex multifactorial disease, is a globally recognized epidemic and a common cause of vision impairment characterized by its increasing prevalence among younger generations and heterogeneity among regions and ethnicities (Holden et al., 2016). Moreover, high myopia also foreshadows the irreversible visual damage caused by its pathological complications, such as retinal detachment, myopia-related retinopathy, and choroidal neovascularization (Wong et al., 2014).

To date, the underlying pathogenesis of myopia is still elusive, and various theories have been proposed to explain its development. The projected mechanisms for myopia are universally considered to be triggered by a combination of genetic susceptibility and environmental elements, among which metabolic factors are the most intricate, with little implications from the available evolutionary analyses (Morgan et al., 2012). Previous practices have attempted to address the impact of retinal defocus, which triggers the retina–choroid pathway, or hypoxia of the sclera, which would cause scleral collagen remodeling (Morgan et al., 2018). The associated mechanisms have been predominantly studied in animal models. Steeper corneas have been implicated in high amounts of form-deprived myopia in experimental animal models (Qiao-Grider et al., 2010). Furthermore, several manipulations justified alterations of the anterior and posterior segments in mammalian and avian ametropia models (Troilo et al., 2019). Nonetheless, the potential roles of the cornea, representing a substantial component of refractive power, and the protective fortress of the eyeball have been underestimated in myopic studies. High-quality analyses conducted in regions with the highest prevalence of myopia could provide useful information using representative clinical ocular samples.

Recent omics studies on myopia have predominantly focused on genomics, in order to identify genetic risk factors. Various international and polycentric genome-wide association studies (GWAS) and meta-analyses have been conducted on refractive phenotypes (Hysi et al., 2014). Proteomic analyses of myopia have hitherto included serum, tear, and aqueous humor samples from humans and retinal, scleral, and vitreous humor samples from animal models, considering sample availability and visually guided structural alterations during model establishment (Grochowski et al., 2020). A recent study first reported differentially abundant corneal proteins in high myopia chick models (Kang et al., 2021). However, no biomarker that corresponds to the diagnosis and classification of human myopia has yet been identified. The exploration of novel biomarkers would provide additional information on disease pathogenesis and related pathways. Therefore, a more comprehensive understanding of the molecular functions and processes involved in the development of high myopia is necessary to promote these interventions.

Small incision lenticule extraction (SMILE) surgery takes advantage of a femtosecond laser to shape a refractive lenticule from the corneal stroma, which is then removed through a particular small incision (Kim et al., 2019). The present study aimed to characterize the potential molecular pattern of the distinct evolution of low versus high myopia in patients scheduled to undergo SMILE surgery for myopia.

MATERIALS AND METHODS

Phase 1: Exploratory Study: Proteomic Approaches to Biomarker Discovery
Subjects Enrollment

The current study acquired approval from the Institutional Review Board of Nankai University and Nankai University Eye Hospital (Ethics Number 201922) and abided by the tenets of the World Medical Association Declaration of Helsinki. The study was case-controlled and cross-sectional and conformed to the Strengthening the Reporting of Observational Studies in Epidemiology (STROBE) guidelines of observational studies. All enrolled participants agreed to the sample collection, and informed consent was obtained. In total, 62 systemically healthy subjects aged 18–34 years (96 eyes), were recruited between 2019 and 2020. Complete general and ophthalmic histories were collected from all participants. Since this study aimed at a proteomic evaluation for low versus high myopia eyes, an individual eye was set as a target, rather than an individual subject, which meant both eyes could be selected from the same subject. The enrolled eyes were divided into the low-myopia and high-myopia groups. The group stratification in our study was determined with respect to the spherical equivalent (SE), which was assessed as sphere + cylinder/2. The SE was defined as less than –3.00D for low myopia and over –6.00D for high myopia (Morgan et al., 2012). The inclusion criteria were as follows: generalized myopic patients scheduled for SMILE surgery with written informed consent; absence of a history or examination evidence of ocular trauma; and absence of unrelated ocular diseases such as cataract, glaucoma, or retinopathy. The systemic exclusion criteria were the presence of systemic disorders such as diabetes mellitus, respiratory or cardiovascular diseases, hypertension, kidney disease, severe infection status, conditions of inflammation or current pregnancy, and not taking any medication such as antimetabolites, immunosuppressants, or steroids.

Sample Collection

Among the 96 eyes of 62 participants, 18—9 eyes with low myopia and 9 eyes with high myopia, respectively, were randomly selected for sample collection. Corneal stroma tissue samples were acquired during VisuMax (Carl Zeiss Meditec, Jena, Germany) SMILE surgery at Nankai University Eye Hospital. Each stroma sample was kept separately in an Eppendorf tube, marked, and frozen in liquid nitrogen immediately after the lenticule extraction procedure. The samples were then stored at –80°C until measurement.

Protein Extraction: Homogenate and SDT Lysis

The nine corneal stroma samples in either group were randomly mixed into three sample mixtures for the tandem mass tag (TMT) proteomic experiment and future validation study. Three mixed samples from low or high myopia eyes were randomly set as one biological parallel (Huang et al., 2020). An equal batch of adequate corneal stroma tissue from each sample was amalgamated and pulverized into a powder. The sorted samples were then homogenized by adding SDT1 buffer [4% sodium dodecyl sulfate (SDS), 1 mmol dithiothreitol (DTT), 100 mmol Tris–HCl, pH 7.6] and transferred to Eppendorf tubes with quartz sand (MP homogenizer, 24 × 2, 6.0 M/S, 60 s, twice). Homogenate of protein extraction was carried out by sonication (power 80 W, worktime 10 s, interval 10 s, cycle 10 times) on ice, and the extractions were then boiled for 15 min. The crude digest was centrifuged for 40 min at 14,000 g, and the supernatant was filtered through 0.22 μm filters. The filtrate was calculated using a BCA Protein Assay Kit (Bio-Rad, United States), and the collection was stored at –80°C for future measurement. Sodium dodecyl sulfate polyacrylamide gel electrophoresis (SDS-PAGE) protein separation was performed. Protein samples (20 μg) were mixed in 5 × loading buffer and boiled for 5 min. Protein separation was performed using a 12.5% SDS-PAGE gel (with 14 mA constant current for 90 min). Coomassie Blue R-250 staining was used to visualize the acquired protein bands (Zhu et al., 2014).

Filter-Aided Sample Preparation Protein Digestion

Protein digestion was performed using filter-aided sample preparation. Briefly, 200 μg of total protein from each sample was incorporated into SDT2 buffer (4% SDS, 100 mmol DTT, 150 mmol Tris–HCl, pH 8.0), boiled for 5 min, and then cooled to 25°C. Excessive DTT, detergents, and other low-molecular-weight components in the protein samples were washed out using UA buffer (8 M urea, 150 mmol Tris–HCl, pH 8.0) by repeated ultrafiltration (Microcon units, 10 kD, 14,000 g, 15 min). Each filter extract was then added to 100 mM iodoacetamide to inhibit the reduced cysteine residues. The extracts were incubated for 30 min in the dark and then centrifuged for 40 min at 14,000 g. The filtrate was discarded, and the filter was washed in 100 μl UA buffer three times and then in 100 μl of 100 mM triethylammonium bicarbonate (TEAB) buffer twice. Subsequently, 4 μg trypsin (Promega, United States) was dissolved in 40 μl TEAB buffer, and protein suspension was added to this buffer and digested overnight at 37°C. Finally, the digested samples were centrifuged to harvest the resulting peptides, and the concentrations of peptide contents were calculated according to 280 nm UV light spectral density by means of an extinction coefficient of 1.1 in 0.1% (g/L) solution measured in the light frequency of tyrosine and tryptophan in the vertebrate protein atlas (Wiśniewski et al., 2009).

Tandem Mass Tag Labeling and High pH Reversed-Phase Fractionation

Each consequent peptide mixture (100 μg) was labeled with TMT reagent (Thermo Fisher Scientific, United States). Principally, the three mixed samples of low myopia were labeled with 126, 127C, and 127N isobaric TMT tags, and the three mixed samples of high myopia were labeled with 129C, 130C, and 130N isobaric TMT tags. After TMT labeling, the labeled digest samples were fractionated, and 10 fractions were obtained. The

surplus labels and salts were diminished using a high reversed-phase fractionation kit (Thermo Fisher Scientific, United States) to increase the acetonitrile step-gradient elution.

Liquid Chromatography–Mass Spectrometry/Mass Spectrometry Analysis

Liquid chromatography–mass spectrometry/mass spectrometry (LC-MS/MS) analysis was performed for each fraction. The peptide compounds were dissolved in buffer A (0.1% formic acid) and then loaded onto a reverse-phase trap column (Thermo Fisher Scientific, PepMap100, 100 μm × 2 cm, nano Viper C18) which was coupled to a C18 reverse-phase analytical column (Thermo Scientific, 75 μm × 10 cm, 3 μm resin) and divided using linear-gradient buffer B (84% acetonitrile + 0.1% formic acid) at a flow rate of 300 nl/min. The linear gradient was processed using the following parameters: 0–55% buffer B for 80 min, 55–100% buffer B for 5 min, and 100% buffer B for 5 min.

LC-MS/MS was performed on a Q Exactive mass spectrometer connected to Easy nLC (Thermo Fisher Scientific) in positive ion mode for 90 min. The procedure was performed in peptide recognition mode. MS data were obtained using a data-dependent top 10 method, which allows dynamic selection of the most copious precursor ions from the 300 to 1,800 m/z survey scan for higher-energy collisional dissociation (HCD) fragmentation. The instrument parameters were set as follows: automatic gain control (AGC) target, 3e6; HCD spectra, 35,000 resolution at m/z 200; survey scans. Seventy thousand resolution at m/z 200; width of resolution, 2 m/z; maximum injection time, 10 ms; and dynamic exclusion duration, 40.0 s. The normalized collision energy was set to 30 eV, and the underfill ratio was defined as 0.1% to allow the minimum percentage of the target value to be accomplished at maximum full time.

Data Analysis and Protein Identification

The acquired LC-MS/MS spectra were searched using the MASCOT engine (version 2.2; Matrix Science, London, United Kingdom) in Proteome Discoverer 1.4 (Thermo Electron, San Jose, CA, United States). The following parameters were selected: the enzyme applied was trypsin, fragment mass tolerance of 0.1 Da, peptide mass tolerance of ± 20 ppm, and maximum missed cleavages of 2. Fixed modifications were set for the TMT-10 plex, and variable modifications were applied for oxidation. The false discovery rate of the peptides was set as < 0.01. Protein quantification was calculated using protein ratios, which were presented as the median of protein unique peptides. The median protein ratio was used to normalize all peptide ratios. The median protein ratio was defined as 1 after normalization for the experimental bias. The D'Agostino and Pearson normality test was used to calculate data normality. Chi-square and Student's t-tests were used to analyze demographic and clinical data. For quantitative protein expression analysis, pair-wise group comparisons were performed using LC-MS, and significant differences between groups were assessed using normalized protein abundances in arcsinh transformation. To distinguish differentially abundant proteins (DAPs), the fold change was set as > 1.2 or < 0.83. A p-value (Student's t-test) of < 0.05 was considered statistically significant (Li et al., 2019).

Bioinformatic Analysis

Hierarchical Clustering Analysis

Hierarchical clustering analysis was performed using protein relative expression data via Cluster 3.0 software[1] and Java Treeview software[2]. The Euclidean distance algorithm for similarity measure and average linkage clustering algorithm using centroids of the observations for clustering were selected. In addition to a dendrogram, a heatmap is often presented as a visual aid. The clustering heatmap and volcano plots of DAPs were visualized using R 3.6.0 software (R: A Language and Environment for Statistical Computing, R Development Core Team).

Gene Ontology and Kyoto Encyclopedia of Genes and Genomes Pathway Annotations

The expression trends of human corneal stromal proteins were searched in the UniProt KB database and retrieved in FASTA format in batches. The retrieved sequences of differentially expressed proteins were searched with reference to the local SwissProt database (human) using NCBI BLAST + client software for homolog sequences from which the gene ontology (GO) functional annotation could be merged. In this procedure, the top 10 blast hits with E-values of $<1e^{-3}$ for every query sequence were restored and loaded into Blast2GO software (Version 3.3.5) (Götz et al., 2008) for GO prognostication and annotation, which was set with default gradual enzyme code (EC) weights, a GO weight of 5, an annotation cutoff of 75, and a filtered E-value of $1e^{-6}$. The unannotated sequences without BLAST hits were re-annotated with more permissive parameters and were then selected to go through InterProScan (Quevillon et al., 2005) meriting comparison with European Bioinformatics Institute (EBI) databases to fetch functional annotations of protein motifs and derive the InterProScan GO annotation terms. The results of the GO annotation sets were mapped using R scripts (R Development Core Team).

The protein sequences in FASTA form of differentially expressed proteins were searched in the Kyoto Encyclopedia of Genes and Genomes (KEGG) database[3]. The corresponding KEGG pathways were retrieved and extracted (Moriya et al., 2007).

Functional Enrichment Analysis

Functional enrichment analysis was carried out to further explore the influence of differentially altered proteins in cellular physio-pathological processes and the discovery of internal connections between the DAPs. The entire protein quantification dataset was set as the background. GO term enrichment on three ontology modules (BP—biological process, MF—molecular function, and CC—cellular component) and KEGG pathway annotation analyses were measured using Fisher's exact test. The derived p-values were further adjusted by the application of Benjamin–Hochberg correction for multiple tests, and only GO functional categories and KEGG pathways with p-values < 0.05 were considered statistically significant.

Protein–Protein Interaction Network

The information of protein–protein interaction (PPI) of the target proteins was searched using the gene symbols and retrieved from the STRING (Search Tool for the Retrieval of Interacting Genes/Proteins) online database[4] or IntAct molecular interaction database[5]. The results were downloaded and imported into Cytoscape software (version 3.2.1)[6]. Visualization and functional analysis of the PPI networks were conducted. Additionally, the degree of interaction of each target protein was calculated to assess its significance in the PPI network.

Phase 2: Validation Study: Parallel Reaction Monitoring Analysis

Parallel Reaction Monitoring Assay Development

Prioritized Target Protein Selection

The next step after the TMT discovery experiment involved an LC-parallel reaction monitoring (PRM)-based workflow to establish sensitive and accurate detection of the relative abundance of the candidate protein markers. Considering the scarcity of clinically available corneal stroma samples, the PRM validation study was carried out using the same cohort in the phase 1 exploratory study to reinforce the consistency between studies. However, reagent costs have limited the possibility of performing analyses for all identified candidate proteins, which necessitates a further step of prioritization. As a result, the identified proteins from the phase 1 TMT experiment were coped with hierarchical clustering, GO functional enrichment, KEGG pathway enrichment, and PPI network analysis for a comprehensive overview of the DAPs between the comparisons.

Peptide Selection

In the next step of targeted PRM assays, the selected proteins were optimized in corneal stroma samples using a set of three proteo-unique peptides. The unique peptides were screened from the phase 1 study. For proteins with fewer than three proteo-unique peptides, extra peptides were searched through the online selected reaction monitoring (SRM) Atlas[7] (Bostanci et al., 2018). All designated peptides ranged from 6 to 20 amino acids in length and contained tryptic ends without any missing cleavages. For the PRM analysis, SPOT synthesis (JPT Peptide Technologies, Germany) was applied to standard stable isotope-labeled peptides that were identical to the proteo-typic peptides and contained either a C-terminal arginine or lysine residue in unpurified form for chemical synthesis.

Sample Preparation and Protein Digestion

The protein expression levels obtained by TMT analysis were further quantified by LC-PRM/MS analysis (Peterson et al., 2012). A portion of 200 μg proteins from each sample was designated for in-solution trypsin digestion following the TMT protocol, and an aqua-stable isotope peptide was spiked per sample as an internal standard reference. Tryptic peptides were loaded on C18

---

[1]http://bonsai.hgc.jp/~mdehoon/software/cluster/software.htm

[2]http://jtreeview.sourceforge.net

[3]https://www.kegg.jp/

[4]http://string-db.org/

[5]http://www.ebi.ac.uk/intact/

[6]http://www.cytoscape.org/

[7]http://www.srmatlas.org

stage tips (Wicom International AG, Maienfeld, Switzerland) for desalting prior to reversed-phase liquid chromatography (RPLC) on the Easy nLC-1200 system (Thermo Fisher Scientific). We proceeded with LC for 1 h with gradients of acetonitrile ranging from 5 to 35% in 45 min.

Parallel Reaction Monitoring Measurements

The succeeding PRM measurements were continued on a Q Exactive Plus mass spectrometer (Thermo Scientific). Highly intensive proteo-unique peptides were utilized for the confidential analysis of each target protein with optimization for charge state, collision time, and retention times. The mass spectrometer was operated in positive ion mode. The following parameters were set: full MS1 scan resolution, 70,000 (at 200 m/z); AGC target, 3.0×10^{-6}; and ion injection time, 200 ms maximum. After the full MS scans, 20 PRM scans were followed at 35,000 resolution (at 200 m/z) with AGC 3.0×10^{-6} and 200 ms maximum injection times. The resulting peptides were consequently isolated in a 2Th window with ion activation/dissociation at a collision energy of 27 within a higher energy dissociation collision cell (Zhang et al., 2019).

Parallel Reaction Monitoring Data Processing

The PRM raw data were processed using the Skyline bioinformatics tool (MacCoss Lab, University of Washington, United States) (MacLean et al., 2010) where the detected signal intensities for individual peptide sequences of each target protein were quantified with standard reference normalization and relative to the respective sample. The Skyline PRM acquisition methods were time-scheduled, and the quantification files contained the results from all selected samples with measurements of the target proteins, including three target proteins and five unique peptide sequences, both heavy and

light. A proper Q-value was selected to filter the results of peptide assays for high data quality, where a Q-value > 0.05 was removed. In addition, assays with reported 0 intensity were removed. Subsequently, the light-to-heavy ratio was programmed as log2 fold change. The correlation between peptide transitions was computed and demanded a quality filter. All peptide transitions with more than 10 nucleic acids and with a Pearson correlation of <0.5 were removed from the dataset. The median of the log2(l/h) ratios for peptide transitions was used to acquire peptide quantification and to obtain the protein log2(l/h) ratios.

Predictive Protein–Protein Interaction Analysis

The STRING functional protein association networks online database (see text footnote 4) and GeneMANIA online database for genes and gene sets functional predictions[8] were used for the critical evaluation and integration of predictive PPI networks based on the PRM validation evidence as well as genomic and proteomic knowledge gained from human studies. The prioritized proteins were mapped individually and integrally to create the predicted images.

RESULTS

Phase 1: Discovery Study—Tandem Mass Tag Proteomic Approach for Quantitative Analysis

Characteristics of the Study Subjects

The present study included 96 eyes of 62 systemically healthy subjects, among which 18 eyes from 13 subjects were randomly

---

[8]http://genemania.org/

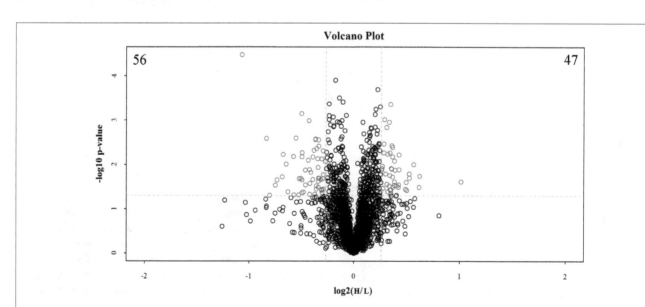

FIGURE 1 | Volcano plot of differentially abundant proteins between the low and high myopia groups. The volcano plot shows a significant difference in differentially abundant proteins (DAPs) between the two groups of samples. The x-axis represents the difference multiple (log2 fold change), and the y-axis represents the p-value of the difference (–log10). The red dots in the figure represent the significant DAPs (multiple changes > 1.2 or < 0.83 and p < 0.05), and the black dots show that there are no differences detected in the proteins between the two groups. H, high myopia group; L, low myopia group.

selected for proteomic discovery analysis. The low myopia group included nine eyes (OD = 4/OS = 5) from seven subjects (six males/one female), aged 24 ± 6.5 years, with an SE of −1.94 ± 0.30D. The high myopia group included nine eyes

(OD = 5/OS = 4) from six subjects (five males/one female), aged 22.6 ± 6.8 years, with an SE of −8.68 ± 0.60D. No significant differences were noted between the two groups in terms of age, gender, and left or right eye selected, but subjects in the low myopia group had a significantly lower SE than did those in the high myopia group ($p < 0.001$).

Protein Identification and Differentially Abundant Protein Analysis

The discovery study was conducted using high-throughput TMT quantitative proteomic techniques. A total of 2,455 different proteins in the *Homo sapiens* protein atlas were identified (**Supplementary Table 1**). Overall, 103 DAPs were confirmed in the comparison between low and high myopic eyes. Among the DAPs, 47 proteins were upregulated, and 56 proteins were downregulated (**Figure 1**). A heat map was plotted for the visualization of the hierarchical clustering analysis of the identified DAPs (**Figure 2**).

Bioinformatic Analysis and Functional Enrichment Analysis

The results of the bioinformatics and functional enrichment analyses are presented in **Table 1**. The significantly altered proteins between the low-myopia and high-myopia groups were further categorized, whereby relevant GO and KEGG term enrichment were prioritized with regard to their *E*-value and *p*-value. The mapped GO function and KEGG pathway demonstrated that the functions of the DAPs were predominantly catalytic activity, binding, molecular function regulator, structural molecule activity, and transporter activity,

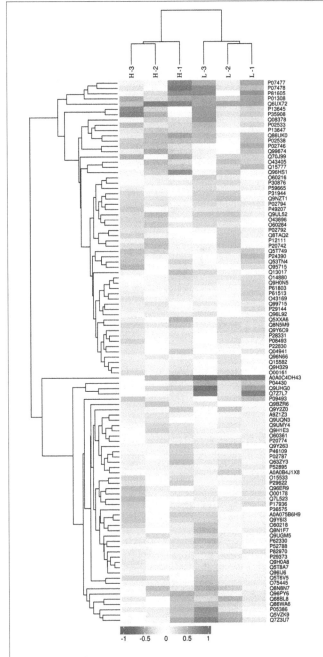

FIGURE 2 | Clustering analysis of differentially abundant proteins. Hierarchical clustering analysis was performed using a tree heat map. In the heat map, each row represents a protein [i.e., the ordinate represents the significant differentially abundant proteins (DAPs)], and each column represents a group of samples (the abscissa is the sample information). The logarithm values (log2 expression) of the significant DAPs are displayed in different colors, where red represents significantly upregulated proteins, purple represents significantly downregulated proteins, and gray represents no available protein quantitative information.

TABLE 1 | Top five ontology terms for GO and KEGG analysis.

Ontology	Description	Adjust *p*-value	RichFactor
BP	Keratinization	< 0.001	0.27
BP	Cornification	< 0.001	0.25
BP	Epidermis development	< 0.001	0.15
BP	Keratinocyte migration	0.001	0.5
BP	Epidermal cell differentiation	0.001	0.15
MF	Ferric iron binding	< 0.001	1
MF	Ferrous iron binding	< 0.001	0.57
MF	Oxidoreductase activity	< 0.001	0.6
MF	Structural constitute of cytoskeleton	0.005	0.15
MF	Ferroxidase activity	0.005	0.67
CC	Keratin filament	< 0.001	0.56
CC	Intermediate filament	< 0.001	0.21
CC	Intracellular ferritin complex	0.002	1
CC	Ferritin complex	0.002	1
CC	Intermediate filament cytoskeleton	0.003	0.17
KEGG	Mineral absorption	< 0.001	0.5
KEGG	Protein digestion and absorption	0.014	0.17
KEGG	Staphylococcus aureus infection	0.018	0.16
KEGG	Ferroptosis	0.026	0.19
KEGG	Viral protein interaction with cytokine	0.042	1

GO, gene ontology; KEGG, Kyoto Encyclopedia of Genes and Genomes; BP, biological process; MF, molecular function; CC, cellular component.

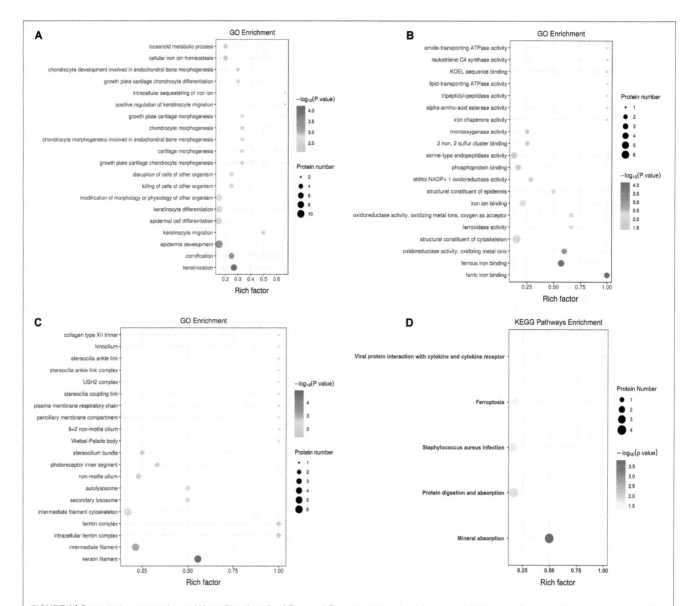

FIGURE 3 | Gene ontology annotation and Kyoto Encyclopedia of Gene and Genomes pathway enrichment analysis between the low and high myopia groups. The ordinate in the figure stands for the enriched gene ontology (GO) functional annotation, which can be divided into **(A)** BP, **(B)** MF, and **(C)** CC or **(D)** enriched Kyoto Encyclopedia of Genes and Genomes (KEGG) pathways. The abscissa stands for enrichment factors (rich factor ≤ 1). The rich factor represents the proportion of DAPs annotated in a functional ontology to the number of all identified proteins annotated in that functional ontology. The size of the bubbles in the figure indicates the number of differentially expressed proteins in each classified functional ontology. The color of the bubbles indicates the significance of the enriched functional categories. The color gradient displays the *p*-value, where the closer to red, the smaller the *p*-value and the higher the significance level of the corresponding ontology.

and the most significantly regulated processes in high myopia compared with low myopia were "metabolic process," "cellular process," "biological regulation," "response to stimulus," and "regulation of biological process."

Figure 3 demonstrates the top 20 enriched GO terms of BP (**Figure 3A**), MF (**Figure 3B**), and CC (**Figure 3C**). The main biological processes of DAPs involved metabolic process, cellular process, biological regulation, and response to stimulus. The main molecular functions were associated with ferric iron binding, ferrous iron binding, structural molecule activity, catalytic activity, and molecular transducer activity. The main

cellular components of these proteins were exhibited as cell and organelle part, ferritin complex, intracellular ferritin complex, and protein-containing complex (**Figure 4**).

Figure 3D shows the KEGG pathway enrichment analysis. The DAPs were enriched into mineral absorption, ferroptosis, staphylococcus aureus infection, protein digestion, and absorption pathways. **Figure 5** demonstrates the top 20 enriched KEGG pathways.

The interaction map of the differentially expressed proteins, which were enriched in a larger interaction network, is presented in **Figure 6**. PPI analysis suggested that the

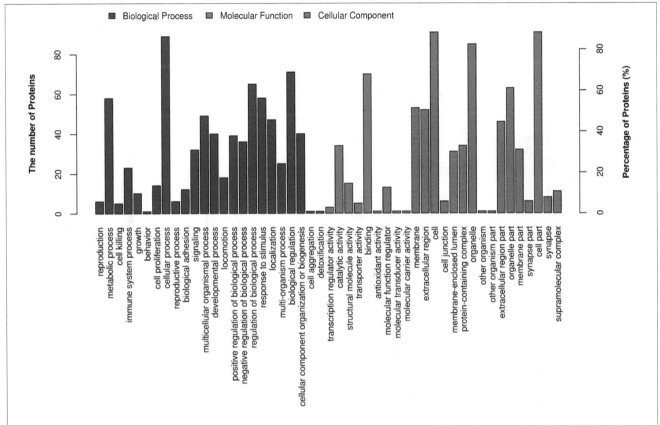

FIGURE 4 | GO level 2 functional analysis. The x-axis shows the enriched GO level 2 functional annotation, which was demonstrated as BP (red), MF (purple), and CC (orange). The y-axis shows the number and percentage of proteins detected. BP, biological process; MF, molecular function; CC, cellular component.

development of myopia could result from the dysfunction of multiple pathways.

Phase 2: Validation Study—Verification of Myopia-Associated Protein Biomarker Candidates via the PRM Approach

Protein Selection and Parallel Reaction Monitoring Measurements

After a thorough evaluation of the GO annotation, KEGG pathway analysis, and PPI network analysis, we focused on the main GO terms "ferric iron binding" and "oxidizing metal irons" and the main KEGG pathways "mineral absorption" and "ferroptosis." Therefore, we further selected three iron- and redox-related DAPs, including serotransferrin (TF, P02787), ferritin light chain (FTL, P02792), and ferritin heavy chain (FTH1, P02794) for validation studies using the PRM approach. TF is a major iron-uptake protein. Ferritin is a major iron-storage protein. Among the validation results, the abundance of TF was increased in the high myopia group, while FTL and FTH1 expression were both reduced in the high myopia group compared to the low myopia group (**Figure 7**). It could be deduced from the PRM results that the selected proteins presented semblable trends, similar to the aforementioned TMT proteomic results. Verification of the candidate DAPs confirmed the credibility of our proteomic research.

Predictive Protein–Protein Interaction Analysis

The STRING and GeneMANIA online tools were further applied for the integration and prediction analysis of PPIs of the validated target proteins. The prioritized proteins—TF, FTL, and FTH1— were mapped, and an integrated predicting PPI network image was created (**Figures 8–11** and **Supplementary Figure 1**).

DISCUSSION

In this study, for the first time, we employed proteomic approaches to investigate the molecular characterization of the human corneal stroma in relation to myopia. The present study has uncovered the broadest human corneal stroma proteome to date, as compared with previous studies (Dyrlund et al., 2012), and discovered different proteomic signatures between low and high myopia eyes. The stroma proteome provides novel biomarker candidates and signaling pathways to further elucidate the mechanisms underlying myopia development.

The pending issue of the complex pathogenesis and lack of adequate treatment has made the prevention and control of myopia difficult. Moreover, the available approaches for differentiating low and high myopia rely primarily on ocular biometric parameters, including SE and axial length. Therefore, the identification of potential molecular patterns is essential for further understanding the mechanism and susceptibility

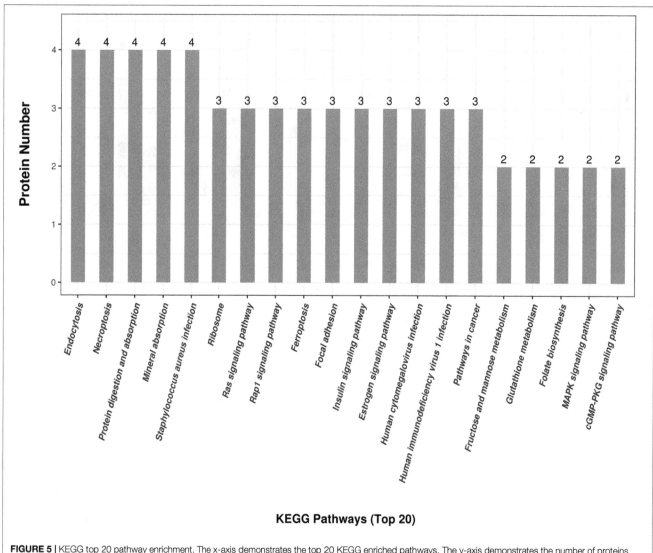

FIGURE 5 | KEGG top 20 pathway enrichment. The x-axis demonstrates the top 20 KEGG enriched pathways. The y-axis demonstrates the number of proteins participating in the enriched pathways.

of myopia and offer new perspectives for early diagnosis and therapeutic targets.

Generally speaking, GWAS are valuable in myopia-associated research but may not succeed in addressing a large portion of genetic variability. Analysis of gene–gene interaction networks and regulation of signaling pathways, rather than studying genes individually, has greater potential for investigating related phenotypes (Lauwen et al., 2017). In the past decade, human proteomic studies have played an essential role in discerning the molecular mechanisms involved in the diagnosis and treatment of different diseases. The high stringency human proteome analysis developed targeted proteomic assays for the investigation of key proteins and signaling pathways (Adhikari et al., 2020). The novel tandem MS methods and PRM assays could permit the identification of peptides from various samples simultaneously according to their relative abundance with better performance, higher sensitivity, and greater accuracy than other proteomic methods (Thompson et al., 2003; Stergachis et al., 2011).

The DAP profiles and functional enrichment analyses of our study revealed novel iron metabolism features of myopic eyes, with implications for corneal reactive oxygen species (ROS) acceleration. The main GO annotations implicated the major biological processes "metabolic process" and "cellular iron ion homeostasis," remarkable molecular functions of "ferric iron binding" and "ferroxidase activity," and an outstanding cellular component of "ferric complex" (**Figures 3A–C**). The KEGG pathways were mainly enriched to "mineral absorption" and "ferroptosis" (**Figure 3D**). Furthermore, the three selected proteins (TF, FTL, and FTH1) associated with iron metabolism and oxidative stress exhibited a similar gradient between the TMT and PRM quantitative results.

Proteins play a significant role in ocular metabolism. The distribution of iron and iron homeostasis proteins in the rodent retina has been reported previously (Yefimova et al., 2000). Iron is an essential biometal and a principal source of nutrients for the eye. Previous studies characterized circulating iron and associated

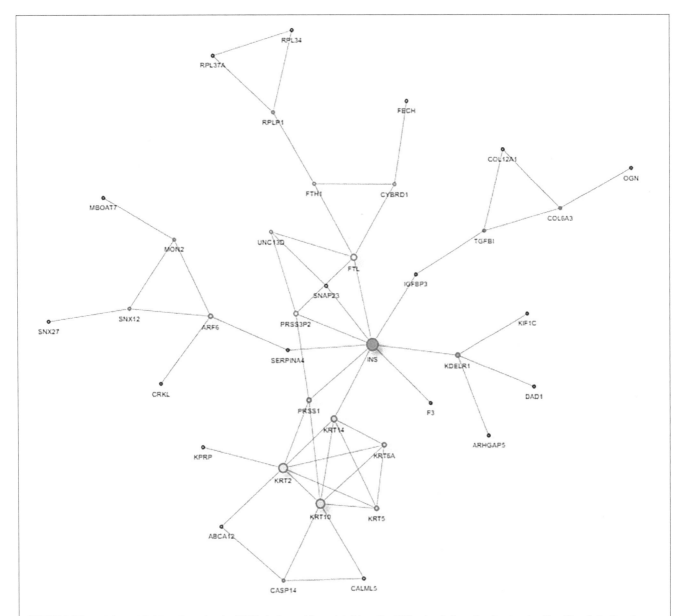

FIGURE 6 | The protein–protein interaction network of DAPs. In the protein–protein interaction (PPI) network, the colored nodes stand for differentially altered proteins, and lines are mapped for the interactions between proteins. Larger nodes correspond to a higher degree of protein aggregation in the PPI network.

homeostasis proteins, such as ferritin and TF, in various ocular tissues, including the cornea (Linsenmayer et al., 2005), aqueous humor (Yu and Okamura, 1988), and lens (Harned et al., 2006).

TFs are iron-binding transport proteins responsible for heme absorption and utilization. TF binds two Fe^{3+} ions together with an anion, most commonly bicarbonate. They are growth factors required for all cells and play a central role in stimulating cell proliferation (Fulcher et al., 1988). It has been demonstrated that proliferating cells are capable of expressing TF receptors with enhanced density, making them preferential targets for the inhibition of malignant cells (Trowbridge and Domingo, 1981). The GO-biological process annotation implicates its role in cellular protein metabolic and iron homeostasis processes. To the best of our knowledge, this is the first study to

illustrate the role of TF in human myopia, which, as an eye disorder, could present with hyperproliferative features. A previous animal quantitative proteomic analysis reported a remarkable upregulation of ovotransferrin, which belongs to the transferrin family in myopic chick vitreous. Ovotransferrin could function as an antioxidant in tissues, and its upregulation in the vitreous chamber indicates increased oxidative stress along with axial elongation (Yu et al., 2017). Future investigation of the mechanism of TF and TF receptors in corneal and other ocular cell divisions could offer further avenues for the study of proliferative conditions in myopic eyes.

Cellular iron is stored as cytosolic ferritin. Ferritins sequester intracellular iron in an innoxious and readily soluble form, which is vital for iron homeostasis. A ferritin molecule can hold up to

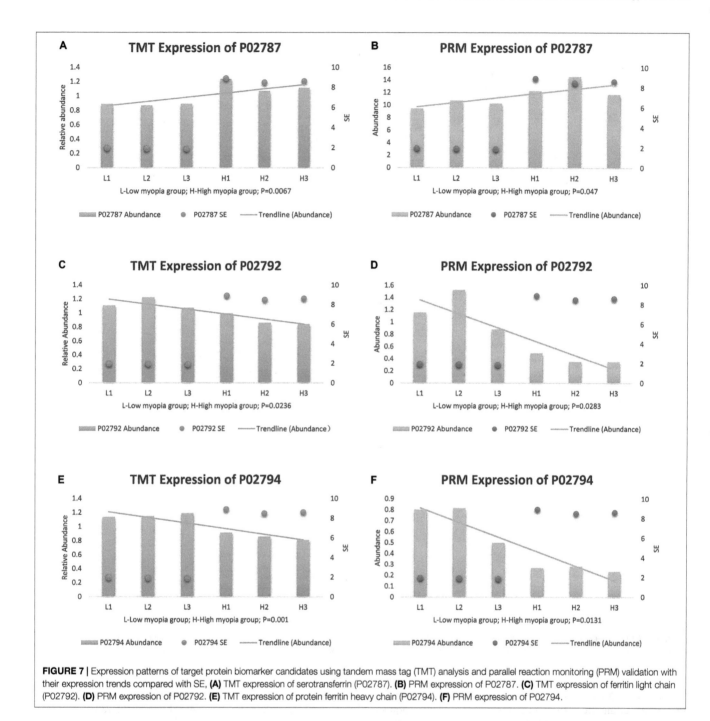

FIGURE 7 | Expression patterns of target protein biomarker candidates using tandem mass tag (TMT) analysis and parallel reaction monitoring (PRM) validation with their expression trends compared with SE, **(A)** TMT expression of serotransferrin (P02787). **(B)** PRM expression of P02787. **(C)** TMT expression of ferritin light chain (P02792). **(D)** PRM expression of P02792. **(E)** TMT expression of protein ferritin heavy chain (P02794). **(F)** PRM expression of P02794.

4,500 ferric-state iron molecules in its center core (Aisen et al., 2001). Iron is ingested in the ferrous form and deposited after oxidation as ferric hydroxides. Human ferritins consist of two types of ferritin subunits: H chain for heavy or heart and L chain for light or liver. A previous proteomic study by Karring et al. (2005) identified the presence of ferritin subunits in the human corneal epithelium. Free iron has the ability to catalyze ultraviolet-induced oxidation reactions via the Fenton reaction. FTH1 is a ferroxidase, and its increase is believed to reduce intracellular free iron oxidation levels and improve cellular resistance against oxidative stress. In contrast, FTL shares 50%

identity with the FTH1 at the amino acid level. The light chain lacks the ferroxidase feature of the heavy chain but can facilitate iron cooperation within the ferritin cavity (Cozzi et al., 2000).

The intracellular iron status is registered by iron-regulatory proteins (IRPs). Regarding the status of intracellular iron deficiency, IRPs would bind to iron-responsive elements (IREs), which are present on the mRNAs of the regulated proteins. The IRE of ferritin lies on the 5′- terminal of ferritin mRNAs, and its binding with IRPs could efficiently obstruct the steric translation of ferritin, thereby inducing iron deficiency with insufficient ferritin levels. Reciprocally, the connection of IRPs with the

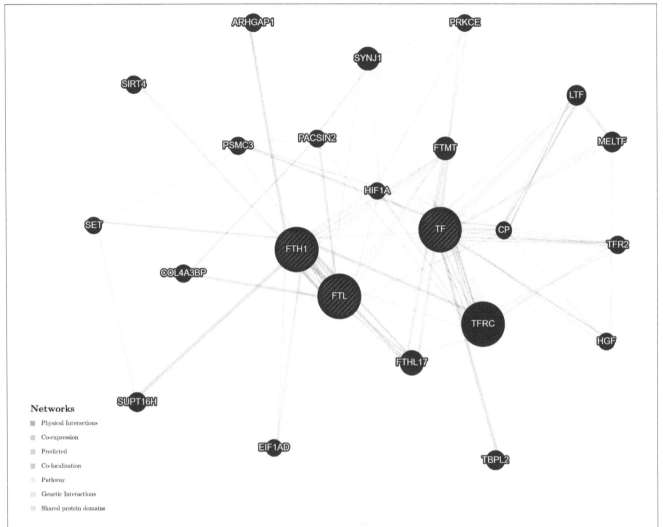

FIGURE 8 | Predictive PPI network of the validated protein biomarker candidates: TF-FTL-FTH1. In the PPI network prediction, the nodes in the middle with bias represent the validated protein biomarkers, and lines are mapped for the interactions between proteins. Larger nodes correspond to a higher degree of protein aggregation in the PPI network, and different colors correspond to various functional networks.

IREs of transferrin and receptors, which lie on the $3'$-portion of the mRNAs, would restrain the process of mRNA degradation, resulting in an increase in transferrin in iron deficiency (Rouault, 2002). In our proteomic study, the expression levels of FTL and FTH1 were both decreased in the high myopia group, while the TF abundance was increased in the high myopia group compared to the low myopia group, indicating the potential impact of iron deficiency on the progression of myopia.

Previous attempts to investigate ferritin metabolism in the cornea have been conducted in avian corneal epithelial cells, where FTH1 was observed to function as a developmentally regulated nuclear protein, although ferritin is one of the cytoplasmic components in most cells. The study revealed the similarity between the structure and biological properties of nuclear and cytoplasmic ferritin. Considering that corneal epithelial cells can be constantly exposed to ultraviolet light, nuclear ferritin is speculated to promote iron sequestration and prevent oxidative damage to cell DNA (Linsenmayer et al., 2005).

Iron has been implicated in a wide range of ophthalmic disorders, such as cataracts, glaucoma, macular degeneration, and intraocular hemorrhage. However, the underlying correlation with myopia was underestimated. The derived PPI networks involved in iron metabolism are intriguing (**Figures 8–11** and **Supplementary Figure 1**). Transferrin and ferritins are circulation proteins and are also considered essential cofactors in the integration of dopamine, neurotransmitters, and norepinephrine (He et al., 2007). Their alterations could suggest an environmental impact on the ocular surface and would in turn represent circulating features shown in the cornea.

Iron is crucial for various metabolic processes but can also cause oxidative stress by functioning as a reactive free radical. Iron ions are redox-active metals that can catalyze the production of OH^- from H_2O_2 (He et al., 2007). Oxidative stress can cause oxidative damage, resulting from the disequilibrium between free radical production and antioxidant defenses, which implicates the interaction of multiple molecular species. Oxidative stress has

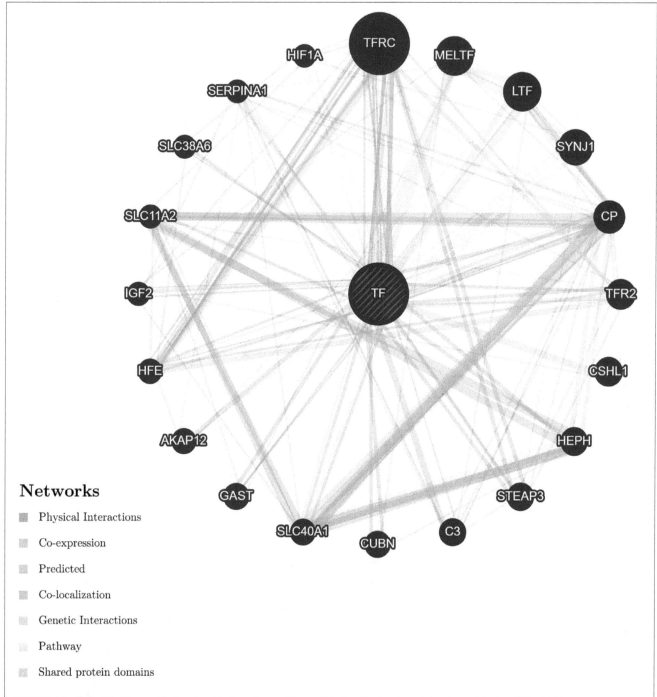

FIGURE 9 | Predictive PPI network of the target protein biomarker candidates: TF. In the PPI network prediction, the node in the middle with bias represents the target protein biomarker, and lines are mapped for the interactions between proteins. Larger nodes correspond to a higher degree of protein aggregation in the PPI network, and different colors correspond to various functional networks.

been described in previous reports of retinal and macular diseases with retinal pigment epithelium or choroidal atrophy. The cornea consumes oxygen mainly from oxygen in the air, and daily light exposure may have an impact on the cornea. Either of these processes could well generate ROS in the cornea (Francisco et al., 2015), which may induce DNA cleavage, protein alterations, and deleterious peroxidation of lipids. Hypoxia has been associated

with various ophthalmic conditions caused by oxidative damage. This could be one of the key targets for myopia study since oxidative circumstances exist chronically (Wu et al., 2018).

Oxidative stress has been implicated in different ocular tissues in myopic eyes, such as the retina and sclera, which can explain the complex signaling pathways involved in the regulation of myopia, particularly the hypoxia-inducible factor-1

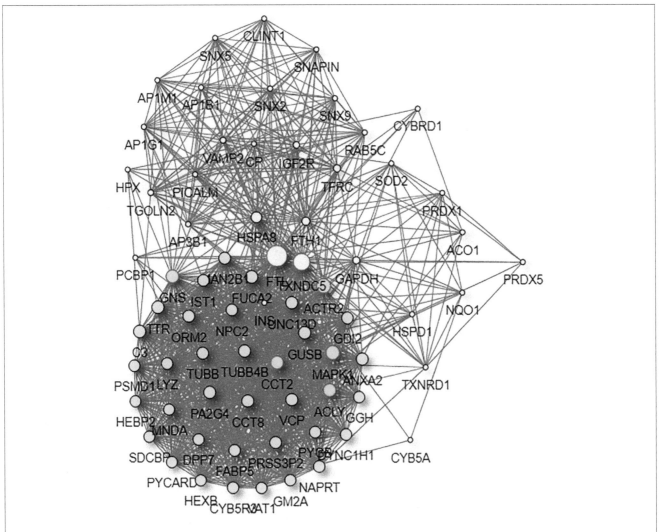

FIGURE 10 | Predictive PPI network of the target protein biomarker candidate: FTL. In the PPI network prediction, the colored node in the middle represents the target protein biomarker, and lines are mapped for the interactions between proteins. Larger nodes correspond to a higher degree of protein aggregation in the PPI network.

alpha (HIF-1α) signaling pathway. The TF gene was implicated in the HIF-1α signaling pathway according to a previous PPI network analysis (Wu et al., 2018). Hypoxia results in imbalanced cellular prooxidants and antioxidants via oxidative stress or ROS accumulation, which is a key mechanism of cytotoxicity (Junk et al., 2002). Oxidative stress leads to higher levels of HIF-1α, a subunit of the heterodimeric basic helix–loop–helix-structured HIF-1. HIF-1α protein is generally undetectable in well-oxygenated cells as it degrades rapidly. Under conditions of normoxia, prolyl hydroxylation is processed at its highly conserved prolyl residues by members of the prolyl hydroxylase domain family (PHD). Prolyl hydroxylases demand Fe^{2+}, O_2, ascorbate, and oxoglutarate for catalytic activity, and when HIF-1α is overexpressed, hydroxylation takes place and polyubiquitylation induces proteasomal degradation. PHD proteins belong to the Fe^{2+}-dependent oxygenase superfamily. Conversely, the HIF-1α hydroxylation rate is suppressed under hypoxic conditions (Kaelin and Ratcliffe, 2008). Furthermore,

the involvement of oxidative stress could implicate the process of chronic inflammation, leading to ocular tissue dysfunction during the progression of myopia.

Iron-associated corneal abnormalities are clinically manifest as corneal iron deposition. Investigations into such abnormalities have hitherto been conducted in physiological and pathological conditions (Yeung et al., 2006). Hudson–Stahli lines are typical in aging corneas, and a Fleischer ring is often suggestive of keratoconus (Gass, 1964). Other pathological conditions include a postoperative paracentral ring (Mannis, 1983) or central spot (Seiler and Holschbach, 1993) following ablative refractive surgery, and a fitting curve ring is observed in orthokeratology (Liang et al., 2003). The pathogenesis of corneal iron deposition has been an issue of major debate in recent decades. Both the epithelium basal cell migration theory and the combination theory of tear desiccation and senescent basal cell mechanism have been proposed (Assil et al., 1993). Previous observations have suggested that iron deposition is consistent with the area

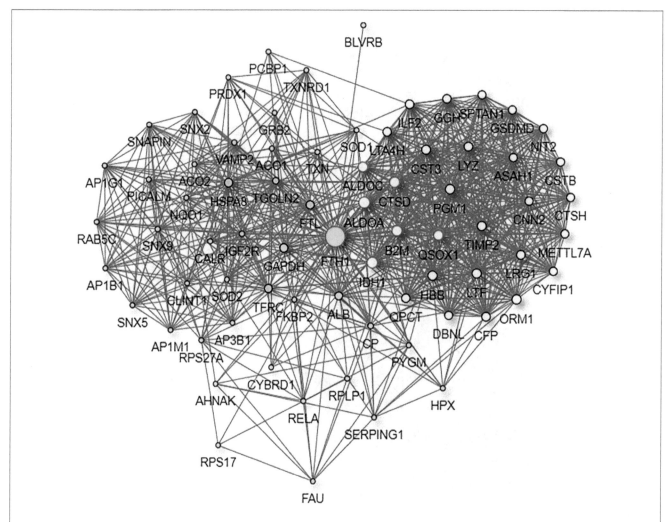

FIGURE 11 | Predictive PPI network of the target protein biomarker candidate: FTH1. In the PPI network prediction, the colored node in the middle represents the target protein biomarker, and lines are mapped for the interactions between proteins. Larger nodes correspond to a higher degree of protein aggregation in the PPI network.

of greatest epithelial hyperplasia, which is promoted by basal cell mitosis and migration (Yeung et al., 2006).

Keratoectasia is considered the most devastating postoperative complication after ablative refractive surgeries because it causes severe vision loss. Fleisher's ring is a typical sign of keratoconus, which represents corneal iron deposition in the epithelial basement membrane. Free iron in tissue can cause oxidative damage via Fenton and Haber-Weiss reactions that transfer hydrogen peroxide to free radicals. Ferritin expression is controlled by erythroid-derived 2. Ferritins block peroxide free radical formation and control the expression of nicotinamide adenine dinucleotide phosphate [NAD(P)H]: quinone oxidoreductase 1, which inhibits free radical formation by quinone redox cycling (Nioi and Hayes, 2004). Ferritin sequesters free iron, and the downregulated ferritin expression reported in corneas with keratoconus could explain the phenomenon of iron accumulation. Ferritins can protect cellular DNA from oxidative stress caused by free radicals or ultraviolet light (Joseph et al., 2011). The decrease in

ferritin levels in the corneal stroma of myopic eyes implies reduced protective effects of the cornea and further increased oxidative damage in the cornea. Previous studies have implicated oxidative damage, metabolic malfunction, and increased cell death of corneal stromal keratocytes in keratoconus (Foster et al., 2014). The discovery of the associations among oxidative stress, alteration of iron metabolism, and myopia may offer further solutions for the identification of patients with potential keratectasia.

After reviewing a wealth of literature, we discovered potential clues between iron uptake and myopia. García-Casal and Leets (2014) investigated ferritin synthesis by Caco-2 cells and found that carotenoids—lycopene, lutein, and zeaxanthin—rather than vitamin A, could improve iron uptake from ferrous fumarate and NaFe-EDTA. Lutein is a major xanthophyll carotenoid found in the human retina at preferentially high concentrations. Various studies have reported its antioxidative and anti-inflammatory properties related to different ocular disorders, indicating a protective effect against oxidative and inflammatory diseases such as diabetic retinopathy, retinopathy of prematurity, and myopia. Furthermore, a significant inverse association was found between axial length and macular pigment levels in the Chinese adult population, including lutein and zeaxanthin (Li et al., 2020).

CONCLUSION

Collectively, our study identified novel corneal protein biomarker candidates in high-myopia eyes, discovering different proteomic profiles between low and high myopia. The results further demonstrate that disturbances in iron homeostasis could be closely implicated in myopia development, and accelerated corneal oxidative stress was induced in the more myopic eyes. The final identification of rigorous biomarkers for high myopia requires further biological and functional experiments, as well as clinical studies. The key protein biomarker candidates identified and hallmark signaling pathways enriched in the study are under investigation to further determine their specific roles in the pathogenesis and development of myopia. Iron metabolism and associated proteins might serve as potential diagnostic or predictive biomarker candidates for high myopia and other conditions characterized by ocular oxidative damage.

ETHICS STATEMENT

The studies involving human participants were reviewed and approved by the Ethical Committee of Nankai University. The patients/participants provided their written informed consent to participate in this study.

AUTHOR CONTRIBUTIONS

YW, JC, and WW designed the research, performed the research, and wrote the manuscript. JC, ZW, CZ, MA, and BD analyzed the data. JC, ZW, and CZ prepared the figures. JC, BD, and YW contributed analytic tools and edited the manuscript. JC and YW critically revised the manuscript and addressed feedbacks. YW acquired the funding. All authors contributed to the article and approved the submitted version.

ACKNOWLEDGMENTS

We gratefully acknowledge Tianjin Key Lab of Ophthalmology and Visual Science (Tianjin, China) and Applied Protein Technology facility (Shanghai, China) for the technical support during the study.

REFERENCES

Adhikari, S., Nice, E. C., Deutsch, E. W., Lane, L., Omenn, G. S., Pennington, S. R., et al. (2020). A high-stringency blueprint of the human proteome. *Nat. Commun.* 11:5301. doi: 10.1038/s41467-020-19045-9

Aisen, P., Enns, C., and Wessling-Resnick, M. (2001). Chemistry and biology of eukaryotic iron metabolism. *Int. J. Biochem. Cell Biol.* 33, 940–959. doi: 10.1016/s1357-2725(01)00063-2

Assil, K. K., Quantock, A. J., Barrett, A. M., and Schanzlin, D. J. (1993). Corneal iron lines associated with the intrastromal corneal ring. *Am. J. Ophthalmol.* 116, 350–356. doi: 10.1016/s0002-9394(14)71353-4

Bostanci, N., Selevsek, N., Wolski, W., Grossmann, J., Bao, K., Wahlander, A., et al. (2018). Targeted proteomics guided by label-free quantitative proteome analysis in saliva reveal transition signatures from health to periodontal disease. *Mol. Cell Proteomics* 17, 1392–1409. doi: 10.1074/mcp.RA118.000718

Cozzi, A., Corsi, B., Levi, S., Santambrogio, P., Albertini, A., and Arosio, P. (2000). Overexpression of wild type and mutated human ferritin H-chain in HeLa cells: in vivo role of ferritin ferroxidase activity. *J. Biol. Chem.* 275, 25122–25129. doi: 10.1074/jbc.M003797200

Dyrlund, T. F., Poulsen, E. T., Scavenius, C., Nikolajsen, C. L., Thøgersen, I. B., Vorum, H., et al. (2012). Human cornea proteome: identification and quantitation of the proteins of the three main layers including epithelium, stroma, and endothelium. *J. Proteome Res.* 11, 4231–4239. doi: 10.1021/pr300358k

Foster, J., Wu, W. H., Scott, S. G., Bassi, M., Mohan, D., Daoud, Y., et al. (2014). Transforming growth factor β and insulin signal changes in stromal fibroblasts of individual keratoconus patients. *PLoS One* 9:e106556. doi: 10.1371/journal.pone.0106556

Francisco, B. M., Salvador, M., and Amparo, N. (2015). Oxidative stress in myopia. *Oxid. Med. Cell. Longev.* 2015:750637. doi: 10.1155/2015/750637

Fulcher, S., Lui, G. M., Houston, L. L., Ramakrishnan, S., Burris, T., Polansky, J., et al. (1988). Use of immunotoxin to inhibit proliferating corneal endothelium. *Invest. Ophthalmol. Vis. Sci.* 29, 755–759.

García-Casal, M. N., and Leets, I. (2014). Carotenoids, but not vitamin A, improve iron uptake and ferritin synthesis by Caco-2 cells from ferrous fumarate and NaFe-EDTA. *J. Food Sci.* 79, H706–H712. doi: 10.1111/1750-3841.12374

Gass, J. D. (1964). The iron lines of the superficial cornea. Hudson-Stahli line. Stocker's line and Fleischer's ring. *Arch. Ophthalmol.* 71, 348–358.

Götz, S., García-Gómez, J. M., Terol, J., Williams, T. D., Nagaraj, S. H., Nueda, M. J., et al. (2008). High-throughput functional annotation and data mining with the Blast2GO suite. *Nucleic Acids Res.* 36, 3420–3435. doi: 10.1093/nar/gkn176

Grochowski, E. T., Pietrowska, K., Kowalczyk, T., Mariak, Z., Kretowski, A., Ciborowski, M., et al. (2020). Omics in myopia. *J. Clin. Med.* 9:3464. doi: 10.3390/jcm9113464

Harned, J., Fleisher, L. N., and McGahan, M. C. (2006). Lens epithelial cells synthesize and secrete ceruloplasmin: effects of ceruloplasmin and transferrin on iron efflux and intracellular iron dynamics. *Exp. Eye Res.* 83, 721–727. doi: 10.1016/j.exer.2006.01.018

He, X., Hahn, P., Iacovelli, J., Wong, R., King, C., Bhisitkul, R., et al. (2007). Iron homeostasis and toxicity in retinal degeneration. *Prog. Retin. Eye Res.* 26, 649–673. doi: 10.1016/j.preteyeres.2007.07.004

Holden, B. A., Fricke, T. R., Wilson, D. A., Jong, M., Naidoo, K. S., Sankaridurg, P., et al. (2016). Global prevalence of myopia and high myopia and temporal trends from 2000 through 2050. *Ophthalmology* 123, 1036–1042. doi: 10.1016/j.ophtha.2016.01.006

Huang, D., Wang, Y., Lv, J., Yan, Y., Hu, Y., Liu, C., et al. (2020). Proteomic profiling analysis of postmenopausal osteoporosis and osteopenia identifies potential proteins associated with low bone mineral density. *PeerJ* 8:e9009. doi: 10.7717/peerj.9009

Hysi, P. G., Wojciechowski, R., Rahi, J. S., and Hammond, C. J. (2014). Genome-wide association studies of refractive error and myopia, lessons learned, and implications for the future. *Invest. Ophthalmol. Vis. Sci.* 55, 3344–3351. doi: 10.1167/iovs.14-14149

Joseph, R., Srivastava, O. P., and Pfister, R. R. (2011). Differential epithelial and stromal protein profiles in keratoconus and normal human corneas. *Exp. Eye Res.* 92, 282–298. doi: 10.1016/j.exer.2011.01.008

Junk, A. K., Mammis, A., Savitz, S. I., Singh, M., Roth, S., Malhotra, S., et al. (2002). Erythropoietin administration protects retinal neurons from acute ischemia-reperfusion injury. *Proc. Natl. Acad. Sci. U.S.A.* 99, 10659–10664. doi: 10.1073/pnas.152321399

Kaelin, W. G., and Ratcliffe, P. J. (2008). Oxygen sensing by metazoans: the central role of the HIF hydroxylase pathway. *Mol. Cell* 30, 393–402. doi: 10.1016/j.molcel.2008.04.009

Kang, B. S., Lam, T. C., Cheung, J. K., Li, K. K., and Kee, C. S. (2021). Corneal proteome and differentially expressed corneal proteins in highly myopic chicks using a label-free SWATH-MS quantification approach. *Sci. Rep.* 11:5495. doi: 10.1038/s41598-021-84904-4

Karring, H., Thøgersen, I. B., Klintworth, G. K., Møller-Pedersen, T., and Enghild, J. J. (2005). A dataset of human cornea proteins identified by peptide mass fingerprinting and tandem mass spectrometry. *Mol. Cell Proteomics* 4, 1406–1408. doi: 10.1074/mcp.D500003-MCP200

Kim, T. I., Alió Del Barrio, J. L., Wilkins, M., Cochener, B., and Ang, M. (2019). Refractive surgery. *Lancet* 393, 2085–2098. doi: 10.1016/S0140-6736(18)33209-4

Lauwen, S., de Jong, E. K., Lefeber, D. J., and den Hollander, A. (2017). Omics biomarkers in ophthalmology. *Invest. Ophthalmol. Vis. Sci.* 58, BIO88–BIO98. doi: 10.1167/iovs.17-21809

Li, J., Liu, X., Zhou, Z., Tan, L., Wang, X., Zheng, Y., et al. (2019). Lysozyme-assisted photothermal eradication of methicillin-resistant *Staphylococcus aureus* infection and accelerated tissue repair with natural melanosome nanostructures. *ACS Nano* 13, 11153–11167. doi: 10.1021/acsnano.9b03982

Li, L. H., Lee, J. C., Leung, H. H., Lam, W. C., Fu, Z., and Lo, A. (2020). Lutein supplementation for eye diseases. *Nutrients* 12:1721. doi: 10.3390/nu12061721

Liang, J. B., Chou, P. I., Wu, R., and Lee, Y. M. (2003). Corneal iron ring associated with orthokeratology. *J. Cataract. Refract. Surg.* 29, 624–626. doi: 10.1016/s0886-3350(02)01458-x

Linsenmayer, T. F., Cai, C. X., Millholland, J. M., Beazley, K. E., and Fitch, J. M. (2005). Nuclear ferritin in corneal epithelial cells: tissue-specific nuclear transport and protection from UV-damage. *Prog. Retin. Eye Res.* 24, 139–159. doi: 10.1016/j.preteyeres.2004.08.004

MacLean, B., Tomazela, D. M., Shulman, N., Chambers, M., Finney, G. L., Frewen, B., et al. (2010). Skyline: an open source document editor for creating and analyzing targeted proteomics experiments. *Bioinformatics* 26, 966–968. doi: 10.1093/bioinformatics/btq054

Mannis, M. J. (1983). Iron deposition in the corneal graft. Another corneal iron line. *Arch. Ophthalmol.* 101, 1858–1861. doi: 10.1001/archopht.1983.01040020860003

Morgan, I. G., French, A. N., Ashby, R. S., Guo, X., Ding, X., He, M., et al. (2018). The epidemics of myopia: aetiology and prevention. *Prog. Retin. Eye Res.* 62, 134–149. doi: 10.1016/j.preteyeres.2017.09.004

Morgan, I. G., Ohno-Matsui, K., and Saw, S. M. (2012). Myopia. *Lancet* 379, 1739–1748. doi: 10.1016/S0140-6736(12)60272-4

Moriya, Y., Itoh, M., Okuda, S., Yoshizawa, A. C., and Kanehisa, M. (2007). KAAS: an automatic genome annotation and pathway reconstruction server. *Nucleic Acids Res.* 35, W182–W185. doi: 10.1093/nar/gkm321

Nioi, P., and Hayes, J. D. (2004). Contribution of NAD(P)H:quinone oxidoreductase 1 to protection against carcinogenesis, and regulation of its gene by the Nrf2 basic-region leucine zipper and the arylhydrocarbon receptor basic helix-loop-helix transcription factors. *Mutat. Res.* 555, 149–171. doi: 10.1016/j.mrfmmm.2004.05.023

Perez-Riverol, Y., Csordas, A., Bai, J., Bernal-Llinares, M., Hewapathirana, S., Kundu, D. J., et al. (2019). The PRIDE database and related tools and resources in 2019: improving support for quantification data. *Nucleic Acids Res.* 47, D442–D450. doi: 10.1093/nar/gky1106

Peterson, A. C., Russell, J. D., Bailey, D. J., Westphall, M. S., and Coon, J. J. (2012). Parallel reaction monitoring for high resolution and high mass accuracy quantitative, targeted proteomics. *Mol. Cell Proteomics* 11, 1475–1488. doi: 10.1074/mcp.O112.020131

Qiao-Grider, Y., Hung, L. F., Kee, C. S., Ramamirtham, R., and Smith, E. L. III (2010). Nature of the refractive errors in rhesus monkeys (*Macaca mulatta*) with experimentally induced ametropias. *Vision Res.* 50, 1867–1881. doi: 10.1016/j.visres.2010.06.008

Quevillon, E., Silventoinen, V., Pillai, S., Harte, N., Mulder, N., Apweiler, R., et al. (2005). InterProScan: protein domains identifier. *Nucleic Acids Res.* 33, W116–W120. doi: 10.1093/nar/gki442

Rouault, T. A. (2002). Post-transcriptional regulation of human iron metabolism by iron regulatory proteins. *Blood Cells Mol. Dis.* 29, 309–314. doi: 10.1006/bcmd.2002.0571

Seiler, T., and Holschbach, A. (1993). Central corneal iron deposit after photorefractive keratectomy. *Ger. J. Ophthalmol.* 2, 143–145.

Stergachis, A. B., MacLean, B., Lee, K., Stamatoyannopoulos, J. A., and MacCoss, M. J. (2011). Rapid empirical discovery of optimal peptides for targeted proteomics. *Nat. Methods* 8, 1041–1043. doi: 10.1038/nmeth.1770

Thompson, A., Schäfer, J., Kuhn, K., Kienle, S., Schwarz, J., Schmidt, G., et al. (2003). Tandem mass tags: a novel quantification strategy for comparative analysis of complex protein mixtures by MS/MS. *Anal. Chem.* 75, 1895–1904. doi: 10.1021/ac0262560

Troilo, D., Smith, E. L. III, Nickla, D. L., Ashby, R., Tkatchenko, A. V., Ostrin, L. A., et al. (2019). IMI – report on experimental models of emmetropization and myopia. *Invest. Ophthalmol. Vis. Sci.* 60, M31–M88. doi: 10.1167/iovs.18-25967

Trowbridge, I. S., and Domingo, D. L. (1981). Anti-transferrin receptor monoclonal antibody and toxin-antibody conjugates affect growth of human tumour cells. *Nature* 294, 171–173. doi: 10.1038/294171a0

Wiśniewski, J. R., Zougman, A., Nagaraj, N., and Mann, M. (2009). Universal sample preparation method for proteome analysis. *Nat. Methods* 6, 359–362. doi: 10.1038/nmeth.1322

Wong, T. Y., Ferreira, A., Hughes, R., Carter, G., and Mitchell, P. (2014). Epidemiology and disease burden of pathologic myopia and myopic choroidal neovascularization: an evidence-based systematic review. *Am. J. Ophthalmol.* 157, 9–25.e12. doi: 10.1016/j.ajo.2013.08.010

Wu, H., Chen, W., Zhao, F., Zhou, Q., Reinach, P. S., Deng, L., et al. (2018). Scleral hypoxia is a target for myopia control. *Proc. Natl. Acad. Sci. U.S.A.* 115, E7091–E7100. doi: 10.1073/pnas.1721443115

Yefimova, M. G., Jeanny, J. C., Guillonneau, X., Keller, N., Nguyen-Legros, J., Sergeant, C., et al. (2000). Iron, ferritin, transferrin, and transferrin receptor in the adult rat retina. *Invest. Ophthalmol. Vis. Sci.* 41, 2343–2351.

Yeung, L., Chen, Y. F., Lin, K. K., Huang, S. C., and Hsiao, C. H. (2006). Central corneal iron deposition after myopic laser-assisted in situ keratomileusis. *Cornea* 25, 291–295. doi: 10.1097/01.ico.0000183532.32825.ce

Yu, F. J., Lam, T. C., Liu, L. Q., Chun, R. K., Cheung, J. K., Li, K. K., et al. (2017). Isotope-coded protein label based quantitative proteomic analysis reveals significant up-regulation of apolipoprotein A1 and ovotransferrin in the myopic chick vitreous. *Sci. Rep.* 7:12649. doi: 10.1038/s41598-017-12650-7

Yu, T. C., and Okamura, R. (1988). Quantitative study of characteristic aqueous humor transferrin, serum transferrin and desialized serum transferrin in aqueous humor. *Jpn. J. Ophthalmol.* 32, 268–274.

Zhang, G., Li, J., Zhang, J., Liang, X., Zhang, X., Wang, T., et al. (2019). Integrated analysis of transcriptomic, miRNA and proteomic changes of a novel hybrid yellow catfish uncovers key roles for miRNAs in heterosis. *Mol. Cell Proteomics* 18, 1437–1453. doi: 10.1074/mcp.RA118.001297

Zhu, Y., Xu, H., Chen, H., Xie, J., Shi, M., Shen, B., et al. (2014). Proteomic analysis of solid pseudopapillary tumor of the pancreas reveals dysfunction of the endoplasmic reticulum protein processing pathway. *Mol. Cell Proteomics* 13, 2593–2603. doi: 10.1074/mcp.M114.038786

Permissions

The contributors of this book come from diverse backgrounds, making this book a truly international effort. This book will bring forth new frontiers with its revolutionizing research information and detailed analysis of the nascent developments around the world.

We would like to thank all the contributing authors for lending their expertise to make the book truly unique. They have played a crucial role in the development of this book. Without their invaluable contributions this book wouldn't have been possible. They have made vital efforts to compile up to date information on the varied aspects of this subject to make this book a valuable addition to the collection of many professionals and students.

This book was conceptualized with the vision of imparting up-to-date information and advanced data in this field. To ensure the same, a matchless editorial board was set up. Every individual on the board went through rigorous rounds of assessment to prove their worth. After which they invested a large part of their time researching and compiling the most relevant data for our readers.

The editorial board has been involved in producing this book since its inception. They have spent rigorous hours researching and exploring the diverse topics which have resulted in the successful publishing of this book. They have passed on their knowledge of decades through this book. To expedite this challenging task, the publisher supported the team at every step. A small team of assistant editors was also appointed to further simplify the editing procedure and attain best results for the readers.

Apart from the editorial board, the designing team has also invested a significant amount of their time in understanding the subject and creating the most relevant covers. They scrutinized every image to scout for the most suitable representation of the subject and create an appropriate cover for the book.

The publishing team has been an ardent support to the editorial, designing and production team. Their endless efforts to recruit the best for this project, has resulted in the accomplishment of this book. They are a veteran in the field of academics and their pool of knowledge is as vast as their experience in printing. Their expertise and guidance has proved useful at every step. Their uncompromising quality standards have made this book an exceptional effort. Their encouragement from time to time has been an inspiration for everyone.

The publisher and the editorial board hope that this book will prove to be a valuable piece of knowledge for researchers, students, practitioners and scholars across the globe.

List of Contributors

Li Dong, Yan Ni Yan, Nan Zhou, Lei Shao, Yin Jun Lan, Yang Li and Wen Bin Wei
Beijing Key Laboratory of Intraocular Tumor Diagnosis and Treatment, Beijing Ophthalmology and Visual Sciences Key Laboratory, Medical Artificial Intelligence Research and Verification Key Laboratory of the Ministry of Industry and Information Technology, Beijing Tongren Eye Center, Beijing Tongren Hospital, Capital Medical University, Beijing, China

Xin Yue Hu, Jian Hao Xiong and Cong Xin Liu
Beijing Eaglevision Technology Co., Ltd., Beijing, China

Qi Zhang, Ya Xing Wang and Jie Xu
Beijing Ophthalmology and Visual Science Key Laboratory, Beijing Tongren Eye Center, Beijing Tongren Hospital, Beijing Institute of Ophthalmology, Capital Medical University, Beijing, China

Zong Yuan Ge
eResearch centre, Monash University, Melbourne, VIC, Australia
ECSE, Faculty of Engineering, Monash University, Melbourne, VIC, Australia

Jost. B. Jonas
Department of Ophthalmology, Medical Faculty Mannheim, Heidelberg University, Mannheim, Germany

Wanyun Zhang, Zhijun Chen, Guannan Su, Lin Chen, Ying Zhu, Qingfeng Cao, Chunjiang Zhou, Yao Wang and Peizeng Yang
The First Affiliated Hospital of Chongqing Medical University, Chongqing Key Laboratory of Ophthalmology and Chongqing Eye Institute, Chongqing Branch of National Clinical Research Center for Ocular Diseases, Chongqing, China

Han Zhang
School of Computer Science and Technology, Harbin Institute of Technology, Harbin, China

Qingfeng Wang, Shenglan Yi, Ziyu Du, Su Pan, Xinyue Huang and Gangxiang Yuan
The First Affiliated Hospital of Chongqing Medical University, Chongqing Key Laboratory of Ophthalmology, Chongqing Eye Institute, Chongqing Branch of National Clinical Research Center for Ocular Diseases, Chongqing, China

Aize Kijlstra
University Eye Clinic Maastricht, Maastricht, Netherlands

Zixi Zhou, Zheng Zheng, Xiaojing Xiong, Xu Chen, Jingying Peng, Hao Yao, Jiaxin Pu, Qingwei Chen and Minming Zheng
The Second Affiliated Hospital of Chongqing Medical University, Chongqing, China

Su Pan, Handan Tan, Rui Chang, Qingfeng Wang and Hongxi Li
The First Affiliated Hospital of Chongqing Medical University, Chongqing Key Lab of Ophthalmology, Chongqing Eye Institute, Chongqing Branch of National Clinical Research Center for Ocular Diseases, Chongqing, China

Jingfei Hu and Hua Wang
School of Biological Science and Medical Engineering, Beihang University, Beijing, China
Hefei Innovation Research Institute, Beihang University, Hefei, China
Beijing Advanced Innovation Centre for Biomedical Engineering, Beihang University, Beijing, China
School of Biomedical Engineering, Anhui Medical University, Hefei, China

Zhaohui Cao and Guang Wu
Hefei Innovation Research Institute, Beihang University, Hefei, China

Jost B. Jonas
Beijing Institute of Ophthalmology, Beijing Tongren Hospital, Capital Medical University, Beijing Ophthalmology and Visual Sciences Key Laboratory, Beijing, China
Department of Ophthalmology, Medical Faculty Mannheim of the Ruprecht-Karls-University Heidelberg, Mannheim, Germany

Ya Xing Wang
Beijing Institute of Ophthalmology, Beijing Tongren Hospital, Capital Medical University, Beijing Ophthalmology and Visual Sciences Key Laboratory, Beijing, China

Jicong Zhang
School of Biological Science and Medical Engineering, Beihang University, Beijing, China
Hefei Innovation Research Institute, Beihang University, Hefei, China
Beijing Advanced Innovation Centre for Biomedical Engineering, Beihang University, Beijing, China
School of Biomedical Engineering, Anhui Medical University, Hefei, China
Beijing Advanced Innovation Centre for Big Data-Based Precision Medicine, Beihang University, Beijing, China

Xu Hou, Hong-Jun Du, Jian Zhou, Dan Hu and Yu-Sheng Wang
Department of Ophthalmology, Eye Institute of Chinese PLA, Xijing Hospital, Fourth Military Medical University, Xi'an, China

Xuri Li
State Key Laboratory of Ophthalmology, Zhongshan Ophthalmic Center, Sun Yat-sen University, Guangzhou, China

Yimeng Sun, Feng Wen, Chun Yan, Lishi Su and Wei Chi
State Key Laboratory of Ophthalmology, Zhongshan Ophthalmic Center, Sun Yat-sen University, Guangzhou, China

Shaochong Zhang
State Key Laboratory of Ophthalmology, Zhongshan Ophthalmic Center, Sun Yat-sen University, Guangzhou, China
Shenzhen Key Laboratory of Ophthalmology, Shenzhen Eye Hospital, Jinan University, Shenzhen, China

Xiaojing Xiong, Huafeng Ma, Yazhu Yang, Zhu Chen and Zixi Zhou
Department of Ophthalmology, Second Affiliated Hospital of Chongqing Medical University, Chongqing, China

Qingwei Chen
Department of general practice, Second Affiliated Hospital of Chongqing Medical University, Chongqing, China

Tian Yuan
Department of Otolaryngology-Head and Neck Surgery, Department of Allergy, The Third Affiliated Hospital of Sun Yat-sen University, Guangzhou, China
Department of Otolaryngology, Yong Loo Lin School of Medicine, National University of Singapore, Singapore, Singapore

Rui Zheng, Qing-wu Wu, Wei-hao Wang, Hui-yi Deng, Wei-feng Kong, Hui-jun Qiu, Xue-kun Huang and Qin-tai Yang
Department of Otolaryngology-Head and Neck Surgery, Department of Allergy, The Third Affiliated Hospital of Sun Yat-sen University, Guangzhou, China

Xiang-min Zhou, Peng Jin, Xiao-xue Zi, Yan-yi Tu, Tao Li and Li Shi
Department of Otolaryngology-Head and Neck Surgery, Shandong Provincial ENT Hospital, Cheeloo College of Medicine, Shandong University, Jinan, China

Zhi-qun Huang
Department of Otolaryngology-Head and Neck Surgery, The First Affiliated Hospital of Nanchang University, Nanchang, China

Sui-zi Zhou and Qian-min Chen
Department of Otolaryngology, Zhujiang Hospital, Southern Medical University, Guangzhou, China

Jing Liu, Hsiao Hui Ong and De-yun Wang
Department of Otolaryngology, Yong Loo Lin School of Medicine, National University of Singapore, Singapore, Singapore
NUHS Infectious Diseases Translational Research Program, Yong Loo Lin School of Medicine, National University of Singapore, Singapore, Singapore

Kai Sen Tan
Department of Otolaryngology, Yong Loo Lin School of Medicine, National University of Singapore, Singapore, Singapore
NUHS Infectious Diseases Translational Research Program, Yong Loo Lin School of Medicine, National University of Singapore, Singapore, Singapore
Department of Microbiology and Immunology, Yong Loo Lin School of Medicine, National University of Singapore, Singapore, Singapore
Biosafety Level 3 Core Facility, Yong Loo Lin School of Medicine, National University Health System, National University of Singapore, Singapore, Singapore

Zhuang-gui Chen
Department of Pediatrics, Department of Allergy, The Third Affiliated Hospital of Sun Yat-sen University, Guangzhou, China

Tian Wang, Yiming Li, Miao Guo and Mengyu Liao
Department of Ophthalmology, Tianjin Medical University General Hospital, Tianjin, China
Laboratory of Molecular Ophthalmology, Tianjin Medical University, Tianjin, China

Xue Dong
Department of Ophthalmology, Tianjin Medical University General Hospital, Tianjin, China
Laboratory of Molecular Ophthalmology, Tianjin Medical University, Tianjin, China
Tianjin Key Laboratory of Inflammation Biology, Department of Pharmacology, School of Basic Medical Sciences, Tianjin Medical University, Tianjin, China

Mei Du and Xiaohong Wang
Laboratory of Molecular Ophthalmology, Tianjin Medical University, Tianjin, China
Tianjin Key Laboratory of Inflammation Biology, Department of Pharmacology, School of Basic Medical Sciences, Tianjin Medical University, Tianjin, China

Haifang Yin
Tianjin Key Laboratory of Cellular Homeostasis and Human Diseases, Department of Cell Biology, Tianjin Medical University, Tianjin, China

Hua Yan
Department of Ophthalmology, Tianjin Medical University General Hospital, Tianjin, China

Haihan Zhang, Yueming Liu, Shiqi Hui, Yu Feng, Jingting Luo and Wenbin Wei
Beijing Tongren Eye Center, Beijing Key Laboratory of Intraocular Tumor Diagnosis and Treatment, Beijing Ophthalmology and Visual Sciences Key Lab, Medical Artificial Intelligence Research and Verification Key Laboratory of the Ministry of Industry and Information Technology, Beijing Tongren Hospital, Capital Medical University, Beijing, China

Kai Zhang
SenseTime Group Ltd., Shanghai, China

Qiaoxing Liang, Jing Li, Xiao Hu, Xiuli Deng, Bin Zou, Yu Liu, Lai Wei, Lingyi Liang and Xiaofeng Wen
State Key Laboratory of Ophthalmology, Guangdong Provincial Key Laboratory of Ophthalmology and Visual Science, Zhongshan Ophthalmic Center, Sun Yat-sen University, Guangzhou, China

Yanli Zou
State Key Laboratory of Ophthalmology, Guangdong Provincial Key Laboratory of Ophthalmology and Visual Science, Zhongshan Ophthalmic Center, Sun Yat-sen University, Guangzhou, China
Department of Ophthalmology, Foshan Hospital Affiliated to Southern Medical University, Foshan, China

Zhen Xiong, Qianqian Wang, Wanhong Li, Lijuan Huang, Jianing Zhang, Juanhua Zhu, Bingbing Xie, Shasha Wang, Haiqing Kuang, Xianchai Lin, Chunsik Lee, Anil Kumar and Xuri Li
State Key Laboratory of Ophthalmology, Zhongshan Ophthalmic Center, Sun Yat-sen University, Guangzhou, China

Ling Wei, Wenwen He, Keke Zhang, Yu Du, Jiao Qi, Jiaqi Meng, Xiaodi Qiu, Lei Cai, Qi Fan, Zhennan Zhao, Yating Tang, Yi Lu and Xiangjia Zhu
Department of Ophthalmology, Eye and ENT Hospital, Eye Institute, Fudan University, Shanghai, China
Key Laboratory of Myopia, NHC Key Laboratory of Myopia, Fudan University, Chinese Academy of Medical Sciences, Shanghai, China
Shanghai Key Laboratory of Visual Impairment and Restoration, Shanghai, China

Jinrui Wang, Xixi He and Dayong Ding
Visionary Intelligence Ltd, Beijing, China

Shuang Ni and Haike Guo
Department of Ophthalmology, Heping Eye Hospital, Shanghai, China

Yunxiao Song
Illinois Computer Science, University of Illinois, Champaign, IL, United States

Jinyan Li, Yijia Chen, Shuai Ouyang, Jingyu Ma, Hui Sun, Lixia Luo, Shuyi Chen and Yizhi Liu
State Key Laboratory of Ophthalmology, Zhongshan Ophthalmic Center, Sun Yat-sen University, Guangzhou, China

Yang Deng, Yunzhao Fu, Longxiang Sheng, Yixin Hu and Jiawen Luo
State Key Laboratory of Ophthalmology, Zhongshan Ophthalmic Center, Sun Yat-sen University, Guangzhou, China

Xiayin Zhang, Ruixin Wang, Ting Wang, Xulin Zhang, Meimei Dongye, Dongni Wang, Jinghui Wang, Wangting Li, Xiaohang Wu and Duoru Lin
State Key Laboratory of Ophthalmology, Zhongshan Ophthalmic Center, Sun Yat-sen University, Guangzhou, China

Haotian Lin
State Key Laboratory of Ophthalmology, Zhongshan Ophthalmic Center, Sun Yat-sen University, Guangzhou, China
Center for Precision Medicine, Sun Yat-sen University, Guangzhou, China

Li Lu, Ming Yang, Minjie Yuan, Wangshu Yu, Jiani Huang and Wei Han
Department of Ophthalmology, Eye Center of the Second Affiliated Hospital, School of Medicine, Zhejiang University, Hangzhou, China

Peifang Ren, Xuyuan Tang, Qin He and Miaomiao Zhu
Department of Ophthalmology, The First Affiliated Hospital, School of Medicine, Zhejiang University, Hangzhou, China

Enliang Zhou and Genjie Ke
Department of Ophthalmology, The First Affiliated Hospital of University of Science and Technology of China, Hefei, China

Lixian Lu
College of Computer Science and Technology, Zhejiang University, Hangzhou, China

Jingyi Chen and Yan Wang
School of Medicine, NanKai University, Tianjin, China
Tianjin Key Lab of Ophthalmology and Visual Science, Tianjin Eye Hospital, Tianjin Eye Institute, Nankai University Eye Hospital, Tianjin, China

Wenjing Wu
Tianjin Key Lab of Ophthalmology and Visual Science, Tianjin Eye Hospital, Tianjin Eye Institute, Nankai University Eye Hospital, Tianjin, China

Zhiqian Wang
Department of Optometry, Shenyang Eye Institute, The 4th People's Hospital of Shenyang, Shenyang, China

Chuannan Zhai
Department of Cardiology, Tianjin Chest Hospital, Tianjin, China

Baocheng Deng
Department of Infectious Disease, The 1st Affiliated Hospital of China Medical University, Shenyang, China

Mohammad Alzogool
School of Medicine, NanKai University, Tianjin, China

Index

Printed in the USA
CPSIA information can be obtained
at www.ICGtesting.com
JSHW051410091023
49903JS00006B/360